Kidney Cancer

Mukul K. Divatia • Ayhan Ozcan
Charles C. Guo • Jae Y. Ro
Editors

Kidney Cancer

Recent Advances in Surgical and Molecular Pathology

Springer

Editors

Mukul K. Divatia
Department of Pathology and Genomic Medicine
Houston Methodist Hospital, Weill Medical College of Cornell University
Houston, TX
USA

Charles C. Guo
Department of Pathology
The University of Texas MD Anderson Cancer Center
Houston, TX
USA

Ayhan Ozcan
Gulhane Military Medical Academy School of Medicine
Department of Pathology
Ankara, Turkey

Yeni Yuzyil University Gaziosmanpasa Hospital
Department of Pathology
Istanbul, Turkey

Jae Y. Ro
Department of Pathology and Genomic Medicine
Houston Methodist Hospital, Weill Medical College of Cornell University
Houston, TX
USA

ISBN 978-3-030-28332-2 ISBN 978-3-030-28333-9 (eBook)
https://doi.org/10.1007/978-3-030-28333-9

This Springer imprint is published by the registered company Springer Nature Switzerland AG
The registered company address is: Gewerbestrasse 11, 6330 Cham, Switzerland

Preface

Conceptual knowledge regarding kidney cancer has been undergoing a paradigm shift over the past few years. Significant advancements have been made in the development of molecular targeted therapies with implications for the role of precise tumor subtyping by the pathologists, progress in molecular diagnostics with cytogenetic analysis, revisions of kidney tumor classification with incorporation of newly recognized and evolving entities, updates in cancer staging systems, and advances in imaging with applied theranostics.

This textbook provides a comprehensive overview of pathology of kidney tumors along with radiological features and up-to-date treatment strategies that enable the readers to avail this information in day-to-day pathology sign-out as well as interaction with clinical colleagues of different disciplines. It also serves as a referral resource for the current medical or surgical practice while preparing for examinations or maintenance of certification. The chapters contain an updated review of important pathologic parameters mandated for diagnosis and reporting with emphasis on updated information regarding new developments in this interesting field. Numerous high-resolution color images aptly illustrate the various pathologic entities and their features as outlined in the text section along with tables that highlight the differential diagnoses and salient ancillary features.

Each chapter is authored by experts with significant experience in the diagnosis and management of kidney cancers. The editors wish to acknowledge their contributions to this book as well as to the ongoing developments in the field of kidney cancers. The goal of this text is to provide up-to-date information on renal tumor pathology, radiology, and management that are required in daily practice. We hope that this book serves as a quick reference for all categories of readers alike.

We are indebted to our colleagues and friends who contributed slides and images to this volume and to clinical colleagues who contribute interesting and challenging cases to our pathology service. As lifelong learners, we continue to be amazed with all the new developments in kidney cancer that prompt us to revisit old concepts and establish newer parameters, allowing our vast field to progress.

Houston, TX, USA — Mukul K. Divatia, MD
Istanbul, Turkey — Ayhan Ozcan, MD
Houston, TX, USA — Charles C. Guo, MD, PhD
Houston, TX, USA — Jae Y. Ro, MD, PhD

Contents

Contributors

Komal Arora, MD Department of Pathology and Genomic Medicine, Houston Methodist Hospital, Weill Medical College of Cornell University, Houston, TX, USA

Nicola Battelli, MD Oncology Unit, Macerata Hospital, Macerata, Italy

Dilek Ertoy Baydar, MD Department of Pathology, Koç University School of Medicine, İstanbul, Turkey

Liang Cheng, MD Departments of Pathology, Urology, and Laboratory Medicine, Indiana University School of Medicine, Indianapolis, IN, USA

Boonyarit Cheunsuchon, MD Department of Pathology, Faculty of Medicine, Siriraj Hospital, Mahidol University, Bangkok, Thailand

Se Young Choi, MD, PhD Department of Urology, Asan Medical Center, University of Ulsan College of Medicine, Seoul, South Korea

Department of Urology, Chung-Ang University Hospital, Chung-Ang University College of Medicine, Seoul, South Korea

Kyoung-Sik Cho, MD, PhD Department of Radiology, Research Institute of Radiology, Asan Medical Center, University of Ulsan College of Medicine, Seoul, South Korea

Alessia Cimadamore, MD Institute of Pathological Anatomy and Histopathology, University of the Marche Region, Ancona, Italy

Suzanne M. Crumley, MD Department of Pathology and Genomic Medicine, Houston Methodist Hospital, Weill Medical College of Cornell University, Houston, TX, USA

Fang-Ming Deng, MD, PhD Department of Pathology, New York University Langone Medical Health, New York, NY, USA

Mukul K. Divatia, MD Department of Pathology and Genomic Medicine, Houston Methodist Hospital, Weill Medical College of Cornell University, Houston, TX, USA

Ziad M. El-Zaatari, MD Department of Pathology and Genomic Medicine, Houston Methodist Hospital, Weill Medical College of Cornell University, Houston, TX, USA

Seyda Erdogan, MD Department of Pathology, Cukurova University, School of Medicine, Adana, Turkey

Maren Y. Fuller, MD Texas Children's Hospital/Baylor College of Medicine, Houston, TX, USA

Lillian W. Gaber, MD Departments of Pathology and Genomic Medicine, The Houston Methodist Hospital, Weill-Cornell Medical College, Houston, TX, USA

Silvia Gasparrini, MD Section of Pathological Anatomy, Polytechnic University of the Marche Region, School of Medicine, Ancona, Italy

Julia T. Geyer, MD Division of Hematopathology, Department of Pathology and Laboratory Medicine, Weill Cornell Medicine, New York, NY, USA

Charles C. Guo, MD Department of Pathology, The University of Texas MD Anderson Cancer Center, Houston, TX, USA

Choung-Soo Kim, MD Department of Urology, Asan Medical Center, University of Ulsan College of Medicine, Seoul, South Korea

Mi-hyun Kim, MD Department of Radiology, Research Institute of Radiology, Asan Medical Center, University of Ulsan College of Medicine, Seoul, South Korea

Antonio Lopez-Beltran, MD Department of Pathology and Surgery, Cordoba University School of Medicine, Córdoba, Spain

Shamlal Mangray, MD Department of Pathology, Lifespan Academic Medical Center and Brown University, Providence, RI, USA

Elizabeth M. Margolskee, MD, MPH Division of Hematopathology, Department of Pathology and Laboratory Medicine, Weill Cornell Medicine, New York, NY, USA

Andres Matoso, MD Department of Pathology, Urology, and Oncology, Johns Hopkins Medical Institutions, Baltimore, MD, USA

Rodolfo Montironi, MD Institute of Pathological Anatomy and Histopathology, United Hospitals, Ancona, Italy

Ayhan Ozcan, MD Gulhane Military Medical Academy, School of Medicine, Department of Pathology, Ankara, Turkey

Yeni Yuzyil University Gaziosmanpasa Hospital, Department of Pathology, Istanbul, Turkey

Priya Rao, MD Department of Pathology, The University of Texas M. D. Anderson Cancer Center, Houston, TX, USA

Maria R. Raspollini, MD Histopathology and Molecular Diagnostics. University Hospital Careggi, Florence, Italy

Aseeb Rehman, MD Department of Pathology and Genomic Medicine, Houston Methodist Hospital, Weill-Cornell Medical College, Houston, TX, USA

Jae Y. Ro, MD, PhD Department of Pathology and Genomic Medicine, Houston Methodist Hospital, Weill Medical College of Cornell University, Houston, TX, USA

Jeman Ryu, MD Department of Urology, Asan Medical Center, University of Ulsan College of Medicine, Seoul, South Korea

Steven P. Salvatore, MD Division of Renal Pathology, Department of Pathology and Laboratory Medicine, Weill Cornell Medicine, New York, NY, USA

Matteo Santoni, MD Oncology Unit, Macerata Hospital, Macerata, Italy

Marina Scarpelli, MD Institute of Pathological Anatomy and Histopathology, United Hospitals, Ancona, Italy

Kanishka Sircar, MD Division of Pathology and Laboratory Medicine, Departments of Pathology and Translational Molecular Pathology, The University of Texas MD Anderson Cancer Center, Houston, TX, USA

Pheroze Tamboli, MBBS Division of Pathology and Laboratory Medicine, Department of Pathology, The University of Texas MD Anderson Cancer Center, Houston, TX, USA

Ngoentra Tantranont, MD Department of Pathology, Faculty of Medicine, Siriraj Hospital, Mahidol University, Bangkok, Thailand

Luan D. Truong, MD Department of Pathology and Genomic Medicine, The Houston Methodist Hospital, Houston, TX, USA

Department of Pathology and Laboratory Medicine, Weill Cornell Medical College of Cornell University, New York, NY, USA

Department of Pathology and Medicine, Baylor College of Medicine, Houston, TX, USA

Evgeny Yakirevich, MD Department of Pathology, Lifespan Academic Medical Center and Brown University, Providence, RI, USA

Dalsan You, MD, PhD Department of Urology, Asan Medical Center, University of Ulsan College of Medicine, Seoul, South Korea

Qihui Jim Zhai, MD Department of Laboratory Medicine and Pathology, Mayo Clinic, Jacksonville, FL, USA

Miao Zhang, MD, PhD Department of Pathology, The University of Texas MD Anderson Cancer Center, Houston, TX, USA

Amado J. Zurita, MD Department of Genitourinary Medical Oncology, The University of Texas MD Anderson Cancer Center, Houston, TX, USA

Part I
Clinical Aspects

Chapter 1
Surgical Consideration in Renal Tumors

Dalsan You, Se Young Choi, Jeman Ryu, and Choung-Soo Kim

Renal cell carcinomas (RCCs) account for approximately 2–3% of adult malignancies and 90–95% of kidney tumors [1, 2]. In 2012, there were approximately 338,000 new cases of RCC, and 143,000 deaths occurred from kidney cancer worldwide [3]. In 2017, there were approximately 64,000 new cases and 14,000 deaths in the United States [4]. As a result of increased utilization and availability of ultrasonography and cross-sectional imaging, more renal masses have been identified and stage migration has occurred; namely, renal masses are detected at much earlier stages. Of 236,975 RCC patients registered in the National Cancer Data Base, the percentage of patients with stage I disease significantly increased from 43.0% in 1993 to 57.1% in 2004, and the proportion of stage IV disease decreased from 27.4% to 18.7% over the 12-year period [5]. Traditionally, partial and radical nephrectomies are therapeutic surgical options for long-term cure in localized RCC. Globally, 25% of patients with RCC have metastatic disease at diagnosis, and 20–40% of patients develop metastatic disease after nephrectomy. The prognosis for patients with metastatic RCC was poor, with a median survival of 1 year and a 2-year survival rate of 10–20% [6]. Since the inception of new systemic agents, the survival of patients with metastatic RCC has been prolonged [7]. However, these new agents rarely provide complete (less than 1%) or long-term responses [8–10]. Therefore, surgical resection of the primary tumor and metastases is considered

D. You · J. Ryu · C.-S. Kim (✉)
Department of Urology, Asan Medical Center, University of Ulsan College of Medicine, Seoul, South Korea
e-mail: cskim@amc.seoul.kr

S. Y. Choi
Department of Urology, Asan Medical Center, University of Ulsan College of Medicine, Seoul, South Korea

Department of Urology, Chung-Ang University Hospital, Chung-Ang University College of Medicine, Seoul, South Korea

M. K. Divatia et al. (eds.), *Kidney Cancer*, https://doi.org/10.1007/978-3-030-28333-9_1

important for cure or long-term survival. In this chapter, we summarize the contemporary surgical management of localized, locally advanced, and metastatic RCC.

Surgical Treatment of Localized Renal Cell Carcinoma

The incidence of localized renal mass detection has increased due to the widespread use of cross-sectional imaging [11]. Clinical T1 renal masses are heterogeneous; 20% of them are benign and only about 20% exhibit potentially aggressive carcinoma at diagnosis [12]. Multiple management options, including surgery, thermal ablation, and active surveillance, are now available [1, 13, 14]. Urologic/non-urologic morbidities of each option, the patient's coexisting conditions, life expectancy, and the treatment provider's experience should be taken into consideration in tumor management [14, 15].

Renal mass biopsy can be used to assess tumor grade and histology, given that clinical and radiographic factors have very limited accuracy in predicting tumor aggressiveness [16, 17].

Partial Nephrectomy

In 1890, Czerny described nephron-sparing surgery for RCC. However, high complication rates were reported in the early years. Partial nephrectomy techniques were developed after taking into consideration detailed renal imaging, various techniques preventing ischemic renal damage, renal vascular surgery expertise, deleterious effects of chronic kidney disease, a large number of incidentally detected low-stage RCCs during medical checkups, and good survival rates after this treatment (Fig. 1.1) [18]. Table 1.1 summarizes the indications of partial nephrectomy (nephron-sparing surgery).

Traditionally, partial nephrectomy is considered in cases where radical nephrectomy can be associated with high risk of chronic kidney disease or dialysis [18]. Patients with bilateral RCC or RCC in a solitary functioning kidney are relevant. Another indication

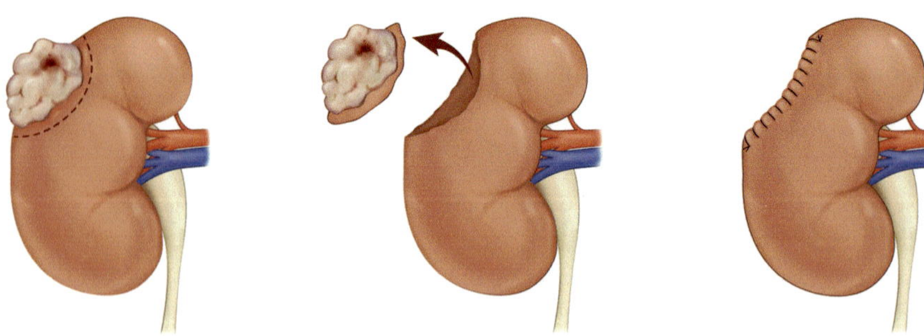

Fig. 1.1 The concept of partial nephrectomy

Table 1.1 Indications for partial nephrectomy (nephron-sparing surgery)

Indication
Absolute
Bilateral tumors
Tumor in single kidney
Poorly functioning or nonfunctioning contralateral kidney
Relative
Renal dysfunction
Hereditary renal cell carcinoma
Genetic predisposition to metachronous renal cell carcinoma
Systemic threats to future renal function (e.g., diabetes mellitus, hypertension)
Local threats to either kidney (e.g., obstructive uropathy, stone disease, renovascular disease)
Elective
Small renal mass and normal contralateral kidney

of partial nephrectomy is unilateral carcinoma when the opposite kidney can potentially have decreased function due to another cause, such as renal artery stenosis [19]. Partial nephrectomy can also preserve functioning renal tissue in patients with bilateral synchronous RCC. If the tumors are large, staged procedures can be performed. However, patients with RCC involving an anatomically or functionally solitary kidney should be warned about the risk of postoperative dialysis. In a previous study, 4.5% of patients were followed up for 3.6 years after surgery [20]. Renal function was preserved in the majority of patients who underwent partial nephrectomy, in accordance with the aforementioned indications [1, 18]. Local recurrence rates of 3–5% were reported after partial nephrectomy, due to many challenges such as hilar tumors, minimized excision of functional parenchyma, or multifocal tumors [1, 18].

Partial nephrectomy presently is the treatment of choice for the management of clinical T1 RCC in patients with a normal contralateral kidney [13, 21]. Several reports comparing partial with radical nephrectomy have showed comparable results in terms of oncologic and renal functional outcomes [1, 22–25]. Previous reports of partial nephrectomy for T1a RCC showed 1–2% local recurrence rates and over 90% cancer-free survival [18]. In addition, similar promising results were reported in clinical T1b tumors [26–28].

To determine the possibility of partial nephrectomy in RCC, the exclusion of locally extensive or metastatic disease with preoperative testing and additional specific renal imaging, identifying the relationship of the tumor with the intrarenal vascular supply and collecting system, is necessary. Renal imaging methods include computed tomography (CT) and renal arteriography/venography, and presently, three-dimensional volume-rendered CT is considered an accurate imaging modality [29].

The performance of partial nephrectomy by minimally invasive methods has recently evolved. Minimally invasive partial nephrectomy is a challenging procedure because poor visualization due to suboptimal hemostasis and the absence of tactile sensation could result in positive resection margins at surgery. However, various techniques, including the occlusion of renal vasculature and intracorporeal suture closing the collecting system and repairing the capsular defect, have been developed to resolve these problems [30, 31]. The oncological outcomes of laparoscopic and open partial nephrectomies were excellent for clinical T1 renal cortical tumors in the previous 10-year follow-up reports of carefully selected patients with limited risk of recurrence [32]. Early unclamping maneuver immediately after running sutures in deep parenchyma across the defect reduced warm ischemic times and postoperative bleeding rates [33, 34].

The relatively small size of remnant renal parenchyma after partial nephrectomy can lead to long-term deterioration of renal function with hyperfiltration renal injury [35]. The occurrence of proteinuria is linearly correlated with the duration of follow-up and depends inversely on the size of remnant renal tissue. Proteinuria should be evaluated annually in patients with a solitary remnant kidney to detect hyperfiltration nephropathy. Angiotensin-converting enzyme inhibitors and protein-restricted diet can improve long-term renal function in patients who underwent partial nephrectomy [36].

There are various partial nephrectomy techniques because it is technically challenging as compared to radical nephrectomy. The selection of the incision site is crucial to expose the tumor, kidney, and renal vasculature. Incision above the 11th rib and the retroperitoneal approach have been predominantly used. The incision level can be adjusted depending on kidney location and the position/size of tumor on preoperative CT. The thoracoabdominal approach is advantageous in upper pole tumors, whereas the subcostal incision is useful in lower pole tumors. After incision, the kidney should be dissected to allow tumor excision. The ureter is encircled with a vessel loop to prevent injury; subsequently, the ureter is dissected superiorly to renal pelvis, and renal pedicles are identified, dissected, and controlled with vessel loops. Perirenal fat is dissected except when overlying the tumor.

Clamping of the renal artery and/or vein is essential to control bleeding during tumor excision. However, the procedure may induce decreased long-term renal function postoperatively [37]. Ischemic time is the most important surgical risk factor affecting decreased renal function after partial nephrectomy, and measures to limit ischemic time and injury should be taken [38]. The non-clamping method can preserve long-term renal function. In non-clamping method, enucleation of tumor can be associated with reduced blood loss and parenchymal damage compared to conventional tumor excision. If abrupt bleeding occurs during tumor excision with non-clamping method, compression of the renal parenchyma near the cut surface with Monocryl sutures into the transected vessels facilitates easy hemostasis.

The conventional process of partial nephrectomy includes the occlusion of the renal artery during tumor excision. The clamping method is advantageous in bleeding control, improved visualization, and decreased expansion of renal tissue [39]. Hypothermia of the kidney with ice slush is often used to prevent ischemic renal injury [40]. Cooling of the entire kidney should begin immediately after the occlusion of the renal artery and before tumor excision. Warm ischemia for ≥25 min caused long-lasting diffuse damage throughout the kidney, whereas cold ischemia for up to 58 min prevented ischemic injury to the kidney [41].

Tumor excision with negative resection margin is crucial for oncological outcomes. However, adjacent parenchyma should be maximally preserved for long-term renal function; the width of tumor-free resection margin is not associated with prognosis [42]. Various techniques of proper resection, such as enucleation, wedge resection, and polar segmental nephrectomy, have been developed. After tumor excision, 4-0 monocryl suture is performed for hemostasis of transected blood vessels, and the argon beam coagulator can also be used. If the collecting system is opened, interrupted or running 4-0 monocryl suture is useful for closure. When leakage of urine is suspected despite suturing collecting system, retrograde ureteral stent insertion should be considered. After closure of the blood vessels and collecting system, hemostatic bolster, composed of Surgicel and Floseal hemostatic matrix, is applied to the defect of the renal tissue. The approximation of cortical edges with a bolster and interrupted 2-0 polyglactin sutures in a tension-free manner is performed. Nephropexy to the posterior muscle can be useful in preventing kidney migration. Jackson-Pratt drain is retroperitoneally placed to drain blood and identify urine leakage by checking creatinine levels.

Thermal Ablative Therapies

Alternative nephron-sparing procedures for patients with localized RCC, thermal ablative therapies, such as radiofrequency ablation and renal cryosurgery, have also emerged (Fig. 1.2) [43–46]. Thermal ablative therapies are useful in old patients or patients with life-threatening comorbidities who are not candidates for partial nephrectomy, patients with local recurrence after prior partial nephrectomy, and multifocal hereditary RCC, where it is not possible to perform multiple partial nephrectomies [12]. Thermal ablative therapies have been associated with decreased

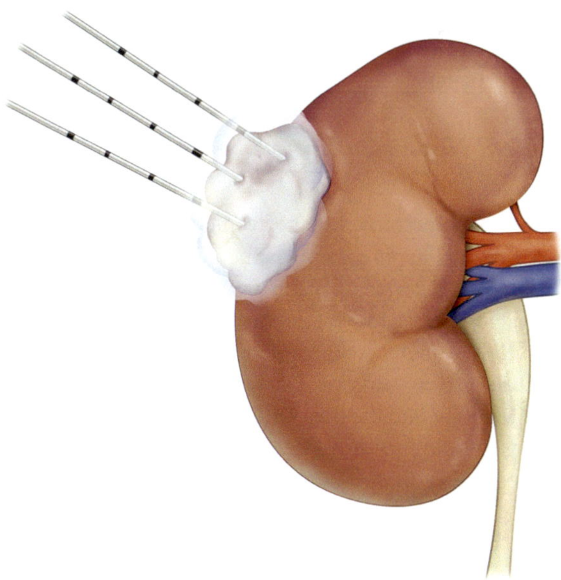

Fig. 1.2 The concept of thermal ablative therapy

Table 1.2 Indications for thermal ablation therapy

Indications
Small tumor (≤3 cm) in elderly, high-risk patients who opt against active surveillance and prefer intervention
Severe renal dysfunction
Previous abdominal surgery
Recurrent small renal mass in a postoperative renal remnant after prior partial nephrectomy

morbidity and faster recovery compared to partial nephrectomy, although long-term oncological outcomes have not been evaluated, and higher local recurrence rates were reported in preliminary studies [12, 45, 47]. Indications for thermal ablative therapy are listed in Table 1.2.

Active Surveillance

Active surveillance is acceptable for localized RCC and should be the first management option for small renal masses <4 cm in unfit patients or those with limited life expectancy [48]. Patients should be counseled in regard to slow and variable rates of tumor progression during observation period. Patients with active surveillance can lose the opportunity for partial nephrectomy and risk metastasis. Active surveillance is not usually recommended in patients with large renal tumors (>3 cm) and a young age or healthy patients with small tumors [12]. Due to lack of long-term data on surveillance, further research is required to define the preferred group of patients for active surveillance.

Surgical Treatment of Locally Advanced Renal Cell Carcinoma

Radical Nephrectomy

Simple nephrectomy was performed for several decades, but Robson et al. introduced radical nephrectomy as the golden standard to eradicate localized RCC [49]. The authors reported 66% and 64% overall survival for stage I and II tumors, respectively. Nowadays, radical nephrectomy is still the first choice for patients with localized RCC, such as large size (mostly T2 stage) or unsuitable location for nephron-sparing surgery. The major concern with radical nephrectomy is decreased renal function and the possibility of chronic kidney disease, which is correlated with increased mortality [50]. Go et al. reported increased rates of cardiovascular events and deaths in correlation with the progression of chronic kidney disease [51]. Proper selection of patients for radical nephrectomy is important, and radical nephrectomy should only be conducted when necessary.

Radical nephrectomy comprises early ligation of the renal artery and vein, removal of the kidney with Gerota's fascia, ipsilateral adrenalectomy, and regional lymph node dissection between the diaphragm and the aortic bifurcation [52]. The procedure of perifascial dissection is very important to prevent postoperative local recurrence because about 25% of clinical T2 renal RCCs displayed perinephric fat involvement [53]. The ipsilateral adrenalectomy is not always necessary if there is no radiologic adrenal involvement or upper pole tumor near the adrenal gland [52, 54]. There is a controversy with respect to complete regional lymphadenectomy in all patients. Randomized control trials, involving lymph node dissection in RCC, have not displayed significant improvement [55, 56]. RCC spreads through both blood and lymphatic system. Many patients with positive lymph nodes eventually show concealed metastases through the blood stream despite lymph node dissection. In addition, several patients with RCC have distant metastases without regional lymph node involvement, and the lymphatic course from the kidney is variable. Lymphadenectomy can be effective in a limited number of patients (about 2%) with micrometastases [52, 55, 57]. Thus, most urologists selectively conduct lymphadenectomy. Blute et al. reported that high-grade, sarcomatoid component, histologic necrosis, large tumors (>10 cm), and pathologic stages T3 or T4 were risk factors for lymph node involvement [57]. Patients with two or more risk factors showed about 10% lymph node involvement [57]. In a previous study, preoperative or intraoperative frozen sections were taken into consideration to decide dissection of hilar and regional lymph nodes [55].

The surgical approach should be considered depending on the size and location of the tumor and body type of patient. The transperitoneal approach is applied to control metastatic lesions and access renal vessels. Thoracoabdominal incision is used for large tumors involving the upper pole. Extraperitoneal flank incision is applied in old patients, but it is difficult for large tumors. Radical nephrectomy using laparoscopy is in the limelight for tumors 10–12 cm or smaller, localized RCCs without local invasion or in the absence of renal hilum infiltration. Laparoscopic radical nephrectomy resulted in less discomfort and fast recovery [58]. In addition, cancer-specific survival periods of laparoscopic and open radical nephrectomies are similar [59]. Nowadays, laparoscopy is applied in patients who are old and obese, and have prior operation history and large tumors, although selection bias should also be considered in each case [60, 61]. However, laparoscopic radical nephrectomy has been excessively conducted even in the cases of small renal tumors [62].

The oncologic outcome of radical nephrectomy depends on the stage of the tumor. Levy et al. reported 7.1%, 26.5%, and 39.4% recurrences for stages T1, T2, and T3, respectively [63]. Stephenson et al. mentioned increased risk of recurrence in pathologic stage T3 compared to stages T1 and T2 [64]. After radical nephrectomy, bone scans and CT should be conducted only in cases with associated symptoms. This follow-up can be cost-effective and is useful to detect recurrence. Monitoring of chronic kidney disease is also important.

Inferior Vena Cava Involvement

A characteristic of RCC during progression is invasion into the renal veins, inducing venous thrombi. In a number of cases, the tumor thrombus grows into the inferior vena cava, and the thrombus can migrate in the brain or heart. Radical nephrectomy and inferior vena cava thrombectomy are possible solutions for RCC and inferior vena cava thrombus, with cure rates of about 45–70%. The invasion of perinephric fat and positive lymph node and direct wall invasion of the inferior vena cava are risk factors indicating poor prognosis [65]. The reported rates of tumor thrombus in the inferior vena cava were about 4–10%. Symptoms are leg edema, varicocele of the right scrotum, and varicose abdominal veins. The stages are divided in accord with the level of inferior vena cava thrombus: levels 1, 2, and 3 involve adjacent to the ostium of the renal vein (level 1), extending up to the lower aspect of the liver (level 2), and involving the intrahepatic portion of the inferior vena cava but below the diaphragm (level 3), respectively (Fig. 1.3) [66]. Level 4 is correlated with extending above the diaphragm [66]. The prognosis of thrombus levels is controversial. Many studies reported that levels 3–4 showed higher recurrence and progression and reduced survival [67, 68]. Other studies reported that node involvement, metastasis, or tumor grade were more important factors than overall survival rates [69, 70]. Surgical resection of the entire tumor, including inferior vena cava thrombus, is a plausible strategy to cure the disease [71].

Magnetic resonance imaging (MRI) is a useful diagnostic tool of inferior vena cava involvement [72]. Gadolinium helps differentiate tumor thrombus by enhancement. Recently, multiplanar CT was used to differentiate tumor thrombus [73]. MRI or CT preoperative images are very important, and shorter times between imaging and surgery are preferred, because tumor thrombus can rapidly progress [74]. Venacavography can provide accurate imaging of inferior vena cava thrombus, but it is generally conducted in patients who cannot be examined by MRI or CT.

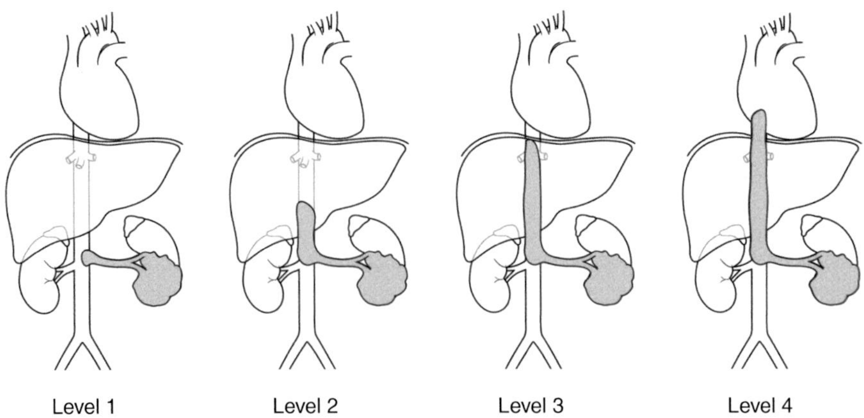

Fig. 1.3 Illustration of inferior vena cava thrombus level

Preoperative embolization of the renal artery can be conducted to reduce thrombus or ease off surgery. However, Subramanian et al. reported that embolization did not reduce blood loss or complications [75]. In cases of thrombus at supradiaphragm, cardiopulmonary bypass can be performed to prevent sudden coronary artery obstruction. Transesophageal sonography is also useful in monitoring thrombus mobilization.

The mobilization of the kidney and ligation of the artery should precede inferior vena cava approach. Level 1 thrombus can be easily removed by using a Satinsky clamp. Level 2 thrombus requires clamping of the caudal inferior vena cava, contralateral renal vessels, cephalad inferior vena cava, and lumbar veins. Subsequently, thrombus can be removed through the opened renal ostium. Levels 3 and 4 require more aggressive extension. Level 3 needs the mobilization of the liver and exposure of the intrahepatic inferior vena cava. In certain cases, clamping the suprahepatic inferior vena cava and Pringle maneuver interrupting blood flow through the hepatic artery and portal vein, thus controlling bleeding from the liver, are necessary. Level 4 has generally been managed by cardiopulmonary bypass with hypothermic circulatory arrest.

Mortality rates for level 4 thrombus surgery as high as 5–10% have been reported; they were related to the patients' comorbidities and tumor characteristics [69]. Thus, the selection of patients and operation planning are important [76]. Good performance status and the absence of lymph node and other metastases are correlated with good prognosis. However, severe edema, ascites, cardiac problems, severe pain, and hematuria can occur after surgery [77]. Therefore, surgery should be avoided in high-risk patients with short life expectancy.

Locally Invasive Renal Cell Carcinoma

Fewer than 2% of nephrectomy cases are at stage T4. Patients with locally invasive RCC have pain due to direct invasion of the abdominal wall, nerve, or paraspinous muscles. Liver invasion is uncommon. Instead, liver metastasis is more common than extension. The capsule of large tumor can press the liver parenchyma. However, direct invasion to the liver is a rare event. Margulis et al. reported that only 40% of patients who were expected to have direct invasion by imaging were confirmed [78]. In cases of direct invasion to the liver, partial hepatectomy is rarely performed. Tumor invasions to the duodenum and pancreas are rare and result in poor prognosis. Rarely do tumors invade the colon or its mesentery. In cases of large masses in the upper abdomen, adrenocortical carcinoma, infiltrative urothelial carcinoma, sarcoma, and lymphoma should be differentially diagnosed and carefully excluded, prior to diagnosis of advanced RCC.

Operation is the only option for locally invasive RCC. Therefore, en bloc resection, including invaded adjacent organs, is conducted in certain cases. Complete elimination of tumor is the goal of treatment. Margulis et al. reported that, despite extensive surgical resection, most patients (83.3%) with pathological stage T4 tumors had recurrences during a median period of 2 months after operation [78]. Karellas et al. reported that 90% of patients with negative resection margins died within a median period of 1 year after operation due to cancer. Preoperative embolization of the renal artery does not provide survival benefit in patients with radical nephrectomy for RCC, but may reduce bleeding [79].

Incomplete resection of large tumors resulted in poor outcomes. Dekernion et al. reported that only 12% of patients who underwent debulking surgery survived at 12 months [80]. Karellas et al. mentioned that positive resection margins of stage T4 tumors showed poor outcomes [81]. The 5-year survival rate was less than 5% in stage T4 tumors that invaded into adjacent organs.

The role of radiotherapy in locally advanced RCC is still questionable. Early studies on radiotherapy reported improved survival [82]. Van der Werf-Messing reported that radiation therapy did not result in survival differences at 5 years [83]. Postoperative radiation therapy can delay progression in cases of residual tumors after surgery of the renal fossa or adjacent lesion [84]. After radiation therapy, complications in small bowel should be considered because it is radiosensitive. Nowadays, radiation therapy is rarely used, and targeted therapy has replaced it in cases of residual or locally recurrent tumors.

Surgical Treatment of Metastatic Renal Cell Carcinoma

Cytoreductive Nephrectomy

Radical nephrectomy in patients initially presenting with metastatic disease, termed cytoreductive nephrectomy, is often indicated as part of a multimodal treatment strategy. The role of cytoreductive nephrectomy preceding cytokine therapy has been extensively studied. It is supported by the results of two prospective clinical trials, in which patients with metastatic RCC were randomly assigned to cytoreductive nephrectomy in combination with interferon-alpha or interferon-alpha treatment only [85, 86]. In a combined analysis, patients treated with cytoreductive nephrectomy followed by interferon-alpha treatment had a survival benefit of 13.6 versus 7.8 months compared to patients taking interferon-alpha alone [87]. A population-based study from the Surveillance, Epidemiology, and End Results database validated these findings and confirmed the survival benefit of cytoreductive nephrectomy relative to no surgery [88]. However, the risk of perioperative morbidity/mortality and the inability of a considerable number of patients undergoing cytoreductive nephrectomy to subsequently receive systemic therapy clearly underscore the need for careful patient selection [89].

The introduction of targeted therapies has prompted reassessment of the role of cytoreductive nephrectomy combined with targeted therapy. Since targeted therapy has a different mechanism of action and produces more robust clinical effects than cytokine therapy, cytoreductive nephrectomy may not increase the clinical efficacy of such drugs [90]. Two randomized prospective trials (CARMENA and SURTIME) were specifically designed to evaluate the survival benefit and appropriate timing of cytoreductive nephrectomy when used in conjunction with targeted therapy [91, 90]. SURTIME trial closed early in July 2016 due to low recruitment and, thus, may not show differences in the primary and secondary endpoints [92]. In CARMENA trial, targeted therapy alone was not inferior to cytoreductive nephrectomy followed by targeted therapy in patients with metastatic RCC who were classified as the Memorial Sloan Kettering Cancer Center intermediate or poor risk [93]. Based on several retrospective series, the role of cytoreductive nephrectomy remains controversial in the era of targeted therapy [94, 95]. Another recent study suggested the potential benefit of cytoreductive nephrectomy in selected patients [96].

Cytoreductive nephrectomy can be performed with palliative intent in patients having intractable pain, hematuria, constitutional symptoms, or paraneoplastic syndrome. Cytoreductive nephrectomy with palliative intent is rarely performed, due to the availability of alternative approaches for symptom palliation and questionable clinical benefit [97].

Metastasectomy in Patients with Metastatic Renal Cell Carcinoma

A complete surgical resection is the only option to cure the disease in patients with metastatic RCC, due to lack of complete or long-term results from currently available systemic agents [8–10]. In 1939, Barney and Churchill first reported a metastatic RCC patient who lived 23 years after undergoing cytoreductive nephrectomy and metastasectomy for lung metastasis [98]. Since then, metastasectomy has become a promising option for treatment of patients with metastatic RCC [99]. However, level 1 evidence showing that metastasectomy improves prognosis and survival is lacking. To date, only one prospective study has evaluated the role of metastasectomy in metastatic RCC patients receiving cytokine, tumor vaccine, or chemotherapy [100]. In this study, the elimination of disease was surgically achieved in 29 out of 38 enrolled patients, and median progression-free and overall survivals were 1.8 and 4.7 years, respectively. Surgically, no evidence of disease was an independent predictor of outcome along with lung metastasectomy. This is consistent with results from large retrospective studies in the cytokine therapy era and a systematic review [67, 101, 102]. Two retrospective studies concluded that complete metastasectomy improved overall survival of metastatic RCC patients who received targeted therapy [103, 104].

Metastasectomies to alleviate pain or prevent potentially life-threatening or debilitating complications are often performed in a variety of situations, including solitary brain metastases, metastatic lesions in weight-bearing bones, or vertebral metastatic lesions with impending cord compression. Metastasectomy is often combined with radiation and/or systemic therapy.

What Information Is Needed from Pathologists? The Urologic Surgeon's Point of View

1. Type of kidney tumor, benign vs. malignant or nonneoplastic
2. In malignant tumors
    - Type of renal cell carcinoma
    - Necrosis, sarcomatoid component (%)
    - Grading [WHO/ISUP grading (Fuhrman nuclear grade) or chromophobe tumor grade]
    - Tumor size
    - Presence or absence of perirenal fat extension or sinus fat invasion
    - Renal vein invasion
    - Extension to pelvicalyceal system or beyond Gerota's fascia or to adrenal gland (direct or noncontiguous)
    - Margins
    - LN status
    - Lymphovascular invasion
    - Tumor synoptic, TNM stage
3. Tissue procurement
4. Any others: Immunohistochemical studies (e.g., VEGF)

References

1. Rini BI, Campbell SC, Escudier B. Renal cell carcinoma. Lancet. 2009;373(9669):1119–32. https://doi.org/10.1016/S0140-6736(09)60229-4.
2. Moch H, Cubilla AL, Humphrey PA, Reuter VE, Ulbright TM. The 2016 WHO classification of tumours of the urinary system and male genital organs-part A: renal, penile, and testicular tumours. Eur Urol. 2016;70(1):93–105. https://doi.org/10.1016/j.eururo.2016.02.029.
3. International Agency for Research on Cancer (IARC). GLOBOCAN database 2012. http://globocan.iarc.fr. Accessed Nov 2017.
4. Siegel RL, Miller KD, Jemal A. Cancer statistics, 2017. CA Cancer J Clin. 2017;67(1):7–30. https://doi.org/10.3322/caac.21387.
5. Kane CJ, Mallin K, Ritchey J, Cooperberg MR, Carroll PR. Renal cell cancer stage migration: analysis of the National Cancer Data Base. Cancer. 2008;113(1):78–83. https://doi.org/10.1002/cncr.23518.
6. Motzer RJ, Mazumdar M, Bacik J, Berg W, Amsterdam A, Ferrara J. Survival and prognostic stratification of 670 patients with advanced renal cell carcinoma. J Clin Oncol Off J Am Soc Clin Oncol. 1999;17(8):2530–40. https://doi.org/10.1200/JCO.1999.17.8.2530.
7. Marchioni M, Bandini M, Pompe RS, Tian Z, Martel T, Kapoor A, et al. Survival of metastatic renal cell carcinoma patients continues to improve over time, even in targeted therapy era. Int Urol Nephrol. 2017;49(12):2143–9. https://doi.org/10.1007/s11255-017-1703-y.
8. Motzer RJ, Hutson TE, Tomczak P, Michaelson MD, Bukowski RM, Rixe O, et al. Sunitinib versus interferon alfa in metastatic renal-cell carcinoma. N Engl J Med. 2007;356(2):115–24. https://doi.org/10.1056/NEJMoa065044.

9. Escudier B, Eisen T, Stadler WM, Szczylik C, Oudard S, Siebels M, et al. Sorafenib in advanced clear-cell renal-cell carcinoma. N Engl J Med. 2007;356(2):125–34. https://doi.org/10.1056/NEJMoa060655.
10. Sternberg CN, Davis ID, Mardiak J, Szczylik C, Lee E, Wagstaff J, et al. Pazopanib in locally advanced or metastatic renal cell carcinoma: results of a randomized phase III trial. J Clin Oncol Off J Am Soc Clin Oncol. 2010;28(6):1061–8. https://doi.org/10.1200/JCO.2009.23.9764.
11. Lipworth L, Tarone RE, McLaughlin JK. The epidemiology of renal cell carcinoma. J Urol. 2006;176(6 Pt 1):2353–8. https://doi.org/10.1016/j.juro.2006.07.130.
12. Russo P, Jang TL, Pettus JA, Huang WC, Eggener SE, O'Brien MF, et al. Survival rates after resection for localized kidney cancer: 1989 to 2004. Cancer. 2008;113(1):84–96. https://doi.org/10.1002/cncr.23520.
13. Kunkle DA, Uzzo RG. Cryoablation or radiofrequency ablation of the small renal mass: a meta-analysis. Cancer. 2008;113(10):2671–80. https://doi.org/10.1002/cncr.23896.
14. Renal mass and localized renal cancer: American Urological Association Guideline. http://www.auanet.org/guidelines/renal-mass-and-localized-renal-cancer-new-(2017). Accessed Nov 2017.
15. Gill IS, Aron M, Gervais DA, Jewett MA. Clinical practice. Small renal mass. N Engl J Med. 2010;362(7):624–34. https://doi.org/10.1056/NEJMcp0910041.
16. Lane BR, Samplaski MK, Herts BR, Zhou M, Novick AC, Campbell SC. Renal mass biopsy--a renaissance? J Urol. 2008;179(1):20–7. https://doi.org/10.1016/j.juro.2007.08.124.
17. Schmidbauer J, Remzi M, Memarsadeghi M, Haitel A, Klingler HC, Katzenbeisser D, et al. Diagnostic accuracy of computed tomography-guided percutaneous biopsy of renal masses. Eur Urol. 2008;53(5):1003–11. https://doi.org/10.1016/j.eururo.2007.11.041.
18. Uzzo RG, Novick AC. Nephron sparing surgery for renal tumors: indications, techniques and outcomes. J Urol. 2001;166(1):6–18.
19. Hafez KS, Krishnamurthi V, Campbell SC, Novick AC. Contemporary management of renal cell carcinoma with coexistent renal artery disease: update of the Cleveland Clinic experience. Urology. 2000;56(3):382–6.
20. Fergany A. Current status and advances in nephron-sparing surgery. Clin Genitourin Cancer. 2006;5(1):26–33. https://doi.org/10.3816/CGC.2006.n.014.
21. Huang Y, Murakami T, Sano F, Kondo K, Nakaigawa N, Kishida T, et al. Expression of aquaporin 1 in primary renal tumors: a prognostic indicator for clear-cell renal cell carcinoma. Eur Urol. 2009;56(4):690–8. https://doi.org/10.1016/j.eururo.2008.10.014.
22. Lau WK, Blute ML, Weaver AL, Torres VE, Zincke H. Matched comparison of radical nephrectomy vs nephron-sparing surgery in patients with unilateral renal cell carcinoma and a normal contralateral kidney. Mayo Clin Proc. 2000;75(12):1236–42.
23. Lee SH, Son HS, Cho S, Kim SJ, Yoo DS, Kang SH, et al. Which patients should we follow up beyond 5 years after definitive therapy for localized renal cell carcinoma? Cancer Res Treat. 2015;47(3):489–94. https://doi.org/10.4143/crt.2014.013.
24. Mitchell RE, Gilbert SM, Murphy AM, Olsson CA, Benson MC, McKiernan JM. Partial nephrectomy and radical nephrectomy offer similar cancer outcomes in renal cortical tumors 4 cm or larger. Urology. 2006;67(2):260–4. https://doi.org/10.1016/j.urology.2005.08.057.
25. Van Poppel H, Joniau S. Is surveillance an option for the treatment of small renal masses? Eur Urol. 2007;52(5):1323–30. https://doi.org/10.1016/j.eururo.2007.07.025.
26. Pahernik S, Roos F, Rohrig B, Wiesner C, Thuroff JW. Elective nephron sparing surgery for renal cell carcinoma larger than 4 cm. J Urol. 2008;179(1):71–4; discussion 4. https://doi.org/10.1016/j.juro.2007.08.165.
27. Peycelon M, Hupertan V, Comperat E, Renard-Penna R, Vaessen C, Conort P, et al. Long-term outcomes after nephron sparing surgery for renal cell carcinoma larger than 4 cm. J Urol. 2009;181(1):35–41. https://doi.org/10.1016/j.juro.2008.09.025.
28. Crispen PL, Wong YN, Greenberg RE, Chen DY, Uzzo RG. Predicting growth of solid renal masses under active surveillance. Urol Oncol. 2008;26(5):555–9. https://doi.org/10.1016/j.urolonc.2008.03.010.

29. VanderBrink BA, Munver R, Tash JA, Sosa RE. Renal angiomyolipoma with contrast-enhancing elements mimicking renal malignancy: radiographic and pathologic evaluation. Urology. 2004;63(3):584–6. https://doi.org/10.1016/j.urology.2003.10.051.
30. Desai MM, Gill IS, Ramani AP, Matin SF, Kaouk JH, Campero JM. Laparoscopic radical nephrectomy for cancer with level I renal vein involvement. J Urol. 2003;169(2):487–91. https://doi.org/10.1097/01.ju.0000041955.93458.f5.
31. Gill IS, Aron M. Against the motion: open partial nephrectomy is the standard of care for small resectable solid renal masses. Eur Urol. 2007;51(2):562–4; discussion 4
32. Lane BR, Campbell SC, Gill IS. 10-year oncologic outcomes after laparoscopic and open partial nephrectomy. J Urol. 2013;190(1):44–9. https://doi.org/10.1016/j.juro.2012.12.102.
33. Bollens R, Rosenblatt A, Espinoza BP, De Groote A, Quackels T, Roumeguere T, et al. Laparoscopic partial nephrectomy with "on-demand" clamping reduces warm ischemia time. Eur Urol. 2007;52(3):804–9. https://doi.org/10.1016/j.eururo.2007.04.011.
34. Breda A, Stepanian SV, Lam JS, Liao JC, Gill IS, Colombo JR, et al. Use of haemostatic agents and glues during laparoscopic partial nephrectomy: a multi-institutional survey from the United States and Europe of 1347 cases. Eur Urol. 2007;52(3):798–803. https://doi.org/10.1016/j.eururo.2007.02.035.
35. Abdi R, Dong VM, Rubel JR, Kittur D, Marshall F, Racusen LC. Correlation between glomerular size and long-term renal function in patients with substantial loss of renal mass. J Urol. 2003;170(1):42–4. https://doi.org/10.1097/01.ju.0000069821.97385.6b.
36. Goldfarb DA. Preservation of renal function and the risk of hyperfiltration nephropathy. Semin Urol Oncol. 1995;13(4):292–5.
37. Thompson RH, Blute ML. At what point does warm ischemia cause permanent renal damage during partial nephrectomy? Eur Urol. 2007;52(4):961–3. https://doi.org/10.1016/j.eururo.2007.04.051.
38. Lane BR, Babineau DC, Poggio ED, Weight CJ, Larson BT, Gill IS, et al. Factors predicting renal functional outcome after partial nephrectomy. J Urol. 2008;180(6):2363–8; discussion 8-9. https://doi.org/10.1016/j.juro.2008.08.036.
39. Lane BR, Novick AC. Nephron-sparing surgery. BJU Int. 2007;99(5 Pt B):1245–50. https://doi.org/10.1111/j.1464-410X.2007.06831.x.
40. Thompson RH, Frank I, Lohse CM, Saad IR, Fergany A, Zincke H, et al. The impact of ischemia time during open nephron sparing surgery on solitary kidneys: a multi-institutional study. J Urol. 2007;177(2):471–6. https://doi.org/10.1016/j.juro.2006.09.036.
41. Funahashi Y, Yoshino Y, Sassa N, Matsukawa Y, Takai S, Gotoh M. Comparison of warm and cold ischemia on renal function after partial nephrectomy. Urology. 2014;84(6):1408–12. https://doi.org/10.1016/j.urology.2014.08.040.
42. Castilla EA, Liou LS, Abrahams NA, Fergany A, Rybicki LA, Myles J, et al. Prognostic importance of resection margin width after nephron-sparing surgery for renal cell carcinoma. Urology. 2002;60(6):993–7.
43. Hinshaw JL, Lee FT Jr. Image-guided ablation of renal cell carcinoma. Magn Reson Imaging Clin N Am. 2004;12(3):429–47, vi. https://doi.org/10.1016/j.mric.2004.03.003.
44. Lowry PS, Nakada SY. Renal cryotherapy: 2003 clinical status. Curr Opin Urol. 2003;13(3):193–7. https://doi.org/10.1097/01.mou.0000068745.22370.75.
45. Raman JD, Raj GV, Lucas SM, Williams SK, Lauer EM, Ahrar K, et al. Renal functional outcomes for tumours in a solitary kidney managed by ablative or extirpative techniques. BJU Int. 2010;105(4):496–500. https://doi.org/10.1111/j.1464-410X.2009.08776.x.
46. Sterrett SP, Nakada SY, Wingo MS, Williams SK, Leveillee RJ. Renal thermal ablative therapy. Urol Clin North Am. 2008;35(3):397–414, viii. https://doi.org/10.1016/j.ucl.2008.05.005.
47. Johnson DB, Solomon SB, Su LM, Matsumoto ED, Kavoussi LR, Nakada SY, et al. Defining the complications of cryoablation and radio frequency ablation of small renal tumors: a multi-institutional review. J Urol. 2004;172(3):874–7. https://doi.org/10.1097/01.ju.0000135833.67906.ec.

48. Beisland C, Hjelle KM, Reisaeter LA, Bostad L. Observation should be considered as an alternative in management of renal masses in older and comorbid patients. Eur Urol. 2009;55(6):1419–27. https://doi.org/10.1016/j.eururo.2008.12.031.
49. Robson CJ, Churchill BM, Anderson W. The results of radical nephrectomy for renal cell carcinoma. J Urol. 1969;101(3):297–301.
50. Choi SY, Yoo S, You D, Jeong IG, Song C, Hong B, et al. Adaptive functional change of the contralateral kidney after partial nephrectomy. Am J Physiol Renal Physiol. 2017;313(2):F192–F8. https://doi.org/10.1152/ajprenal.00058.2017.
51. Go AS, Chertow GM, Fan D, McCulloch CE, Hsu CY. Chronic kidney disease and the risks of death, cardiovascular events, and hospitalization. N Engl J Med. 2004;351(13):1296–305. https://doi.org/10.1056/NEJMoa041031.
52. O'Malley RL, Godoy G, Kanofsky JA, Taneja SS. The necessity of adrenalectomy at the time of radical nephrectomy: a systematic review. J Urol. 2009;181(5):2009–17. https://doi.org/10.1016/j.juro.2009.01.018.
53. Lam JS, Klatte T, Patard JJ, Goel RH, Guille F, Lobel B, et al. Prognostic relevance of tumour size in T3a renal cell carcinoma: a multicentre experience. Eur Urol. 2007;52(1):155–62. https://doi.org/10.1016/j.eururo.2007.01.106.
54. Lane BR, Tiong HY, Campbell SC, Fergany AF, Weight CJ, Larson BT, et al. Management of the adrenal gland during partial nephrectomy. J Urol. 2009;181(6):2430–6; discussion 6-7. https://doi.org/10.1016/j.juro.2009.02.027.
55. Leibovich BC, Blute ML. Lymph node dissection in the management of renal cell carcinoma. Urol Clin North Am. 2008;35(4):673–8; viii. https://doi.org/10.1016/j.ucl.2008.07.011.
56. Blom JH, van Poppel H, Marechal JM, Jacqmin D, Schroder FH, de Prijck L, et al. Radical nephrectomy with and without lymph-node dissection: final results of European Organization for Research and Treatment of Cancer (EORTC) randomized phase 3 trial 30881. Eur Urol. 2009;55(1):28–34. https://doi.org/10.1016/j.eururo.2008.09.052.
57. Blute ML, Leibovich BC, Cheville JC, Lohse CM, Zincke H. A protocol for performing extended lymph node dissection using primary tumor pathological features for patients treated with radical nephrectomy for clear cell renal cell carcinoma. J Urol. 2004;172(2):465–9. https://doi.org/10.1097/01.ju.0000129815.91927.85.
58. Hemal AK, Kumar A, Kumar R, Wadhwa P, Seth A, Gupta NP. Laparoscopic versus open radical nephrectomy for large renal tumors: a long-term prospective comparison. J Urol. 2007;177(3):862–6. https://doi.org/10.1016/j.juro.2006.10.053.
59. Hemal AK, Kumar A, Gupta NP, Kumar R. Oncologic outcome of 132 cases of laparoscopic radical nephrectomy with intact specimen removal for T1-2N0M0 renal cell carcinoma. World J Urol. 2007;25(6):619–26. https://doi.org/10.1007/s00345-007-0210-7.
60. Fugita OE, Chan DY, Roberts WW, Kavoussi LR, Jarrett TW. Laparoscopic radical nephrectomy in obese patients: outcomes and technical considerations. Urology. 2004;63(2):247–52; discussion 52. https://doi.org/10.1016/j.urology.2003.09.077.
61. Gabr AH, Elsayed ER, Gdor Y, Roberts WW, Wolf JS Jr. Obesity and morbid obesity are associated with a greater conversion rate to open surgery for standard but not hand assisted laparoscopic radical nephrectomy. J Urol. 2008;180(6):2357–62; discussion 62. https://doi.org/10.1016/j.juro.2008.08.077.
62. Porter MP, Lin DW. Trends in renal cancer surgery and patient provider characteristics associated with partial nephrectomy in the United States. Urol Oncol. 2007;25(4):298–302. https://doi.org/10.1016/j.urolonc.2006.07.016.
63. Levy DA, Slaton JW, Swanson DA, Dinney CP. Stage specific guidelines for surveillance after radical nephrectomy for local renal cell carcinoma. J Urol. 1998;159(4):1163–7.
64. Stephenson AJ, Chetner MP, Rourke K, Gleave ME, Signaevsky M, Palmer B, et al. Guidelines for the surveillance of localized renal cell carcinoma based on the patterns of relapse after nephrectomy. J Urol. 2004;172(1):58–62. https://doi.org/10.1097/01.ju.0000132126.85812.7d.
65. Zini L, Destrieux-Garnier L, Leroy X, Villers A, Haulon S, Lemaitre L, et al. Renal vein ostium wall invasion of renal cell carcinoma with an inferior vena cava tumor thrombus: prediction by

renal and vena caval vein diameters and prognostic significance. J Urol. 2008;179(2):450–4; discussion 4. https://doi.org/10.1016/j.juro.2007.09.042.
66. Wein AJ, Kavoussi LR, Partin AW, Peters CA. Campbell-Walsh urology. Philadelphia, PA : Elsevier; Vol. 4. 2016.
67. Leibovich BC, Cheville JC, Lohse CM, Zincke H, Frank I, Kwon ED, et al. A scoring algorithm to predict survival for patients with metastatic clear cell renal cell carcinoma: a stratification tool for prospective clinical trials. J Urol. 2005;174(5):1759–63; discussion 63. https://doi.org/10.1097/01.ju.0000177487.64651.3a.
68. Kim HL, Zisman A, Han KR, Figlin RA, Belldegrun AS. Prognostic significance of venous thrombus in renal cell carcinoma. Are renal vein and inferior vena cava involvement different? J Urol. 2004;171(2 Pt 1):588–91. https://doi.org/10.1097/01.ju.0000104672.37029.4b.
69. Blute ML, Leibovich BC, Lohse CM, Cheville JC, Zincke H. The Mayo Clinic experience with surgical management, complications and outcome for patients with renal cell carcinoma and venous tumour thrombus. BJU Int. 2004;94(1):33–41. https://doi.org/10.1111/j.1464-410X.2004.04897.x.
70. Terakawa T, Miyake H, Takenaka A, Hara I, Fujisawa M. Clinical outcome of surgical management for patients with renal cell carcinoma involving the inferior vena cava. Int J Urol. 2007;14(9):781–4. https://doi.org/10.1111/j.1442-2042.2007.01749.x.
71. Granberg CF, Boorjian SA, Schaff HV, Orszulak TA, Leibovich BC, Lohse CM, et al. Surgical management, complications, and outcome of radical nephrectomy with inferior vena cava tumor thrombectomy facilitated by vascular bypass. Urology. 2008;72(1):148–52. https://doi.org/10.1016/j.urology.2008.01.006.
72. Oto A, Herts BR, Remer EM, Novick AC. Inferior vena cava tumor thrombus in renal cell carcinoma: staging by MR imaging and impact on surgical treatment. AJR Am J Roentgenol. 1998;171(6):1619–24. https://doi.org/10.2214/ajr.171.6.9843299.
73. Tsili AC, Argyropoulou MI. Advances of multidetector computed tomography in the characterization and staging of renal cell carcinoma. World J Radiol. 2015;7(6):110–27. https://doi.org/10.4329/wjr.v7.i6.110.
74. Wotkowicz C, Wszolek MF, Libertino JA. Resection of renal tumors invading the vena cava. Urol Clin North Am. 2008;35(4):657–71. ; viii. https://doi.org/10.1016/j.ucl.2008.07.013.
75. Subramanian VS, Stephenson AJ, Goldfarb DA, Fergany AF, Novick AC, Krishnamurthi V. Utility of preoperative renal artery embolization for management of renal tumors with inferior vena caval thrombi. Urology. 2009;74(1):154–9. https://doi.org/10.1016/j.urology.2008.12.084.
76. Gettman MT, Boelter CW, Cheville JC, Zincke H, Bryant SC, Blute ML. Charlson comorbidity index as a predictor of outcome after surgery for renal cell carcinoma with renal vein, vena cava or right atrium extension. J Urol. 2003;169(4):1282–6. https://doi.org/10.1097/01.ju.0000049093.03392.cc.
77. Slaton JW, Balbay MD, Levy DA, Pisters LL, Nesbitt JC, Swanson DA, et al. Nephrectomy and vena caval thrombectomy in patients with metastatic renal cell carcinoma. Urology. 1997;50(5):673–7.
78. Margulis V, Sanchez-Ortiz RF, Tamboli P, Cohen DD, Swanson DA, Wood CG. Renal cell carcinoma clinically involving adjacent organs: experience with aggressive surgical management. Cancer. 2007;109(10):2025–30. https://doi.org/10.1002/cncr.22629.
79. May M, Brookman-Amissah S, Pflanz S, Roigas J, Hoschke B, Kendel F. Pre-operative renal arterial embolisation does not provide survival benefit in patients with radical nephrectomy for renal cell carcinoma. Br J Radiol. 2009;82(981):724–31. https://doi.org/10.1259/bjr/17514226.
80. Dekernion JB, Ramming KP, Smith RB. The natural history of metastatic renal cell carcinoma: a computer analysis. J Urol. 1978;120(2):148–52.
81. Karellas ME, Jang TL, Kagiwada MA, Kinnaman MD, Jarnagin WR, Russo P. Advanced-stage renal cell carcinoma treated by radical nephrectomy and adjacent organ or structure resection. BJU Int. 2009;103(2):160–4. https://doi.org/10.1111/j.1464-410X.2008.08025.x.

82. Cox CE, Lacy SS, Montgomery WG, Boyce WH. Renal adenocarcinoma: 28-year review, with emphasis on rationale and feasibility of preoperative radiotherapy. J Urol. 1970;104(1):53–61.
83. van der Werf-Messing B. Proceedings: carcinoma of the kidney. Cancer. 1973;32(5): 1056–61.
84. Kao GD, Malkowicz SB, Whittington R, D'Amico AV, Wein AJ. Locally advanced renal cell carcinoma: low complication rate and efficacy of postnephrectomy radiation therapy planned with CT. Radiology. 1994;193(3):725–30. https://doi.org/10.1148/radiology.193.3.7972814.
85. Mickisch GH, Garin A, van Poppel H, de Prijck L, Sylvester R, European Organisation for R, et al. Radical nephrectomy plus interferon-alfa-based immunotherapy compared with interferon alfa alone in metastatic renal-cell carcinoma: a randomised trial. Lancet. 2001;358(9286):966–70.
86. Flanigan RC, Salmon SE, Blumenstein BA, Bearman SI, Roy V, McGrath PC, et al. Nephrectomy followed by interferon alfa-2b compared with interferon alfa-2b alone for metastatic renal-cell cancer. N Engl J Med. 2001;345(23):1655–9. https://doi.org/10.1056/NEJMoa003013.
87. Flanigan RC, Mickisch G, Sylvester R, Tangen C, Van Poppel H, Crawford ED. Cytoreductive nephrectomy in patients with metastatic renal cancer: a combined analysis. J Urol. 2004;171(3):1071–6. https://doi.org/10.1097/01.ju.0000110610.61545.ae.
88. Zini L, Capitanio U, Perrotte P, Jeldres C, Shariat SF, Arjane P, et al. Population-based assessment of survival after cytoreductive nephrectomy versus no surgery in patients with metastatic renal cell carcinoma. Urology. 2009;73(2):342–6. https://doi.org/10.1016/j.urology.2008.09.022.
89. Trinh QD, Bianchi M, Hansen J, Tian Z, Abdollah F, Shariat SF, et al. In-hospital mortality and failure to rescue after cytoreductive nephrectomy. Eur Urol. 2013;63(6):1107–14. https://doi.org/10.1016/j.eururo.2012.08.069.
90. Immediate surgery or surgery after sunitinib malate in treating patients with metastatic kidney cancer (SURTIME). Available at http://clinicaltrials.gov/ct2/show/NCT01099423. Accessed Nov 2017.
91. Clinical trial to assess the importance of nephrectomy (CARMENA). Available at http://clinicaltrials.gov/ct2/show/NCT00930033. Accessed Nov 2017.
92. Stewart GD, Aitchison M, Bex A, Larkin J, Lawless C, Mejean A, et al. Cytoreductive nephrectomy in the tyrosine kinase inhibitor era: a question that may never be answered. Eur Urol. 2017;71(6):845–7. https://doi.org/10.1016/j.eururo.2016.10.029.
93. Mejean A, Ravaud A, Thezenas S, Colas S, Beauval JB, Bensalah K, et al. Sunitinib alone or after nephrectomy in metastatic renal-cell carcinoma. N Engl J Med. 2018;379(5):417–27. https://doi.org/10.1056/NEJMoa1803675.
94. You D, Jeong IG, Ahn JH, Lee DH, Lee JL, Hong JH, et al. The value of cytoreductive nephrectomy for metastatic renal cell carcinoma in the era of targeted therapy. J Urol. 2011;185(1):54–9. https://doi.org/10.1016/j.juro.2010.09.018.
95. Choueiri TK, Xie W, Kollmannsberger C, North S, Knox JJ, Lampard JG, et al. The impact of cytoreductive nephrectomy on survival of patients with metastatic renal cell carcinoma receiving vascular endothelial growth factor targeted therapy. J Urol. 2011;185(1):60–6. https://doi.org/10.1016/j.juro.2010.09.012.
96. You D, Jeong IG, Song C, Lee JL, Hong B, Hong JH, et al. Analysis of pre-operative variables for identifying patients who might benefit from upfront cytoreductive nephrectomy for metastatic renal cell carcinoma in the targeted therapy era. Jpn J Clin Oncol. 2015;45(1):96–102. https://doi.org/10.1093/jjco/hyu171.
97. Walther MM, Patel B, Choyke PL, Lubensky IA, Vocke CD, Harris C, et al. Hypercalcemia in patients with metastatic renal cell carcinoma: effect of nephrectomy and metabolic evaluation. J Urol. 1997;158(3 Pt 1):733–9.
98. Barney JD, Churchill BM. Adenocarcinoma of the kidney with metastasis to the lung. J Urol. 1939;42:269–76.

99. Kim DY, Karam JA, Wood CG. Role of metastasectomy for metastatic renal cell carcinoma in the era of targeted therapy. World J Urol. 2014;32(3):631–42. https://doi.org/10.1007/s00345-014-1293-6.
100. Daliani DD, Tannir NM, Papandreou CN, Wang X, Swisher S, Wood CG, et al. Prospective assessment of systemic therapy followed by surgical removal of metastases in selected patients with renal cell carcinoma. BJU Int. 2009;104(4):456–60. https://doi.org/10.1111/j.1464-410X.2009.08490.x.
101. Alt AL, Boorjian SA, Lohse CM, Costello BA, Leibovich BC, Blute ML. Survival after complete surgical resection of multiple metastases from renal cell carcinoma. Cancer. 2011;117(13):2873–82. https://doi.org/10.1002/cncr.25836.
102. Dabestani S, Marconi L, Hofmann F, Stewart F, Lam TB, Canfield SE, et al. Local treatments for metastases of renal cell carcinoma: a systematic review. Lancet Oncol. 2014;15(12):e549–61. https://doi.org/10.1016/S1470-2045(14)70235-9.
103. Yu X, Wang B, Li X, Lin G, Zhang C, Yang Y, et al. The significance of metastasectomy in patients with metastatic renal cell carcinoma in the era of targeted therapy. Biomed Res Int. 2015;2015:176373. https://doi.org/10.1155/2015/176373.
104. You D, Lee C, Jeong IG, Song C, Lee JL, Hong B, et al. Impact of metastasectomy on prognosis in patients treated with targeted therapy for metastatic renal cell carcinoma. J Cancer Res Clin Oncol. 2016;142(11):2331–8. https://doi.org/10.1007/s00432-016-2217-1.

Chapter 2
Renal Cell Carcinoma: Oncologist Point of View

Amado J. Zurita

Kidney cancer is among the ten most frequently diagnosed cancers in the United States, with more than an estimated 65,000 new cases and 14,900 deaths in 2018 [1]. Per the Surveillance, Epidemiology, and End Results Program database of the National Institutes of Health, the median age at diagnosis of kidney cancer is 64 years. It is more common in men than in women and among African Americans and American Indian and Alaska Native populations [2]. Kidney cancer's incidence has increased on average 0.7% each year over the last 10 years, while death rates declined on average 0.9% each year over 2005–2014 [2]. Screening for the disease is not standard. Current 5-year survival rates are 76% overall, including 66.7% among patients with regional disease and 11.7% among patients with metastatic disease [2]. Renal cell carcinoma (RCC), the most common form of kidney cancer arising from the nephron and the subject of this chapter, occurs in approximately 90% of cases, and 70–80% of these are clear cell tumors. Other less common cell types with different histologic, molecular, and genetic alterations include papillary, chromophobe, translocation, Bellini duct (collecting duct), and medullary tumors.

Patients with RCC usually present with a mass in the kidney that has been visualized using an imaging study, often a CT scan. The widespread availability of CT and ultrasound has resulted in increased detection of incidental lesions, so that presentations based on the typical triad of symptoms (hematuria, flank mass, and/or flank pain) are nowadays relatively rare. Approximately one third of patients with RCC present with a disease that is no longer localized [2], and of those with localized RCC treated with curative intent, approximately one quarter have distant relapses [3]. Metastases occur most often in the lungs, lymph nodes, liver, bone, and brain. Tumor stage (TNM), defined by the anatomic involvement of disease, remains one

A. J. Zurita (✉)
Department of Genitourinary Medical Oncology, The University of Texas MD Anderson Cancer Center, Houston, TX, USA
e-mail: azurita@mdanderson.org

M. K. Divatia et al. (eds.), *Kidney Cancer*, https://doi.org/10.1007/978-3-030-28333-9_2

of the strongest prognostic factors in the clinical outcome of patients with RCC. Because surgical resection is curative for a proportion of patients with localized RCC, several models have been developed to predict outcomes after surgery. Those most studied, such as the SSIGN or the UISS, include clinicopathologic characteristics (stage, tumor size, nuclear grade, the presence of tumor necrosis, or the Eastern Cooperative Oncology Group performance status) [4, 5], but recent work has also identified prognostically important genomic markers and molecular signatures. Mutations of tumor suppressor genes on chromosome 3p21, including those of BRCA1-associated protein-1 (BAP1) and the histone-lysine N-methyltransferase enzyme SETD2, have been linked to worse prognosis [6]. Conversely, mutations involving polybromo-1 (PBRM1) had a more favorable prognosis [7]. A gene expression panel that included 16 genes was found to independently predict increased risk of recurrence in patients undergoing radical nephrectomy for stage I to III clear cell RCC [8]. Moreover, comprehensive genomic and proteomic profiling of more than 400 primary clear cell RCC tumors from The Cancer Genome Atlas (TCGA) identified four prognostic signatures for clear cell RCC, which appear to represent the variable usage of key pathways and metabolites by tumors [9]. None of these factors or signatures has yet reached clinical application for patient care.

The past 15 years have brought considerable progress in the systemic treatment of RCC, mostly in relation to increasing understanding of the pathogenesis of clear cell renal cell carcinoma. Treatments targeting the vascular endothelial growth factor (VEGF) as a critical mediator of tumor angiogenesis, the negative regulator of the immune response programmed cell death protein 1 (PD-1), and the mechanistic target of rapamycin (mTOR), a central regulator of cellular metabolism, growth, and survival, have significantly increased survival rates in this disease.

Treatment of Localized Disease

Surgical resection remains an effective therapy for clinically localized and locally advanced RCC. The choice of surgical procedure depends upon the extent of disease and patient-specific factors such as age and comorbidity. Options include radical nephrectomy and nephron-sparing surgery through a conventional or a minimally invasive approach such as laparoscopy, aiming to optimize long-term renal function and cancer-free survival. Ablative procedures such as cryotherapy and radiofrequency ablation are alternatives for patients with relatively small renal masses who are not surgical candidates. Disease monitoring typically includes at least history and physical exam, a comprehensive metabolic panel, and imaging of the chest and abdomen. The median time to relapse after surgery is 1–2 years, and most relapses occur within the first 3 years [10].

Any Role for Adjuvant Therapy?

Before the targeted therapies became available, randomized trials comparing adjuvant or complementary high-dose interleukin-2 (IL-2), interferon alpha (IFN-α), or other immune therapy combinations with observation alone showed no delay in time to relapse or improvement in survival in patients with locally advanced, completely resected RCC [11]. An antibody targeting carbonic anhydrase IX [12], hormone therapy, chemotherapy, or radiation treatment was not found efficacious either [11]. Since then, several clinical trials have explored the role of antiangiogenic therapies and mTOR inhibitors, which are known active drugs in the advanced disease setting. The results of S-TRAC, one of those studies, showing an improvement in disease-free survival (DFS) of approximately 1.2 years compared with placebo in patients with clear cell RCC of higher risk, led to the approval of the angiogenesis inhibitor agent sunitinib (54 weeks in 6-week cycles, 4 weeks on and 2 weeks off) for adjuvant therapy [13]. However, the still immature data suggests that the difference in DFS will not translate in overall survival (OS) benefit [13]. Two other large phase 3 trials (ASSURE, testing 1 year of sunitinib, the first-generation antiangiogenic sorafenib, or placebo in patients with intermediate or high risk for recurrence; and PROTECT, evaluating pazopanib, an alternative antiangiogenic, vs. placebo for 1 year) failed to identify important differences in DFS [14–16]. Because of the overall questionable benefit, cost, and the significant and potentially serious side effects of VEGF inhibitors, observation remains the standard of care after nephrectomy for most patients. Those eligible should be offered enrollment in randomized clinical trials, the most widely available of which are evaluating novel immunotherapy agents targeting PD-1.

Indications for Surgery and Radiation in Advanced Disease

Patients with metastasis or unresectable primary disease may also benefit from surgery. Randomized clinical trials showed that cytoreductive nephrectomy performed prior to IFN-α immunotherapy resulted in improved survival compared with no surgery [17, 18], but similar prospective data are not available in the era of angiogenesis inhibitors and more current types of immunotherapy. However, retrospective analyses suggest that cytoreductive nephrectomy continues to play a role in these settings as well [19, 20], and therefore resection of the primary tumor is typically part of the care of patients with known metastatic disease and a good performance status, a limited amount of metastases, and no or little symptoms from them, if the surgery is technically feasible.

Patients who present with primary RCC and a solitary site of metastasis in the lung, bone, or brain, or limited lymphadenopathy, are candidates for nephrectomy and surgical metastasectomy. Similarly, those who develop a solitary recurrence after a prolonged disease-free interval from nephrectomy may benefit from metastasis resection. Most of these patients experience disease recurrence, but prolonged disease control is not uncommon [21].

Conventional and stereotactic modalities of radiation therapy are typically used to treat bone and brain metastases [22]. In particular the stereotactic modality can result in high rates of local control with relatively minimal toxicity [23].

Systemic Therapy for Advanced Disease

Systemic treatment options for metastatic kidney cancer have expanded substantially in the past 12 years. Antiangiogenic drugs targeting VEGF and its receptors (bevacizumab, sorafenib, sunitinib, pazopanib, axitinib, cabozantinib, and lenvatinib), mTOR inhibitors (temsirolimus and everolimus), and an immune checkpoint inhibitor (nivolumab) have resulted in higher rates of response, longer progression-free survival (PFS), and in some cases OS than IFN-α and IL-2, the previously used immunotherapies, and have consequently been approved for use [24]. Treatment decisions are based on the available evidence, the individual characteristics of the disease and the patient including comorbid conditions, and the toxicity profiles of specific agents. Since not all of the drugs have been directly compared, several options exist for both first- and second- and later-line therapies [25].

Clinical factors associated with reduced OS have been integrated into prognostic models, which separate patients according to their expected outcomes and help stratify risk and select therapy. The most widely used are those of the Memorial Sloan Kettering Cancer Center (MSKCC) [26] and the International Metastatic Renal Cell Carcinoma Database Consortium (IMDC) [27], which share four factors—poor performance status, less than a 1-year interval from diagnosis to treatment, a high serum calcium level, and a low hemoglobin concentration—and differ in one: a high serum lactate dehydrogenase level in the MSKCC model is replaced by high neutrophil or platelet count in the IMDC's. The IMDC model was developed after the VEGF-targeted therapies became widely available and stratifies patients into three risk categories on the basis of the number of risk factors, with estimated median OS of 43 months (favorable), 22 months (intermediate), and 8 months (poor risk) [27]. Multiple candidate predictive molecular biomarkers from the blood and tissue have been explored to guide the application of therapy in RCC, but none have been validated for clinical use [28].

In general, systemic therapy is initiated promptly in patients with metastasis or locally advanced RCC, but studies have shown that those asymptomatic with favorable risk and limited disease burden and number of organ sites involved can safely defer treatment until more compelling disease progression is documented [29].

Clear Cell Renal Cell Carcinoma

Molecularly targeted antiangiogenic therapy and increasingly immunotherapy with checkpoint inhibitors are the main systemic treatment options for patients with advanced clear cell RCC. Treatments with level 1 evidence frontline include sunitinib and pazopanib, oral drugs that inhibit the tyrosine kinases of the VEGF and other receptors and are the most commonly used agents; bevacizumab, a monoclonal antibody that blocks VEGF, in combination with IFN-α; and the mTOR inhibitor temsirolimus for the poor risk group. A phase 3 trial compared sunitinib to pazopanib as first-line treatment and found that pazopanib has similar efficacy but less negative effects on quality of life parameters [30]. Common and potentially severe side effects of both such as fatigue, anorexia, nausea, diarrhea, hypertension, and bone marrow toxicity frequently require adjustments in dose and schedule. For the approximately 20% of patients who present with poor-risk clear cell RCC, weekly intravenous temsirolimus is an alternative option with very limited efficacy [31]. However, two recently presented studies are changing the status quo for the patients presenting with the more aggressive disease. CABOSUN was a randomized open-label phase 2 study that compared the VEGF receptor, c-MET, and AXL inhibitor cabozantinib to sunitinib in patients with previously untreated IMDC intermediate and poor-risk RCC [32]. Cabozantinib demonstrated longer PFS (median 3.3 months) and higher objective response rate (ORR) than sunitinib [33] and was approved in the first-line setting by the Food and Drug Administration in December 2017. The second of the trials was the randomized open-label phase 3 CHECKMATE-214 study, which evaluated the combination of the immune checkpoint inhibitors nivolumab (anti-PD-1) and ipilimumab (anti-cytotoxic T lymphocyte-associated antigen 4, CTLA-4) in comparison to sunitinib. The combination of immunotherapies resulted in improved PFS (median 3.2 months), OS (37% decreased risk of death), and higher rates of response (15% difference) than sunitinib in previously untreated patients with IMDC intermediate and poor-risk disease (especially in tumors with ≥1% PD-L1 expression), and therefore it is likely to become a new standard for those patients [34]. Interestingly, IMDC favorable-risk patients achieved higher ORR and longer PFS with sunitinib [34].

In second and later lines of treatment after first-line VEGF-targeted therapy, the results of phase 3 trials provide the highest support for the use of axitinib [35, 36], cabozantinib [37, 38], nivolumab [39], and the combination of everolimus with lenvatinib (an inhibitor of the VEGF receptors, fibroblast growth factor receptors (FGFR) 1–4, and other receptors) [40]. Both cabozantinib and nivolumab demonstrated significantly longer OS (median 4.9 months and 5.4 months, respectively) [38, 39] than the mTOR inhibitor everolimus, which had previously proven to result in longer PFS than placebo in patients with advanced clear cell RCC refractory to antiangiogenic therapy.

Although clearly effective, all these medications can result in important toxicities leading to dose reductions, changes in schedule, and even discontinuation in 7–24% of the patients that take them.

Since options increase and head-to-head comparisons between the best therapies are generally not available, no good data exists to guide how to sequence therapies in the individual patient.

Non-clear Cell Renal Cell Carcinoma

The histologic and molecular characteristics and the clinical outcomes of non-clear cell RCC are heterogeneous and differ from clear cell RCC. Still, available data shows that albeit less effective, targeted therapies approved for clear cell RCC, particularly VEGF inhibitors, may also be beneficial. Two randomized phase 2 trials compared sunitinib with everolimus specifically in patients with non-clear cell RCC, primarily the papillary cell type (the most frequent non-clear cell subtype), and found that sunitinib resulted in better survival outcomes [41, 42]. Other agents showing responses as single agent in papillary RCC include inhibitors of c-MET (sporadic papillary RCC and hereditary papillary type 1 RCC are associated with alterations in *MET*) [43] and erlotinib (an epidermal growth factor receptor inhibitor) [44]. Cytotoxic chemotherapies such as gemcitabine and platinum derivatives are active especially for collecting duct RCC and renal medullary carcinomas [45] and are sometimes used in the treatment of RCC with sarcomatoid features [46]. Data from prospective studies investigating the activity of immunotherapy with checkpoint inhibitors for non-clear cell RCC are still missing.

What Is Next?

Preclinical data suggests synergy between angiogenesis inhibition and immune system activation [47]. This, together with phase 1/2 studies [48] showing promising ORR with manageable toxicities, has led to the development of several phase 3 trials combining anti-VEGF agents with checkpoint inhibitors. The results of these studies are expected to become available within the next 2 years and may well lead to new treatment indications.

Integration of the increasing knowledge on molecular RCC subtypes derived from investigations of somatic mutations, gene expression, and DNA methylation in human samples into the design of clinical trials, and the rationale clinical development of novel drugs in the pipeline targeting pathways relevant to RCC biology, will get us closer toward personalized therapy selection and the definitive goal of cure, even for patients with metastasis.

References

1. Siegel RL, Miller KD, Jemal A. Cancer statistics. CA Cancer J Clin. 2018;68(4):284–96.
2. SEER Cancer stat facts: kidney and renal pelvis cancer. National Cancer Institute. Bethesda, MD. http://seer.cancer.gov/statfacts/html/kidrp.html.

3. Dabestani S, Thorstenson A, Lindblad P, Harmenberg U, Ljungberg B, Lundstam S. Renal cell carcinoma recurrences and metastases in primary non-metastatic patients: a population-based study. World J Urol. 2016;34:1081–6.
4. Beisland C, Gudbrandsdottir G, Reisaeter LA, Bostad L, Wentzel-Larsen T, Hjelle KM. Contemporary external validation of the Leibovich model for prediction of progression after radical surgery for clear cell renal cell carcinoma. Scand J Urol. 2015;49:205–10.
5. Han KR, Bleumer I, Pantuck AJ, Kim HL, Dorey FJ, Janzen NK, et al. Validation of an integrated staging system toward improved prognostication of patients with localized renal cell carcinoma in an international population. J Urol. 2003;170:2221–4.
6. Hakimi AA, Ostrovnaya I, Reva B, Schultz N, Chen YB, Gonen M, et al. Adverse outcomes in clear cell renal cell carcinoma with mutations of 3p21 epigenetic regulators BAP1 and SETD2: a report by MSKCC and the KIRC TCGA research network. Clin Cancer Res. 2013;19:3259–67.
7. Kapur P, Pena-Llopis S, Christie A, Zhrebker L, Pavia-Jimenez A, Rathmell WK, et al. Effects on survival of BAP1 and PBRM1 mutations in sporadic clear-cell renal-cell carcinoma: a retrospective analysis with independent validation. Lancet Oncol. 2013;14:159–67.
8. Rini B, Goddard A, Knezevic D, Maddala T, Zhou M, Aydin H, et al. A 16-gene assay to predict recurrence after surgery in localised renal cell carcinoma: development and validation studies. Lancet Oncol. 2015;16:676–85.
9. Cancer Genome Atlas Research N. Comprehensive molecular characterization of clear cell renal cell carcinoma. Nature. 2013;499:43–9.
10. Eggener SE, Yossepowitch O, Pettus JA, Snyder ME, Motzer RJ, Russo P. Renal cell carcinoma recurrence after nephrectomy for localized disease: predicting survival from time of recurrence. J Clin Oncol. 2006;24:3101–6.
11. Pal SK, Haas NB. Adjuvant therapy for renal cell carcinoma: past, present, and future. Oncologist. 2014;19:851–9.
12. Chamie K, Donin NM, Klopfer P, Bevan P, Fall B, Wilhelm O, et al. Adjuvant weekly girentuximab following nephrectomy for high-risk renal cell carcinoma: the ARISER randomized clinical trial. JAMA Oncol. 2017;3:913–20.
13. Ravaud A. Adjuvant sunitinib in renal-cell carcinoma. N Engl J Med. 2017;376:893.
14. Haas NB, Manola J, Uzzo RG, Flaherty KT, Wood CG, Kane C, et al. Adjuvant sunitinib or sorafenib for high-risk, non-metastatic renal-cell carcinoma (ECOG-ACRIN E2805): a double-blind, placebo-controlled, randomised, phase 3 trial. Lancet. 2016;387:2008–16.
15. Haas NB, Manola J, Dutcher JP, Flaherty KT, Uzzo RG, Atkins MB, et al. Adjuvant treatment for high-risk clear cell renal cancer: updated results of a high-risk subset of the ASSURE randomized trial. JAMA Oncol. 2017;3:1249–52.
16. Motzer RJ, Haas NB, Donskov F, Gross-Goupil M, Varlamov S, Kopyltsov E, et al. Randomized phase III trial of adjuvant pazopanib versus placebo after nephrectomy in patients with localized or locally advanced renal cell carcinoma. J Clin Oncol. 2017;35:3916–23.
17. Flanigan RC, Salmon SE, Blumenstein BA, Bearman SI, Roy V, McGrath PC, et al. Nephrectomy followed by interferon alfa-2b compared with interferon alfa-2b alone for metastatic renal-cell cancer. N Engl J Med. 2001;345:1655–9.
18. Mickisch GH, Garin A, van Poppel H, de Prijck L, Sylvester R, European Organisation for R, et al. Radical nephrectomy plus interferon-alfa-based immunotherapy compared with interferon alfa alone in metastatic renal-cell carcinoma: a randomised trial. Lancet. 2001;358:966–70.
19. Choueiri TK, Xie W, Kollmannsberger C, North S, Knox JJ, Lampard JG, et al. The impact of cytoreductive nephrectomy on survival of patients with metastatic renal cell carcinoma receiving vascular endothelial growth factor targeted therapy. J Urol. 2011;185:60–6.
20. Petrelli F, Coinu A, Vavassori I, Cabiddu M, Borgonovo K, Ghilardi M, et al. Cytoreductive nephrectomy in metastatic renal cell carcinoma treated with targeted therapies: a systematic review with a meta-analysis. Clin Genitourin Cancer. 2016;14:465–72.
21. Alt AL, Boorjian SA, Lohse CM, Costello BA, Leibovich BC, Blute ML. Survival after complete surgical resection of multiple metastases from renal cell carcinoma. Cancer. 2011;117:2873–82.

22. Shaikh T, Handorf EA, Murphy CT, Kutikov A, Uzzo RG, Hallman M, et al. Contemporary trends in the utilization of radiotherapy in patients with renal cell carcinoma. Urology. 2015;86:1165–73.
23. Siva S, Kothari G, Muacevic A, Louie AV, Slotman BJ, Teh BS, et al. Radiotherapy for renal cell carcinoma: renaissance of an overlooked approach. Nat Rev Urol. 2017;14:549–63.
24. Choueiri TK, Motzer RJ. Systemic therapy for metastatic renal-cell carcinoma. N Engl J Med. 2017;376:354–66.
25. National Comprehensive Cancer Network. NCCN clinical practice guidelines in oncology: kidney cancer, version 2. 2018. https://www.nccn.org/professionals/physician_gls/pdf/kidney.pdf.
26. Motzer RJ, Bacik J, Murphy BA, Russo P, Mazumdar M. Interferon-alfa as a comparative treatment for clinical trials of new therapies against advanced renal cell carcinoma. J Clin Oncol. 2002;20:289–96.
27. Heng DY, Xie W, Regan MM, Harshman LC, Bjarnason GA, Vaishampayan UN, et al. External validation and comparison with other models of the International Metastatic Renal-Cell Carcinoma Database Consortium prognostic model: a population-based study. Lancet Oncol. 2013;14:141–8.
28. Maroto P, Rini B. Molecular biomarkers in advanced renal cell carcinoma. Clin Cancer Res. 2014;20:2060–71.
29. Rini BI, Dorff TB, Elson P, Rodriguez CS, Shepard D, Wood L, et al. Active surveillance in metastatic renal-cell carcinoma: a prospective, phase 2 trial. Lancet Oncol. 2016;17:1317–24.
30. Motzer RJ, McCann L, Deen K. Pazopanib versus sunitinib in renal cancer. N Engl J Med. 2013;369:1970.
31. Hudes G, Carducci M, Tomczak P, Dutcher J, Figlin R, Kapoor A, et al. Temsirolimus, interferon alfa, or both for advanced renal-cell carcinoma. N Engl J Med. 2007;356:2271–81.
32. Choueiri TK, Halabi S, Sanford BL, Hahn O, Michaelson MD, Walsh MK, et al. Cabozantinib versus sunitinib as initial targeted therapy for patients with metastatic renal cell carcinoma of poor or intermediate risk: the alliance A031203 CABOSUN trial. J Clin Oncol. 2017;35:591–7.
33. Choueiri TK, Hessel C, Halabi S, Sandford B, Hahn O, Michaelson MD, et al. Progression-free survival (PFS) by independent review and updated overall survival (OS) results from Alliance A031203 trial (CABOSUN): cabozantinib versus sunitinib as initial targeted therapy for patients (pts) with metastatic renal cell carcinoma (mRCC). Ann Oncol. 2017;28(Suppl_5):v605–49. https://doi.org/10.1093/annonc/mdx440.
34. Escudier B, Tannir N, McDermott D, Frontera OA, Melichar B, Plimack ER, et al. Efficacy and safety of nivolumab + ipilimumab (N+I) v sunitinib (S) for treatment-naïve advanced or metastatic renal cell carcinoma (mRCC), including IMDC risk and PD-L1 expression subgroups (abstract LBA5). Ann Oncol. 2017;28(Suppl_5):v605–49. https://doi.org/10.1093/annonc/mdx440.
35. Rini BI, Escudier B, Tomczak P, Kaprin A, Szczylik C, Hutson TE, et al. Comparative effectiveness of axitinib versus sorafenib in advanced renal cell carcinoma (AXIS): a randomised phase 3 trial. Lancet. 2011;378:1931–9.
36. Motzer RJ, Escudier B, Tomczak P, Hutson TE, Michaelson MD, Negrier S, et al. Axitinib versus sorafenib as second-line treatment for advanced renal cell carcinoma: overall survival analysis and updated results from a randomised phase 3 trial. Lancet Oncol. 2013;14:552–62.
37. Choueiri TK, Escudier B, Powles T, Mainwaring PN, Rini BI, Donskov F, et al. Cabozantinib versus everolimus in advanced renal-cell carcinoma. N Engl J Med. 2015;373:1814–23.
38. Choueiri TK, Escudier B, Powles T, Tannir NM, Mainwaring PN, Rini BI, et al. Cabozantinib versus everolimus in advanced renal cell carcinoma (METEOR): final results from a randomised, open-label, phase 3 trial. Lancet Oncol. 2016;17:917–27.
39. Motzer RJ, Escudier B, McDermott DF, George S, Hammers HJ, Srinivas S, et al. Nivolumab versus everolimus in advanced renal-cell carcinoma. N Engl J Med. 2015;373:1803–13.

40. Motzer RJ, Hutson TE, Glen H, Michaelson MD, Molina A, Eisen T, et al. Lenvatinib, everolimus, and the combination in patients with metastatic renal cell carcinoma: a randomised, phase 2, open-label, multicentre trial. Lancet Oncol. 2015;16:1473–82.
41. Tannir NM, Jonasch E, Albiges L, Altinmakas E, Ng CS, Matin SF, et al. Everolimus versus sunitinib prospective evaluation in metastatic non-clear cell renal cell carcinoma (ESPN): a randomized multicenter phase 2 trial. Eur Urol. 2016;69:866–74.
42. Armstrong AJ, Halabi S, Eisen T, Broderick S, Stadler WM, Jones RJ, et al. Everolimus versus sunitinib for patients with metastatic non-clear cell renal cell carcinoma (ASPEN): a multicentre, open-label, randomised phase 2 trial. Lancet Oncol. 2016;17:378–88.
43. Cancer Genome Atlas Research N, Linehan WM, Spellman PT, Ricketts CJ, Creighton CJ, Fei SS, et al. Comprehensive molecular characterization of papillary renal-cell carcinoma. N Engl J Med. 2016;374:135–45.
44. Gordon MS, Hussey M, Nagle RB, Lara PN Jr, Mack PC, Dutcher J, et al. Phase II study of erlotinib in patients with locally advanced or metastatic papillary histology renal cell cancer: SWOG S0317. J Clin Oncol. 2009;27:5788–93.
45. Oudard S, Banu E, Vieillefond A, Fournier L, Priou F, Medioni J, et al. Prospective multicenter phase II study of gemcitabine plus platinum salt for metastatic collecting duct carcinoma: results of a GETUG (Groupe d'Etudes des Tumeurs Uro-Genitales) study. J Urol. 2007;177:1698–702.
46. Diamond E, Molina AM, Carbonaro M, Akhtar NH, Giannakakou P, Tagawa ST, et al. Cytotoxic chemotherapy in the treatment of advanced renal cell carcinoma in the era of targeted therapy. Crit Rev Oncol Hematol. 2015;96:518–26.
47. Vanneman M, Dranoff G. Combining immunotherapy and targeted therapies in cancer treatment. Nat Rev Cancer. 2012;12:237–51.
48. Wallin JJ, Bendell JC, Funke R, Sznol M, Korski K, Jones S, et al. Atezolizumab in combination with bevacizumab enhances antigen-specific T-cell migration in metastatic renal cell carcinoma. Nat Commun. 2016;7:12624.

Part II
Histopathology and Cytology

Chapter 3
Normal Anatomy and Histology of the Kidney: Importance for Kidney Tumors

Ziad M. El-Zaatari, Komal Arora, Mukul K. Divatia, and Jae Y. Ro

The kidneys are a pair of bean-shaped organs located in the upper retroperitoneal cavity. For kidney tumors, a clear understanding of embryology, normal anatomy, and histology is important. In this chapter, we will discuss the embryonic development of the kidney and its normal anatomy and histology, in relation to surgical kidney diseases, especially tumor pathology.

Embryologic Development

Kidney development progresses through three stages: pronephros, mesonephros, and metanephros. The pronephros develops in the lower cervical and upper thoracic regions during the third gestational week as a condensation of the intermediate mesoderm. The pronephros regresses by the fourth gestational week; however, the pronephric duct is preserved and ultimately gives rise to the mesonephric duct. The mesonephros develops more caudally, from the intermediate mesoderm during the fourth week of gestation, before the pronephros regresses. The mesonephros contains 20–40 nephrons, comprising glomeruli that are directly connected to tubules, some of which connect directly to the mesonephric duct. Most tubules degenerate but the mesonephric duct persists bilaterally. The ureters, renal pelvis, and bladder trigone are derived from the mesonephric duct in both sexes. In males, the mesonephric duct also gives rise to the vasa deferentia, epididymis, and seminal vesicles. The mesonephric duct comes in

Z. M. El-Zaatari · K. Arora · M. K. Divatia · J. Y. Ro (✉)
Department of Pathology and Genomic Medicine, Houston Methodist Hospital, Weill Medical College of Cornell University, Houston, TX, USA
e-mail: JaeRo@houstonmethodist.org

M. K. Divatia et al. (eds.), *Kidney Cancer*, https://doi.org/10.1007/978-3-030-28333-9_3

contact with the cloaca, a precursor of the urinary bladder at the caudal aspect. It then grows cranially as the ureteric bud until it comes in contact with the metanephric mesenchyme or blastema. The ureteric bud and metanephric mesenchyme reciprocally induce growth, forming the metanephros or the mature kidney. The ureteric bud branches to form the renal pelvis, major and minor calyces, and collecting ducts. The ureteric bud secretes growth factors that induce blastema to undergo mesenchymal-to-epithelial transition. The metanephric mesenchyme develops into glomeruli, proximal and distal tubules, and the loops of Henle. The process of nephrogenesis continues until the 32nd gestational week. After the metanephros forms, it gradually rises from the pelvis to a higher position in the abdomen, a process referred to as "ascent." As ascent occurs, the vascular supply to the kidney moves from the common iliac arteries to higher branches of the abdominal aorta. Older arteries supplying the kidney successively involute until the final renal arteries are established [1–3].

Perturbations of normal embryologic development can explain the origin of some tumors and anomalies encountered in the kidney. Wilms tumor arises from retained primitive kidney tissues, or nephrogenic rests, and often harbors mutations in genes important for kidney development including the WT1 gene [4]. Metanephric adenoma, which may occur in children to elderly individuals, and more commonly in females, may arise from nephrogenic rests or maturation of Wilms tumor [5]. Premature division of the ureteric bud can give rise to duplications of the ureter, the renal pelvis, or the entire kidney. Duplication of the ureter is the most common malformation of the urinary tract and is associated with urinary tract infections, vesicoureteral reflux, ectopic ureterocele, and poor renal function [6–8]. Renal dysplasia may result from failure of proper differentiation of the nephron and collecting duct [9]. Fusion giving rise to a "horseshoe" kidney results from abnormal migration during kidney ascent [3]. Failure of involution of the developing renal vasculature may lead to the formation of accessory renal arteries [1].

Anatomic Features

The kidneys are retroperitoneal organs that extend from the 12th thoracic vertebra to the 3rd lumbar vertebra and along the borders of the psoas muscles. The kidneys are positioned obliquely with a slight tilt of the upper poles toward the midline. The adult kidney is about 10–12 cm in length, 5.0–7.5 cm in width, and 2.5–3.0 cm thick. The right kidney is slightly shorter than the left one due to downward compression by the liver. Based on a sonographic study, in adults, the medial length is 11.2 cm (4.4 in) for the left kidney and 10.9 cm (4.3 in) for the right one [10]. The normal adult kidney weighs 125–170 g in males and 115–155 g in females [11, 12].

An understanding of the gross anatomic features and anatomic relationships of the kidneys to surrounding organs is essential for accurate gross evaluation of renal tumors and staging of renal cell carcinoma (RCC). Each kidney is enclosed by two layers of fascia and two layers of fat, which are the following (from innermost to outer): the renal capsule, the perirenal fat, the renal fascia (Gerota's fascia), and the pararenal fat [13]. RCC confined to the renal parenchyma without extension beyond the renal capsule is staged as T1 or T2, depending on tumor size. Stage T1 comprises tumors that are 7 cm or less in the greatest dimension, and T2 comprises tumors that are more than 7 cm in the greatest dimension. Extension of RCC beyond the renal parenchyma and into the perirenal fat constitutes T3 disease, whereas extension beyond Gerota's fascia is considered T4 disease [14].

The kidneys are related posteriorly to the diaphragm, muscles of the posterior abdominal wall, and the 11th and 12th ribs. Anteriorly, the right kidney is related to the liver, the second part of the duodenum, and the ascending colon. The left kidney is anteriorly related to the stomach, pancreas, spleen, and descending colon. The adrenal glands cap the kidneys superiorly [13]. Contiguous extension of a primary RCC from the upper pole to the ipsilateral adrenal gland is considered as T4 disease. RCC of the middle or lower pole of the kidney involving the adrenal in a discontinuous manner is considered metastatic (M1) disease [14].

The kidneys are grossly composed of the renal cortex, medulla, major and minor calyces, pelvis, and hilum (Fig. 3.1). The cortex is approximately 1 cm thick and con-

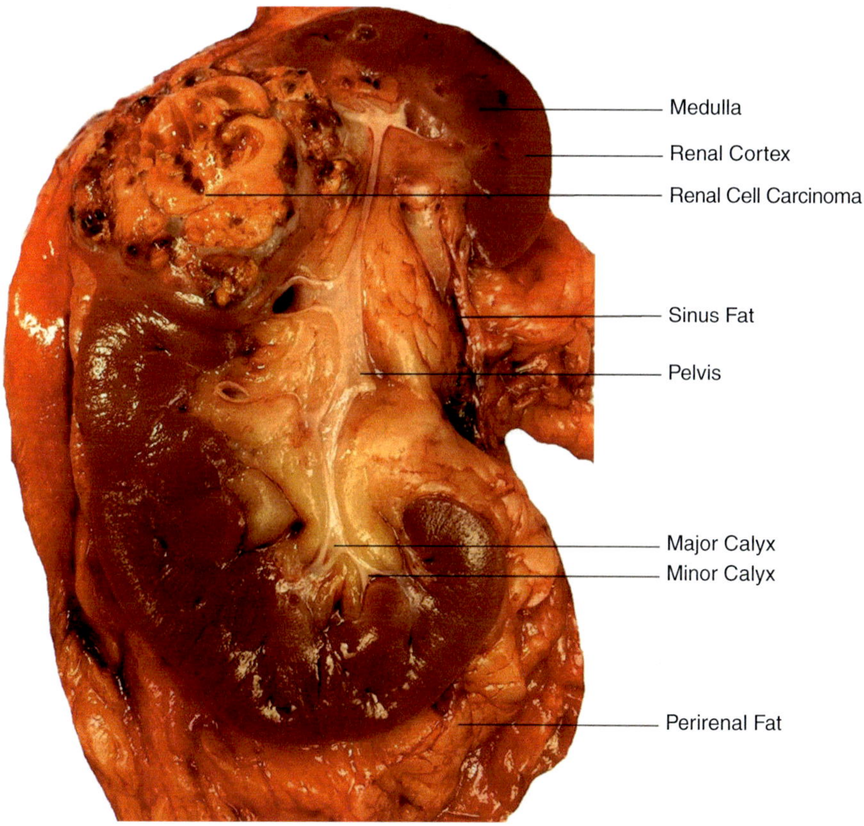

Fig. 3.1 Gross anatomy of the kidney as seen on a nephrectomy specimen with renal cell carcinoma. The knowledge of the various anatomic structures and their relationship to kidney tumors are essential for accurate cancer staging. (Courtesy of Monica B. Lemos, Pathologists' Assistant)

tains the nephrons, which are the units of filtration, in addition to the renal tubules. The medulla is the inner layer and contains the renal tubules and collecting ducts. The pyramids are extensions of the renal cortex between the medulla with tips that end at a minor calyx. Urine is passed to the minor calyces, which drain into a major calyx. The renal pelvis is the confluence of the major calyces and conveys urine to the proximal portion of the ureter. The pelvis exits the kidney through the hilum, which is also the region where arteries, veins, nerves, and lymphatics enter or exit the kidney. The structures of the hilum are surrounded by a portion of the perirenal fat named the renal sinus fat [12, 13]. Invasion of RCC of the renal sinus fat corresponds to pT3a disease [14].

The vascular supply of the kidneys originates from the abdominal aorta, which gives rise to the left and right main renal arteries. These arteries branch into anterior and posterior divisions from which segmental arteries, most commonly five, are derived. The segmental arteries give rise to interlobar arteries, which pass between two renal pyramids (these areas are referred to as the columns of Bertin), and then give rise to arcuate arteries that travel along the corticomedullary junction. The interlobular arteries then rise approximately perpendicular to the arcuate arteries and end in afferent arterioles that enter glomeruli. Exiting each glomerulus is an efferent arteriole that supplies nearby tubules. Most of the blood supply of the medulla also originates from juxtamedullary efferent arterioles that give off long and thin branches, the vasa recta. The remainder of the blood supply to the medulla comes from branches of the interlobar arteries. The venous and lymphatic drainage of the kidney mostly follows the arterial anatomy. The venous drainage terminates in the renal vein, which drains into the vena cava.

The lymphatic vessels drain into the paraaortic lymph nodes [13]. In cases of nephrectomies performed for RCC, lymph node dissection is not routinely performed by the surgeon in many cases, especially in cases of limited disease, as the clinical benefit of this procedure is still contentious [15, 16]. The prosector of a radical nephrectomy specimen may occasionally find lymph nodes within the renal adipose tissue, especially in the renal hilum close to major vessels [14]. Unlike carcinomas of other organs, lymphatic spread of RCC is unusual. Therefore, usually it is not necessary to perform an extensive search for renal hilar lymph nodes, as at least one study showed that positive hilar lymph nodes are almost always grossly visible [17]. In RCC, blood-borne metastasis is usual and more common. The involvement by RCC of the renal vein or its muscle-containing branches is considered stage pT3a, whereas the involvement of the vena cava below or above the diaphragm is defined as pT3b or pT3c disease, respectively. Invasion into the wall of the vena cava is also considered pT3c. Thus, it is important to document the vascular involvement of RCCs in the kidney both macroscopically and microscopically [14].

The kidney receives parasympathetic innervation originating from the vagus nerve and sympathetic innervation supplied by the lesser and least splanchnic nerves in addition to the lumbar splanchnic nerves [13]. Neural invasion is not commonly found in cases of RCC, and the significance of such a finding has not been extensively studied.

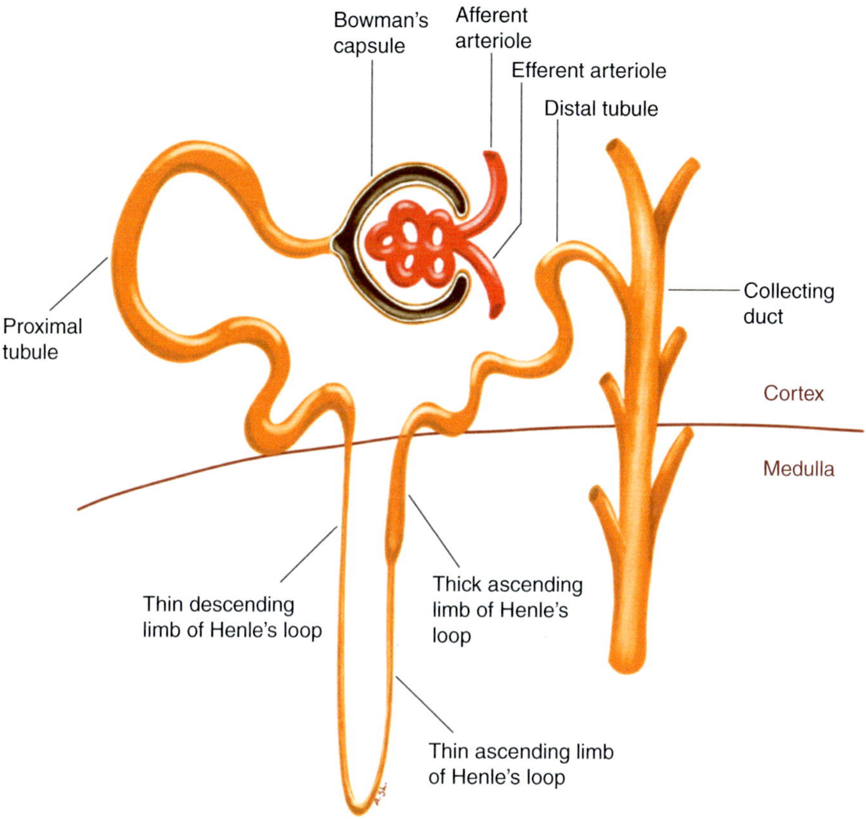

Fig. 3.2 Anatomy of the nephron, the basic structural and functional unit of the kidney. (Courtesy of Ahmed Shehabeldin, MD)

Histology

Understanding normal kidney histology is more essential in nontumoral kidney diseases and less so for mass-forming surgical kidney diseases. Nonetheless, the knowledge of normal histology is relevant to kidney tumor histogenesis and is valuable in assessing renal parenchymal changes in the uninvolved kidney in association with RCC. The principal structural and functional unit of the kidney is the nephron (Fig. 3.2), which is composed of a continuum of microscopic structures through which blood is filtered and urine is formed. The structures of the nephron are ordered topographically within the cortex and medulla and consist of glomeruli and a connected system of tubules that begin with the proximal tubules and end in the distal collecting ducts.

General Nephron Structure

The nephron begins with the glomeruli, which are located within the kidney cortex. Cortical nephrons have glomeruli located more superficially within the cortex, whereas juxtaglomerular nephrons have glomeruli closer to the medulla and course deeper into the medulla. Blood flowing through the convoluted glomerular tuft is filtered, and the filtrate is collected in Bowman's space and passed on to the proximal convoluted tubule. The convoluted proximal tubule is located within the cortex and continues as a straight segment extending from the cortex to the medulla. The loop of Henle is a "U" or hairpin-shaped loop located exclusively within the medulla and connects the proximal tubule with the distal convoluted tubule in the cortex. The distal convoluted tubule connects with the collecting duct, where urine is passed to the renal papilla and collected in the renal pelvis [18].

Glomerulus

The glomerulus is composed of a complex tuft of capillaries, originating from the afferent arteriole, and is surrounded by Bowman's capsule. The term renal corpuscle describes these structures more accurately; however, the term glomerulus is often used interchangeably. In the adult kidney, glomeruli are distributed throughout the cortex, whereas in pediatric kidneys glomeruli are concentrated beneath the capsule and are smaller in size with prominent podocytes and a more clouded appearance. The endothelial cells lining the glomerular capillaries have light eosinophilic cytoplasm and oval-round nuclei. The cytoplasm of each endothelial cell is very thinly stretched around the capillary lumen, with a thicker portion at one pole containing the nucleus. In between capillary loops are mesangial cells and an associated mesangial matrix. Mesangial cell nuclei stain more darkly basophilic than the endothelial cells [1]. Some mesangial cells are located just outside the glomerulus adjacent to the afferent and efferent arterioles and form part of the juxtaglomerular apparatus, a structure that secretes renin and has hormonal control of blood pressure [18].

Juxtaglomerular cell tumor is a rare neoplasm originating from smooth muscle cells within the juxtaglomerular apparatus [19]. Specialized cells referred to as podocytes surround the outer surface of glomerular capillary loops. Under the light microscope, podocytes have oval, round nuclei and abundant pink cytoplasm [1]. The space between the outer surface of capillaries and Bowman's capsule is called urinary space. Finally, Bowman's capsule is lined by a simple squamous epithelium, a fact that can be difficult to demonstrate on H&E-stained sections but is more easily demonstrated with keratin immunostaining [1, 18].

Proximal Tubular System

The proximal tubules are lined with a single layer of cuboidal to low columnar cells with eosinophilic to slightly granular cytoplasm. Each cell includes a round nucleus found in the center or close to the epithelial base. On light microscopy, the borders between tubular epithelial cells are indistinct. On the luminal aspect of the proximal tubule, there is a brush border, which can be highlighted with PAS staining. In cross-sections of the cortex, the proximal tubules occupy the majority of the cortical area with interspersed glomeruli and distal tubules. Compared to the cells lining the distal tubules, those of the proximal tubule appear plumper with more abundant cytoplasm and a higher degree of eosinophilic staining. Also, more nuclei per cross-section are seen in the distal tubules as compared to the proximal tubules [1]. The proximal tubule epithelium is thought to be the origin of conventional (clear cell) and papillary renal cell carcinomas [20].

Loop of Henle

The loop of Henle is composed of thin descending limb, ascending limb, and a thick ascending limb. The straight segment of the proximal convoluted tubule abruptly narrows to transition to the thin descending limb of Henle's loop. The thin limbs of Henle's loop are lined by simple squamous epithelium. The lining epithelium is markedly attenuated with flattened lining cells, scant cytoplasm, and lenticular-shaped nuclei that can be seen slightly protruding into the lumen. The thin limb epithelia have been shown to be positive for keratins 7, 8, 18, and 19 [21, 22]. The thick ascending limb is lined with a single layer of cuboidal cells with more abundant eosinophilic cytoplasm and round nuclei that are apically located and bulge slightly into the lumen.

Distal Convoluted Tubule and Collecting Duct

The distal convoluted tubule begins in the cortex where the thick ascending limb of Henle's loop ends. The lining epithelium is similar to that of the thick ascending limb; however, the cells are taller with nuclei positioned closer to the lumen. The distal convoluted tubule is connected to the collecting duct by a connecting segment. Cells lining the connecting segment are mixed and are similar to either those of the distal convoluted tubule or the collecting duct. In juxtamedullary nephrons, the connecting segments from several nephrons combine to form an arcade that drains into an initial collecting tubule that finally empties into a collecting duct. In most nephrons, however, the connecting segment does not form an arcade and drains directly into an initial collecting tubule before joining the collecting duct. The collecting duct extends from the cortex to the tip of the renal papilla in three segments: cortical, outer medullary, and inner medullary. The collecting ducts progressively join and form ducts with larger lumens as they pass toward the papilla. The ducts of Bellini are the final distal and terminal portions of the collecting ducts. Each renal papilla includes 20–70 of these terminal ducts. The cells lining the collecting ducts are cuboidal proximally and transition to a taller columnar lining distally. Urothelial carcinoma spreading within the collecting ducts, unlike direct invasion of carcinoma of the renal

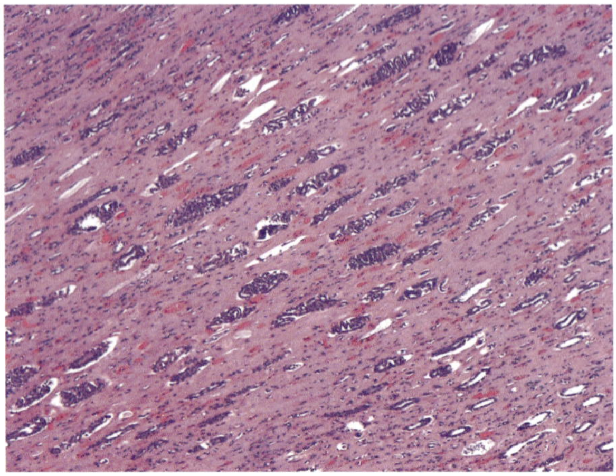

Fig. 3.3 Intratubular spread of urothelial carcinoma through the distal kidney tubules. This type of spread alone does not affect the stage of such tumors. Only the invasion of the renal parenchyma outside the tubules increases the stage

parenchyma, does not affect the T-stage of these tumors [14] (Fig. 3.3). The distal nephron and collecting duct is thought to be the origin of oncocytoma, chromophobe renal cell carcinoma, and collecting duct carcinoma [19].

Interstitium

The kidney interstitium is composed of a loose matrix that increases in quantity from the cortex to medulla. The cortical interstitium is scanty with a nearly back-to-back arrangement of cortical tubules and arteries.

Renomedullary interstitial cell tumor is a benign tumor originating from renomedullary interstitial cells (Fig. 3.4). These tumors are often found incidentally in autopsies or nephrectomies performed for other tumors or conditions [19]. Most of these tumors are small; however, large-sized tumors with symptomatic presentation have been reported in the literature [23, 24].

Renal Pelvis

The human kidney is composed of multiple papillae, where each papilla is surrounded by a funnel-shaped calyx. Each papilla opens into the minor calyces, which in turn unite into major calyces and drain into the renal pelvis. The pelvis is a sac-like compartment between the calyces and the ureter [25]. The pelvicalyceal system is lined with normal urothelial cells (transitional epithelium). The pelvis wall contains smooth muscle that is continuous with that of the ureter.

The renal sinus is located on the medial aspect of the kidney and contains the renal pelvis, the major renal vessels, the lymphatics, and the nerves, all of which are surrounded by fat. The renal hilum is the portal of entry into the sinus. The renal capsule does not enclose the cortical parenchymal surface within the renal sinus, and the fat filling the renal sinus is contiguous with the perirenal fat. Since the venous and lymphatic drainage of the kidney passes through the renal sinus, this

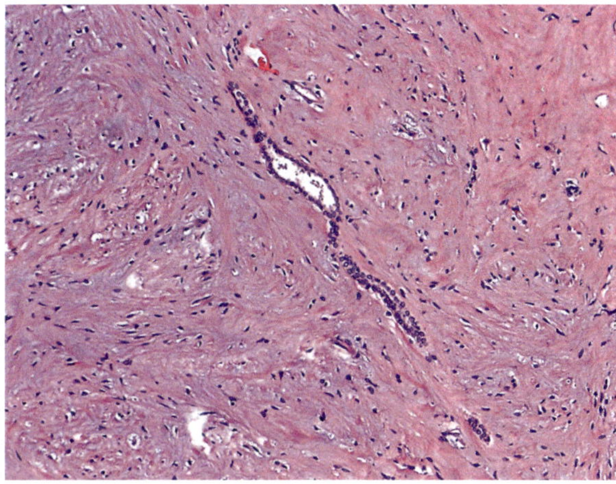

Fig. 3.4 Renal medullary interstitial cell tumor is a benign, often incidental finding, in nephrectomy specimens. The neoplasm originates from interstitial cells of the renal medulla. Entrapped normal kidney tubules, characteristic of this tumor, can be seen in this photograph

region is the portal of exit for tumor cells departing the kidney. Studies have shown that the renal sinus is the main pathway for dissemination in Wilms tumor and RCC [26, 27]. Invasion of the pelvicalyceal system and/or renal sinus fat by RCC is included under stage pT3a.

Gross Examination of Nephrectomy Specimens

Proper gross examination of the kidney is essential for accurate diagnosis and staging. Additionally, gross features, including whether kidney tumors are simple and nodular or have irregular outlines, are indicators of prognosis [28], making detailed gross description essential.

The nephrectomy specimen should be handled in a standardized fashion for accurate pathologic assessment and staging. The International Society of Urological Pathology (ISUP) have established guidelines for handling of kidney tumor specimens [29]. The following outlines recommendations from this document:

1. *Initial sectioning and inking of renal specimens*
    - Both radical and partial nephrectomy specimens should be inked.
    - The initial cut in radical nephrectomy specimen should be along the long axis, followed by additional perpendicular or parallel cuts to identify the tumor (Fig. 3.5). Perirenal fat should not be removed for gross cutting (unlike handling of autopsy kidneys). Renal capsule should not be stripped.
2. *Tumor location and relation to anatomic structures should be noted as follows:*
    - Poles (upper vs. lower pole) vs. hilar
    - Cortical vs. medullary
    - Pelvis involvement
    - Major vein involvement

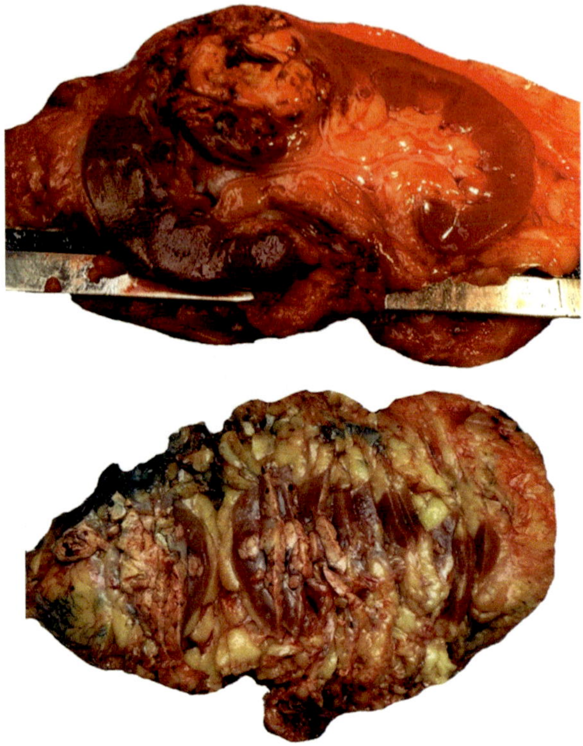

Fig. 3.5 During grossing nephrectomy specimens, a parallel cut to the long axis of the kidney should first be made (top). Following the parallel cut, serial perpendicular sections (bottom) should be made to assess the extent of tumor invasion. (Courtesy of Monica B. Lemos, Pathologists' Assistant)

- Solitary vs. multiple
- Relationship with perirenal or sinus fat and adrenal

3. *Tumor measurement*
   - Greatest tumor dimension in three dimensions should be recorded with special attention given to cutoff points of 4, 7, and 10 cm as they are crucial for accurate staging.
   - The measurement of any tumor invading into the peripheral extracapsular tissue and the renal sinus should be included with the main tumor.
   - The length of the renal vein or caval thrombus and smaller satellite nodules should not be included as part of the main tumor dimensions.
   - In the case of multiple tumors, at least five should be measured and sampled.
4. *Number of blocks for tumor sampling*
   - One block/cm with a minimum of three blocks (subject to modification as needed in individual cases)
5. *Assessment of perinephric fat invasion*
   - RCC growing in a circumscribed manner with pushing borders into the perinephric fat, even if extending well beyond the normal outline of the renal cortex, should not be mistaken as perinephric fat invasion.

- Infiltration into the perinephric fat can be established on gross examination when the tumor loses its rounded and smooth interface with the capsule and the perinephric fat or when visible as nodules or irregular tumor masses protruding within the perinephric fat.

6. *Assessment of renal sinus invasion*
   - When renal sinus invasion is uncertain on gross examination, at least three blocks of the tumor-renal sinus interface should be submitted.
   - When renal sinus invasion is grossly evident, only one block is needed to confirm the gross impression.
7. *Sampling of the renal vein, vena cava invasion, and renal vein margin*
   - The renal vein and its branches should be carefully examined for the presence of tumor.
   - When a specimen is submitted separately as "caval thrombus," at least two sections should be submitted to search for adherent caval wall tissue and possible caval vein invasion.
8. *Sampling of the uninvolved renal parenchyma*
   - The uninvolved renal parenchyma should also be routinely evaluated by including both normal parenchyma adjacent to the tumor and renal parenchyma distant from the tumor.
9. *Adrenal gland involvement*
   - When the adrenal gland is involved by RCC, careful gross examination should determine whether this represents contiguous spread (pT4 disease) or a metastasis (pM1) in the current AJCC/UICC TNM staging system [14].
10. *Assessment of lymph nodes*
    - Renal hilar fat should be palpated and dissected for presence of lymph nodes.
11. *The following sections should be submitted for radical nephrectomy specimens:*
    - Margins (ureter, renal vein, perinephric fat, or Gerota's fascia, if applicable). Take ureter and vein margins first.
    - Tumor sections: with perinephric or sinus fat; tumor sections, one section per centimeter of tumor and different gross appearance. Sarcomatoid components and percentage of tumor necrosis are important prognostic parameters. Therefore, grossly different appearing areas, particularly areas with a "fish flesh" appearance (representing potentially sarcomatoid areas), and necrotic areas should be included for microscopic examination. Gross estimation of necrotic areas should be documented.
    - Sections of grossly normal kidney (1–2).
    - Adrenal gland (1 or more).
    - Lymph node(s), including possible hilar lymph nodes.

References

1. Clapp W, Croker B. Kidney. In: Mills SE, editor. Histology for pathologists. Philadelphia: Lippincott Williams & Wilkins; 2012. p. 891–970.
2. Moore K, Persaud T. The developing human: clinically oriented embryology. 8th ed. Philadelphia: Saunders; 2003. p. 243–83.
3. Scott R, Maezawa Y, Kreidberg J, Quaggin S. Brenner and Rector's the kidney. 10th ed. Philadelphia: Elsevier Health Sciences; 2015.
4. Van den Neuvel-Eibrink M, editor. Wilms tumor. Brisbane: Codon Publications; 2016.
5. Muir TE, Cheville JC, Langer DJ. Metanephric adenoma, nephrogenic rests, and Wilms' tumor: a histologic and immunophenotypic comparison. Am J Surg Pathol. 2001;25:1290–6.
6. Nordmark B. Double formations of the pelves of the kidney and ureters: embryology, occurrence and clinical significance. Acta Radiol. 1948;30:267–78.
7. Siomou E, Papadopoulou F, Kollios K, et al. Duplex collecting system diagnosed during the first 6 years of life after a first urinary tract infection: a study of 63 children. J Urol. 2006;175(2):678–81.
8. Fernbach S, Feinstein K, Spencer K, Lindstrom C. Ureteral duplication and its complications. Radiographics. 1997;17:109–27.
9. Woolf AS, Price KL, Scrambler PJ, Winyard PJD. Evolving concepts in human renal dysplasia. J Am Soc Nephrol. 2004;15:998–1007.
10. Emamian SA, Nielsen MB, Pedersen JF, Ytte L. Kidney dimensions at sonography: correlation with age, sex, and habitus in 665 adult volunteers. Am J Roentgenol. 1993;160(1):83–6.
11. Tanagho E, Lue T. Chapter 1. Anatomy of the genitourinary tract. In: McAninch JW, Lue TF, editors. Smith and Tanagho's general urology. New York: McGraw-Hill; 2013.
12. Bosnib S. Nonneoplastic diseases of the kidney. In: Bostwick DG, Cheng L, editors. Urologic surgical pathology. Philadelphia: Saunders Elsevier; 2014.
13. Hansen J. Netter's clinical anatomy. 3rd ed. Philadelphia: Elsevier Health Sciences; 2014.
14. Amin MB, editor-in-chief. American Joint Committee on Cancer (AJCC) Cancer staging manual. 8th ed. Chicago: Springer International Publishing; 2017.
15. Klatte T, Ficarra V, Gratzke C, et al. A literature review of renal surgical anatomy and surgical strategies for partial nephrectomy. Eur Urol. 2015;68(6):980–92.
16. Alexander R, Sung M, Cheng L. Lymphadenectomy in urologic oncology: pathologic considerations. Urol Clin North Am. 2011;3(4):483–95.
17. Mehta V, Mudaliar K, Ghai R, et al. Renal lymph nodes for RCC staging: appraisal of 871 adult nephrectomies with microscopic examination of hilar fat. Arch Pathol Lab Med. 2013;137(11):1584–90.
18. Ross M, Pawlina W. Histology: a text and atlas with correlated cell and molecular biology. 5th ed. Philadelphia: Lippincott Williams & Wilkins; 2006. p. 646–85.
19. Moch H, Amin MB, Argani P, Cheville J, Delahunt B, Martignoni G, Medeiros LJ, Srigley JR, Tan PH, Tickoo SK. Renal cell tumors. In: Moch H, Humphrey PA, Tomas MU, Reuter VE, editors. WHO classification of tumours of the urinary system and male genital organs. Lyon: IARC; 2016.
20. Cairns P. Renal cell carcinoma. Cancer Biomark. 2011;9(1–6):461–73.
21. Moll R, Hage C, Thoenes W. Expression of intermediate filament proteins in fetal and adult human kidney: modulation of intermediate filament patterns during development and in damaged tissue. Lab Investig. 1991;65:74–86.
22. Oosterwijk E, van Muijen GNP, Oosterwijk-Wakka JC, et al. Expression of intermediate-sized filaments in developing and adult human kidney and in renal cell carcinoma. J Histochem Cytochem. 1990;38:385–92.
23. Kumar S, Choudhary GR, Nanjappa B, Bal A. Benign medullary fibroma of the kidney: a rare diagnostic dilemma. J Clin Imaging Sci. 2013;3:43–6.
24. Magro G, Lopes M, Giannone G. Benign fibromatous tumor (fibroma) of the kidney: a case report. Pathol Res Pract. 1998;194:123–7.

25. Schmidt-Nielsen B. The renal pelvis. Kidney Int. 1987;31(2):621–8.
26. Beckwith JB. National Wilms tumor study: an update for pathologists. Pediatr Dev Pathol. 1998;1:79–84.
27. Bonsib SM. The renal sinus is the principal invasive pathway: a prospective study of 100 renal cell carcinomas. Am J Surg Pathol. 2004;28:1594–600.
28. Jeong SU, Park JM, Shin SJ, Lee J, Song C, Go H, Cho NH, Ro JY, Cho YM. Prognostic significance of macroscopic appearance in clear cell renal cell carcinoma and its metastasis-predicting model. Pathol Int. 2017;67(12):610–9.
29. Trpkov K, Grignon DJ, Bonsib SM, Amin MB, Billis A, Lopez-Beltran A, Samaratunga H, Tamboli P, Delahunt B, Egevad L, Montironi R, Srigley JR. Handling and staging of renal cell carcinoma. The International Society of Urological Pathology Consensus (ISUP) conference recommendations. Am J Surg Pathol. 2013;37:1505–17.

Chapter 4
Benign Renal Epithelial / Epithelial and Stromal Tumors

Dilek Ertoy Baydar

A significant proportion of kidney masses (approximately 20% of surgically resected tumors) are histologically benign. Benign renal neoplasms constitute a heterogeneous group of a broad spectrum with distinctive ontogeny, morphology, and tumor biology. They are categorically renal cell tumors, metanephric tumors, mesenchymal tumors, and mixed epithelial and stromal tumors. Most are asymptomatic and discovered incidentally and are not immediately life threatening. Some exhibit characteristic anatomic distribution and imaging features. However, histologic evaluation is usually required to reach a definitive diagnosis because of overlapping findings between benign and malignant renal proliferations. Percutaneous renal mass biopsy is being increasingly performed to preoperatively characterize the nature of renal masses.

Papillary Adenoma of the Kidney

In the recent World Health Organization (WHO) classification of kidney tumors, papillary adenomas are defined as uncapsulated epithelial lesions with papillary or tubular architecture, low WHO/International Society Urological Pathology (ISUP) grade, and a diameter of ≤15 mm [1]. In the previous WHO classification of renal tumors, the size cut-off was 5 mm for papillary adenoma of the kidney. The decision to increase the threshold has been based on the available data showing that uncapsulated WHO/ISUP grade 1–2 tumors have no capacity to metastasize.

D. Ertoy Baydar (✉)
Department of Pathology, Koç University School of Medicine, İstanbul, Turkey

M. K. Divatia et al. (eds.), *Kidney Cancer*, https://doi.org/10.1007/978-3-030-28333-9_4

Clinical Features

Almost all papillary adenomas are clinically silent and discovered incidentally, either in nephrectomy specimens or at autopsy. They are the commonest neoplasms of the renal tubular epithelium with an incidence as high as 22% in some autopsy studies, although their true incidence is not explicit due to the difficulty to identify the lesion grossly. The frequency of small papillary tumors steadily increases with age to approximately 40% in the population older than 65 years [2]. An incidence of 7% has been encountered in nephrectomy specimens in which surgery was undertaken for either benign or malignant disease [3]. They are more frequently detected in kidneys with chronic pyelonephritis, long-term dialysis, or arteriosclerotic renal vascular disease. They have been reported in 14% of patients undergoing transplantation for terminal stage kidney disease and in up to 33% of patients with acquired renal cystic disease [4, 5].

Macroscopy

Papillary adenomas are nonencapsulated but well-delineated yellow to grayish white cortical nodules (Fig. 4.1). Most occur subcapsularly, and by definition, they are 15 mm or less in largest dimension. The smaller adenomas are usually spherical, but larger ones are often wedge-shaped with the base close to the cortical surface. The majority of the patients have solitary lesion, but multiple and bilateral adenomas can occur. Adenomas associated with papillary renal cell carcinoma (PRCC) tend to be multiple in number [3]. The presence of very numerous or miliary papillary adenomas has been called "renal adenomatosis."

Microscopy

Papillary adenomas generally have a seamless interface with the adjacent renal parenchyma and blend with nonneoplastic renal elements (Fig. 4.2). They are characterized by papillary, tubular, or tubulopapillary architecture. In most of the cases, tumor histology resembles that of type 1 papillary renal cell carcinoma (PRCC). Neoplastic cells are often cuboidal while they have round to oval occasionally grooved uniform small nuclei with stippled to clumped chromatin and inconspicuous ISUP/WHO grades 1 and 2 nucleoli (Fig. 4.3). The cytoplasm is scant that varies from pale to eosinophilic to basophilic. Infrequently, tumor cells resemble those of type 2 PRCC, exhibiting prominent nucleoli and voluminous eosinophilic cytoplasm. Mitotic figures are absent or very rare. Psammoma bodies and foamy macrophages are commonly found.

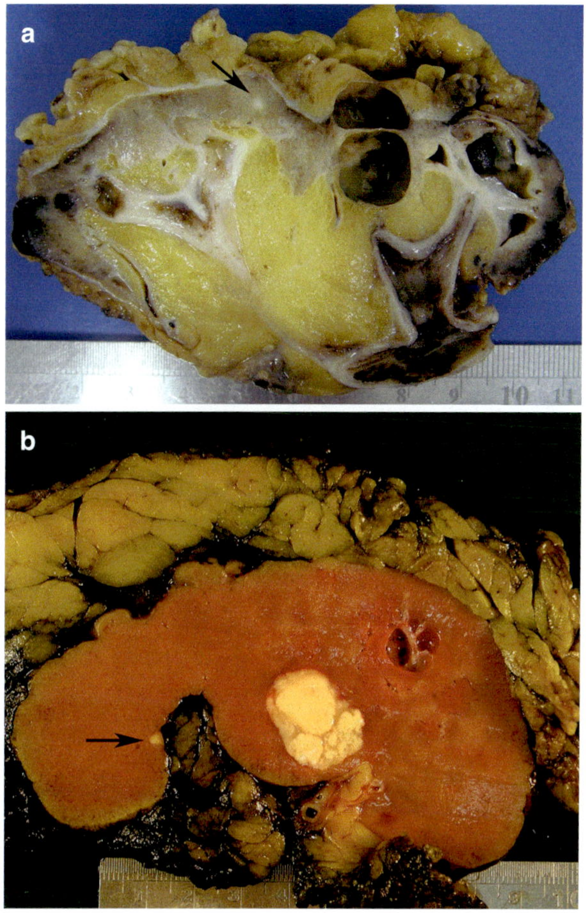

Fig. 4.1 Papillary adenomas incidentally detected in two kidneys; one kidney was removed due to chronic pyelonephritis (**a**) and the other due to papillary renal cell carcinoma (**b**)

Immunohistochemistry

Almost all papillary adenomas react with antibodies to epithelial membrane antigen and low molecular weight cytokeratins [6]. Most of the adenomas stain strongly for AMACR [3].

Molecular/Genetic Findings

The most common genetic changes observed in papillary adenomas are combined tri- or tetrasomy 7 and 17 and loss of chromosome Y [7]. These changes are also present in PRCC, and additional genetic alterations have seem to accumulate as they

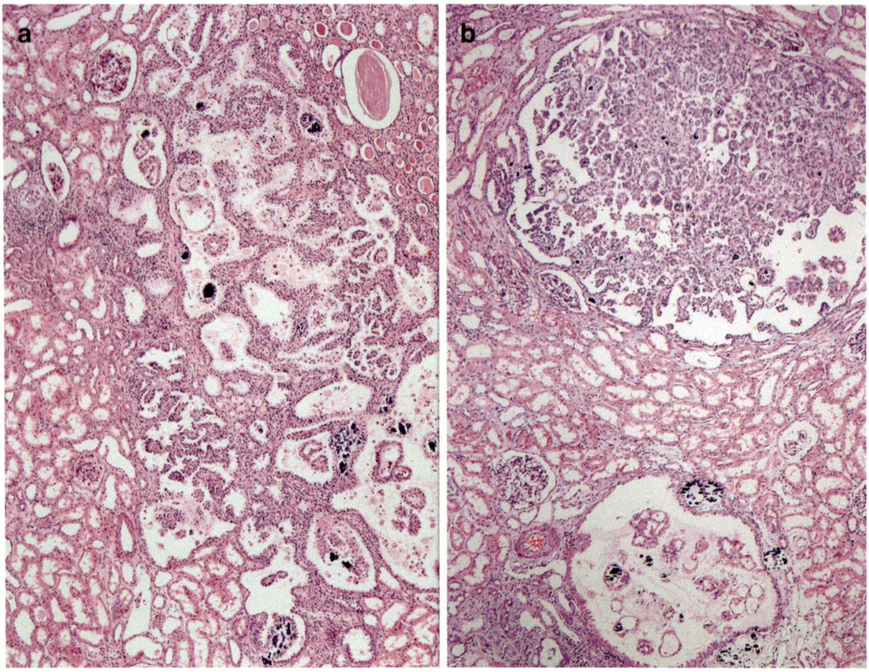

Fig. 4.2 (**a**) Papillary adenoma as a small uncapsulated tumor in the kidney with frequent calcifications and psammomas. (**b**) Multiple (two) lesions are seen in the right panel

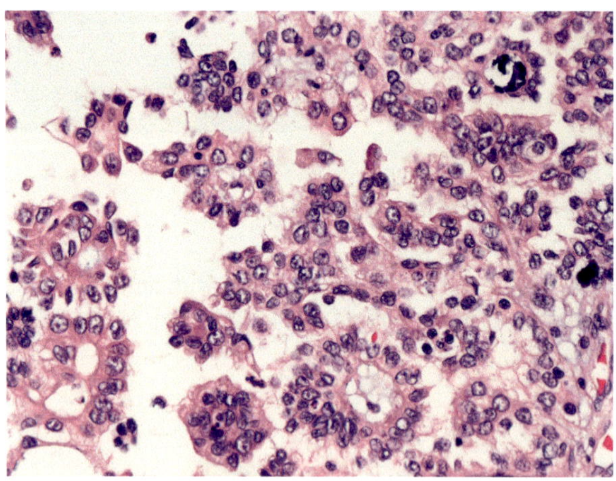

Fig. 4.3 Neoplastic cells of papillary adenoma with small round to oval, occasionally grooved low-grade nuclei and narrow cytoplasm

evolve. Therefore, and also considering histologic and immunohistochemical similarities, papillary adenoma is postulated to be the precursor lesion to PRCC.

Differential Diagnosis

These neoplasms may be indistinguishable histologically from low-grade papillary renal cell carcinoma, so that size becomes the sole criterion that separates the two. Histological resemblance to clear cell, chromophobe, or collecting duct renal cell carcinomas must exclude the diagnosis of papillary adenoma.

Oncocytoma

Oncocytomas are benign renal epithelial tumors that account for approximately 5–9% of all renal cell neoplasms. They have been postulated to arise from the intercalated cells of collecting tubules.

Clinical Features

The age range at the diagnosis of oncocytoma is broad that varies from 25 to 91 with a peak incidence in the seventh decade of life [8, 9]. Men are affected two times more often than women. The majority are asymptomatic and discovered incidentally during radiological workup for unrelated conditions. About a third of patients present with hematuria, flank pain, weight loss, dysuria, or palpable mass. Most cases are sporadic, although rare familial cases have been described and many of these patients have Birt-Hogg-Dubé syndrome.

Macroscopy

Oncocytoma is usually an uncapsulated but well-circumscribed solid cortical mass with a median diameter of 6–7 cm (range: less than 1 cm up to 26 cm). Some may show, however, infiltrative margins, even with extension into perirenal or peripelvic

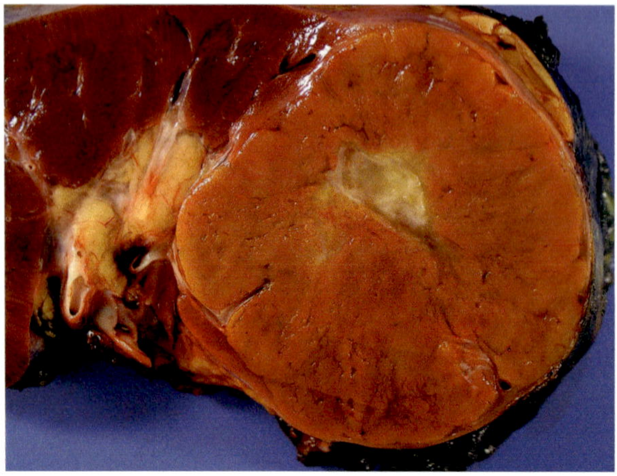

Fig. 4.4 Oncocytoma with typical mahogany brown color and central scar

fat tissue. In most cases, oncocytomas are solitary but approximately 5–13% involve multiple or bilateral tumors. The cut surfaces are characteristically mahogany brown, although they can also be red, tan, or pale yellow (Fig. 4.4). A stellate scar is observed in one third of the tumors, tends to be seen in larger tumors, and can be central or located eccentrically. A diagnosis of oncocytoma may be advocated by the presence of stellate scar when visualized on radiological studies, but this feature is not specific for oncocytoma and can be seen with slow growing low-grade renal cell carcinomas. Hemorrhage may be present in oncocytoma. But grossly visible necrosis should not be evident. Cystic change and calcifications are rare. Tumor extension into the renal vein branches and sometimes in the renal vein itself may occur and does not alter favorable prognosis [10].

Microscopy

Oncocytoma is composed of round to polygonal cells (oncocytes) with swollen acidophilic granular cytoplasm, arranged in an organoid architecture as solid nests/islands or acini growing in an edematous loose hypocellular connective tissue (Fig. 4.5). Microcystic formation or tubulocystic pattern is frequent and occasionally extensive. Papillary architecture should not be seen in oncocytoma, with the exception of minimal short, degenerate appearing papillae or rare papillary formations in the dilated cysts. The neoplastic cells have regular round nuclei with nucleoli that frequently are visible with the 10x objective. Intranuclear inclusions and binucleated cells can be present. Some otherwise typical oncocytomas may contain clusters of bizarre cells with marked nuclear pleomorphism, hyperchromasia with smudged chromatin, and/or multinucleation (Fig. 4.6). These changes are regarded as degenerative type atypia. Occasionally, so-called oncoblasts, which are small cells with scanty cytoplasm and dark monomorphic nuclei lacking nucleoli, are found here

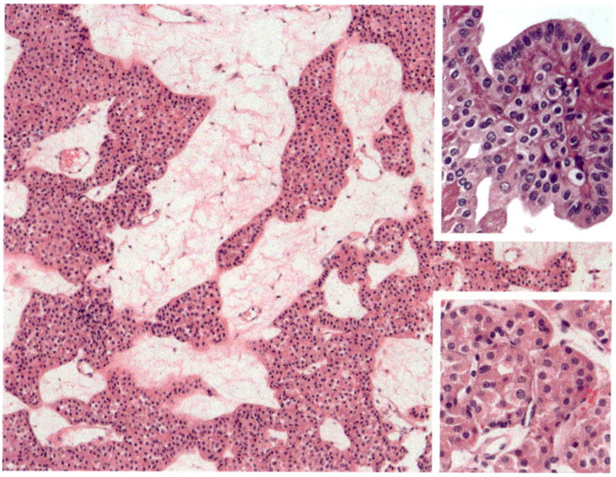

Fig. 4.5 Typical oncocytoma showing nests of deeply eosinophilic large cells with edematous loose stroma. Nuclei are round and regular, some with prominent nucleoli. Upper inset shows a blunt papillary protrusion projecting into a cystic cavity

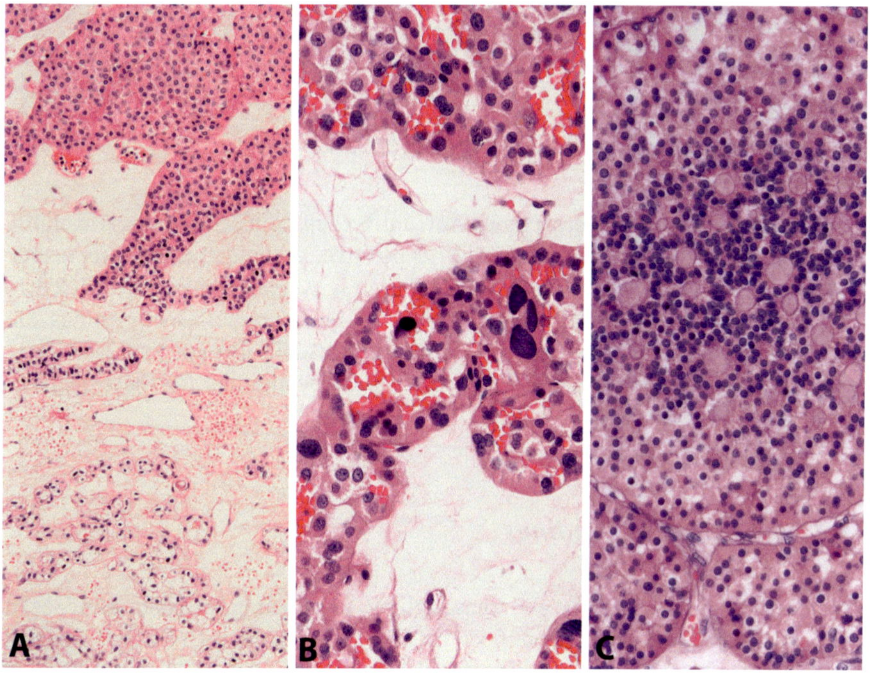

Fig. 4.6 Oncocytomas featuring clear cells in the scarred area (**a**), degenerative type atypia (**b**), and oncoblastic cells with scant cytoplasm and rosette-like arrangements around hyaline basement membrane material (**c**)

and there. In fact, a rare subtype of renal oncocytoma consisting of exclusively oncoblasts has been described [11]. These cases reveal a varying number of pseudorosettes that are composed of small globules of periodic acid-Schiff-positive hyaline basal membrane-like material surrounded by small oncoblastic cells.

Oncocytoma may entrap normal renal tubules at its periphery. Microscopic infiltration into perirenal fat occasionally is present and does not imply an adverse prognostic significance. Mitotic activity is unexpected in oncocytoma; however isolated mitotic figures are identified in rare cases. Tumor stroma may contain rare foam cells, psammoma bodies, dystrophic calcification, or ossification. Focal clear cell changes were found in a small group of oncocytomas, typically within hyalinized scar-like areas.

Histological features considered impermissible for oncocytoma are extensive papillary architecture, sheet-like growth pattern, areas of clear cell carcinoma (except focal clear cells, typically in hyalinized areas), sarcomatoid or spindle cell areas, frequent mitoses including atypical mitosis, and gross or prominent microscopic necrosis. Oncocytoma can be confidently ruled out if a neoplasm demonstrates dominant or significant papillary growth.

Electron microscopy shows abundant mitochondria packed within the cytoplasm of oncocytes. Mitochondria are predominantly uniform and round with stacked parallel (lamellar) cristae. Hale's colloidal iron stain either gives negative result or is only positive at the luminal site of oncocytes.

Immunohistochemistry

Oncocytomas are immunoreactive with antibodies to EMA, pan-cytokeratin, PAX8, E-cadherin, and S100A1. CD117 is positive, showing diffuse cytoplasmic and membranous staining (Fig. 4.7). CK7 reactivity is negative or restricted to only scattered rare cells or small clusters in oncocytoma. Oncocytomas are generally negative for CA9 and vimentin. They usually do not express CD10, RCC antigen, and racemase although occasional positivities for these markers have been reported.

Molecular/Genetic Findings

In a recent study using exome and transcriptome sequencing, two main subtypes of renal oncocytoma have been identified [12]. Type 1 is diploid with CCND1 (located at 11q13) rearrangements, whereas type 2 is aneuploid with recurrent loss of chromosome 1, X or Y, and/or 14 and 21, which may proceed to eosinophilic chromophobe renal cell carcinoma upon acquiring *p53*, *PTEN*, and other mutations. Two subtypes share recurrent inactivating mutations in mitochondrial genes encoded by both nuclear and mitochondrial genomes.

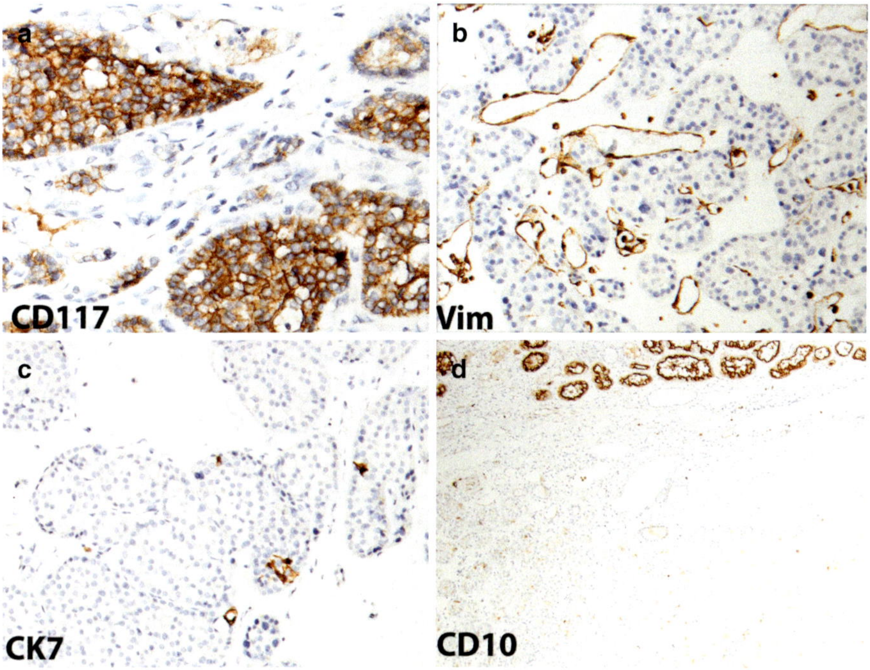

Fig. 4.7 (**a–d**) Immunohistochemistry. Oncocytomas diffusely express CD117, whereas they are usually negative for vimentin and CD10. Cytokeratin 7 is either negative or stains scattered rare cells

Differential Diagnosis

The main differential diagnosis of oncocytoma is the eosinophilic variant of chromophobe renal cell carcinoma (RCC). The cells in chromophobe RCC exhibit extensive nuclear irregularities with a "raisinoid" nuclear shape, perinuclear halo, more frequent mitoses, and prominent cell membranes giving "plant-like" or "cobblestone" appearance. Diffuse and strong cytoplasmic staining for colloidal iron indicate the presence of cytoplasmic acid mucopolysaccharides in chromophobe RCC. It is diffusely and strongly positive in chromophobe RCC, while negative or faintly positive in oncocytoma (usually only at luminal surface). Diffuse membranous staining for CK7 is seen in the majority of chromophobe RCC, whereas CK7 staining is negative or restricted to only rare cells in oncocytoma. S100A1 has been suggested as a useful marker as it is shown positive in oncocytoma and negative in chromophobe RCC.

Conventional (clear cell) RCC with granular or eosinophilic cytoplasm is another entity which may rarely enter into differential diagnosis with oncocytoma. Conventional RCC can readily be distinguished from oncocytoma, based on its gross appearance, higher grade, mitotic activity, delicate vascular network, and its immune profile being CD117 negative, CA9, vimentin, and CD10 positive.

It might be worth reminding that oncocytoma can be found as a coexisting lesion to RCC within the same or opposite kidney, or collision tumors that contain both RCC and oncocytoma may occur rarely [13].

Prognosis and Treatment

Oncocytomas are benign neoplasms that show no progression or metastasis. The management of solid renal masses had until recently involved surgical excision for both diagnostic and therapeutic purposes. Nowadays, diagnostic percutaneous biopsy for preoperative diagnosis has been increasingly offered in many countries to patients presenting with asymptomatic localized renal masses. The majority of oncocytomas show minimal growth rate or even regression. It has been suggested that patients with biopsy-proven oncocytoma can be conservatively managed with active surveillance [14].

Renal Oncocytosis (Oncocytomatosis)

Renal oncocytosis is a rare condition characterized by the presence of oncocytic changes scattered throughout the renal parenchyma and oncocytic tumors [15]. Benign renal tubules show oncocytic change; cysts lined by oncocytic cells and oncocytic cell groups in the interstitium are present (Fig. 4.8). In the largest cohort

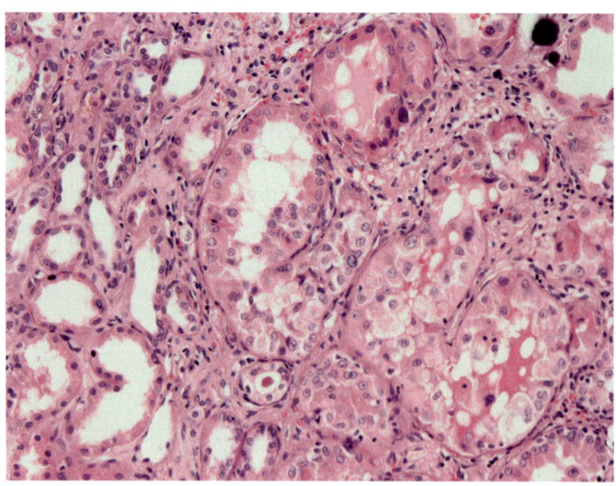

Fig. 4.8 Renal oncocytosis characterized by clusters of tubules with oncocytic change

of oncocytosis [16] consisting of 20 individuals, 50% of patients already had chronic kidney disease (CKD) at the time of diagnosis with 5 additional patients developing CKD after surgery. Hybrid tumors with features between oncocytoma and chromophobe RCC have been the most common histology associated with renal oncocytosis, followed by chromophobe RCC and oncocytoma [16]. The majority of patients had multiple nodules with different histologies in the same kidney. No patient developed distant metastasis during follow-up of median 35 months.

More than a half of the patients affected by Birt-Hogg-Dube (BHD) syndrome show features of renal oncocytosis [17, 18]. The most common kidney tumor histology in patients with BHD syndrome is hybrid oncocytic tumors, and 58–86% of the patients have multiple nodules. Gobbo et al. using selective centromeric probes did not find genetic similarities between oncocytosis, oncocytoma, and chromophobe RCC, and they suggested that these three tumor types represent independent entities with genotypic alterations [19].

Metanephric Tumors

The World Health Organization recognizes three members in the family of benign metanephric neoplasms of the kidney: metanephric adenoma (MA), metanephric adenofibroma (MAF), and metanephric stromal tumor (MST). MA is a highly cellular epithelial neoplasm composed of small, uniform embryonal looking cells but without notable proliferative activity or mitosis. MST stays at the other end of the spectrum being a pure spindle cell neoplasm. MAF lies in between the first two and is a biphasic neoplasm that contains areas morphologically identical to MST and MA.

The histology of MA closely resembles differentiated epithelial Wilms' tumor (nephroblastoma), and the neoplastic cells consistently label for WT1 protein on immunohistochemistry. MST from the other side may show heterologous stromal differentiation, including glial and chondroid elements, again similar to Wilms' tumor. Primarily based on these overlapping morphologic features, metanephric neoplasms have long been postulated to potentially represent the differentiated end of the Wilms' tumor spectrum. However, recent investigations identifying mutations in the *BRAF* gene in all three members of metanephric tumor family suggest that their molecular pathogenesis is probably distinct from that of Wilms' tumor.

Metanephric Adenoma

Metanephric adenoma (MA) is a rare neoplasm composed of tubular and tubulopapillary structures and glomeruloid bodies reminiscent of Wilms' tumor, but with a high degree of maturation and differentiation. It has a wide age range distribution despite being the most common benign renal epithelial tumor of children and young adults.

Clinical Features

MAs occur at all ages (range 5–83 years), but most develop in adults in the fifth or sixth decade of life (median age is about 50 years) with a 2:1 female preponderance [20]. Approximately 50% are discovered incidentally, and others manifest with polycythemia, abdominal or flank pain, mass, or hematuria. Polycythemia, found in 10–15% of patients, is thought to be induced by erythropoietin or cytokines secreted by neoplastic cells. It is usually cured by tumor removal.

Macroscopy

MAs vary widely in size. The largest tumor reported is 15 cm in diameter [20], while the most lesions lie between 3 and 6 cm. They are well-circumscribed and uncapsulated lesions; however a thin and discontinuous pseudocapsule can be seen rarely (Fig. 4.9). Bilaterality has not been reported. Multifocality is also unusual, but has been encountered. Their cut surfaces are gray to tan to yellow and soft to firm. Foci of hemorrhage and necrosis are often present, particularly in large masses. Cystic degeneration and calcification within the solid or cystic areas may be noted.

Microscopy

Metanephric adenomas appear as hypercellular proliferations under the microscope. They consist of closely spaced, often overlapping uniform epithelial cells that are small, and cytologically bland, with scant pale to light pink cytoplasm, round to oval, hyperchromatic nuclei slightly larger than lymphocytes. Chromatin is finely distributed and their nucleoli are invisible. Neoplastic cells form tightly packed small round acini, tubules with narrow lumina, and glomeruloid bodies without capillary tufts, giving the tumor a characteristic fetal nephron-like appearance (Fig. 4.10). Long branching and angulated tubular formations are also seen. Papillary architecture is common and may be noted in the form of polypoid fronds within cystic spaces in addition to short stubby glomeruloid infoldings within the tubules.

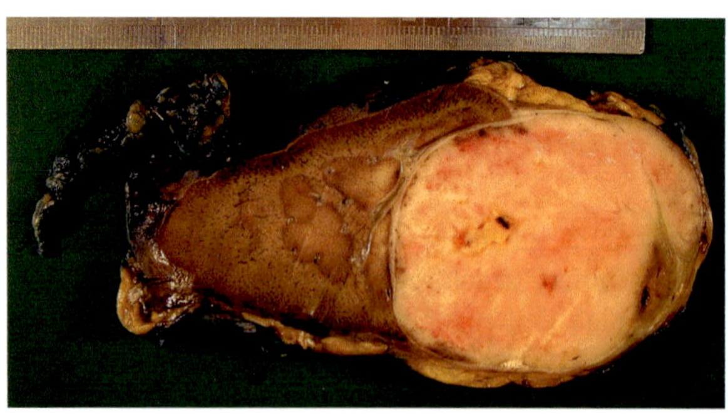

Fig. 4.9 Metanephric adenoma as a well-delineated mass from surrounding parenchyma. A focal area of intratumoral necrosis is evident

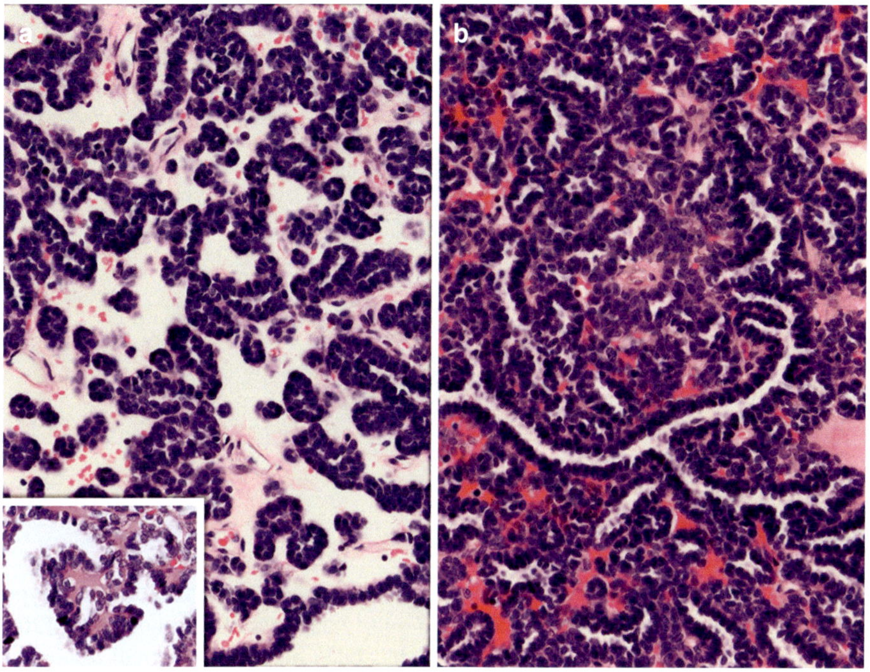

Fig. 4.10 (**a**, **b**) Metanephric adenoma formed by small round crowded acini and branching tubules in a hyalinized or edematous hypocellular stroma. Inset shows a small papillary infolding within tubular space producing a glomeruloid appearance

Microcysts lined by flattened cells can be seen infrequently. Stroma is loose and paucicellular and variable in amount from scant to large areas of scar-like hyalinization. Psammoma bodies are common and may be a few or numerous. Some tumors contain dystrophic calcifications in the hyalinized areas or focal osseous metaplasia in the stroma. Mitotic figures are absent or rare.

Metanephric adenomas are sharply demarcated from the adjacent renal parenchyma (Fig. 4.11). They are usually uncapsulated lesions although some may show a thin discontinuous fibrous capsule. Renal capsular or vascular invasion does not occur. There have been reports of composite metanephric adenoma with coexisting renal cell carcinoma [21, 22].

MA does not contain blastema and is not associated with nephrogenic rests.

Immunohistochemistry

WT1 is diffusely detectable in the nuclei of metanephric adenomas [23]. CD57, vimentin, and S100 are also commonly expressed [23, 24]. The cells of MA are typically negative for EMA, AMACR, CD56, CD10, and desmin. CK7 is either negative or focally (<5% of the tumor cells) positive, usually in the elongate tubules.

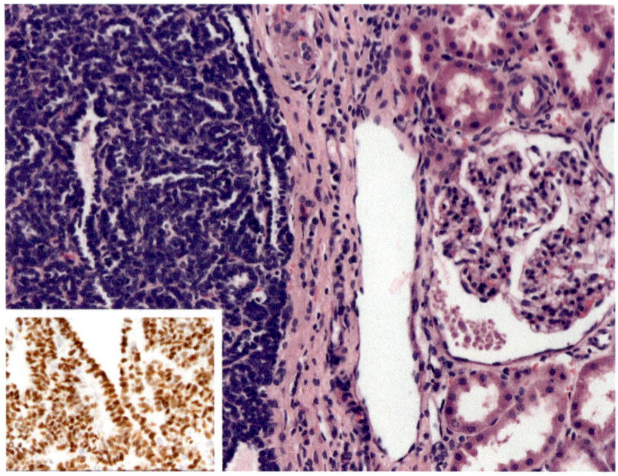

Fig. 4.11 Metanephric adenoma that directly abuts the renal parenchyma. Neoplastic cells have nuclei slightly bigger than lymphocytes with no nucleoli or mitosis. Cytoplasm is minimal. Inset shows nuclear WT1 expression

Molecular/Genetic Findings

Most studies confirm normal chromosome copy numbers and a diploid karyotype [25]. MA lacks the gains of chromosomes 7 and 17 and loss of chromosome Y [26]. A candidate tumor suppressor gene in MA has been mapped to a small region on chromosome 2p [27]. Choueiri et al. have demonstrated that approximately 90% of MAs harbor *BRAF* V600E mutations [28]. All epithelial predominant nephroblastomas have been found *BRAF* wild type.

Differential Diagnosis

The differential diagnosis of metanephric adenoma includes the solid variant of type 1 papillary renal cell carcinoma (PRCC), as well as epithelial predominant Wilms' tumor (WT) given that its histological characteristics often overlap with PRCC and WT, especially when the tumor morphology is not typical. Lack of encapsulation, sharp interface between the tumor and the kidney, absence of nucleoli, and relative lack of mitotic activity are helpful features of MA that can be used to rule out PRCC. Additionally, metanephric adenomas often have elongate, pointed, branching channels lined by epithelial cells that are not found in PRCC or WT. PRCC does not react with antibody to WT1 and S100. CK7, AMACR, EMA, and CD10 are usually present in type 1 PRCC, but largely absent in MA.

Nephroblastoma is usually triphasic, with epithelial, blastemal, and stromal components. However, a monophasic WT rarely can occur. The presence of cytologic atypia, mitoses, and anaplastic foci favors the diagnosis of WT. Metanephric adenomas express CD57, but not CD56 which is positive in WT. Positive IHC staining for BRAF V600E supports the diagnosis of MA [29].

Prognosis and Treatment

Metanephric adenoma is almost always cured by excision. Hilar lymph node involvement was reported, but this was regarded as passive mechanical seeding, not true metastasis [30]. A few case reports suggest that metanephric adenomas can rarely metastasize [31], but this is not completely clear.

Metanephric Adenofibroma

In 1992, Hennigar and Beckwith described five cases of a biphasic neoplasm with an epithelial component identical to metanephric adenoma and a stromal component of spindle cells [32]. They proposed the name nephrogenic adenofibroma, but today metanephric adenofibroma (MAF) is favored to emphasize its close relationship with metanephric adenoma.

Clinical Features

MAF is a rare tumor that appears to affect predominantly children and teenagers. Patients' age has ranged from 13 months to 36 years [32, 33]. There is a male predominance. Gross hematuria is a common presentation, but a significant proportion of patients are asymptomatic. Other symptoms seen in some patients include polycythemia, hematuria, and hypertension which resolve following nephrectomy. The tumors can achieve a substantial size, up to 19 cm [34].

Macroscopy

MAFs are solitary tumors which tend to be centered in medulla. They are firm masses without capsule and with indistinct borders. The lesions are often partially cystic and have tan, white-gray or yellow cut surface. Necrosis is unusual and arises the suspicion of an associating nephroblastoma.

Microscopy

MAF is a biphasic tumor that spans the morphologic spectrum between metanephric adenoma which is a pure epithelial lesion and metanephric stromal tumor which is a pure stromal lesion (Fig. 4.12). Epithelial and stromal components are variable in proportions. The epithelial nodules identical to metanephric adenoma are embedded in the moderately cellular stroma. Stroma is composed of fibroblast-like bland spindle cells with pale eosinophilic cytoplasm, oval to fusiform nuclei, and

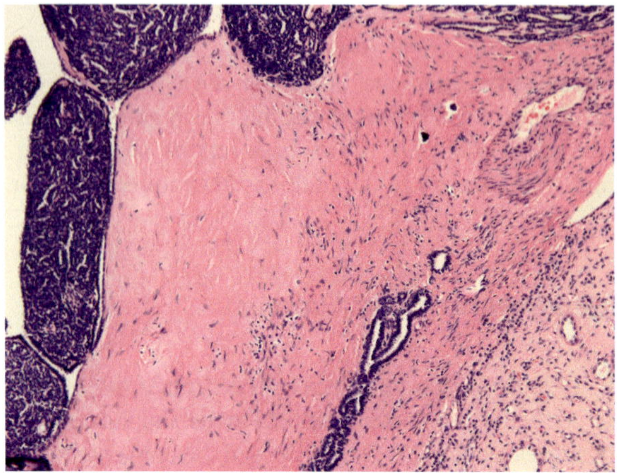

Fig. 4.12 Metanephric adenofibroma as a biphasic tumor having an epithelial component identical to metanephric adenoma in addition to a stromal component

inconspicuous nucleoli. Mitotic figures are absent or rare. Hyalinization and myxoid change can be found. The boundary of the tumor with nonneoplastic kidney parenchyma is typically irregular as the stromal component may entrap renal structures as it grows. Spindle cells may form concentric onion skin-like cuffings or collarettes around entrapped tubules and blood vessels. Angiodysplasia (epithelioid transformation of the medial smooth muscle cells in the tumor arterioles) are noted in two thirds of MAFs, and heterologous elements (glia, fat, or cartilage) can be seen in a subset of these tumors [33]. Unlike metanephric stromal tumor, juxtaglomerular cell hyperplasia is not observed.

Composite tumors composed of MAF and Wilms' tumor or MAF and renal cell carcinoma have been described [33, 35].

Immunohistochemistry

The stromal component of metanephric adenofibroma is immunoreactive for CD34 and vimentin and negative for S100 and desmin. Heterologous glial elements will stain for S100 and GFAP. The epithelial component has a similar immunohistochemical profile to metanephric adenoma.

Molecular/Genetic Findings

Metanephric adenofibroma was thought to represent a well-differentiated, mature form of Wilms' tumor [36]. However similar to metanephric adenoma, *BRAF* V600E mutations have been described both in epithelial and stromal components of MAF [37, 38]. This finding argues against a common origin for MAF and Wilms' tumor. In one case studied, MAF has displayed a normal karyotype [39].

Differential Diagnosis

The main differential diagnoses are classic congenital mesoblastic nephroma and Wilms' tumor. Congenital mesoblastic nephroma (CMN) typically occurs before the age of 3 months, whereas MAF tends to involve older children and young adults. MAF is usually well demarcated, whereas CMN has an infiltrative growth pattern. Intratumoral angiodysplasia, concentric cuffing around entrapped tubules, and heterologous differentiation are useful histological features when seen in MAF. Immunohistochemically, the spindle cells of MAF are negative for actin and positive for CD34, while spindle cells in CMN are vice versa.

MAF can potentially be mistaken as Wilms' tumor. The presence of cytologic atypia, numerous mitotic figures, and blastemal elements found in Wilms' tumors should rule out MAF.

Prognosis and Treatment

Tumors follow benign course. However, the ultimate management of MAF will be complete surgical resection because of the description of composite examples of MAF and WT or renal cell carcinoma with regional lymph node metastasis.

There are also reported adult cases of metanephric adenosarcoma that contain a benign-appearing epithelial component of metanephric adenoma and a malignant stromal part [40, 41]. It might be suggested that these could represent examples of dedifferentiated MAF in which its benign stromal component was overgrown by sarcomatous transformation. However, Su et al. could not detect *BRAF* mutation in their case [41].

Metanephric Stromal Tumor

Metanephric stromal tumor (MST) is a recently recognized entity which was mislabeled as mesoblastic nephroma previously [42]. It is primarily a pediatric renal neoplasm occurring in infants and very young children.

Clinical Features

Most MSTs occur in early infancy and childhood (range, from a few days to 15 years; median age, 13 months and peak at 2 years). Only two adult cases (females at 53 and 55 years of age) have been reported so far [43, 44]. The most common presentation in children is an abdominal mass. This is followed by hematuria, recurrent urinary tract infection, incontinence, fever, anemia, and hypertension. A small number of patients may experience the consequences of extrarenal angiodysplasia that can result in significant morbidity and mortality. Some tumors are found incidentally while examining the individual for other medical conditions.

Macroscopy

Metanephric stromal tumors appear as nonencapsulated solid or cystic masses with indistinct borders and yellow-tan fibrous appearing firm lobulated cut surface. They are centered in the renal medulla and have an average diameter of approximately 5 cm. In the series of Argani et al., the largest was measured 10 cm in diameter [42]. Multifocality is seen in about one sixth of the cases.

Microscopy

MSTs are identical to stromal component of metanephric adenofibroma and composed of spindle and epithelioid cells that have elongated hyperchromatic tapered thin nuclei and indistinct cytoplasm (Fig. 4.13). They lack a fibrous capsule and have infiltrative scalloped borders. Neoplastic cells entrap native kidney constituents and nerves and usually undermine calyceal or pelvic urothelium. The most characteristic histologic finding is the presence of onion skin-like concentric encirclement of entrapped renal tubules and vessels by spindle tumor cells with a myxoid background (Fig. 4.14a). The periphery of these laminations is hypercellular and less myxoid compared with the surrounding stroma, leading to a typical vaguely nodular appearance. Most MSTs induce angiodysplasia in the entrapped intratumoral arterioles, which is characterized by epithelioid transformation of the medial smooth muscle cells and myxoid changes (Fig. 4.14b). A unique but less frequent feature is the presence of juxtaglomerular

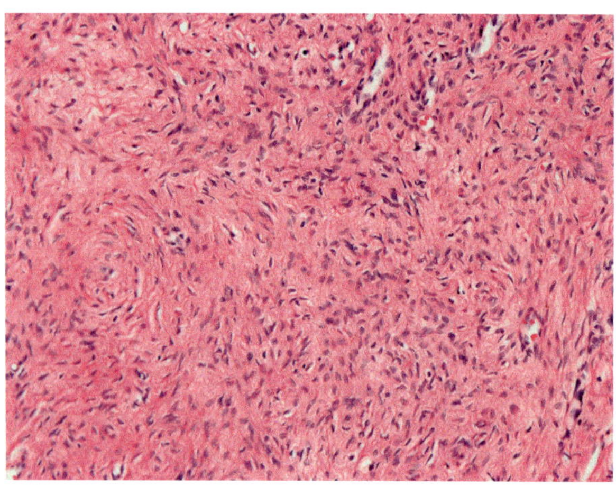

Fig. 4.13 Metanephric stromal tumor composed of spindle cells with indistinct cytoplasmic borders

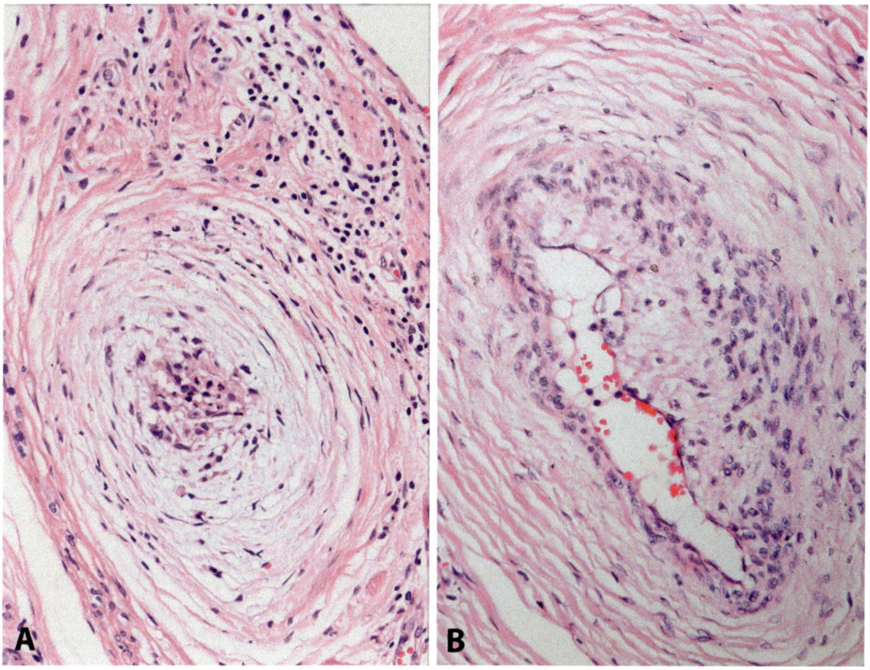

Fig. 4.14 Concentric "onion skin" ring or collarette formed by neoplastic cells in a myxoid background around a blood vessel (**a**) and angiodysplasia (**b**) in metanephric stromal tumor

cell hyperplasia within the entrapped glomeruli, which may lead to elevated renin levels and hypertension in some patients. Heterologous elements in the form of glia, cartilage, or fat are seen in about one fifth of metanephric stromal tumors. Mitosis and necrosis are unusual.

Immunohistochemistry

The spindle tumor cells are immunoreactive for CD34 and vimentin. They are negative for desmin, smooth muscle actin, cytokeratins, EMA, CD117, and S100, although heterologous glial elements may stain for S100 and glial fibrillary acidic protein (GFAP).

Molecular/Genetic Findings

Similar to other metanephric tumors, *BRAF* V600E mutations are common in MSTs as documented by two different studies, found in 6 of 7 cases and in 11 of 16 cases [45, 46].

Differential Diagnosis

MST is often difficult to distinguish from classic type congenital mesoblastic nephroma (CMN), as both are centered around renal medulla and feature bland spindle cells. However, subtly infiltrative scalloped margins in MST contrast with deeply invasive nature of CMN. Moreover, low power nodularity, the presence of peritubular or perivascular concentric onion skinning/cuffing, juxtaglomerular cell hyperplasia, and angiodysplasia indicate MST. Detection of heterologous elements, positive staining with anti-CD34 antibodies, and negativity for actin and desmin are diagnostic of MST.

The wide variety of architectural patterns seen in MST yields resemblance to primary sarcomas such as clear cell sarcoma of the kidney (CCSK). In contrast to renal sarcomas, necrosis and mitoses are usually absent in MST as well as vascular invasion. Regular branching capillary vascular pattern is characteristic of CCSK but not found in MST. CD34 immunoreactivity is also helpful.

Prognosis and Treatment

Metanephric stromal tumors are benign neoplasms with excellent prognostic outcome. No distant metastasis has been documented. Recurrence has been reported only in one case which was not given any further treatment and is still surviving years later [46]. Associating renal angiodysplasia may cause morbidity due to vascular complication. Surgical resection is the preferred treatment modality.

Mixed Epithelial and Stromal Tumor Family

Mixed epithelial and stromal tumor (MEST) family encompasses a spectrum including predominantly cystic tumors (adult cystic nephromas) and tumors that are more solid. They are rare tumors of biphasic morphology with a spindle cell stroma and an epithelial component consisting of glands and cysts.

Adult cystic nephroma (CN) is a benign cystic renal neoplasm of adults which has also been called multilocular cyst or multilocular cystic nephroma. It was previously grouped with pediatric cystic nephroma. Depending on the similar age and sex distributions, a similar immunohistochemical profile, and overlapping morphology, adult cystic nephroma is now classified within the spectrum of MEST family. Pediatric cystic nephroma is indeed a disparate entity with specific DICER1 mutations which are not found in adult cystic nephroma.

Clinical Features

Neoplasms of MEST family predominantly occur in middle-aged women, and a correlation with hormonal imbalance, menopausal status, or other hormonal factors has been hypothesized [47, 48]. They show a striking predilection toward females, with a 7:1 female-to-male ratio. The history of hormonal ablation treatment has been described in some male patients [47–49]. Patients are usually asymptomatic, and most lesions are found incidentally [47, 48, 50]. Other described symptoms include abdominal pain, hematuria, and urinary tract infections. Radiologic appearance of MEST is of a complex cystic renal mass, usually sorting these tumors as Bosniak class III to IV lesions, indistinguishable from cystic RCC. Although the diagnosis of CN can be suggested by a typical round or oval appearance and multiple thin septations in radiological imagings, these findings are not specific.

Macroscopic Findings

Tumors are solitary, nonencapsulated, but generally well-demarcated lesions that may be located in medulla or cortex and medulla. They can be centered within the renal pelvis and can prolapse or project into the collecting system. Their size varies largely and may reach up to 25 cm [51]. CNs are diffusely cystic tumors with typically less than 5 mm thick fibrous septae but without expansile solid areas (Fig. 4.15). On the other hand, MESTs show an admixture of cysts and solid component (Fig. 4.16). The cysts range from small to large, and the content is typically clear yellow fluid. The solid areas have a firm, white cut surface.

Microscopic Findings

Tumors are characterized by an admixture of variably sized cysts, microcysts, and tubules with stroma that varies in cellularity. In CNs, epithelial component constitutes the larger proportion of the tumor and is mainly represented by cysts (Fig. 4.17). MESTs tend to have a more complex epithelial architecture, as shown

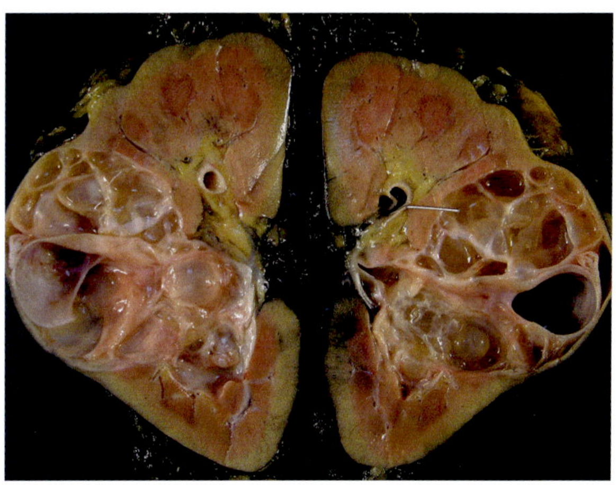

Fig. 4.15 Cystic nephroma. Cystic nephromas are well-circumscribed, multilocular cystic lesions with no discernible solid areas. Internal surfaces of the cysts are characteristically smooth

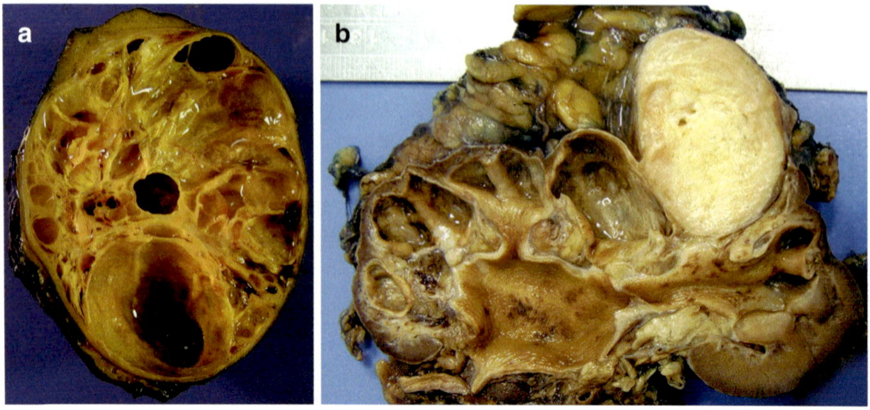

Fig. 4.16 Mixed epithelial and stromal tumor. Tumors can be predominantly cystic (**a**) or predominantly solid (**b**)

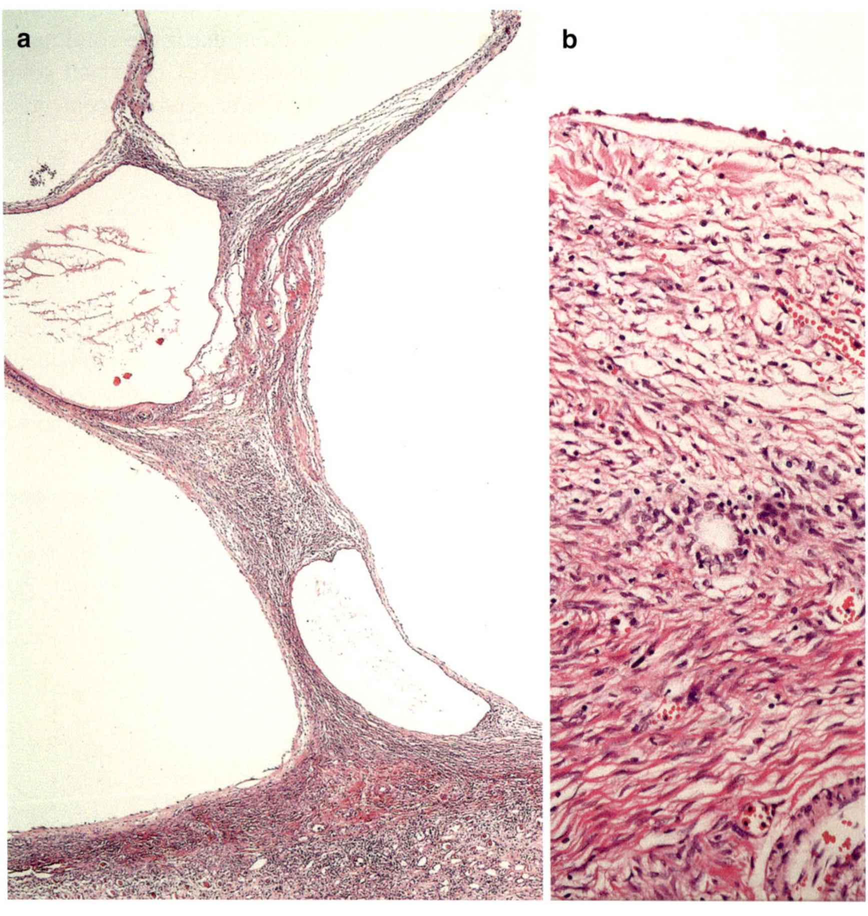

Fig. 4.17 (**a**, **b**) Cystic nephroma as a multilocular cystic lesion septated by thin fibrous tissue that may resemble ovarian stroma. Cysts are lined by hobnail or flattened cells

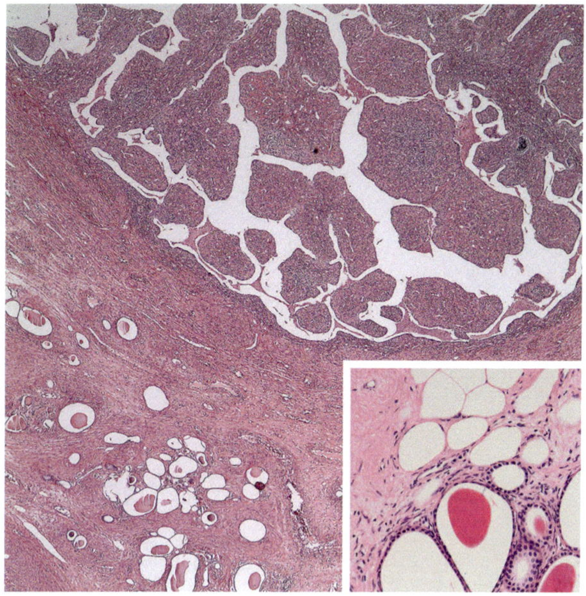

Fig. 4.18 Mixed epithelial and stromal tumor. The epithelial component consists of variably sized tubules and intracystic broad papillary projections. Fat cell metaplasia may be present in the stroma, as shown by the inset

by a higher percentage of crowded small- to medium-sized glands, branching glands and ducts, sometimes complex tubulopapillary structures, as well as phyllodes-type morphology (Fig. 4.18). These varying elements often are intermingled in the same tumor.

The cysts and glands are typically lined by a single layer of flattened, hobnail, cuboidal, or low columnar epithelial cells with pale, acidophilic, amphophilic, or vacuolated cytoplasm (Fig. 4.19). Epithelium sometimes has Müllerian characteristics with focal endometrioid and tubal appearance; infrequently it may be squamous, pyloric, intestinal, or urothelial [52]. The stromal component of both CN and MEST is a fibrous tissue that is composed of slender to plump spindle cells with low to moderate to marked cellularity and varies from edematous to collagenous, rarely myxoid. It may show condensation around epithelial elements. Smooth muscle metaplasia is commonly observed, sometimes in the form of large nodules (Fig. 4.19). Spindle-shaped cells with scant cytoplasm, arranged in whorls or a storiform pattern resembling ovarian stroma, are often present, which may undergo secondary luteinization [48]. Scattered fat cells and small clusters of adipocytes were a frequent feature in one study, seen in 34% of cases [53]. In approximately one fourth of the cases, stroma may contain unusual blood vessels, either slit-like or thick-walled or both.

Mitotic figures are seldom and necrosis is very uncommon. The majority of tumors have very bland cytology both in epithelial and stromal cells. Rarely, focal areas with increased nuclear/cytoplasmic ratio, nuclear atypia, and prominent nucleoli can be found that may be interpreted as reactive [48]. Majority of tumors lack pseudocapsule and have pushing borders. Renal parenchymal tubules can be entrapped at the periphery of the tumor.

A few cases of MEST with malignant transformation have been reported [54–60]. Morphology in these tumors may resemble rhabdomyosarcoma,

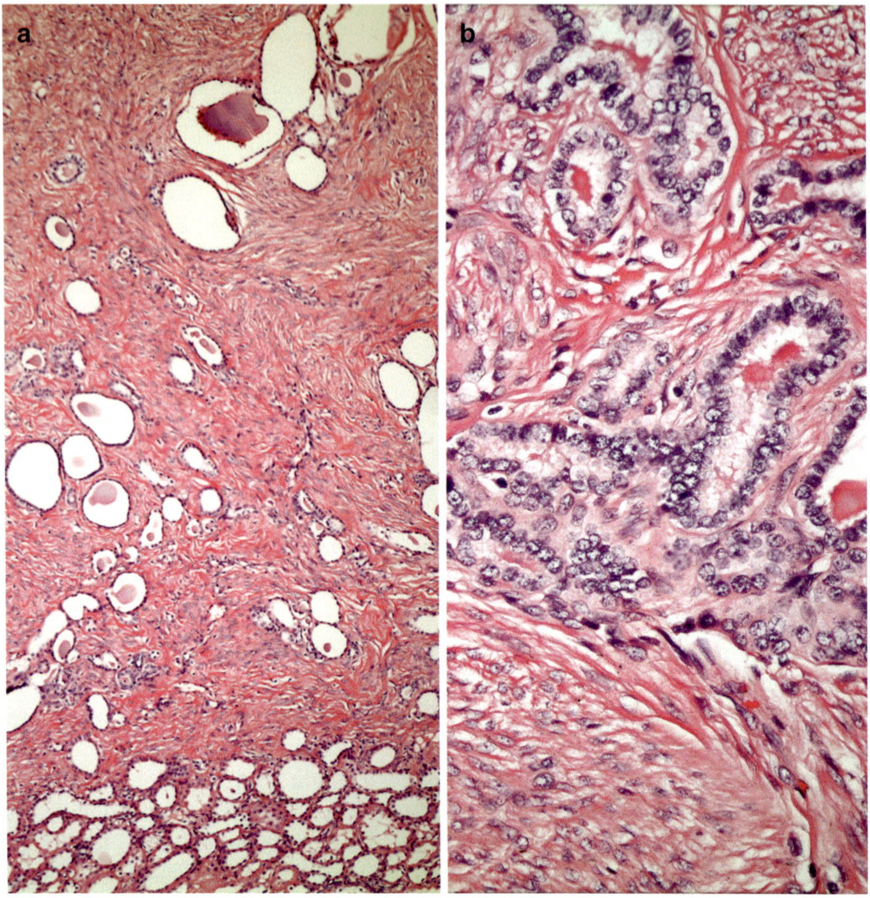

Fig. 4.19 (**a**, **b**) Mixed epithelial and stromal tumor with smooth muscle stroma. Single layer of cuboidal cells line the tubules seen in the right panel

chondrosarcoma, undifferentiated sarcoma, carcinosarcoma, or malignant neoplasm with rhabdoid features. Rarely, MEST may coexist with renal cell carcinoma [61].

Immunohistochemistry

The stromal component reacts for vimentin and smooth muscle actin diffusely and strongly in most cases. The immunoreactivity for desmin is also common, but can be variable and patchy (Fig. 4.20). Their nuclei frequently express progesterone and estrogen receptors, being strongest in the more cellular zones adjacent to cysts. Ovarian type stroma may express inhibin and calretinin, particularly if there is luteinization. The stromal cells surrounding the cystic spaces have been shown

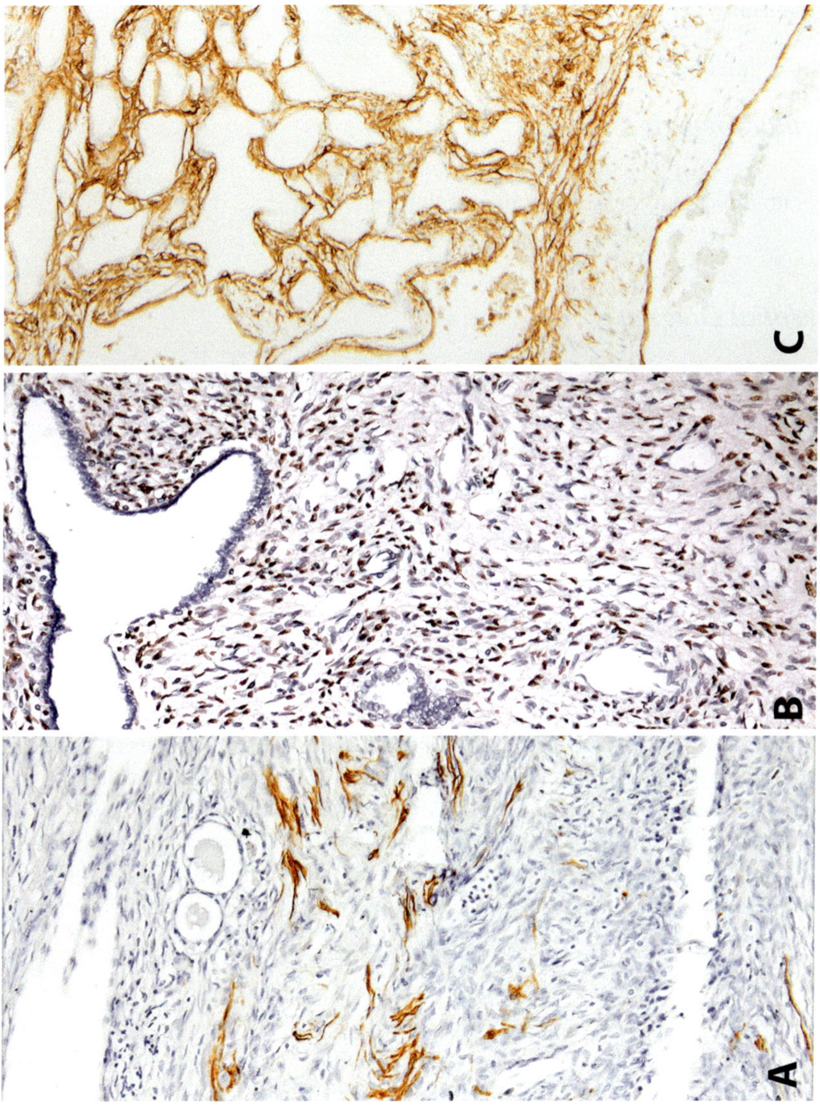

Fig. 4.20 Mixed epithelial and stromal tumor with patchy reactivity for desmin (**a**), diffuse staining for progesterone receptors in the stroma (**b**), and CD34 expression around epithelial component (**c**)

positive for CD34 in 47% and for CD10 in 90% of cases [53]. Stromal nuclear WT1 immunolabeling has been observed in 26% of tumors in one study [53]. The epithelial elements react with cytokeratins, PAX8, and often with vimentin. The coexpression of PAX8 and GATA3 can be focally found in the epithelium. Estrogen and progesterone receptor immunolabeling in the epithelial component is rarer than in stromal cells.

Molecular/Genetic Findings

There is no molecular marker specific for these entities.

Differential Diagnosis

In contrast to CN, nonneoplastic pluricystic renal lesions contain remnants of nephrons in the septae between adjacent cysts. Multilocular cystic renal neoplasm of low malignant potential is distinguished from CN by the presence of intraseptal clusters of clear cells identical to low-grade clear cell carcinoma, which are not present in the latter. Tubulocystic renal cell carcinoma is another well-circumscribed, predominantly cystic neoplasm of kidney that may enter into the differential diagnosis of MEST. However, it is made up of cells with high-grade nuclear features and does not enclose a neoplastic stroma.

MEST with extensive solid areas can be confused with other biphasic lesions of the kidney such as metanephric adenofibroma (MAF). The epithelial components of MEST and MAF are quite distinct. MAF is typically composed of tightly packed small uniform acini with an embryonal appearance embedded in spindle cell stroma. Cystic partially differentiated nephroblastoma (CPDN) is a multilocular cystic neoplasm, composed of epithelial and stromal elements like MEST. However, it possesses nephroblastematous tissue, such as blastema, immature stromal cells, and primitive epithelium. Furthermore, the vast majority of CPDN patients are younger than 24 months of age, whereas MEST is a disease of adults.

Prognosis and Treatment

These are generally benign lesions that are cured by excision. Conservative surgery is usually adequate, but incomplete removal may result in tumor recurrence [62]. An aggressive clinical course causing death has been reported in a few patients, whom sarcoma has arisen in the renal tumor. In these cases, the morphology in stromal component was obviously malignant (sarcomatoid). Histologically benign MESTs have an uneventful course.

References

1. Moch H, Humprey PA, Ulbrignt TM, Reuter VE. WHO classification of tumours of the urinary system and male genital organs. Lyon: IARC Press; 2016.
2. Grignon DJ, Eble JN. Papillary and metanephric adenomas of the kidney. Semin Diagn Pathol. 1998;15:41–53.
3. Wang KL, Weinrach DM, Luan C, et al. Renal papillary adenoma--a putative precursor of papillary renal cell carcinoma. Hum Pathol. 2007;38:239–46.
4. Denton MD, Magee CC, Ovuworie C, et al. Prevalence of renal cell carcinoma in patients with ESRD pre-transplantation: a pathologic analysis. Kidney Int. 2002;61:2201–9.
5. Hughson MD, Buchwald D, Fox M. Renal neoplasia and acquired cystic kidney disease in patients receiving long-term dialysis. Arch Pathol Lab Med. 1986;110:592–601.
6. Cohen C, McCue PA, DeRose PB. Immunohistochemistry of renal adenomas and carcinomas. J Urol Pathol. 1995;3:61–71.
7. Kovacs G, Fuzesi L, Emanual E, et al. Cytogenetics of papillary renal cell tumors. Genes Chromosomes Cancer. 1991;3:249–55.
8. Trpkov K, Yilmaz A, Uzer D, et al. Renal oncocytoma revisited: a clinicopathologic study of 109 cases with emphasis on problematic diagnostic features. Histopathology. 2010;57:893–906.
9. Perez-Ordonez B, Hamed G, et al. Renal oncocytoma: a clinicopathologic study of 70 cases. Am J Surg Pathol. 1997;21:871–83.
10. Wobker SE, Przybycin CG, Sircar K, Epstein JI. Renal oncocytoma with vascular invasion: a series of 22 cases. Hum Pathol. 2016;58:1–6.
11. Petersson F, Síma R, Grossmann P, et al. Renal small cell oncocytoma with pseudorosettes A histomorphologic, immunohistochemical, and molecular genetic study of 10 cases. Hum Pathol. 2011;42:1751–60.
12. Joshi S, Tolkunov D, Aviv H, et al. The genomic landscape of renal oncocytoma identifies a metabolic barrier to tumorigenesis. Cell Rep. 2015;13:1895–908.
13. Goyal R, Parwani AV, Gellert L, et al. A collision tumor of papillary renal cell carcinoma and oncocytoma: case report and literature review. Am J Clin Pathol. 2015;144:811–6.
14. Liu S, Lee S, Rashid P, et al. Active surveillance is suitable for intermediate term follow-up of renal oncocytoma diagnosed by percutaneous core biopsy. BJU Int. 2016;118(Suppl 3):30–4.
15. Tickoo SK, Reuter VE, Amin MB, et al. Renal oncocytosis: a morphologic study of fourteen cases. Am J Surg Pathol. 1999;23:1094–101.
16. Adamy A, Lowrance WT, Yee DS, et al. Renal oncocytosis: management and clinical outcomes. J Urol. 2011;185:795–801.
17. Pavlovich CP, Grubb RL 3rd, Hurley K, et al. Evaluation and management of renal tumors in the Birt-Hogg-Dube syndrome. J Urol. 2005;173:1482–6.
18. Pavlovich CP, Walther MM, Eyler RA, et al. Renal tumors in the Birt-Hogg- Dube syndrome. Am J Surg Pathol. 2002;26:1542–52.
19. Gobbo S, Eble JN, Delahunt B, et al. Renal cell neoplasms of oncocytosis have distinct morphologic, immunohistochemical, and cytogenetic profiles. Am J Surg Pathol. 2010;34:620–6.
20. Davis CJ Jr, Barton JH, Sesterhenn IA, Mostofi FK. Metanephric adenoma: clinicopathological study of fifty patients. Am J Surg Pathol. 1995;19:1101–14.
21. Drut R, Drut RM, Ortolani C. Metastatic metanephric adenoma with foci of papillary carcinoma in a child: a combined histologic, immunohistochemical, and FISH study. Int J Surg Pathol. 2001;9:241–7.
22. Li G, Tang Y, Zhang R, et al. Adult metanephric adenoma presumed to be all benign? A clinical perspective. BMC Cancer. 2015;15:310.
23. Muir TE, Cheville JC, Lager DJ. Metanephric adenoma, nephrogenic rests, and Wilms' tumor: a histologic and immunophenotypic comparison. Am J Surg Pathol. 2001;25:1290–6.
24. Sun Z, Kan S, Zhang L, et al. Immunohistochemical phenotype and molecular pathological characteristics of metanephric adenoma. Int J Clin Exp Pathol. 2015;8:6031–6.

25. Kato H, Suzuki M, Aizawa S, Hano H. Metanephric adenoma of the kidney with massive hemorrhage and necrosis: immunohistochemical, ultrastructural, and flow cytometric studies. Int J Surg Pathol. 2003;11:345–52.
26. Kinney SN, Eble JN, Hes O, et al. Metanephric adenoma: the utility of immunohistochemical and cytogenetic analyses in differential diagnosis, including solid variant papillary renal cell carcinoma and epithelial-predominant nephroblastoma. Mod Pathol. 2015;28:1236–48.
27. Pesti T, Sukosd F, Jones EC, et al. Mapping a tumor suppressor gene to chromosome 2p13 in metanephric adenoma by microsatellite allelotyping. Hum Pathol. 2001;32:101–4.
28. Choueiri TK, Cheville J, Palescandolo E, et al. BRAF mutations in metanephric adenoma of the kidney. Eur Urol. 2012;62:917–22.
29. Udager AM, Pan J, Magers MJ, et al. Molecular and immunohistochemical characterization reveals novel BRAF mutations in metanephric adenoma. Am J Surg Pathol. 2015;39:549–57.
30. Paner GP, Turk TM, Clark JI, et al. Passive seeding in metanephric adenoma: a review of pseudometastatic lesions in perinephric lymph nodes. Arch Pathol Lab Med. 2005;129:1317–21.
31. Renshaw AA, Freyer DR, Hammers YA. Metastatic metanephric adenoma in a child. Am J Surg Pathol. 2000;24:570–4.
32. Hennigar RA, Beckwith JB. Nephrogenic adenofibroma: a novel kidney tumor of young people. Am J Surg Pathol. 1992;16:325–34.
33. Arroyo MR, Green DM, Perlman EJ, et al. The spectrum of metanephric adenofibroma and related lesions: clinicopathologic study of 25 cases from the National Wilms Tumor Study Group Pathology Center. Am J Surg Pathol. 2001;25:433–44.
34. Piotrowski Z, Canter DJ, Kutikov A, et al. Metanephric adenofibroma: robotic partial nephrectomy of a large Wilms' tumor variant. Can J Urol. 2010;17:5309–12.
35. Galluzzo ML, Garcia de Davila MT, Vujanić GM. A composite renal tumor: metanephric adenofibroma, Wilms tumor, and renal cell carcinoma: a missing link? Pediatr Dev Pathol. 2012;15:65–70.
36. Argani P. Metanephric neoplasms: the hyperdifferentiated, benign end of the Wilms tumor spectrum. Clin Lab Med. 2005;25:379–92.
37. Mangray S, Breese V, Jackson CL, et al. Application of BRAF V600E mutation analysis for the diagnosis of metanephric adenofibroma. Am J Surg Pathol. 2015;39:1301–4.
38. Chami R, Yin M, Marrano P, et al. BRAF mutations in pediatric metanephric tumors. Hum Pathol. 2015;46:1153–61.
39. Yao DW, Qu F, Hu SW, et al. Metanephric adenofibroma in a 10-year-old boy: report of a case and review of the literature. Int J Clin Exp Pathol. 2015;8:3250–6.
40. Picken MM, Curry JL, Lindgren V, et al. Metanephric adenosarcoma in a young adult: morphologic, immunophenotypic, ultrastructural and fluorescence in situ hybridization analyses. Am J Surg Pathol. 2001;25:1451–7.
41. Tiefen S, Yan F, Zhu P. Metanephric adenosarcoma: a rare case with immunohistochemistry and molecular analysis. Diagn Pathol. 2014;9:179.
42. Argani P, Beckwith JB. Metanephric stromal tumor: report of 31 cases of a distinctive pediatric pediatric renal neoplasm. Am J Surg Pathol. 2000;24:917–26.
43. Bluebond-Langner R, Pinto PA, Argani P, et al. Adult presentation of metanephric stromal tumour. J Urol. 2002;168:1482–3.
44. McDonald OG, Rodriguez R, Bergner A, et al. Metanephric stromal tumour arising in a patient with neurofibromatosis type 1 syndrome. Int J Surg Pathol. 2011;19:667–71.
45. Argani P, Lee J, Netto GJ, et al. Frequent *BRAF* V600E mutations in metanephric stromal tumor. Am J Surg Pathol. 2016;40:719–22.
46. De Pasquale MD, Diomedi-Camassei F, Serra A, et al. Recurrent metanephric stromal tumor in an infant. Urology. 2011;78:1411–3.
47. Adsay NV, Eble JN, Srigley JR, et al. Mixed epithelial and stromal tumor of the kidney. Am J Surg Pathol. 2000;24:958–70.

48. Turbiner J, Amin MB, Humphrey PA, et al. Cystic nephroma and mixed epithelial and stromal tumor of kidney: a detailed clinicopathologic analysis of 34 cases and proposal for renal epithelial and stromal tumor (REST) as a unifying term. Am J Surg Pathol. 2007;31:489–500.
49. Michal M, Hes O, Bisceglia M, et al. Mixed epithelial and stromal tumors of the kidney. A report of 22 cases. Virchows Arch. 2004;445:359–67.
50. Montironi R, Mazzucchelli R, Lopez-Beltran A, et al. Cystic nephroma and mixed epithelial and stromal tumour of the kidney: opposite ends of the spectrum of the same entity? Eur Urol. 2008;54:1237–46.
51. Kalra S, Manikandan R, Dorairajan LN. Giant renal mixed epithelial and stromal tumour in a young female: a rare presentation. J Clin Diagn Res. 2015;9:XD01–2.
52. Yang Y, Ondrej H, Zhang L, et al. Mixed epithelial and stromal tumor of the kidney with cervical and intestinal differentiation. Virchows Arch. 2005;447:669–71.
53. Caliò A, Eble JN, Grignon DJ, Delahunt B. Mixed epithelial and stromal tumor of the kidney: a clinicopathologic study of 53 cases. Am J Surg Pathol. 2016;40:1538–49.
54. Svec A, Hes O, Michal M, Zachoval R. Malignant mixed epithelial and stromal tumor of the kidney. Virchows Arch. 2001;439:700–2.
55. Nakagawa T, Kanai Y, Fujimoto H, et al. Malignant mixed epithelial and stromal tumours of the kidney: a report of the first two cases with a fatal clinical outcome. Histopathology. 2004;44:302–4.
56. Jung SJ, Shen SS, Tran T, et al. Mixed epithelial and stromal tumor of kidney with malignant transformation: report of two cases and review of literature. Hum Pathol. 2008;39:463–8.
57. Zou L, Zhang X, Xiang H. Malignant mixed epithelial and stromal tumor of the kidney: the second male case and review of literature. Int J Clin Exp Pathol. 2014;7:2658–63.
58. Suzuki T, Hiragata S, Hosaka K, et al. Malignant mixed epithelial and stromal tumor of the kidney: report of the first male case. Int J Urol. 2013;20:448–50.
59. Menéndez CL, Rodríguez VD, Fernández-Pello S, et al. A new case of malignant mixed epithelial and stromal tumor of the kidney with rhabdomyosarcomatous transformation. Anal Quant Cytopathol Histpathol. 2012;34:331–4.
60. Sukov WR, Cheville JC, Lager DJ, et al. Malignant mixed epithelial and stromal tumor of the kidney with rhabdoid features: report of a case including immunohistochemical, molecular genetic studies and comparison to morphologically similar renal tumors. Hum Pathol. 2007;38:1432–7.
61. Mudaliar KM, Mehta V, Gupta GN, Picken MM. Expanding the morphologic spectrum of adult biphasic renal tumors – mixed epithelial and stromal tumor of the kidney with focal papillary renal cell carcinoma: case report and review of the literature. Int J Surg Pathol. 2014;22:266–71.
62. Farias JA, Laryea J, Gokden N, Kamel MH. Peritoneal seeding following incomplete resection of mixed epithelial stromal tumor of the kidney: first case report. Urol Ann. 2016;8:114–7.

Chapter 5
Major Subtypes of Renal Cell Carcinoma

Mukul K. Divatia, Charles C. Guo, Aseeb Rehman, and Jae Y. Ro

Renal cell carcinoma (RCC) and its treatment have consistently remained in the foreground as one of the most rapidly evolving areas in the ever-expanding field of solid tumor oncology. Significant developments have occurred over the past two decades in the clinical landscape that have vastly enhanced comprehension of etiopathogenesis of RCC and its modalities of management including advancements in minimally invasive surgical techniques, employment of focal therapy, increased renal biopsy-based approach, advancements in immunotherapy, adoption of active surveillance strategies, and the use of targeted treatment strategies for patients with advanced disease. Efforts aimed at morphologically grouping specific cancers into distinct pathologic subtypes have not only allowed a common descriptive language, but are helping to crystallize the understanding of RCC's molecular origins and its clinical behavior. It is these improved insights into the similarities and differences among RCC variants that offer clinical and therapeutic opportunities to improve patient care.

Renal neoplasms represent a group of heterogeneous tumors with various genetic and epigenetic abnormalities that are reflected in their histopathologic features and

M. K. Divatia (✉) · J. Y. Ro
Department of Pathology and Genomic Medicine, Houston Methodist Hospital, Weill Medical College of Cornell University, Houston, TX, USA
e-mail: mdivatia@houstonmethodist.org; JaeRo@houstonmethodist.org

C. C. Guo
Department of Pathology, The University of Texas MD Anderson Cancer Center, Houston, TX, USA
e-mail: ccguo@mdanderson.org

A. Rehman
Department of Pathology and Genomic Medicine, Houston Methodist Hospital, Weill-Cornell Medical College, Houston, TX, USA

M. K. Divatia et al. (eds.), *Kidney Cancer*, https://doi.org/10.1007/978-3-030-28333-9_5

molecular profiles [1–16]. Improved comprehension of the morphology, immunohistochemistry, genomics, and epidemiology of renal cell tumors has resulted in the identification of novel morphologic as well as molecular features. Therefore, the classification of renal cell tumors has recently been revised and published in the 2016 World Health Organization (WHO) classification [1]. This review briefly summarizes the pathologic, molecular, and epidemiologic features of the major subtypes of renal cell tumors.

WHO 2016 Classification of Renal Tumors

The revised WHO classification is based on advances in the understanding of newly identified characteristics of the molecular pathological epidemiology of renal cell tumors. The majority of the International Society of Urological Pathology (ISUP) Vancouver classification of renal neoplasia [17] was adopted for the revised 2016 WHO classification of renal cell tumors [1].

The various subtypes of renal cell tumors are based on characteristic morphologic features (Table 5.1) [1]. The major subtypes are clear cell RCC (CCRCC) (Fig. 5.1a), papillary RCC (PRCC) (Fig. 5.1b), and chromophobe RCC (ChRCC) (Fig. 5.1c) comprising 65–70%, 15–20%, and 5–7% of all RCCs, respectively. The designations of these various subtypes are based on their predominant cytoplasmic staining and cellular features (e.g., CCRCC, ChRCC, and renal oncocytoma), architectural features (e.g., PRCC), and combinations of these features (e.g., clear cell papillary RCC [CCPRCC]). Other subtypes of renal cell tumors are based on the anatomical location of the tumor (e.g., collecting duct and renal medullary carcinomas), association with renal disease (e.g., acquired cystic disease-associated RCC [ACD-associated RCC]), defining molecular alterations (e.g., microphthalmia transcription factor [MiT] family translocation RCC and succinate dehydrogenase-deficient RCC [SDH-deficient RCC]), and familial predisposition (e.g., hereditary leiomyomatosis and RCC-associated RCC [HLRCC-associated RCC]) [1].

Table 5.1 Classification of renal cell tumors according to the 2016 WHO classification

Current renal cell tumor subtypes	New renal cell tumor subtypes
Clear cell RCC	Multilocular cystic renal neoplasm of low malignant potential
Papillary RCC	MiT family translocation RCC
Chromophobe RCC	Tubulocystic RCC
Collecting duct car carcinoma	Acquired cystic disease-associated RCC
Renal medullary carcinoma	Clear cell papillary RCC
Mucinous spindle and tubular cell carcinoma	Succinate dehydrogenase-deficient RCC
RCC, unclassified	Hereditary leiomyomatosis and RCC-associated RCC
Papillary adenoma	
Oncocytoma	

MiT microphthalmia transcription factor, *RCC* renal cell carcinoma, *WHO* World Health Organization
From Moch et al. [18], with permission

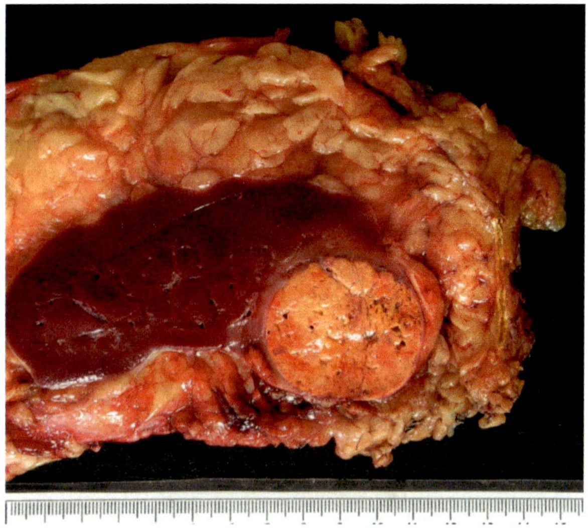

Fig. 5.1 Well-circumscribed clear cell renal cell carcinoma confined to kidney parenchyma

Clear Cell Renal Cell Carcinoma

CCRCC arises in epithelial cells lining the proximal tubule [19]. Although it can affect people of all ages including children, most of these tumors develop in patients older than 40 years of age with a male predominance and a male-to-female ratio of approximately 1.5: 1 [20].

The vast majority of cases of CCRCC have characteristic cytogenetic abnormalities that involve loss of genetic material from the short arm of chromosome 3 (3p) and mutations in the VHL gene [21–27]. The VHL gene, which is located at 3p25-26 and serves as a tumor suppressor gene, has been identified through studies of patients with VHL disease [23, 27–29]. One copy of VHL is either mutated or silenced in 90% of sporadic CCRCCs, whereas another copy is typically lost through 3p deletions, according to the comprehensive molecular profiling of CCRCCs by The Cancer Genome Atlas (TCGA) [2]. The biallelic loss of VHL allows for the inappropriate stabilization of hypoxia-inducible factors (HIFs), which results in a proangiogenic gene expression signature that is an important step in the carcinogenesis of CCRCC [30, 31].

According to the TCGA, CCRCCs are characterized by recurrent mutations in the PI3K/AKT/MTOR pathway (a potential therapeutic target), mutations in SETD2 (associated with widespread DNA hypomethylation), and mutations involving the SWI/SNF chromatin remodeling complex (PBRM1, ARID1A, and SMARCA4). Aggressive CCRCCs demonstrate a metabolic shift [2]. Other genes may be involved as tumor suppressors and lead to development of CCRCC, particularly 3p14.2 deletions, likely resulting in inactivation of the FHIT gene, as well as tumor suppressor genes at 3p12.176. A continuous deletion from 3p14.2-p25, including the FHIT and VHL genes, can be identified in up to 96% of cases [32].

Following the initiating event involving the 3p gene, additional genetic alterations occur in clonal tumor cell populations resulting in tumor progression and metastatic disease. Consequently, these additional genetic abnormalities, when detectable, are often associated with higher histologic grade, higher pathologic stage, and an adverse prognosis. The genetic abnormalities associated with these effects are loss of 9p, 14q, and loss of heterozygosity on chromosome 10q around the PTEN/MAC locus [33].

CCRCC may arise in a familial setting, especially in cases of VHL disease. In addition, 35–45% of affected patients with VHL disease develop bilateral multifocal CCRCC. Onset of renal carcinoma in patients with VHL disease is often early; clinically evident renal cancer has been reported in adolescence, and the mean age at diagnosis is 39 years. Historically, without treatment, up to 40% of patients with VHL disease died of advanced renal carcinoma. In VHL disease, patients are born with a germline defect in one of the two alleles of the VHL gene, located on chromosome 3p9.25-26, which functions as a tumor suppressor. Loss of the second allele results in clinical disease expression [34]. Additional heritable settings in which clear cell RCC may develop include families segregating constitutional chromosome 3 translocations as well as families with succinate dehydrogenase B (SDHB)-associated heritable paraganglioma [35, 36].

On gross examination, CCRCC ranges in size from subcentimeter lesions to large masses weighing several kilograms and an average diameter of 7 cm. These tumors are usually unilateral and solitary; bilaterality and multicentricity are reported in familial cases. Imaging studies frequently show a bosselated mass protruding from the external surface. The cut surface often demonstrates a characteristic golden-yellow appearance due to abundant cholesterol and other phospholipids within the tumor cells. The cut surface is typically heterogeneous with areas of gray-white fibrosis and recent or remote hemorrhage. These tumors exhibit an expansile pushing growth pattern and are either well demarcated from the adjacent uninvolved parenchyma by a variably thick fibrous pseudocapsule or widely infiltrate the adjacent renal parenchyma. Cystic change and foci of calcification are commonly present, often in association with areas of necrosis. Figures 5.1, 5.2, 5.3, 5.4, 5.5, 5.6, and 5.7 illustrate different growth patterns and gross features that are helpful in staging renal carcinomas in nephrectomy specimens.

The microscopic appearance of CCRCC includes a variety of architectural patterns; tumor cells are arranged in a variable combination of compact nests, alveolar, acinar, solid sheet-like and cystic patterns, separated by an arborizing network of thin-walled blood vessels (Fig. 5.8). Cystic areas are filled with extravasated erythrocytes or eosinophilic fluid. Occasional, small papillary structures lined by clear cells may be present focally, but they almost always represent a minor component of the tumor.

In CCRCC, the tumor cells contain distinct cell membranes and optically clear cytoplasm owing to loss of cytoplasmic lipids and glycogen during histologic processing. Some cases of CCRCC comprise of varying areas demonstrating tumor cells with granular eosinophilic cytoplasm; such foci are more often seen in high-

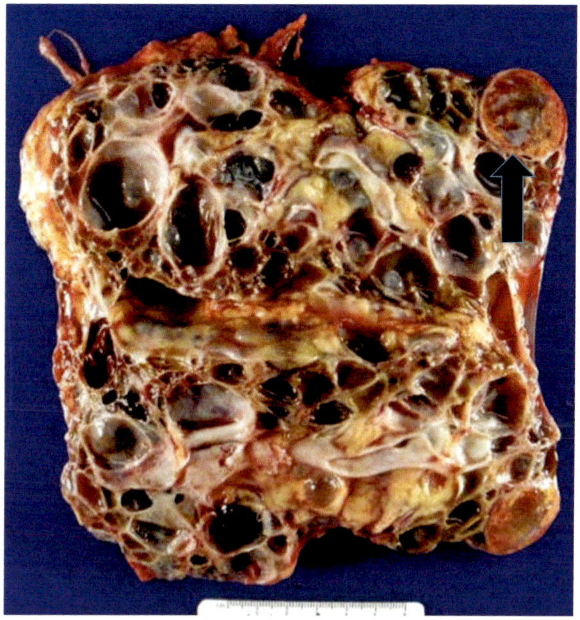

Fig. 5.2 Polycystic disease with characteristic gross appearance of bivalved kidney and solitary circumscribed clear cell renal cell carcinoma identified in upper right corner

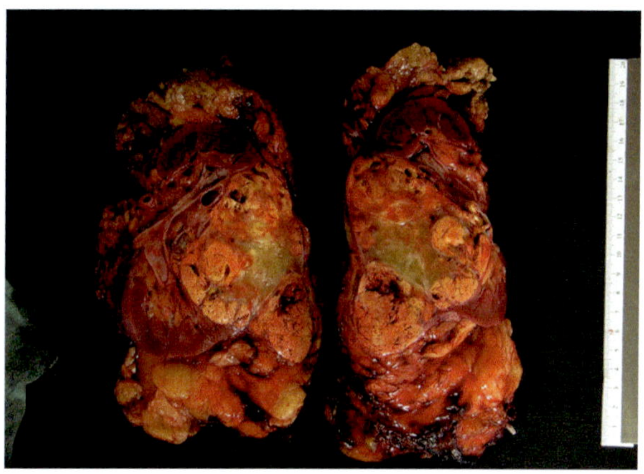

Fig. 5.3 Clear cell renal cell carcinoma widely infiltrating kidney parenchyma with invasion into perinephric adipose tissue

grade cancer or near areas of hemorrhage or necrosis. The nuclei of CCRCC show considerable variation in size, shape, and nucleolar prominence, as discussed in the section on grading, and these features are assessed when assigning a nuclear grade to an individual tumor.

Sarcomatoid and rhabdoid differentiation are seen in approximately 5% of cases and carry prognostic significance (Figs. 5.9, 5.10, and 5.11) [37–39]. Other uncommon histologic variations with unknown prognostic significance have been described in RCC, including intra- or extracellular hyaline globules, basophilic cytoplasmic inclusions, abundant multinucleated giant cells, sarcoid-like granulomas, myospherulosis, and dense inflammation [40–44].

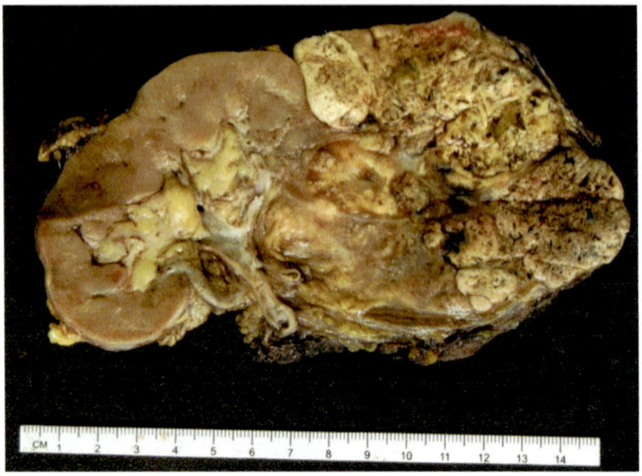

Fig. 5.4 High-grade clear cell renal cell carcinoma with direct invasion and effacement of overlying adrenal gland

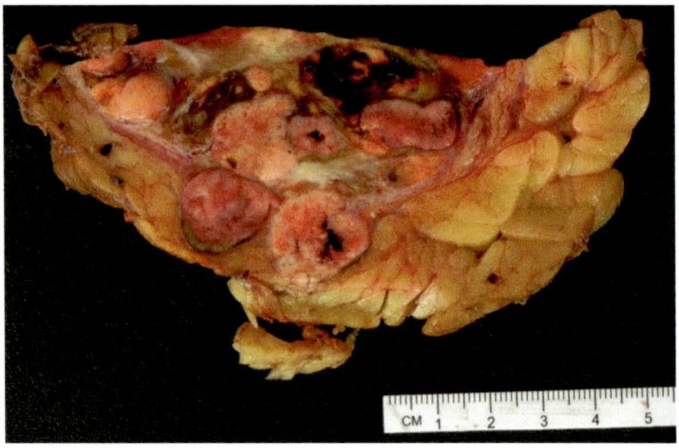

Fig. 5.5 Clear cell renal cell carcinoma penetrating through capsular surface and extending into perinephric adipose tissue (pT3)

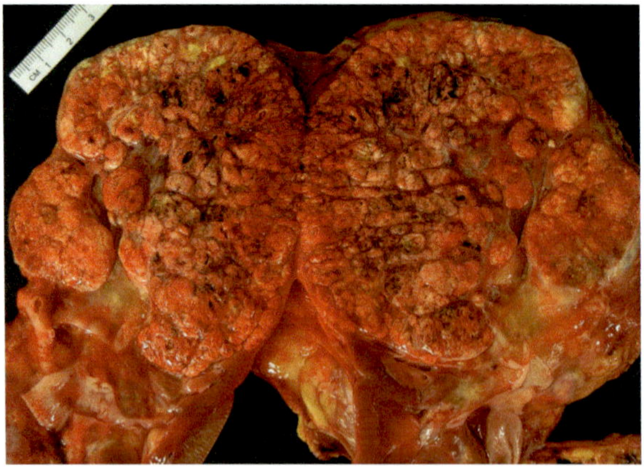

Fig. 5.6 Widespread invasion of renal sinus adipose tissue in clear cell renal cell carcinoma (pT3)

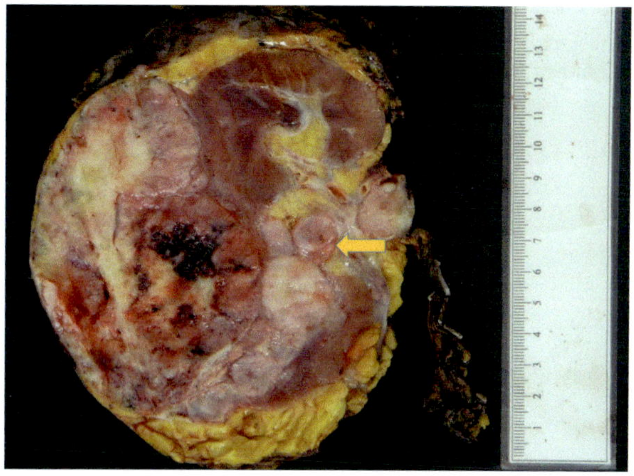

Fig. 5.7 Large tumor thrombus occluding lumen of renal vein (arrow) in a case of clear cell renal cell carcinoma

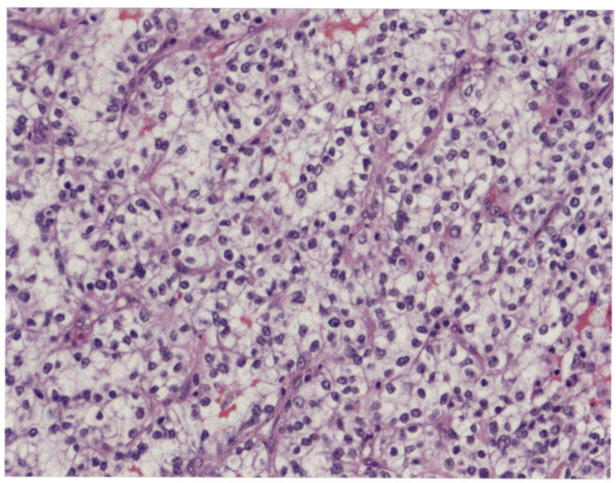

Fig. 5.8 Clear cell renal cell carcinoma demonstrating characteristic features with nests of tumor cells containing clear cytoplasm and an arborizing network of thin-walled blood vessels

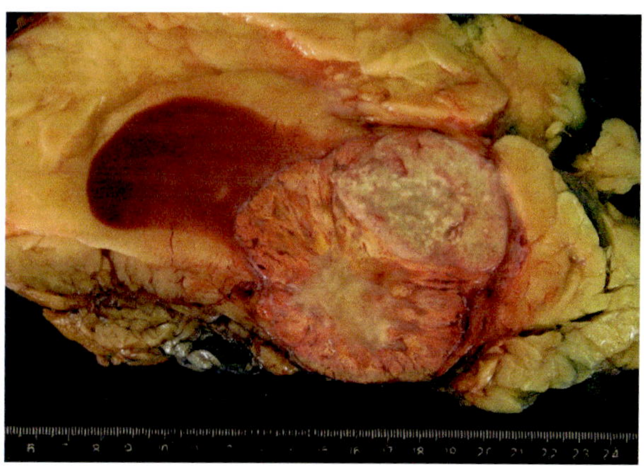

Fig. 5.9 Clear cell renal cell carcinoma with sarcomatoid and rhabdoid growth patterns as demonstrated by the presence of fleshy nodular areas in the tumor on gross examination

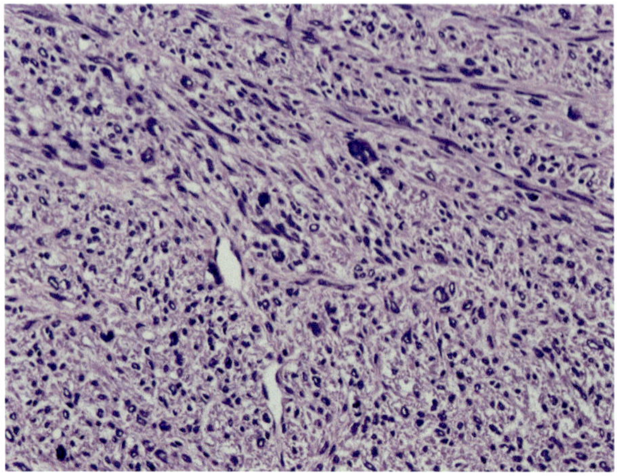

Fig. 5.10 Sarcomatoid RCC with a malignant spindled-tumor cell morphology

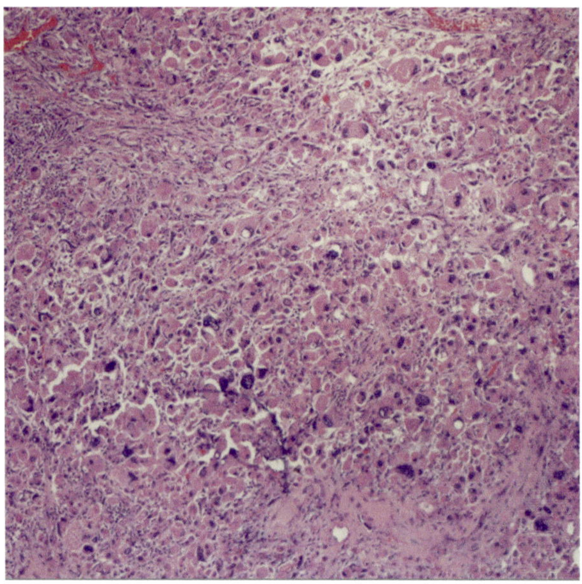

Fig. 5.11 Rhabdoid differentiation in renal cell carcinoma with tumor cells containing eccentric nuclei and abundant eosinophilic cytoplasm

Immunohistochemically, clear cell carcinoma typically shows positive immunostaining for vimentin, cytokeratin (CK) AE1/AE3, RCC antigen, CD10, PAX2, PAX8, and carbonic anhydrase-IX (CA IX). Immunostaining reactions for HMWCK, CK7, CK20, mucin 1, cell surface associated (MUC1), parvalbumin, AMACR, kidney-specific cadherin, and CD117 are negative in most cases [45–57].

Pathologic staging most accurately predicts the prognosis for patients with CCRCC [58–60]. Major factors outlining the prognosis in tumors with same stage include tumor grade, tumor necrosis, and the presence or absence of sarcomatoid or rhabdoid differentiation. Tumors with higher grades are associated with progressively worsening prognosis [58]. Tumor necrosis accounting for more than 10% of the total tumor volume is more likely to have an adverse outcome. Sarcomatoid and rhabdoid differentiation are seen in less than 10% of cases of CCRCC and associated with a worse prognosis [59, 60]. Cases with sarcomatoid differentiation have a 5-year survival rate of 15–22%, and in cases with rhabdoid differentiation, the median survival ranges from 8 to 31 months [59, 60].

Multilocular Cystic Renal Neoplasm of Low Malignant Potential

This tumor was previously referred to as multilocular cystic RCC and encompasses renal neoplasms with a fibrous pseudocapsule that are composed entirely of cysts and septa with no expansile solid nodules; the septa should contain aggregates of low-grade tumor cells with clear cytoplasm [61–66]. Combined experience with more than 200 patients with follow-up times longer than 5 years indicates no recurrence or cancer-related mortality in these patients; however, the natural history of this tumor is unknown because all these reported cases were treated with definitive surgery. Consequently, multilocular cystic renal neoplasm of low malignant potential (MCRNLMP) is now the WHO-recommended term for this lesion.

It constitutes approximately up to 5% of all RCCs and has a male predominance with a male-to-female ratio of 2–3: 1. The age ranges from 20 to 76 years; most patients are above 50 years of age, and women tend to present at a younger age than do men [61–66].

Most patients in this cohort are asymptomatic and these neoplasms are incidental lesions with few cases presenting with a palpable mass, gross hematuria, abdominal or back pain. Most patients have no biochemical abnormalities. Imaging studies usually outline a complex cystic mass that may have focal calcification.

Grossly, MCRNLMP ranges from subcentimeter lesions to large tumors measuring over 10 cm in greatest dimension. The tumor is usually a unilateral and solitary well-circumscribed mass composed entirely of variably sized cysts separated from each other by thin fibrous septae and from adjacent renal parenchyma by a fibrous wall (Fig. 5.12); however, it can be multifocal as well as bilateral [61–66]. The cysts contain clear or hemorrhagic fluid. Necrosis is not seen and there are no grossly identifiable nodules expanding the septa, a feature that differentiates this tumor from extensively cystic conventional CCRCC.

Microscopically, the cysts are lined by a single layer of clear tumor cells with occasional multilayered epithelium and rare papillary structures; some cysts lack any lining epithelium (Fig. 5.13a, b). The tumor cells have variable amounts of cytoplasm that may be clear or lightly eosinophilic. Many of these tumors show calcifications within the septa, and metaplastic bone formation is occasionally encountered. Within the septa in all cases are clusters of low-grade tumor cells with clear cytoplasm (Fig. 5.13b). These cells are often difficult to distinguish from histiocytes or from lymphocytes with surrounding retraction artifact. Increased vascularity is sometimes

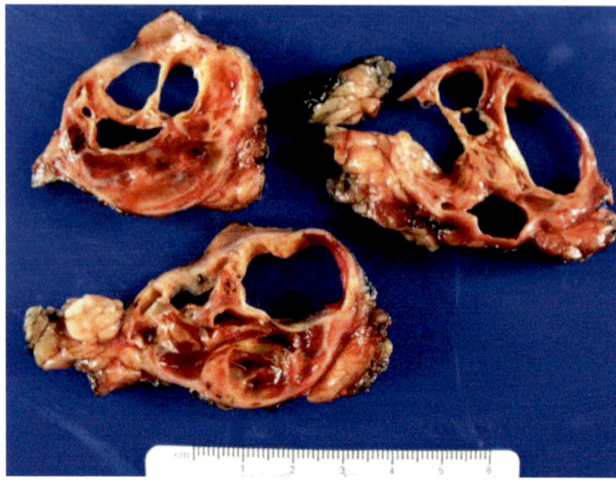

Fig. 5.12 Multilocular cystic renal cell neoplasm of low malignant potential, a well-circumscribed tumor composed entirely of variably sized cysts

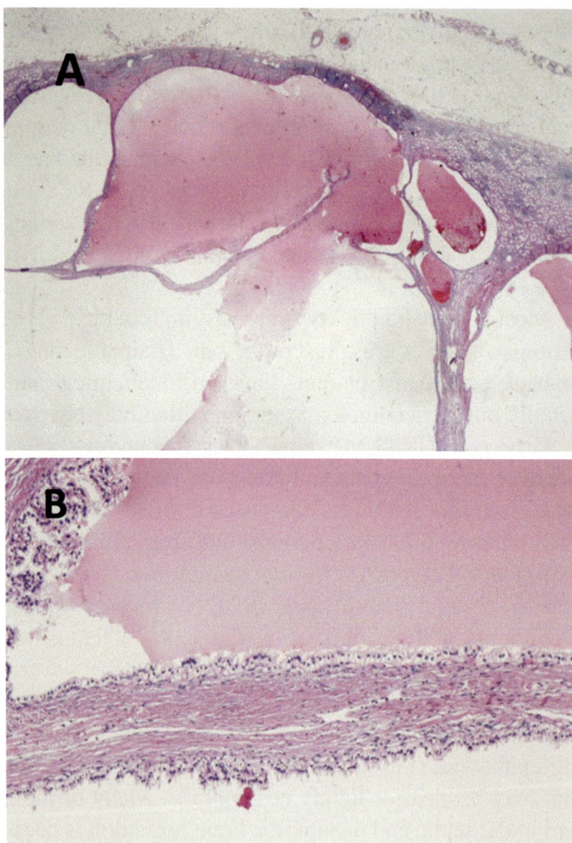

Fig. 5.13 Multilocular cystic renal neoplasm of low malignant potential. Note the low-power appearance of variably sized cysts filled with eosinophilic fluid (**a**) and clusters of low-grade tumor cells with clear cytoplasm within the septae (**b**)

associated with septal tumor cell clusters, and this feature may be helpful in recognition of this entity. There should be no nodular expansion of clear tumor cells in the septa, a feature that serves to mainly distinguish it from extenisvely cystic CCRCC. In challenging cases, the epithelial nature of the tumor cells can be confirmed by their immunoreactivity to antibodies against cytokeratin and EMA; results of immunostains for histiocytic markers are negative. Tumor cells are also strongly immunoreactive for PAX8 and CA-IX aiding in this diagnosis [61–66].

VHL gene mutations have been reported in about 25% in MCRNLMP, and there is no difference in the status of chromosome 3p deletion between low-grade CCRCC and this neoplasm, supporting the hypothesis that it is a subtype of CCRCC [64–66].

Papillary Renal Cell Carcinoma

PRCC, the second most common type of RCC, bears characteristic cytogenetic, gross, and histologic features that distinguish it from other types of RCC [67].

Most of these tumors are sporadic, but some occur in a familial setting with hereditary papillary renal carcinoma (HPRCC), an inherited renal cancer characterized by mutations in the *MET* oncogene at 7q31 and by a predisposition to develop multiple bilateral papillary renal tumors. *MET* mutations have been detected in approximately 13% of patients with PRCC who have no family history of renal tumors [68–71].

The mean age of patients with PRCC ranges from 52 to 66 years and the male-to-female ratio of 2.4: 1 [67, 72]. The common presenting signs and symptoms of RCC are noted. PRCC is more likely to be multifocal and necrotic than other common RCC subtypes and exhibits an association with end-stage renal disease. Each papillary tumor arises independently in cases of multiple PRCCs without a family history of renal tumors [73].

Grossly, PRCC is typically well circumscribed, the vast majority of cases are confined to the renal parenchyma [67, 72–74]. Multifocality is identified particularly in cases of HPRC [68–71]. A thick fibrous pseudocapsule is present in up to two-thirds of mirroring the extent of hemorrhage and necrosis present in the tumor. The cut surface ranges from light gray tan to golden yellow to red brown, depending upon the hemorrhage and hemosiderin accumulation in accompanying macrophages as well as stroma (Fig. 5.14) [67, 72–74].

Microscopically, PRCC is composed of varying proportions of papillary and tubular structures and also contains variable cystic change with papillary excrescences or with tumor infiltrating the cyst wall [67, 72–74]. “Papillary” morphology is also encountered in a host of other kidney tumors and is thus not specific or entirely representative of this neoplasm. Papillae are lined by a single layer of tumor cells with variable pseudostratification [74]. The papillary stalks contain fibrovascular cores and a variable degree of macrophages that is not linked to the extent of accompanying hemorrhage and/or necrosis. The tumor papillae may be slender and easily recognizable or compact and tightly packed resulting in a solid appearance;

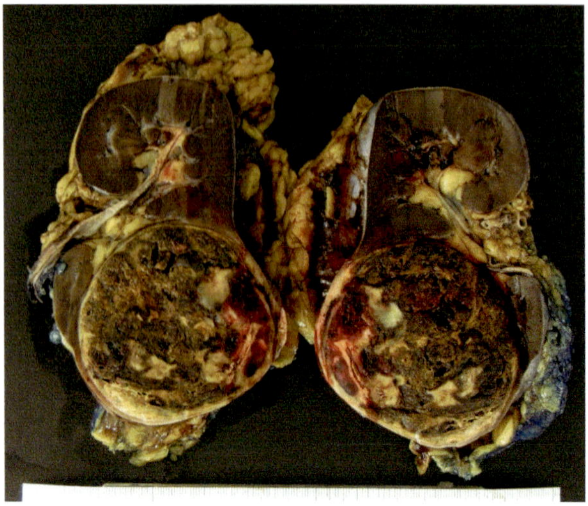

Fig. 5.14 Well-circumscribed papillary renal cell carcinoma with hemorrhage and hemosiderin deposition grossly imparting a brown appearance to the cut surface

and in some tumors, the papillae are arranged in long parallel arrays, imparting a trabecular appearance [72].

A few cases of papillary carcinoma exhibit solid areas composed of spindle cells with low-grade nuclear features, admixed with variable amounts of tumor with tubular or papillary architecture [75, 76]. In one series of such cases, all were confirmed as PRCC by molecular studies [75]. The spindle cell components of such tumors do not meet the criteria for sarcomatoid differentiation and are therefore not associated with a worse prognosis.

PRCC can be categorized into two morphologic classes, which have been designated types 1 and 2, based on morphologic criteria, immunohistochemical staining, clinicopathologic staging parameters, and survival outcome analysis [74, 77–79]. Tumors in both categories share several features including tumor-associated inflammatory infiltrate, extensive necrosis, psammoma bodies, cholesterol clefts, hemorrhagic background, and foci of dystrophic calcification yet exhibit significant differences in molecular profiles and overall outcomes [74, 78].

Type 1 PRCC is composed of papillae covered by a single layer of low-grade tumor cells containing small round to ovoid nuclei with inconspicuous nucleoli and minimal pale to clear cytoplasm (Fig. 5.15). Tubular profiles in these neoplasms have similar lining cells. The short, complex papillae sometimes impart a glomeruloid appearance. The papillae of type 1 tumors are usually thin, delicate, and often short and are frequently edematous [74, 78]. Aggregates of foamy macrophages are commonly seen within the papillary cores or in between aggregates of tumor cells. This morphological pattern is seen in both sporadic and in HPRC cases [71].

Type 2 PRCC demonstrates significantly higher nucleolar grade and overall larger tumor size [74, 78]. In these cases, tumor cells exhibit prominent nucleoli and varying degrees of nuclear pseudostratification with abundant eosinophilic cyto-

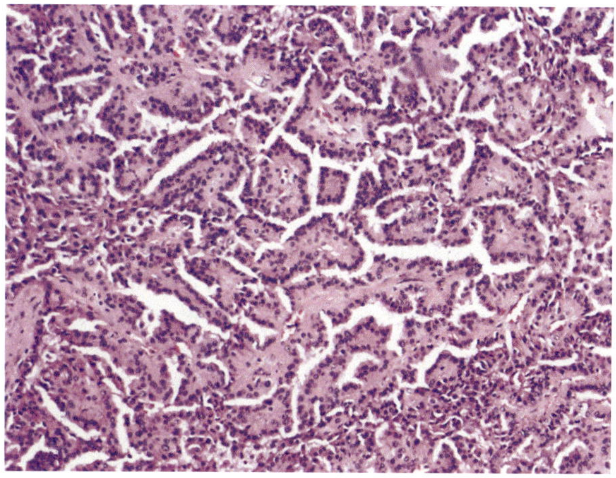

Fig. 5.15 Papillary renal carcinoma type 1 with characteristic morphologic features including delicate fibrovascular cores lined by single layer of tumor cells

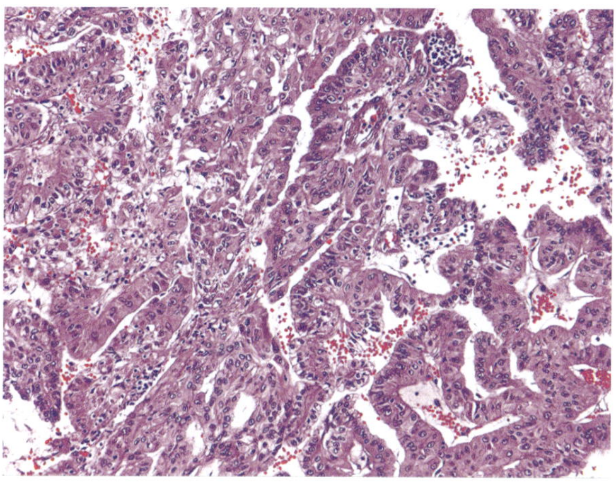

Fig. 5.16 Papillary renal cell carcinoma type 2 with broad papillae containing tumor cells exhibiting prominent nucleoli and nuclear pseudostratification with abundant eosinophilic cytoplasm

plasm (Fig. 5.16). The fibrovascular cores of most cases of type 2 PRCC tend to be dense and fibrous instead of thin and delicate, and edema and glomeruloid bodies are less prevalent than in type 1 tumors. Macrophages are more likely identified near necrotic tumor foci. ISUP nucleolar grading system is validated for reporting of PRCCs. Sarcomatoid and rhabdoid changes are categorized as grade 4 tumors, usually associated with an adverse prognosis.

Type 1 PRCC reveals loss of Y chromosome and gains in chromosomes 7, 17, 16, and 20 [79]. Activation of the MET pathway is a recognized finding in up to 80% of type 1 PRCC tumors [80, 81]. Type 2 PRCC tumors demonstrate a heterogeneous pattern of chromosomal gains and losses, involving chromosomes 1, 3, 4, 5, 6, 8q, 9, 14, and 15 [80–84]. Type 2 PRCCs are more frequently associated with aggressive clinicopathologic parameters than type 1 PRCCs, including higher TNM stage, larger tumor size, and an overall worse prognosis [77, 78, 85]. Although some studies have documented a worse prognosis in type 2 PRCCs based on univariate analysis, other studies have not reported the same findings on multivariate analysis upon factoring of tumor grade and stage [77, 78, 82, 85–87].

PRCCs exhibit positivity for cytokeratin AE1/AE3, CK7, CAM5.2, EMA, high-molecular-weight cytokeratin, racemase (AMACR), CA-IX, RCC antigen, CD10, and vimentin. Type 2 PRCC demonstrates more variable immunoreactivity for the above markers, including reduced expression of CK7.

Subtyping PRCCs is difficult in a notable subset of cases, further complicating the classification schemata as some examples exhibit nuclear features typical of type 1 PRCC, but cytoplasmic features characteristic of type 2 PRCC, whereas other cases comprised tumor cells with high nuclear grade with variable cytoplasmic features [77–87]. Across the board, the proportion of both type 1 and type 2 PRCC tumors varies between 30% and 70% [77–87]. A significant proportion of PRCC cases do not meet the documented histologic parameters for typing in either category, and such tumors have been designated as mixed, unclassified, overlapping, or not otherwise specified tumors [77–87]. Additionally, an oncocytic low-grade variant of PRCC has been identified, composed predominantly of tumor cells with oncocytic cytoplasm and round, nonoverlapping low-grade nuclei with inconspicuous nucleoli and a linear arrangement toward cell apices (Fig. 5.17). These tumors exhibit molecular features akin to type 1 PRCC, with gains in chromosomes 7 and 17. These tumors carry a good prognosis owing to their indolent behavior [88–92].

The Cancer Genome Atlas (TCGA) Research Network showed that types 1 and 2 PRCCs are actually different types of renal cancer based on comprehensive molecular analysis of a cohort of 161 tumors. PRCC1 is associated with MET alterations. Multiple molecular subgroups were identified within the type 2 PRCC cohort that was otherwise characterized by CDKN2A silencing, SETD2 mutations, transcription factor E3 (TFE3) fusions, and increased expression of the NrF2-antioxidant response element pathway. A CpG island methylator phenotype was observed in a distinct subgroup of type 2 PRCC that was characterized by poor survival and muta-

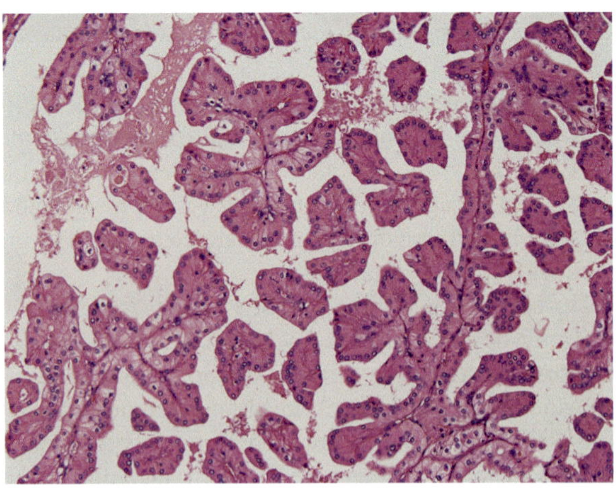

Fig. 5.17 Oncocytic low-grade variant of papillary RCC composed of tumor cells with oncocytic cytoplasm, papillary architecture, and round, nonoverlapping low-grade nuclei

tion of the gene-encoding fumarate hydratase (FH) [81]. It is now established that type 2 PRCCs represent a heterogeneous group of tumors that requires better characterization based on molecular characterization and morphologic correlates.

The cancer-specific survival rates at 5 years after surgery for a large series of patients with CCRCC, PRCC, and chromophobe RCC were 72%, 91%, and 88%, respectively [93]. PRCC has a more favorable outcome than other aggressive subtypes like collecting duct carcinoma and HLRCC-RCC [94, 95]. Type 1 PRCC cases are associated with a significantly better survival rate than type 2 PRCCs, though this difference is linked to the grade and stage at presentation rather than tumor subtyping [86].

Chromophobe Renal Cell Carcinoma

ChRCC was first reported in 1985 and derived its name from the morphologically similar tumor cells identified in the experimentally produced rat kidney tumor [96]. The eosinophilic variant of ChRCC was described in 1988 [97]. ChRCC has its postulated origin in the intercalated cells of the collecting duct system [98]. Most of these tumors are sporadic, but also occur in a familial setting in patients with Birt–Hogg–Dubé syndrome [99]. A germline mutation of PTEN in Cowden syndrome also predisposes to development of ChRCC [100].

Patients range in age from 23 to 86 years, and a slight male preponderance is seen with a greater incidence in Middle Eastern nations [101–106]. The presenting signs and symptoms are not different from other renal tumors and a palpable mass is rarely noted. Radiologically, no features reliably distinguish chromophobe RCC from other kidney tumors, including oncocytoma.

Tumors are well circumscribed and vary widely in size, from 1.5 to 25 cm in diameter, mean diameter ranges from 6.9 to 8.5 cm [101–106]. The cut surface is usually solid, homogeneous, and tan brown (Fig. 5.18). Hemorrhage and necrosis, when present, are limited and seen in a minority of cases. Central scar formation is infrequently present.

Microscopically, the tumor cells are typically arranged in solid sheets with focal tubulocystic pattern in some cases. There are fibrous septa of variable thickness with relatively larger caliber blood vessels in contrast to the delicate vasculature seen in clear cell carcinoma. Variable populations of two types of tumor cells are seen – the typical ChRCC tumor cell is a large polygonal cell with abundant, almost transparent, and slightly flocculent cytoplasm and prominent plant-like cell membranes that is commonly seen abutting vascular channels (Fig. 5.19a). Usually these are admixed with a second population of smaller cells with less abundant cytoplasm that is granular and eosinophilic (Fig. 5.19b) [101–106].

A variant of ChRCC that is virtually entirely composed of intensely eosinophilic cells with prominent cell membranes has been designated the eosinophilic variant of this neoplasm (Fig. 5.20a) [101–106]. The nuclei of both cell types are typically hyperchromatic with irregular wrinkled nuclear contours; binucleation is commonly present. Perinuclear halos are more commonly identified in the

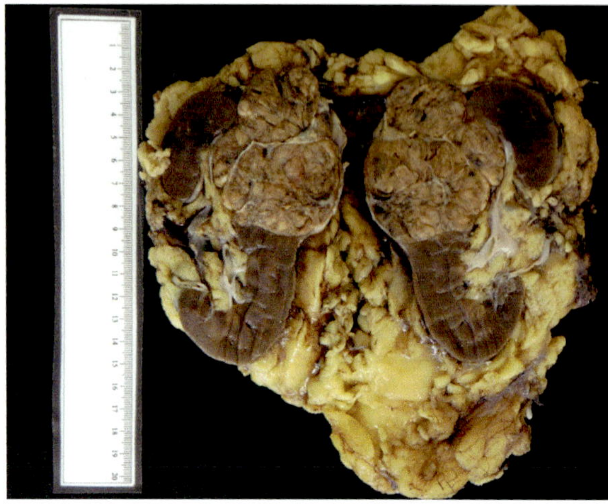

Fig. 5.18 Chromophobe renal cell carcinoma. Note the well-circumscribed tumor with a characteristic tan brown appearance

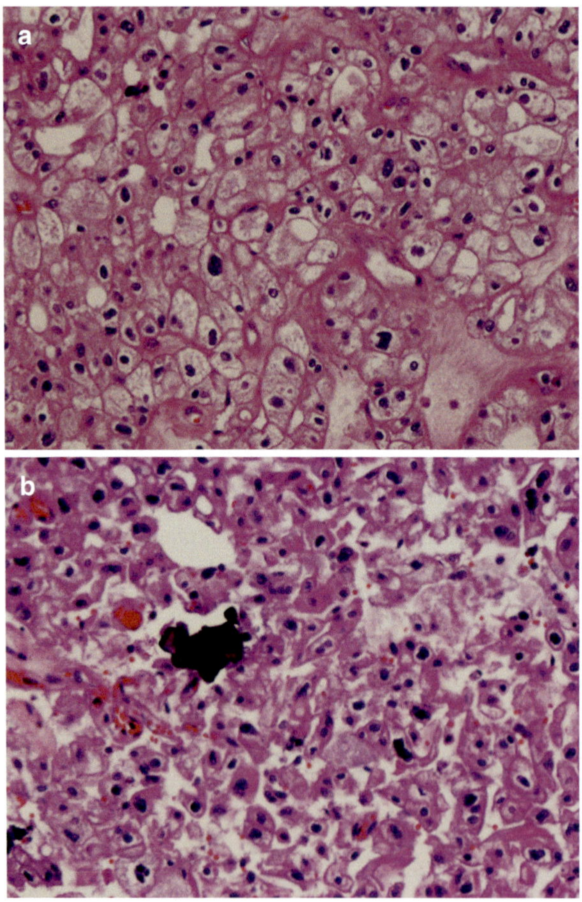

Fig. 5.19 Chromophobe renal cell carcinoma with (**a**) tumor cells containing abundant flocculent cytoplasm and well-defined plant-like cell membranes and (**b**) tumor cells with more granular eosinophilic calcification, perinuclear haloes, and raisinoid nuclei. Microcalcifications are frequently seen in these tumors

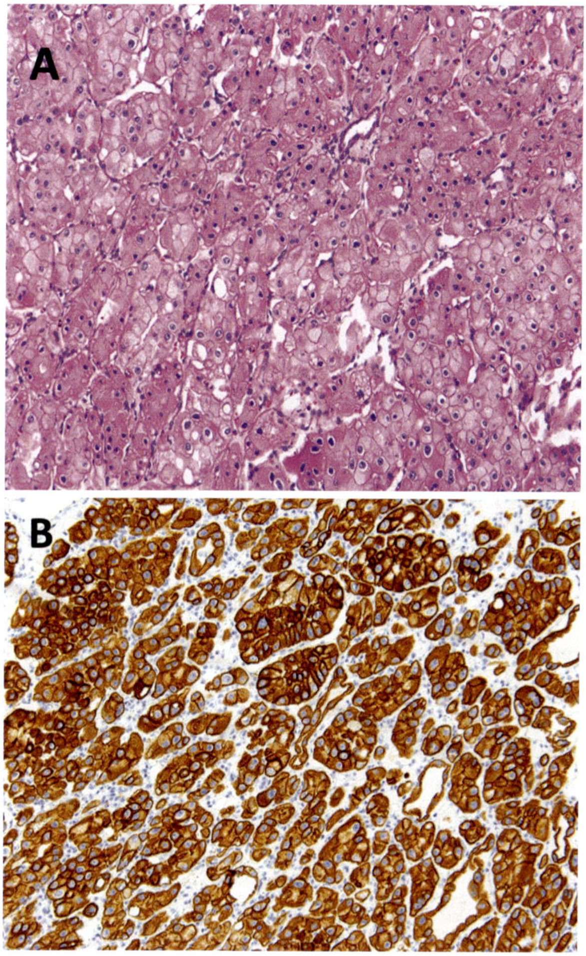

Fig. 5.20 (**a**) Eosinophilic variant of chromophobe renal cell carcinoma with sheets of tumor cells resembling an oncocytoma. (**b**) Strong and diffuse cytokeratin 7 expression on immunostaining serves to distinguish this tumor from oncocytoma

eosinophilic cells, a diagnostically helpful finding, but often it is not possible to distinguish eosinophilic ChRCC from oncocytoma particularly in biopsy specimens. Immunostaining for CK7 showing strong and diffuse positivity in tumor cells is noted in eosinophilic variant of ChRCC (Fig. 5.20b) [101–107]. Sarcomatoid transformation, a feature common to other types of RCC, may be identified in less than 10% of cases [37, 38, 108, 109]. Rare cases with osteosarcoma-like differentiation, rhabdoid morphology, or extensive calcification and ossification have been reported [110, 111].

Some kidney tumors demonstrate mixed morphologic patterns, with features overlapping between oncocytoma and ChRCC in the same tumor, and are designated hybrid oncocytic chromophobe tumors [112–115]. Such tumors may arise in different settings: as tumors present in cases of renal oncocytosis, as tumors arising in patients with Birt–Hogg–Dubé syndrome, and as sporadic tumors [112–115]. These tumors either show a gradual transition from one pattern to another or appear as distinctly separate areas adjacent to one another, or the two patterns are intimately admixed with one another. In spite of overlapping morphologies, tumors from all three groups have different molecular genetic makeup, and their molecular features are different from those of oncocytoma and ChRCC. The tumors in all three groups exhibit indolent behavior in the reported literature and are currently subcategorized under ChRCC [112–115].

The genetic abnormality most frequently identified in ChRCC has been loss of one copy of the entire chromosome for most or all of the chromosomes 1, 2, 6, 10, 13, 17, and 21 (in >80% of cases), as well as losses of various other chromosomes [98, 116, 117]. In regard to the eosinophilic variant of ChRCC, approximately 50% of cases have different chromosomal abnormalities than the classic type [98]. Sarcomatoid ChRCC analysis often shows multiple gains (polysomy) of chromosomes 1, 2, 6, 10, and 17, and distant metastases in ChRCC cases show the same genetic alterations as reported in the primary tumors [118].

ChRCC demonstrates positive immunohistochemical staining for PAX8, CD117 (c-kit), pancytokeratin, and EMA and negative immunostaining for vimentin, CK20, and racemase. The most helpful immunostain in distinguishing between oncocytoma and ChRCC is CK7 that is very frequently diffusely positive in ChRCC, in contrast with oncocytomas, which usually show focal scattered positivity in tumor cells [101–106].

Renal oncocytomas do not demonstrate combined losses of heterozygosity at chromosomes 1, 2, 6, 10, 13, 17, and 21 that are characteristically associated with ChRCC. Fluorescence in situ hybridization (FISH) studies detect the aforementioned cytogenetic findings and therefore are helpful distinguishing between the two entities [119].

A recent study demonstrated that approximately 70% of ChRCCs carry either a hemizygous deletion of RB1 or ERBB4, and oncocytomas do not show deletions of these genes. FISH testing may therefore be useful to detect deletion of these genes and furnish an assay with high sensitivity and specify to distinguish between ChRCC and oncocytoma [120].

The prognosis for ChRCC has been shown in several sizable case series to be significantly better than for CCRCC. There is no significant difference in outcome between the classical and the eosinophilic variants of this neoplasm [101–106]. Stage at presentation with ChRCC is significantly lower than with CCRCC. Metastatic ChRCC is seen in less than 5% of cases at presentation compared with one-fourth of cases of CCRCC. Sarcomatoid differentiation and histologic tumor necrosis confer a worse prognosis. The cancer-specific 5-year survival rate for ChRCC postnephrectomy is about 90% [28]. Median cancer-specific survival for patients with metastatic ChRCC is 0.6 years, which is not unlike cases of metastatic RCC of other subtypes. Metastatic ChRCCs demonstrate the presence of TP53 and PTEN mutations apart from imbalanced chromosome duplications (duplication of three or more chromosomes) [121].

Collecting Duct Carcinoma

Collecting duct carcinoma (CDC) is an uncommon albeit well-recognized aggressive subtype of RCC that has its purported origin from the principal cells in the collecting ducts of Bellini. It comprises less than 1% of renal malignancies with over 250 reported cases in the literature, the first case being reported in 1986 [122].

This RCC affects all ages, with a mean age of 55 years, and occurs more commonly in male patients, with a male-to-female ratio of 2: 1 [123–132]. Although up to a quarter of cases are discovered incidentally, most patients present with abdominal or constitutional symptoms or even with metastatic disease [123–132]. Radiological examination reveals a predominantly solid kidney mass. Urine cytology can also rarely be positive for malignancy in these cases [128].

CDC arises at any location in the renal parenchyma, and identification of a particular site of origin is difficult, especially as the tumor increases in size. Tumor size is variable with cases ranging up to 16 cm in greatest dimension. The cut surface of CDC is usually gray white and firm, and foci of overt necrosis are often present. Tumors are frequently infiltrative and multifocal involvement of the kidney may be exhibited as satellite tumor nodules (Fig. 5.21). Involvement of the adrenal gland, perinephric fat, renal sinus fat, renal pelvis, Gerota's fascia, renal vein, and regional lymph nodes is grossly identified in the majority of cases on radiological and/or pathologic examination [123–132].

Microscopically, CDC shows ill-defined borders with prominent infiltration of adjacent parenchyma and an interstitial growth pattern with relatively preserved glomeruli is commonly noted. Marked stromal desmoplasia is almost always present [94]. It is frequently accompanied by an acute and chronic inflammatory cell infiltrate at the interface between tumor and normal parenchyma. A number of different growth patterns may be seen within the same tumor including solid sheets/cords/nests, tubulopapillary structures, or infiltrating small- to medium-sized malig-

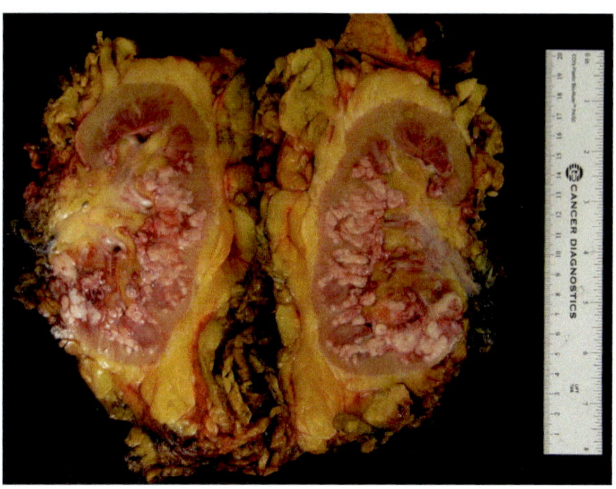

Fig. 5.21 Collecting duct carcinoma demonstrating an infiltrative growth pattern comprising multiple tumor nodules with irregular borders invading the renal medulla

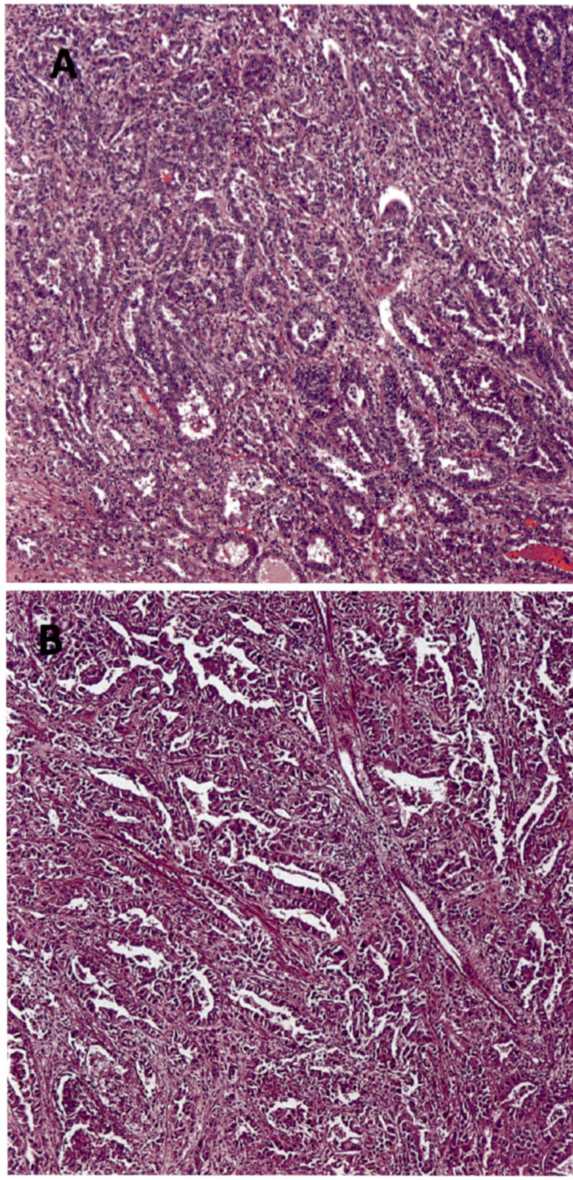
A
B

Fig. 5.22 Collecting duct carcinoma composed of high-grade carcinoma demonstrating areas of distinctly tubular (**a**) and tubulopapillary (**b**) growth patterns with a prominent admixed inflammatory infiltrate

nant glands/tubules (Fig. 5.22a, b) along with surrounding desmoplastic stroma (Fig. 5.23). An extensive component of tubulocystic growth pattern that typifies tubulocystic carcinoma excludes tumors from being considered as CDC [94]. Some cases demonstrate a microcystic pattern with intracystic high-grade malignant papillary proliferations. Another pattern is characterized by intratubular extension with microscopic subcapsular deposits distant from the main tumor. The epithelium lining uninvolved ducts adjacent to or far from the main tumor may exhibit severe cytologic atypia amounting to carcinoma in situ-like growth. Tumor cells are uni-

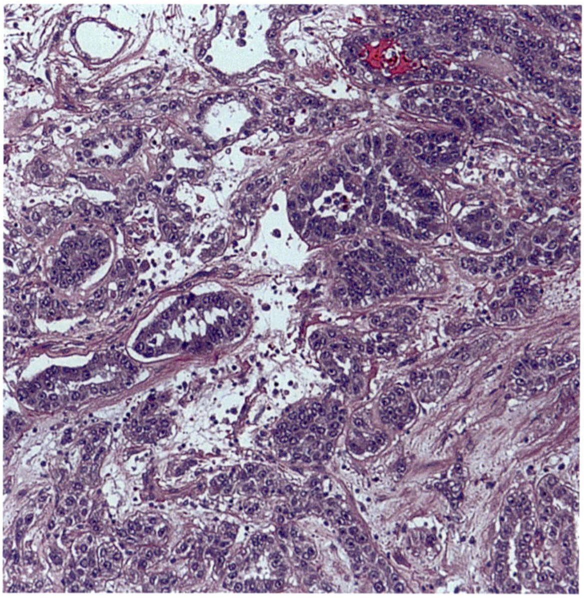

Fig. 5.23 Malignant glandular differentiation in collecting duct carcinoma-exhibiting presence of tumor cells with high-grade nuclei, prominent nucleoli, and an accompanying desmoplastic stromal reaction

formly high cytologic grade, with nuclear pleomorphism and prominent nucleoli and varying amounts of eosinophilic cytoplasm. Cells lining malignant tubular profiles may often exhibit hobnailing, a finding that is not usually encountered in other RCC subtypes. Sarcomatoid differentiation is identified in up to one-third of the cases. Lymphovascular invasion is frequently seen, and renal vein invasion is present in a significant number of cases (20–44%) [94, 123–132].

Intra- or extracellular mucin production in these tumors can often be demonstrated using mucicarmine, Alcian blue, or PAS stains [132, 133]. Exclusion of metastatic adenocarcinoma and high-grade urothelial carcinoma by obtaining clinical history of extrarenal primary tumor and extensive sampling of the pelvicalyceal system is crucial prior to making a diagnosis of CDC, as these are the major entities in the differential diagnosis. To that effect, an immunohistochemical panel including PAX8, GATA3, and p63 is helpful as urothelial carcinomas are more likely to be positive for GATA3 and p63, whereas CDC does not stain with these markers [134, 135]. Of note, PAX8 may be positive in both urothelial carcinomas involving the renal pelvis and CDCs, a finding that should be considered prior to establishing any further diagnosis [136].

The reported molecular features in CDC are notably variable and limited, and no distinctive molecular mechanism or pathway has been proposed for collecting duct carcinoma [130]. A recent study highlights that a significant number of cases (up to 25%) previously reported as CDC are in fact examples of fumarate hydratase (FH)-deficient RCC [94]. These tumors are described in further detail in the Hereditary Leiomyomatosis and Renal Cell Carcinoma-Associated RCC section. Therefore, immunohistochemical stains for FH and 2SC should be performed in high-grade carcinomas with a diagnostic consideration of CDC, along with germline mutational testing for FH mutations, if deemed clinically necessary. Another entity in the differential diagnosis is renal medullary carcinoma that is discussed in the section below. CDC is thus diagnosed upon excluding the aforementioned entities in the differential diagnosis.

CDC cases often present at an advanced disease stage and the overall prognosis is poor. Almost 50% of patients have regional nodal and/or distant metastases at the time of initial diagnosis [94, 123–132]. Approximately two-thirds of patients with CDC die of disease-related causes within 2 years and mortality rates are extremely high. Chemotherapy and immunotherapy are of very little benefit in managing collecting duct carcinoma [94, 123–132].

Renal Medullary Carcinoma

Renal medullary carcinoma (RMC) is a relatively rare and highly aggressive renal malignancy, first reported in 1995. The terminal collecting duct epithelium is the proposed site of origin [137–140]. There is a very strong association of this tumor occurring in conjunction with sickle cell hemoglobinopathies, and according to various hypotheses it is the terminal collecting duct epithelium that undergoes chronic ischemic damage due to accumulating drepanocytes (sickled erythrocytes) resulting in tumorigenesis. Most affected patients have been African Americans with sickle cell trait (HbAS) or hemoglobin SC disease (HbSC), but this tumor has also been reported in a patient with sickle cell disease (HbSS) as well as in white patients without evidence of sickle cell hemoglobinopathies [96, 137–141].

Most patients are diagnosed in the second or third decades of life, ranging from 5 to 58 years, with a mean age at diagnosis of 20 years. The male-to-female ratio is at least 2: 1, and approximately 75% of tumors occur in the right kidney and 25% occur on the left. The vast majority of cases occur in those with African ancestry, but Central and South American and Mediterranean individuals are also at risk for RMC. Almost 90% of reported cases occurred in patients with sickle cell trait. Common presenting symptoms include abdominal or flank pain, gross hematuria, weight loss with constitutional symptoms of relatively short duration, and a minority of patients (10%) have a palpable abdominal mass [137–143].

Grossly, these tumors usually involve the renal medulla and are poorly circumscribed, lobulated, firm, gray-tan, with variable hemorrhage and necrosis. They range widely in size (1.8–13 cm in greatest dimension, with a mean of 7 cm) and frequently present at an advanced stage with satellite nodules, perinephric extension, and sinus fat invasion (Fig. 5.24) [137–144]. A host of morphologic patterns is noted on microscopic examination including the characteristic finding of a reticular or microcystic growth pattern resembling yolk sac tumor of the testis (Fig. 5.25). Areas similar to adenoid cystic carcinoma of salivary glands with a cribriform or sieve-like growth are often noted (Fig. 5.26). Drepanocytes (sickled erythrocytes) are also seen within and surrounding the tumors. Other common patterns include

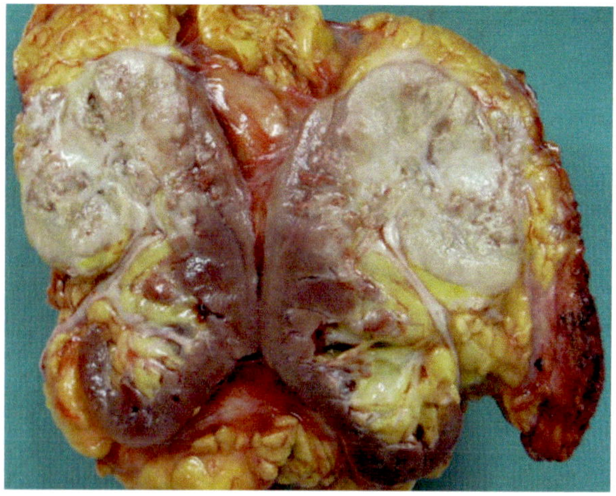

Fig. 5.24 Renal medullary carcinoma with sinus fat invasion and perinephric extension in an African American patient with sickle cell trait

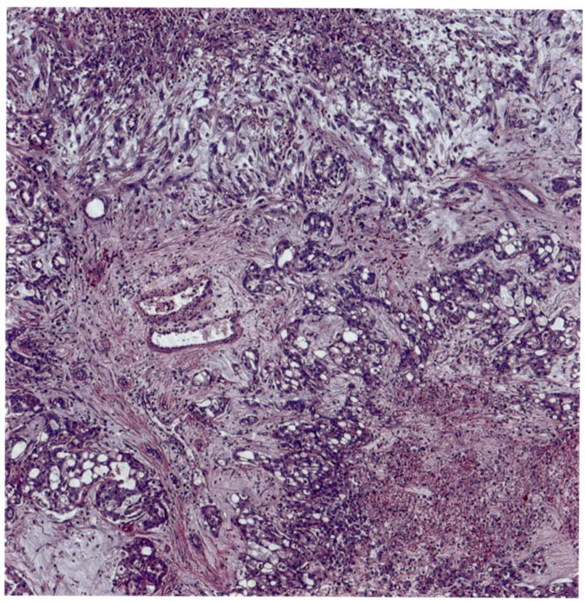

Fig. 5.25 Renal medullary carcinoma with a microcystic growth pattern and marked stromal desmoplasia

tubule formation and growth in diffuse sheets or solid nodules. Tumor cells are commonly pleomorphic with enlarged nuclei, prominent nucleoli, and variable amounts of eosinophilic cytoplasm. Squamoid or rhabdoid appearance of tumor cells in solid sheet-like areas is often noted. Numerous aggregates of neutrophils may be seen within the tumor (Fig. 5.27), and there is often a dense inflammatory response at the interface between tumor and the adjacent renal parenchyma. A prominent desmoplastic stromal reaction is another constant feature seen in most cases (Fig. 5.25). Mucin production is variably seen in most of these tumors (Fig. 5.26).

Renal origin of this tumor is confirmed by positive immunostaining for PAX8 in all cases. Loss of expression of SMARCB1 (INI1), a nuclear transcription regulator encoded on chromosome 22, is now a mandatory criterion to make a diagnosis of RMC [94]. It occurs as a result of a loss of heterozygosity or hemizygous deletions at the SMARCB1 locus, rarely due to loss of chromosome 22 or balanced translocation involving chromosome 22 [145, 146]. Another unique finding is that up to two-thirds of RMCs show positive immunostaining for OCT3/4 (POU5F1) [94, 147]. Variable degrees of positive immunostaining are reported for cytokeratins AE1/AE3 and CAM5.2, CK7, CK20, polyclonal carcinoembryonic antigen (CEA), and EMA [94, 130, 145–148].

This tumor carries a very dismal prognosis with almost all patients presenting with metastatic disease at the time of diagnosis. Common sites of metastasis are lymph nodes, lung, liver, and adrenal glands. Long-term disease-free survival rates are very low; average survival is between 2 and 68 weeks, with a mean survival duration of 19 weeks [130, 143, 144]. Neoadjuvant therapy prolongs survival by a limited duration, but tumor recurrence and death inevitably occur even after a period of remission [149, 150].

There are notable overlapping clinical and pathologic features between collecting duct carcinoma and RMC, raising a consideration that RMC is a subtype of collecting duct carcinoma [130, 151]. Loss of SMARCB1 (INI1) immunostaining and presence of hemoglobinopathy by history and laboratory test confirmation, with accompanying drepanocytes in tumor stroma and/or blood vessels, are required to establish a diagnosis of RMC [94]. On the other hand, rare tumors demonstrating RMC-like histology, INI1-deficient immunophenotype, but arising in patients in whom sickle cell trait or disease has been definitively excluded are designated as RCC, unclassified, with medullary phenotype in the present scenario [94].

Mucinous Tubular and Spindle Cell Carcinoma

This entity was initially described in 1997 by MacLennan et al. and designated as "low-grade collecting duct carcinoma." Other subsequently reported them as "low-grade myxoid renal epithelial neoplasms" and "low-grade tubular mucinous renal neoplasms" in 2001–2002 [152–154]. Most of these tumors are identified incidentally. The tumor is far more commonly seen in females with a ratio of 3:1. The age range is wide (13–82 years, mean age of 58 years).

Tumors range in diameter from 2.2 to 12 cm (average 6.5 cm). They are well circumscribed, gray white, tan, or yellow, with focal hemorrhage or necrosis (Fig. 5.28). Histologic examination of classic tumors shows tightly packed, small elongated tubules separated by abundant basophilic extracellular mucin, sometimes with a "bubbly" myxoid consistency (Fig. 5.29a) [152–154]. Areas of spindled cells are also seen more prominently in some of these tumors (Fig. 5.29b) [155]. The mucin stains strongly with Alcian blue at pH 2.5. Tubules are lined by uniform low cuboidal cells with scant cytoplasm and round nuclei of low nuclear grade with absent or inconspicuous nucleoli. Mitotic activity is not significantly elevated.

There are several morphologic variations associated with this tumor including relative lack of mucinous matrix, small well-formed papillae, presence of foamy

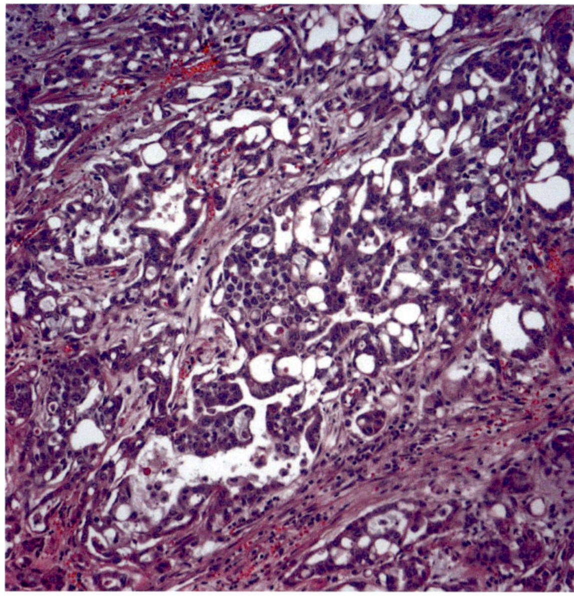

Fig. 5.26 Microcystic cribriform or sieve-like growth pattern with wispy blue mucin secretion in renal medullary carcinoma. Scattered sickled erythrocytes are present in the background

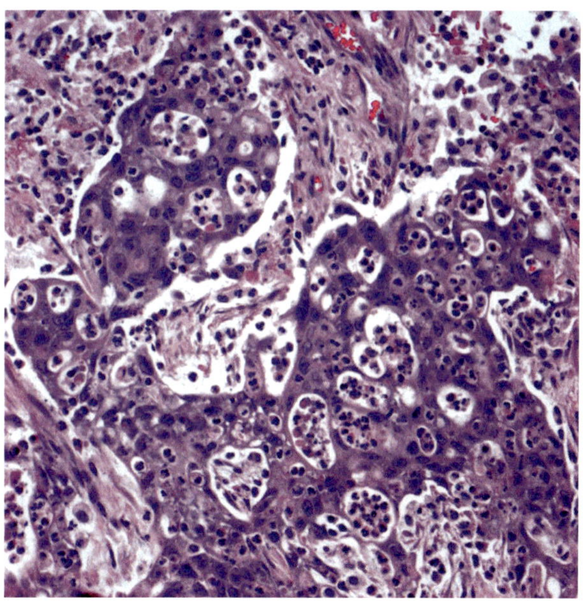

Fig. 5.27 Renal medullary carcinoma with tubular differentiation, tumor cells with high-grade nuclei containing prominent nucleoli, and a dense neutrophilic inflammatory infiltrate

macrophages, focal clear cell change in tubular component, focal necrosis, oncocytic change, small vacuolations, psammomatous calcification, or heterotopic bone formation [156]. High nuclear grade, areas of coagulative tumor necrosis, sarcomatoid differentiation, and aggressive behavior have been documented in a small cohort of these tumors [157–160]. Tumor cells have a variable immunophenotype, but are usually immunoreactive for CK7, AMACR, and PAX8 (Fig. 5.30) [161–163].

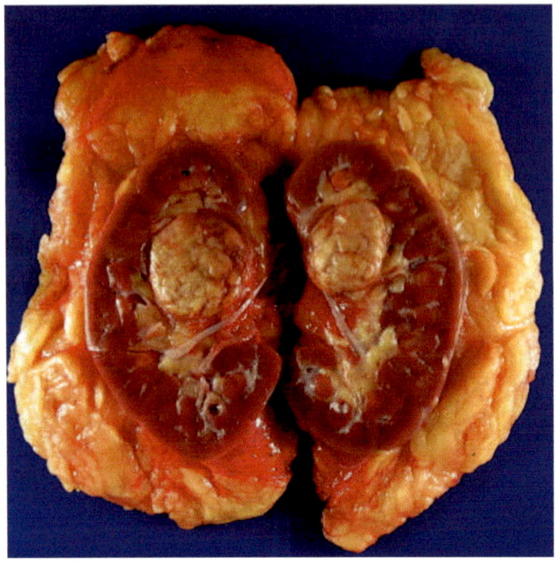

Fig. 5.28 Mucinous tubular and spindle cell carcinoma of kidney. Note the tan yellow tumor with well-circumscribed borders and a glistening cut surface with bulging contours

The characteristic gains of chromosomes 7 and 17 and loss of Y chromosome that are seen in papillary RCC are not seen in mucinous tubular and spindle cell carcinoma [164]. Alterations in the Hippo pathway are present in mucinous tubular and spindle cell carcinoma, but are not seen in PRCC [165]. Cytogenetic analyses and comparative genomic hybridization studies demonstrated multiple genetic alterations that include loss of chromosomes 1, 4, 6, 8, 9, 13, 14, 15, 18, and 22 [166, 167].

Most of these tumors with classic histologic findings are indolent, and surgical excision is curative as they are low stage at the time of resection. However, high nuclear grade and sarcomatoid change in a few cases have been associated with adverse outcomes [168, 169].

Renal Cell Carcinoma, Unclassified

RCC, unclassified, is a diagnostic category for the designation of RCCs that have histologic features that cannot be categorized under any of the well-characterized RCC subtypes. These tumors represent up to 5–6% of RCC cases [1]. Morphologic patterns falling under this category include tumors that show a composite mixture of recognized types, novel or unrecognized cell types, tumors with mucin production, and renal carcinomas with entirely sarcomatoid morphology, lacking recognizable epithelial elements [170]. Low- or high-grade unclassifiable oncocytic neoplasms were also included in this category [1]. However, most genitourinary pathologists including this author team do not classify an RCC with a composite mixture of recognized subypes as an unclassified RCC. We designate such tumors as a composite RCC and list the subtypes identified therein.

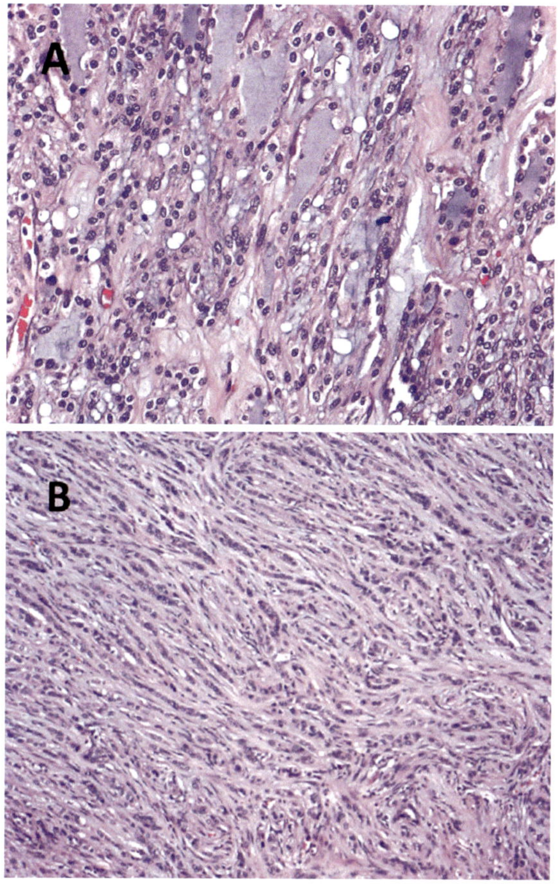

Fig. 5.29 Mucinous tubular and spindle cell carcinoma composed of closely packed elongated tubules in a background of “bubbly mucin” (**a**) with some cases demonstrating prominent spindling of tumor cells (**b**)

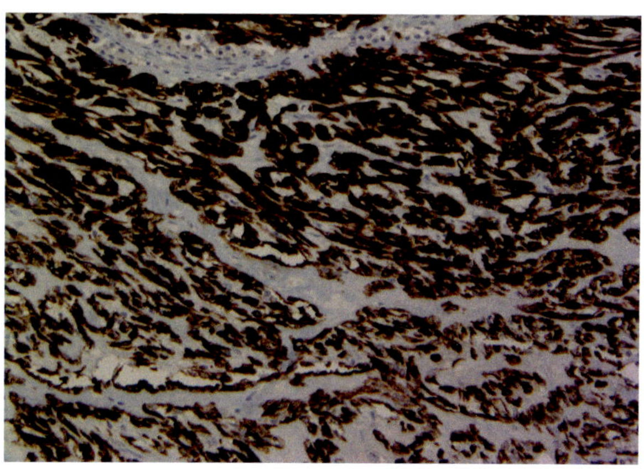

Fig. 5.30 Diffuse and strong cytokeratin 7 immunohistochemical staining of tumor cells in mucinous tubular and spindle cell carcinoma, a feature in common with papillary renal cell carcinoma

Patients of any age can be affected (range: 21–91 years) [21–23, 171–174]. These tumors usually present at an advanced stage, are large, and demonstrate histologic features that correlate with an adverse prognosis including high nuclear grade, tumor necrosis, and lymphovascular invasion [21–23, 170, 174]. Data from limited analysis of these tumors show that they exhibit marked genetic instability [21]. In a molecular study of 62 unclassified RCC, approximately 75% of cases were categorized into several subsets of abnormalities of variable prognostic significance that might be useful for either diagnostic or therapeutic implications [23].

Unclassified RCC is a histologically and clinically heterogeneous group of tumors, wherein prognosis depends upon similar clinical and pathologic findings determining outcome in conventional RCCs [21, 170, 173, 174].

Grading and Staging Renal Cell Carcinoma

Cytologic grading is one of the most essential parameters that aid in predicting the biologic behavior of RCC [24–29]. The Fuhrman system was widely used up until recently for grading RCCs and presently the four-tiered WHO/International Society of Urologic Pathology (ISUP) grading system has been recommended for use in grading clear cell and papillary RCCs in view of the fact that there is sufficient evidence-based data that can be used for predicting prognosis [175, 176]. Grades 1–3 are based on prominence of nucleoli and grade 4 includes pronounced nuclear pleomorphism, tumor giant cells, and rhabdoid or sarcomatoid changes (Table 5.2) [175]. Grading is performed after assessing the aforementioned criteria within a single high-power field showing the highest nucleolar grade or greatest degree of nuclear pleomorphism. The WHO/ISUP grading system is not currently applicable for predicting prognosis for other types of RCC due to a lack of outcome data for these different subtypes [175, 176].

Incorporation of tumor necrosis, defined as homogeneous aggregates and sheets of nonviable tumor cells, or coalescing groups of cells containing nuclear and cytoplasmic debris is another feature that has been studied as a possible factor that can be included in the grading criteria. Some published studies have indicated that including tumor necrosis in CCRCC cases furnishes additional prognostic information in comparison to sole inclusion of WHO/ISUP nucleolar grade [177].

Tumor stage indicates the extent of involvement by disease and represents the most important factor in predicting the clinical behavior and prognosis of RCC [32].

Table 5.2 International society of urologic pathology grading for clear cell and papillary renal cell carcinoma

1. Nucleoli are inconspicuous or absent at 400× magnification.
2. Nucleoli are distinctly visible at 400× magnification, but inconspicuous or invisible at 100 × magnification.
3. Nucleoli are distinctly visible at 100× magnification.
4. Tumor exhibits the presence of tumor giant cells and/or extreme nuclear pleomorphism and/or sarcomatoid differentiation and/or rhabdoid differentiation.

Adapted from Delahunt et al. [59]

Currently, the tumor, nodes, and metastasis (TNM) staging system is used all across the world for RCC staging [178]. The eighth edition of the *AJCC Cancer Staging Manual* was published in 2017 and criteria listed in this latest update to the staging system are being reported [179]. Staging parameters for carcinomas arising in the kidney are provided, and definitions for primary tumor (T), regional lymph nodes (N), and distant metastasis (M) are established in this staging system (Table 5.3).

Table 5.3 American Joint Committee on Cancer 2017 TNM staging of carcinomas arising in the kidney (8th edition)

Definition of primary tumor (T)			
1. TX: Primary tumor cannot be assessed			
2. T0: No evidence of primary tumor			
3. T1: Tumor ≤7 cm in greatest dimension, limited to the kidney			
1. T1a: Tumor ≤4 cm in greatest dimension, limited to the kidney			
2. T1b: Tumor >4 cm, but ≤7 cm in greatest dimension, limited to the kidney			
4. T2: Tumor >7 cm in greatest dimension, limited to the kidney			
1. T2a: Tumor >7 cm, but ≤10 cm in greatest dimension, limited to the kidney			
2. T2b: Tumor >10 cm, limited to the kidney			
5. T3: Tumor extends into major veins or perinephric tissues, but not into the ipsilateral adrenal gland and not beyond Gerota fascia			
1. T3a: Tumor extends into the renal vein or its segmental branches, or invades the pelvicaliceal system, or invades perirenal and/or renal sinus fat, but not beyond Gerota fascia			
2. T3b: Tumor extends into the vena cava below the diaphragm			
3. T3c: Tumor extends into the vena cava above the diaphragm or invades the wall of the vena cava			
6. T4: Tumor invades beyond Gerota fascia (including contiguous extension into the ipsilateral adrenal gland)			
Definition of regional lymph node (N)			
1. NX: Regional lymph nodes cannot be assessed			
2. N0: No regional lymph node metastasis			
3. N1: Metastasis in regional lymph node(s)			
Definition of distant metastasis (M)			
1. M0: No distant metastasis			
2. M1: Distant metastasis			
American Joint Committee on Cancer (AJCC) Prognostic Stage Groups			
When T is…	And N is…	And M is…	Stage group is:
T1	N0	M0	I
T1	N1	M0	III
T2	N0	M0	II
T2	N1	M0	III
T3	N0	M0	III
T3	N1	M0	III
T4	Any N	M0	IV
Any T	Any N	M1	IV

Used with permission of the American College of Surgeons, Chicago, Illinois. The original source for this information is the AJCC Cancer Staging Manual, Eighth Edition (2017) published by Springer International Publishing

References

1. Moch H, Humphrey PA, Ulbright TM, Reuter VE. WHO classification of tumours of the urinary system and male genital organs. 4th ed. Lyon: IARC Press; 2016.
2. The Cancer Genome Atlas Research Network. Comprehensive molecular characterization of clear cell renal cell carcinoma. Nature. 2013;499:43–9.
3. Linehan WM, Spellman PT, Ricketts CJ, Creighton CJ, Fei SS, Davis C, Wheeler DA, Murray BA, Schmidt L, Vocke CD, et al. Comprehensive molecular characterization of papillary renal-cell carcinoma. N Engl J Med. 2016;374:135–45.
4. Davis CF, Ricketts CJ, Wang M, Yang L, Cherniack AD, Shen H, Buhay C, Kang H, Kim SC, Fahey CC, et al. The somatic genomic landscape of chromophobe renal cell carcinoma. Cancer Cell. 2014;26:319–30.
5. Durinck S, Stawiski EW, Pavia-Jimenez A, Modrusan Z, Kapur P, Jaiswal BS, Zhang N, Toffessi-Tcheuyap V, Nguyen TT, Pahuja KB, et al. Spectrum of diverse genomic alterations define non-clear cell renal carcinoma subtypes. Nat Genet. 2015;47:13–21.
6. Hakimi AA, Reznik E, Lee CH, Creighton CJ, Brannon AR, Luna A, Aksoy BA, Liu EM, Shen R, Lee W, et al. An integrated metabolic atlas of clear cell renal cell carcinoma. Cancer Cell. 2016;29:104–16.
7. Gotoh M, Ichikawa H, Arai E, Chiku S, Sakamoto H, Fujimoto H, Hiramoto M, Nammo T, Yasuda K, Yoshida T, et al. Comprehensive exploration of novel chimeric transcripts in clear cell renal cell carcinomas using whole transcriptome analysis. Genes Chromosomes Cancer. 2014;53:1018–32.
8. Malouf GG, Zhang J, Yuan Y, Comperat E, Roupret M, Cussenot O, Chen Y, Thompson EJ, Tannir NM, Weinstein JN, et al. Characterization of long non-coding RNA transcriptome in clear-cell renal cell carcinoma by next-generation deep sequencing. Mol Oncol. 2015;9:32–43.
9. Gowrishankar B, Przybycin CG, Ma C, Nandula SV, Rini B, Campbell S, Klein E, Chaganti RS, Magi-Galluzzi C, Houldsworth J. A genomic algorithm for the molecular classification of common renal cortical neoplasms: development and validation. J Urol. 2015;193:1479–85.
10. Christinat Y, Krek W. Integrated genomic analysis identifies subclasses and prognosis signatures of kidney cancer. Oncotarget. 2015;6:10521–31.
11. Eckel-Passow JE, Igel DA, Serie DJ, Joseph RW, Ho TH, Cheville JC, Parker AS. Assessing the clinical use of clear cell renal cell carcinoma molecular subtypes identified by RNA expression analysis. Urol Oncol. 2015;33:17–23.
12. Rathmell KW, Chen F, Creighton CJ. Genomics of chromophobe renal cell carcinoma: implications from a rare tumor for pan-cancer studies. Oncoscience. 2015;2:81–90.
13. Malouf GG, Ali SM, Wang K, Balasubramanian S, Ross JS, Miller VA, Stephens PJ, Khayat D, Pal SK, Su X, et al. Genomic characterization of renal cell carcinoma with sarcomatoid dedifferentiation pinpoints recurrent genomic alterations. Eur Urol. 2016;70:348–57.
14. Chen YB, Xu J, Skanderup AJ, Dong Y, Brannon AR, Wang L, Won HH, Wang PI, Nanjangud GJ, Jungbluth AA, et al. Molecular analysis of aggressive renal cell carcinoma with unclassified histology reveals distinct subsets. Nat Commun. 2016;7:13131.
15. De Velasco G, Culhane AC, Fay AP, Hakimi AA, Voss MH, Tannir NM, Tamboli P, Appleman LJ, Bellmunt J, Kimryn Rathmell W, et al. Molecular subtypes improve prognostic value of international metastatic renal cell carcinoma database consortium prognostic model. Oncologist. 2017;22:286–92.
16. Seles M, Hutterer GC, Kiesslich T, Pummer K, Berindan-Neagoe I, Perakis S, Schwarzenbacher D, Stotz M, Gerger A, Pichler M. Current insights into long non-coding RNAs in renal cell carcinoma. Int J Mol Sci. 2016;17:573.
17. Srigley JR, Delahunt B, Eble JN, Egevad L, Epstein JI, Grignon D, Hes O, Moch H, Montironi R, Tickoo SK, et al. The International Society of Urological Pathology (ISUP) Vancouver classification of renal neoplasia. Am J Surg Pathol. 2013;37:1469–89.

18. Moch H, Cubilla AL, Humphrey PA, Reuter VE, Ulbright TM. The 2016 WHO classification of tumours of the urinary system and male genital organs-part A: renal, penile, and testicular tumours. Eur Urol. 2016;70(1):93–105.
19. Yoshida SO, Imam A, Olson CA, et al. Proximal renal tubular surface membrane antigens identified in primary and metastatic renal cell carcinomas. Arch Pathol Lab Med. 1986;110:825–32.
20. Bruder E, Passera O, Harms D, et al. Morphologic and molecular characterization of renal cell carcinoma in children and young adults. Am J Surg Pathol. 2004;28:1117–32.
21. Hu ZY, Pang LJ, Qi Y, et al. Unclassified renal cell carcinoma: a clinicopathological, comparative genomic hybridization, and whole-genome exon sequencing study. Int J Clin Exp Pathol. 2014;7:3865–75.
22. Li Y, Reuter VE, Matoso A, et al. Re-evaluation of 33 'unclassified' eosinophilic renal cell carcinomas in young patients. Histopathology. 2018;72:588–600.
23. Chen YB, Xu J, Skanderup AJ, et al. Molecular analysis of aggressive renal cell carcinoma with unclassified histology reveals distinct subsets. Nat Commun. 2016;7:13131.
24. Fuhrman SA, Lasky LC, Limas C. Prognostic significance of morphologic parameters in renal cell carcinoma. Am J Surg Pathol. 1982;6:655–63.
25. Goldstein NS. The current state of renal cell carcinoma grading. Union Internationale Contre le Cancer (UICC) and the American Joint Committee on Cancer (AJCC). Cancer. 1997;80:977–80.
26. Usubutun A, Uygur MC, Ayhan A, et al. Comparison of grading systems for estimating the prognosis of renal cell carcinoma. Int Urol Nephrol. 1998;30:391–7.
27. Ficarra V, Righetti R, Martignoni G, et al. Prognostic value of renal cell carcinoma nuclear grading: multivariate analysis of 333 cases. Urol Int. 2001;67:130–4.
28. Lohse CM, Cheville JC. A review of prognostic pathologic features and algorithms for patients treated surgically for renal cell carcinoma. Clin Lab Med. 2005;25:433–64.
29. Lohse CM, Blute ML, Zincke H, et al. Comparison of standardized and nonstandardized nuclear grade of renal cell carcinoma to predict outcome among 2,042 patients. Am J Clin Pathol. 2002;118:877–86.
30. Shen C, Kaelin WG Jr. The VHL/HIF axis in clear cell renal carcinoma. Semin Cancer Biol. 2013;23:18–25.
31. Haake SM, Rathmell WK. Renal cancer subtypes: should we be lumping or splitting for therapeutic decision making? Cancer. 2017;123:200–9.
32. Thrasher JB, Paulson DF. Prognostic factors in renal cancer. Urol Clin North Am. 1993;20:247–62.
33. Velickovic M, Delahunt B, McIver B, et al. Intragenic PTEN/MMAC1 loss of heterozygosity in conventional (clear-cell) renal cell carcinoma is associated with poor patient prognosis. Mod Pathol. 2002;15:479–85.
34. Linehan WM, Walther MM, Zbar B. The genetic basis of cancer of the kidney. J Urol. 2003;170:2163–72.
35. Van EF, Van RC, Bodmer D, et al. Chromosome 3 translocations and the risk to develop renal cell cancer: a Dutch intergroup study. Genet Couns. 2003;14:149–54.
36. Vanharanta S, Buchta M, McWhinney SR, et al. Early-onset renal cell carcinoma as a novel extraparaganglial component of SDHB-associated heritable paraganglioma. Am J Hum Genet. 2004;74:153–9.
37. Cheville JC, Lohse CM, Zincke H, et al. Sarcomatoid renal cell carcinoma: an examination of underlying histologic subtype and an analysis of associations with patient outcome. Am J Surg Pathol. 2004;28:435–41.
38. de Peralta-Venturina M, Moch H, Amin M, et al. Sarcomatoid differentiation in renal cell carcinoma: a study of 101 cases. Am J Surg Pathol. 2001;25:275–84.
39. Gokden N, Nappi O, Swanson PE, et al. Renal cell carcinoma with rhabdoid features. Am J Surg Pathol. 2000;24:1329–38.

40. Haddad FS, Shah IA, Manne RK, et al. Renal cell carcinoma insulated in the renal capsule with calcification and ossification. Urol Int. 1993;51:97–101.
41. Bonsib SM. Renal cell carcinoma with lymphomatoid features. J Urol Pathol. 1997;6:109–18.
42. Jagirdar J, Irie T, French SW, et al. Globular Mallory-like bodies in renal cell carcinoma: report of a case and review of cytoplasmic eosinophilic globules. Hum Pathol. 1985;16:949–52.
43. Arora K, Divatia MK, Truong L, Shen SS, Ayala AG, Ro JY. Sarcoid-like granulomas in renal cell carcinoma: the Houston Methodist Hospital experience. Ann Diagn Pathol. 2017;31:62–5.
44. Chau KY, Pretorius JM, Stewart AW. Myospherulosis in renal cell carcinoma. Arch Pathol Lab Med. 2000;124:1476–9.
45. Mathers ME, Pollock AM, Marsh C, et al. Cytokeratin 7: a useful adjunct in the diagnosis of chromophobe renal cell carcinoma. Histopathology. 2002;40:563–7.
46. Wu SL, Kothari P, Wheeler TM, et al. Cytokeratins 7 and 20 immunoreactivity in chromophobe renal cell carcinomas and renal oncocytomas. Mod Pathol. 2002;15:712–7.
47. McGregor DK, Khurana KK, Cao C, et al. Diagnosing primary and metastatic renal cell carcinoma: the use of the monoclonal antibody 'Renal Cell Carcinoma Marker'. Am J Surg Pathol. 2001;25:1485–92.
48. Avery AK, Beckstead J, Renshaw AA, et al. Use of antibodies to RCC and CD10 in the differential diagnosis of renal neoplasms. Am J Surg Pathol. 2000;24:203–10.
49. Ordonez NG. The diagnostic utility of immunohistochemistry in distinguishing between mesothelioma and renal cell carcinoma: a comparative study. Hum Pathol. 2004;35:697–710.
50. Kim MK, Kim S. Immunohistochemical profile of common epithelial neoplasms arising in the kidney. Appl Immunohistochem Mol Morphol. 2002;10:332–8.
51. Langner C, Wegscheider BJ, Ratschek M, et al. Keratin immunohistochemistry in renal cell carcinoma subtypes and renal oncocytomas: a systematic analysis of 233 tumors. Virchows Arch. 2004;444:127–34.
52. Young AN, Amin MB, Moreno CS, et al. Expression profiling of renal epithelial neoplasms: a method for tumor classification and discovery of diagnostic molecular markers. Am J Pathol. 2001;158:1639–51.
53. Tretiakova MS, Sahoo S, Takahashi M, et al. Expression of alpha-methylacyl-CoA racemase in papillary renal cell carcinoma. Am J Surg Pathol. 2004;28:69–76.
54. Petit A, Castillo M, Santos M, et al. KIT expression in chromophobe renal cell carcinoma: comparative immunohistochemical analysis of KIT expression in different renal cell neoplasms. Am J Surg Pathol. 2004;28:676–8.
55. Langner C, Ratschek M, Rehak P, et al. Expression of MUC1 (EMA) and E-cadherin in renal cell carcinoma: a systematic immunohistochemical analysis of 188 cases. Mod Pathol. 2004;17:180–8.
56. Zhou M, Roma A, Magi-Galluzzi C. The usefulness of immunohistochemical markers in the differential diagnosis of renal neoplasms. Clin Lab Med. 2005;25:247–57.
57. Gobbo S, Eble JN, MacLennan GT, et al. Renal cell carcinomas with papillary architecture and clear cell components: the utility of immunohistochemical and cytogenetical analyses in differential diagnosis. Am J Surg Pathol. 2008;32:1780–6.
58. Shuch BM, Lam JS, Belldegrun AS, et al. Prognostic factors in renal cell carcinoma. Semin Oncol. 2006;33:563–75.
59. Delahunt B, Cheville JC, Martignoni G, et al. The International Society of Urological Pathology (ISUP) grading system for renal cell carcinoma and other prognostic parameters. Am J Surg Pathol. 2013;37:1490–504.
60. Leroy X, Zini L, Buob D, et al. Renal cell carcinoma with rhabdoid features: an aggressive neoplasm with overexpression of p53. Arch Pathol Lab Med. 2007;131:102–6.
61. Nassir A, Jollimore J, Gupta R, et al. Multilocular cystic renal cell carcinoma: a series of 12 cases and review of the literature. Urology. 2002;60:421–7.
62. Suzigan S, Lopez-Beltran A, Montironi R, et al. Multilocular cystic renal cell carcinoma: a report of 45 cases of a kidney tumor of low malignant potential. Am J Clin Pathol. 2006;125:217–22.

63. Williamson SR, MacLennan GT, Lopez-Beltran A, et al. Cystic partially regressed clear cell renal cell carcinoma: a potential mimic of multilocular cystic renal cell carcinoma. Histopathology. 2013;63:767–79.
64. von Teichman A, Comperat E, Behnke S, et al. VHL mutations and dysregulation of pVHL- and PTEN-controlled pathways in multilocular cystic renal cell carcinoma. Mod Pathol. 2011;24:571–8.
65. Halat S, Eble JN, Grignon DJ, et al. Multilocular cystic renal cell carcinoma is a subtype of clear cell renal cell carcinoma. Mod Pathol. 2010;23:931–6.
66. Williamson SR, Halat S, Eble JN, et al. Multilocular cystic renal cell carcinoma: similarities and differences in immunoprofile compared with clear cell renal cell carcinoma. Am J Surg Pathol. 2012;36:1425–33.
67. Amin MB, Amin MB, Tamboli P, et al. Prognostic impact of histologic subtyping of adult renal epithelial neoplasms: an experience of 405 cases. Am J Surg Pathol. 2002;26:281–91.
68. Zbar B, Tory K, Merino M, et al. Hereditary papillary renal cell carcinoma. J Urol. 1994;151:561–6.
69. Ornstein DK, Lubensky IA, Venzon D, et al. Prevalence of microscopic tumors in normal appearing renal parenchyma of patients with hereditary papillary renal cancer. J Urol. 2000;163:431–3.
70. Fischer J, Palmedo G, von Knobloch R, et al. Duplication and overexpression of the mutant allele of the MET proto-oncogene in multiple hereditary papillary renal cell tumours. Oncogene. 1998;17:733–9.
71. Lubensky IA, Schmidt L, Zhuang Z, et al. Hereditary and sporadic papillary renal carcinomas with c-met mutations share a distinct morphological phenotype. Am J Pathol. 1999;155:517–26.
72. Amin MB, Corless CL, Renshaw AA, et al. Papillary (chromophil) renal cell carcinoma: histomorphologic characteristics and evaluation of conventional pathologic prognostic parameters in 62 cases. Am J Surg Pathol. 1997;21:621–35.
73. Schraml P, Muller D, Bednar R, et al. Allelic loss at the D9S171 locus on chromosome 9p13 is associated with progression of papillary renal cell carcinoma. J Pathol. 2000;190:457–61.
74. Delahunt B, Eble JN. Papillary renal cell carcinoma: a clinicopathologic and immunohistochemical study of 105 tumors. Mod Pathol. 1997;10:537–44.
75. Argani P, Netto GJ, Parwani AV. Papillary renal cell carcinoma with low-grade spindle cell foci: a mimic of mucinous tubular and spindle cell carcinoma. Am J Surg Pathol. 2008;32:1353–9.
76. Cantley R, Gattuso P, Cimbaluk D. Solid variant of papillary renal cell carcinoma with spindle cell and tubular components. Arch Pathol Lab Med. 2010;134:1210–4.
77. Delahunt B, Eble JN, McCredie MR, et al. Morphologic typing of papillary renal cell carcinoma: comparison of growth kinetics and patient survival in 66 cases. Hum Pathol. 2001;32:590–5.
78. Allory Y, Ouazana D, Boucher E, et al. Papillary renal cell carcinoma. Prognostic value of morphological subtypes in a clinicopathologic study of 43 cases. Virchows Arch. 2003;442:336–42.
79. Brunelli M, Eble JN, Zhang S, et al. Gains of chromosomes 7, 17, 12, 16, and 20 and loss of Y occur early in the evolution of papillary renal cell neoplasia: a fluorescent in situ hybridization study. Mod Pathol. 2003;16:1053–9.
80. Chevarie-Davis M, Riazalhosseini Y, Arseneault M, et al. The morphologic and immunohistochemical spectrum of papillary renal cell carcinoma: study including 132 cases with pure type 1 and type 2 morphology as well as tumors with overlapping features. Am J Surg Pathol. 2014;38:887–94.
81. Cancer Genome Atlas Research N, Linehan WM, Spellman PT, et al. Comprehensive molecular characterization of papillary renal-cell carcinoma. N Engl J Med. 2016;374:135–45.
82. Klatte T, Pantuck AJ, Said JW, et al. Cytogenetic and molecular tumor profiling for type 1 and type 2 papillary renal cell carcinoma. Clin Cancer Res. 2009;15:1162–9.

83. Marsaud A, Dadone B, Ambrosetti D, et al. Dismantling papillary renal cell carcinoma classification: the heterogeneity of genetic profiles suggests several independent diseases. Genes Chromosomes Cancer. 2015;54:369–82.
84. Yang XJ, Tan MH, Kim HL, et al. A molecular classification of papillary renal cell carcinoma. Cancer Res. 2005;65:5628–37.
85. Mejean A, Hopirtean V, Bazin JP, et al. Prognostic factors for the survival of patients with papillary renal cell carcinoma: meaning of histological typing and multifocality. J Urol. 2003;170:764–7.
86. Saleeb RM, Brimo F, Farag M, et al. Toward biological subtyping of papillary renal cell carcinoma with clinical implications through histologic, immunohistochemical, and molecular analysis. Am J Surg Pathol. 2017;41:1618–29.
87. Sukov WR, Lohse CM, Leibovich BC, et al. Clinical and pathological features associated with prognosis in patients with papillary renal cell carcinoma. J Urol. 2012;187:54–9.
88. Lefevre M, Couturier J, Sibony M, et al. Adult papillary renal tumor with oncocytic cells: clinicopathologic, immunohistochemical, and cytogenetic features of 10 cases. Am J Surg Pathol. 2005;29:1576–81.
89. Furge KA, Chen J, Koeman J, et al. Detection of DNA copy number changes and oncogenic signaling abnormalities from gene expression data reveals MYC activation in high-grade papillary renal cell carcinoma. Cancer Res. 2007;67:3171–6.
90. Saleeb RM, Plant P, Tawedrous E, et al. Integrated phenotypic/genotypic analysis of papillary renal cell carcinoma subtypes: identification of prognostic markers, cancer-related pathways, and implications for therapy. Eur Urol Focus. 2018;4:740–8.
91. Kunju LP, Wojno K, Wolf JS Jr, et al. Papillary renal cell carcinoma with oncocytic cells and nonoverlapping low grade nuclei: expanding the morphologic spectrum with emphasis on clinicopathologic, immunohistochemical and molecular features. Hum Pathol. 2008;39:96–101.
92. Park BH, Ro JY, Park WS, et al. Oncocytic papillary renal cell carcinoma with inverted nuclear pattern: distinct subtype with an indolent clinical course. Pathol Int. 2009;59:137–46.
93. Leibovich BC, Lohse CM, Crispen PL, et al. Histological subtype is an independent predictor of outcome for patients with renal cell carcinoma. J Urol. 2010;183:1309–15.
94. Ohe C, Smith SC, Sirohi D, et al. Reappraisal of morphologic differences between renal medullary carcinoma, collecting duct carcinoma, and fumarate hydratase-deficient renal cell carcinoma. Am J Surg Pathol. 2018;42:279–92.
95. Merino MJ, Torres-Cabala C, Pinto P, et al. The morphologic spectrum of kidney tumors in hereditary leiomyomatosis and renal cell carcinoma (HLRCC) syndrome. Am J Surg Pathol. 2007;31:1578–85.
96. Thoenes W, Storkel S, Rumpelt HJ. Human chromophobe cell renal carcinoma. Virchows Arch B Cell Pathol Incl Mol Pathol. 1985;48:207–17.
97. Thoenes W, Storkel S, Rumpelt HJ, et al. Chromophobe cell renal carcinoma and its variants—a report on 32 cases. J Pathol. 1988;155:277–87.
98. Davis CF, Ricketts CJ, Wang M, et al. The somatic genomic landscape of chromophobe renal cell carcinoma. Cancer Cell. 2014;26:319–30.
99. Zbar B, Alvord WG, Glenn G, et al. Risk of renal and colonic neoplasms and spontaneous pneumothorax in the Birt-Hogg-Dube syndrome. Cancer Epidemiol Biomark Prev. 2002;11:393–400.
100. Shuch B, Ricketts CJ, Vocke CD, et al. Germline PTEN mutation Cowden syndrome: an underappreciated form of hereditary kidney cancer. J Urol. 2013;190:1990–8.
101. Akhtar M, Kardar H, Linjawi T, et al. Chromophobe cell carcinoma of the kidney. A clinicopathologic study of 21 cases. Am J Surg Pathol. 1995;19:1245–56.
102. Crotty TB, Farrow GM, Lieber MM. Chromophobe cell renal carcinoma: clinicopathological features of 50 cases. J Urol. 1995;154:964–7.
103. Moch H, Gasser T, Amin MB, et al. Prognostic utility of the recently recommended histologic classification and revised TNM staging system of renal cell carcinoma: a Swiss experience with 588 tumors. Cancer. 2000;89:604–14.

104. Onishi T, Oishi Y, Yanada S, et al. Prognostic implications of histological features in patients with chromophobe cell renal carcinoma. BJU Int. 2002;90:529–32.
105. Peyromaure M, Misrai V, Thiounn N, et al. Chromophobe renal cell carcinoma: analysis of 61 cases. Cancer. 2004;100:1406–10.
106. Abrahams NA, MacLennan GT, Khoury JD, et al. Chromophobe renal cell carcinoma: a comparative study of histological, immunohistochemical and ultrastructural features using high throughput tissue microarray. Histopathology. 2004;45:593–602.
107. Abrahams NA, Tamboli P. Oncocytic renal neoplasms: diagnostic considerations. Clin Lab Med. 2005;25:317–39.
108. Abrahams NA, Ayala AG, Czerniak B. Chromophobe renal cell carcinoma with sarcomatoid transformation. Ann Diagn Pathol. 2003;7:296–9.
109. Akhtar M, Tulbah A, Kardar AH, et al. Sarcomatoid renal cell carcinoma: the chromophobe connection. Am J Surg Pathol. 1997;21:1188–95.
110. Itoh T, Chikai K, Ota S, et al. Chromophobe renal cell carcinoma with osteosarcoma-like differentiation. Am J Surg Pathol. 2002;26:1358–62.
111. Shannon BA, Cohen RJ. Rhabdoid differentiation of chromophobe renal cell carcinoma. Pathology. 2003;35:228–30.
112. Gobbo S, Eble JN, Delahunt B, et al. Renal cell neoplasms of oncocytosis have distinct morphologic, immunohistochemical, and cytogenetic profiles. Am J Surg Pathol. 2010;34:620–6.
113. Petersson F, Gatalica Z, Grossmann P, et al. Sporadic hybrid oncocytic/chromophobe tumor of the kidney: a clinicopathologic, histomorphologic, immunohistochemical, ultrastructural, and molecular cytogenetic study of 14 cases. Virchows Arch. 2010;456:355–65.
114. Klomp JA, Petillo D, Niemi NM, et al. Birt-Hogg-Dube renal tumors are genetically distinct from other renal neoplasias and are associated with up-regulation of mitochondrial gene expression. BMC Med Genet. 2010;3:59.
115. Latham B, Dickersin GR, Oliva E. Subtypes of chromophobe cell renal carcinoma: an ultrastructural and histochemical study of 13 cases. Am J Surg Pathol. 1999;23:530–5.
116. Brunelli M, Eble JN, Zhang S, et al. Eosinophilic and classic chromophobe renal cell carcinomas have similar frequent losses of multiple chromosomes from among chromosomes 1, 2, 6, 10, and 17, and this pattern of genetic abnormality is not present in renal oncocytoma. Mod Pathol. 2005;18:161–9.
117. Speicher MR, Schoell B, du Manoir S, et al. Specific loss of chromosomes 1, 2, 6, 10, 13, 17, and 21 in chromophobe renal cell carcinomas revealed by comparative genomic hybridization. Am J Pathol. 1994;145:356–64.
118. Brunelli M, Gobbo S, Cossu-Rocca P, et al. Chromosomal gains in the sarcomatoid transformation of chromophobe renal cell carcinoma. Mod Pathol. 2007;20:303–9.
119. Herbers J, Schullerus D, Chudek J, et al. Lack of genetic changes at specific genomic sites separates renal oncocytomas from renal cell carcinomas. J Pathol. 1998;184:58–62.
120. Liu Q, Cornejo KM, Cheng L, et al. Next-generation sequencing to detect deletion of RB1 and ERBB4 genes in chromophobe renal cell carcinoma: a potential role in distinguishing chromophobe renal cell carcinoma from renal oncocytoma. Am J Pathol. 2018;188:846–52.
121. Casuscelli J, Weinhold N, Gundem G, et al. Genomic landscape and evolution of metastatic chromophobe renal cell carcinoma. JCI Insight. 2017;2 https://doi.org/10.1172/jci.insight.92688.
122. Fleming S, Lewi HJ. Collecting duct carcinoma of the kidney. Histopathology. 1986;10:1131–41.
123. Chao D, Zisman A, Pantuck AJ, et al. Collecting duct renal cell carcinoma: clinical study of a rare tumor. J Urol. 2002;167:71–4.
124. Srigley JR, Eble JN. Collecting duct carcinoma of kidney. Semin Diagn Pathol. 1998;15:54–67.
125. Olivere JW, Cina SJ, Rastogi P, et al. Collecting duct meningeal carcinomatosis. Arch Pathol Lab Med. 1999;123:638–41.
126. Dimopoulos MA, Logothetis CJ, Markowitz A, et al. Collecting duct carcinoma of the kidney. Br J Urol. 1993;71:388–91.

127. Peyromaure M, Thiounn N, Scotte F, et al. Collecting duct carcinoma of the kidney: a clinicopathological study of 9 cases. J Urol. 2003;170:1138–40.
128. Mauri MF, Bonzanini M, Luciani L, et al. Renal collecting duct carcinoma. Report of a case with urinary cytologic findings. Acta Cytol. 1994;38:755–8.
129. Parker R, Reeves HM, Sudarshan S, et al. Abnormal fluorescence in situ hybridization analysis in collecting duct carcinoma. Urology. 2005;66:1110.
130. Gupta R, Billis A, Shah RB, et al. Carcinoma of the collecting ducts of Bellini and renal medullary carcinoma: clinicopathologic analysis of 52 cases of rare aggressive subtypes of renal cell carcinoma with a focus on their interrelationship. Am J Surg Pathol. 2012;36:1265–78.
131. Baer SC, Ro JY, Ordonez NG, et al. Sarcomatoid collecting duct carcinoma: a clinicopathologic and immunohistochemical study of five cases. Hum Pathol. 1993;24:1017–22.
132. Kennedy SM, Merino MJ, Linehan WM, et al. Collecting duct carcinoma of the kidney. Hum Pathol. 1990;21:449–56.
133. Halenda G, Sees JN Jr, Belis JA, et al. Atypical renal adenocarcinoma with features suggesting collecting duct origin and mimicking a mucinous adenocarcinoma. Urology. 1993;41:165–8.
134. Albadine R, Schultz L, Illei P, et al. PAX8 (+)/p63 (−) immunostaining pattern in renal collecting duct carcinoma (CDC): a useful immunoprofile in the differential diagnosis of CDC versus urothelial carcinoma of upper urinary tract. Am J Surg Pathol. 2010;34:965–9.
135. Gonzalez-Roibon N, Albadine R, Sharma R, et al. The role of GATA binding protein 3 in the differential diagnosis of collecting duct and upper tract urothelial carcinomas. Hum Pathol. 2013;44:2651–7.
136. Tong GX, Yu WM, Beaubier NT, et al. Expression of PAX8 in normal and neoplastic renal tissues: an immunohistochemical study. Mod Pathol. 2009;22:1218–27.
137. Davis CJ Jr, Mostofi FK, Sesterhenn IA. Renal medullary carcinoma. The seventh sickle cell nephropathy. Am J Surg Pathol. 1995;19:1–11.
138. Adsay NV, de Roux SJ, Sakr W, et al. Cancer as a marker of genetic medical disease: an unusual case of medullary carcinoma of the kidney. Am J Surg Pathol. 1998;22:260–4.
139. Dimashkieh H, Choe J, Mutema G. Renal medullary carcinoma: a report of 2 cases and review of the literature. Arch Pathol Lab Med. 2003;127:e135–8.
140. Yang XJ, Sugimura J, Tretiakova MS, et al. Gene expression profiling of renal medullary carcinoma: potential clinical relevance. Cancer. 2004;100:976–85.
141. Kalyanpur A, Schwartz DS, Fields JM, et al. Renal medulla carcinoma in a white adolescent. AJR Am J Roentgenol. 1997;169:1037–8.
142. Simpson L, He X, Pins M, et al. Renal medullary carcinoma and ABL gene amplification. J Urol. 2005;173:1883–8.
143. Khan A, Thomas N, Costello B, et al. Renal medullary carcinoma: sonographic, computed tomography, magnetic resonance and angiographic findings. Eur J Radiol. 2000;35:1–7.
144. Selby DM, Simon C, Foley JP, et al. Renal medullary carcinoma: can early diagnosis lead to long-term survival? J Urol. 2000;163:1238.
145. Amin MB, Smith SC, Agaimy A, et al. Collecting duct carcinoma versus renal medullary carcinoma: an appeal for nosologic and biological clarity. Am J Surg Pathol. 2014;38:871–4.
146. Calderaro J, Masliah-Planchon J, Richer W, et al. Balanced translocations disrupting SMARCB1 are hallmark recurrent genetic alterations in renal medullary carcinomas. Eur Urol. 2016;69:1055–61.
147. Rao P, Tannir NM, Tamboli P. Expression of OCT3/4 in renal medullary carcinoma represents a potential diagnostic pitfall. Am J Surg Pathol. 2012;36:583–8.
148. Liu Q, Galli S, Srinivasan R, et al. Renal medullary carcinoma: molecular, immunohistochemistry, and morphologic correlation. Am J Surg Pathol. 2013;37:368–74.
149. Pirich LM, Chou P, Walterhouse DO. Prolonged survival of a patient with sickle cell trait and metastatic renal medullary carcinoma. J Pediatr Hematol Oncol. 1999;21:67–9.
150. Stahlschmidt J, Cullinane C, Roberts P, et al. Renal medullary carcinoma: prolonged remission with chemotherapy, immunohistochemical characterisation and evidence of bcr/abl rearrangement. Med Pediatr Oncol. 1999;33:551–7.

151. Lopez-Beltran A, Cheng L, Raspollini MR, et al. SMARCB1/INI1 genetic alterations in renal medullary carcinomas. Eur Urol. 2016;69:1062–4.
152. MacLennan GT, Farrow GM, Bostwick DG. Low-grade collecting duct carcinoma of the kidney: report of 13 cases of low-grade mucinous tubulocystic renal carcinoma of possible collecting duct origin. Urology. 1997;50:679–84.
153. Parwani AV, Husain AN, Epstein JI, et al. Low-grade myxoid renal epithelial neoplasms with distal nephron differentiation. Hum Pathol. 2001;32:506–12.
154. Rakozy C, Schmahl GE, Bogner S, et al. Low-grade tubular-mucinous renal neoplasms: morphologic, immunohistochemical, and genetic features. Mod Pathol. 2002;15:1162–71.
155. Ferlicot S, Allory Y, Comperat E, et al. Mucinous tubular and spindle cell carcinoma: a report of 15 cases and a review of the literature. Virchows Arch. 2005;447:978–83.
156. Fine SW, Argani P, DeMarzo AM, et al. Expanding the histologic spectrum of mucinous tubular and spindle cell carcinoma of the kidney. Am J Surg Pathol. 2006;30:1554–60.
157. Dhillon J, Amin MB, Selbs E, et al. Mucinous tubular and spindle cell carcinoma of the kidney with sarcomatoid change. Am J Surg Pathol. 2009;33:44–9.
158. Bulimbasic S, Ljubanovic D, Sima R, et al. Aggressive high-grade mucinous tubular and spindle cell carcinoma. Hum Pathol. 2009;40:906–7.
159. Pillay N, Ramdial PK, Cooper K, et al. Mucinous tubular and spindle cell carcinoma with aggressive histomorphology—a sarcomatoid variant. Hum Pathol. 2008;39:966–9.
160. Sadimin ET, Chen YB, Wang L, et al. Chromosomal abnormalities of high-grade mucinous tubular and spindle cell carcinoma of the kidney. Histopathology. 2017;71:719–24.
161. Paner GP, Srigley JR, Radhakrishnan A, et al. Immunohistochemical analysis of mucinous tubular and spindle cell carcinoma and papillary renal cell carcinoma of the kidney: significant immunophenotypic overlap warrants diagnostic caution. Am J Surg Pathol. 2006;30:13–9.
162. Gupta R, Balzer B, Picken M, et al. Diagnostic implications of transcription factor Pax 2 protein and transmembrane enzyme complex carbonic anhydrase IX immunoreactivity in adult renal epithelial neoplasms. Am J Surg Pathol. 2009;33:241–7.
163. Molinie V, Balaton A, Rotman S, et al. Alpha-methyl CoA racemase expression in renal cell carcinomas. Hum Pathol. 2006;37:698–703.
164. Cossu-Rocca P, Eble JN, Delahunt B, et al. Renal mucinous tubular and spindle carcinoma lacks the gains of chromosomes 7 and 17 and losses of chromosome Y that are prevalent in papillary renal cell carcinoma. Mod Pathol. 2006;19:488–93.
165. Mehra R, Vats P, Cieslik M, et al. Biallelic alteration and dysregulation of the hippo pathway in mucinous tubular and spindle cell carcinoma of the kidney. Cancer Discov. 2016;6:1258–66.
166. Brandal P, Lie AK, Bassarova A, et al. Genomic aberrations in mucinous tubular and spindle cell renal cell carcinomas. Mod Pathol. 2006;19:186–94.
167. Ren Q, Wang L, Al-Ahmadie HA, et al. Distinct genomic copy number alterations distinguish mucinous tubular and spindle cell carcinoma of the kidney from papillary renal cell carcinoma with overlapping histologic features. Am J Surg Pathol. 2018;42:767–77.
168. Kuroda N, Hes O, Michal M, et al. Mucinous tubular and spindle cell carcinoma with Fuhrman nuclear grade 3: a histological, immunohistochemical, ultrastructural and FISH study. Histol Histopathol. 2008;23:1517–23.
169. Simon RA, di Sant'agnese PA, Palapattu GS, et al. Mucinous tubular and spindle cell carcinoma of the kidney with sarcomatoid differentiation. Int J Clin Exp Pathol. 2008;1:180–4.
170. Perrino CM, Grignon DJ, Williamson SR, et al. Morphological spectrum of renal cell carcinoma, unclassified: an analysis of 136 cases. Histopathology. 2018;72:305–19.
171. Storkel S, Eble JN, Adlakha K, et al. Classification of renal cell carcinoma: workgroup no. 1. Union Internationale Contre le Cancer (UICC) and the American Joint Committee on Cancer (AJCC). Cancer. 1997;80:987–9.
172. Karakiewicz PI, Hutterer GC, Trinh QD, et al. Unclassified renal cell carcinoma: an analysis of 85 cases. BJU Int. 2007;100:802–8.
173. Lopez-Beltran A, Kirkali Z, Montironi R, et al. Unclassified renal cell carcinoma: a report of 56 cases. BJU Int. 2012;110:786–93.

174. Crispen PL, Tabidian MR, Allmer C, et al. Unclassified renal cell carcinoma: impact on survival following nephrectomy. Urology. 2010;76:580–6.
175. Delahunt B, Sika-Paotonu D, Bethwaite PB, et al. Grading of clear cell renal cell carcinoma should be based on nucleolar prominence. Am J Surg Pathol. 2011;35:1134–9.
176. Dagher J, Delahunt B, Rioux-Leclercq N, et al. Clear cell renal cell carcinoma: validation of World Health Organization/International Society of Urological Pathology grading. Histopathology. 2017;71:918–25.
177. Khor LY, Dhakal HP, Jia X, et al. Tumor necrosis adds prognostically significant information to grade in clear cell renal cell carcinoma: a study of 842 consecutive cases from a single institution. Am J Surg Pathol. 2016;40:1224–31.
178. Leibovich BC, Blute ML, Cheville JC, et al. Prediction of progression after radical nephrectomy for patients with clear cell renal cell carcinoma: a stratification tool for prospective clinical trials. Cancer. 2003;97:1663–71.
179. Amin MB, Edge S, Greene FL, et al. AJCC Cancer staging manual. 8th ed. New York: Springer International Publishing; 2017.

Chapter 6
New and Emerging Subtypes of Renal Cell Carcinoma

Priya Rao and Jae Y. Ro

New Entities

Tubulocystic Renal Cell Carcinoma

Tubulocystic renal cell carcinoma (RCC) was first described in 1956 by Masson and designated as Bellinien epithelioma. Tumors occur in adults in age range of 30–80 years (mean 57 years) with a strong male predominance (7:1 or greater). So far, there are approximately 100 cases reported in the literature [1, 2].

Macroscopic Appearance

Grossly, tumors are well circumscribed, but unencapsulated with a unique sponge-like or "bubble wrap" cut surface that results from the presence of macro- and microscopic cysts. Hemorrhage and necrosis are uncommon. It is not uncommon for these tumors to grow to large sizes, while still remaining organ confined, making them amenable to surgical resection. Although the majority of cases follow an indolent clinical course, cases with metastasis to the lymph nodes, bone, and liver have been reported [3].

P. Rao
Department of Pathology, The University of Texas M. D. Anderson Cancer Center, Houston, TX, USA

J. Y. Ro (✉)
Department of Pathology and Genomic Medicine, Houston Methodist Hospital, Weill Medical College of Cornell University, Houston, TX, USA
e-mail: JaeRo@houstonmethodist.org

M. K. Divatia et al. (eds.), *Kidney Cancer*, https://doi.org/10.1007/978-3-030-28333-9_6

Histologic Appearance

Microscopically, the tumor is composed of small- to medium-sized cysts and tubules that are lined by large eosinophilic cells. Tumor cells show a characteristic hobnail morphology with a high Fuhrman nuclear grade (grade 3 or 4 with a prominent nucleolus). The intervening stroma is composed of dense fibroconnective tissue, imparting the spongy, gross appearance of these tumors (Fig. 6.1).

Immunohistochemical Findings

Immunohistochemistry is not usually required for diagnosis due to the classic gross and microscopic appearance of these tumors. By immunohistochemistry, tumors are positive for CK8, CK18, CK19, AMACR, and CD10. CK7 positivity is variable and can show weak and patchy staining. PAX2 and CAIX may be positive in about half of the cases.

Differential Diagnosis

Differential diagnostic considerations include collecting duct carcinoma, papillary RCC, and hereditary leiomyomatosis and RCC (HLRCC). The diagnosis of tubulocystic carcinoma should be reserved only for those tumors that show classic gross

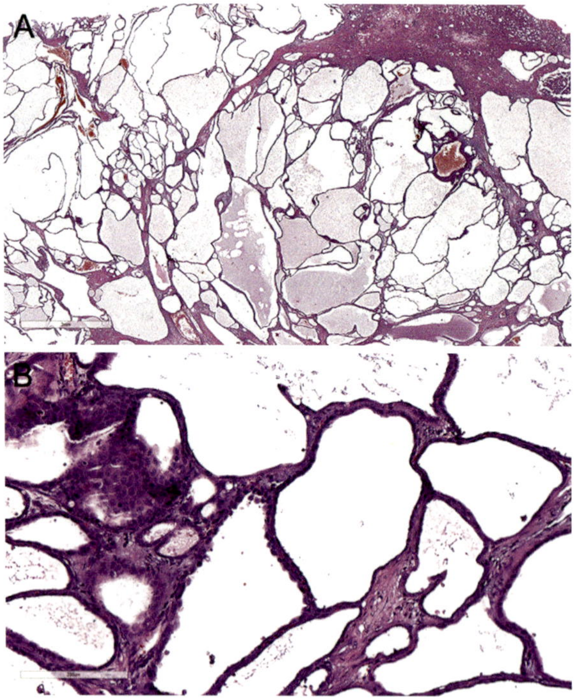

Fig. 6.1 Tubulocystic renal cell carcinoma. (**a**) Low-power view showing an extensively cystic architecture. (**b**) Cysts are lined by hobnailed eosinophilic cells with a high Fuhrman nuclear grade

morphology and microscopic features. Another differential diagnostic consideration is cystic nephroma, which is a biphasic tumor with both epithelial and mesenchymal components. The presence of a high nuclear grade that defines tubulocystic RCC helps in the distinction from cystic nephroma, which shows bland nuclear features in addition to an ovarian type stoma that is lacking in the former. Special attention must be taken to not misdiagnose these tumors as multilocular cystic renal cell neoplasm, simply due to the cystic nature. Multilocular cystic renal neoplasm is typically lined by clear cells with a low nuclear grade that lacks a solid mass of clear cells, and is now widely considered to be an indolent neoplasm with no significant metastatic potential. HLRCC can be virtually indistinguishable from tubulocystic RCC, especially in small biopsy specimens, as the latter can frequently show areas of tubulocystic morphology and shows a similarly high nuclear grade with prominent nucleolus. While the presence of perinucleolar halos in HLRCC may serve as a clue, this feature is by no means diagnostic in itself, and genetic counseling should be considered if clinical suspicion persists. In HLRCC, immunohistochemistry for loss of fumarate hydratase and overexpression of S-(2-succinyl)cysteine (2SC) is of diagnostic utility.

Molecular Findings

Molecular studies show that these tumors are similar to papillary RCC, which demonstrate gain of chromosomes 17p and 17q (trisomy 17). However, trisomy 7, which is also characteristic for papillary RCC, has not been identified in tubulocystic RCC, indicating differential genetic makeup in these two tumors.

MiT Family Translocation Renal Cell Carcinoma

Gene fusions involving the microphthalmia (MiT) family of transcription factors, which include TFE3, TFEB, TFC, and MiTF, have been implicated in the development of RCC. Xp11 translocation RCC was first formally recognized as a variant in the 2004 WHO classification of renal tumors.

Xp11 translocation RCCs are a subset of tumors that are characterized by translocations involving the TFE3 gene, which maps to the Xp11.2 locus. This results in the fusion of the TFE3 gene to any one of multiple partner genes, including ASPL, PRCC, SFPQ, CLTC, Non-O, and a variety of unknown gene fusion partners. Xp11.2 translocation RCC was first recognized in children and it accounts for approximately 40% of all RCCs diagnosed in this age group [4]. The tumor also occurs in adults, with reported incidences varying from 1.6% to 4.2% of all RCCs, making the absolute numbers in adults much higher than in children due to the higher incidence of RCC in the adult population [5, 6].

t(6;11) renal cell carcinoma that harbors the t(6;11) (p21;q12) translocation has now been formally recognized by the 2012 Vancouver classification of renal neoplasia as a subtype of MiT family RCCs. These tumors result from the fusion of the *transcription factor EB* (TFEB) gene, a transcription factor related to microphthalmia transcription factor (MiTF), with *alpha (MALAT1)*, thus resulting in overexpression of native TFEB [4]. These tumors are rare with less than a hundred cases being reported in the literature. Like Xp11.2 RCCs, t(6;11) RCCs can also occur in any age group, though the mean reported age is 31 years.

Macroscopic Appearance

Grossly, Xp11.2 RCCs resemble conventional clear cell RCC (ccRCC), often present as large tumors with areas of necrosis. These tumors are usually of high stage at diagnosis and have a propensity for lymph node metastasis.

Histologic Appearance

The striking microscopic feature is the presence of a neoplasm with papillary architecture, lined by predominantly clear cells with abundant voluminous cytoplasm. Often, there may be admixed solid or nested areas that mimic ccRCC. Other frequent histologic features include psammoma bodies within the tumor and absence of the "chicken wire" vasculature that surrounds the tumor nests that is described in ccRCC. Clues to the fusion gene partner involved may be apparent on microscopy. Tumors with the *ASPSCR1–TFE3* gene fusion typically show larger tumor cells with voluminous cytoplasm, discrete cell borders, and prominent nucleoli and are associated with more extensive psammomatous calcification. In contrast, tumors harboring the *PRCC–TFE3* gene fusion tend to be composed of tumor cells with a more nested growth pattern, less abundant cytoplasm, and less frequent psammoma bodies [4] (Fig. 6.2).

The microscopic appearance of t(6;11) RCC is that of a biphasic tumor that is composed of larger epithelioid cells with clear cytoplasm at the periphery and a second population of centrally located smaller cells clustered around pink hyaline or basement membrane material, resembling Call–Exner bodies. Nuclear atypia is uncommon, and cells show low-grade cytology. Entrapped single renal tubules at the periphery of the tumor are a common histologic finding (Fig. 6.3).

Immunohistochemical Findings

These tumors characteristically show only focal staining or absent staining with epithelial markers such as EMA and cytokeratins, which is helpful in the distinction from ccRCC. Tumors also express PAX2, PAX8, and occasionally may show focal expression of melanocytic markers [4]. The most specific immunohistochemical marker is the strong nuclear expression of TFE3 using an antibody

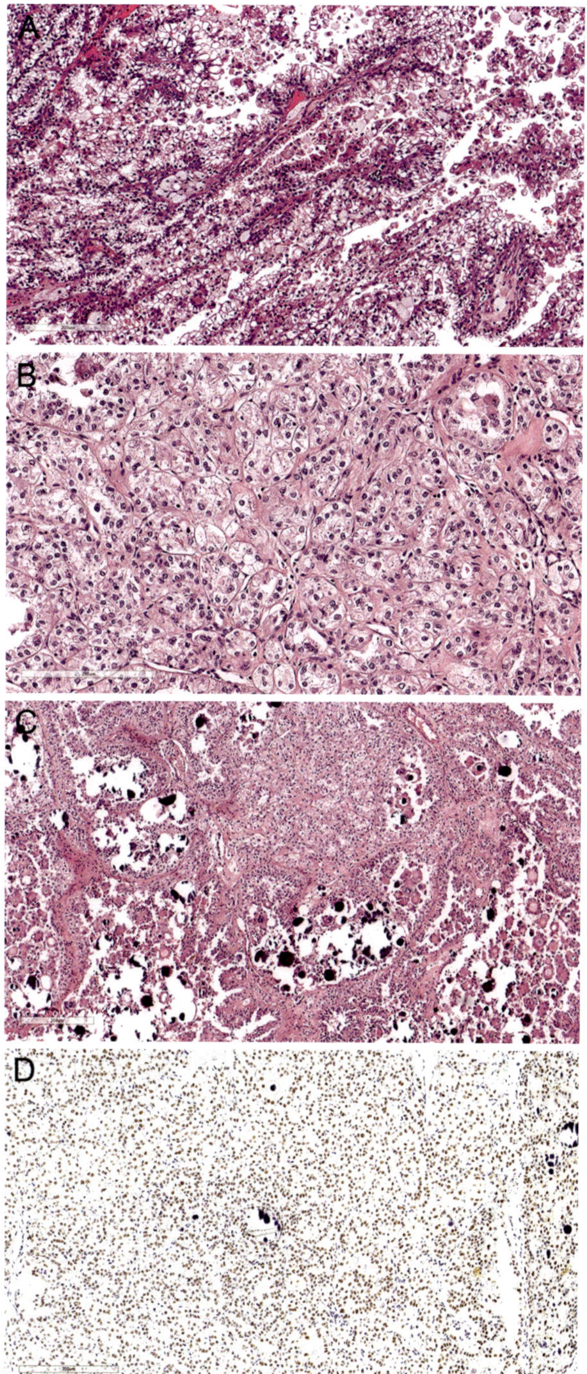

Fig. 6.2 MiT family translocation-associated renal cell carcinoma associated with TFE3 gene fusion. (**a**) Tumors cells show papillary architecture. Papillae are lined by large clear cell with abundant voluminous cytoplasm. (**b**) Tumors may also show nested architecture resembling clear cell renal cell carcinoma. (**c**) Areas of psammomatous calcification are common and may present a diagnostic clue. (**d**) Nuclear expression of TFE3 is the diagnostic hallmark

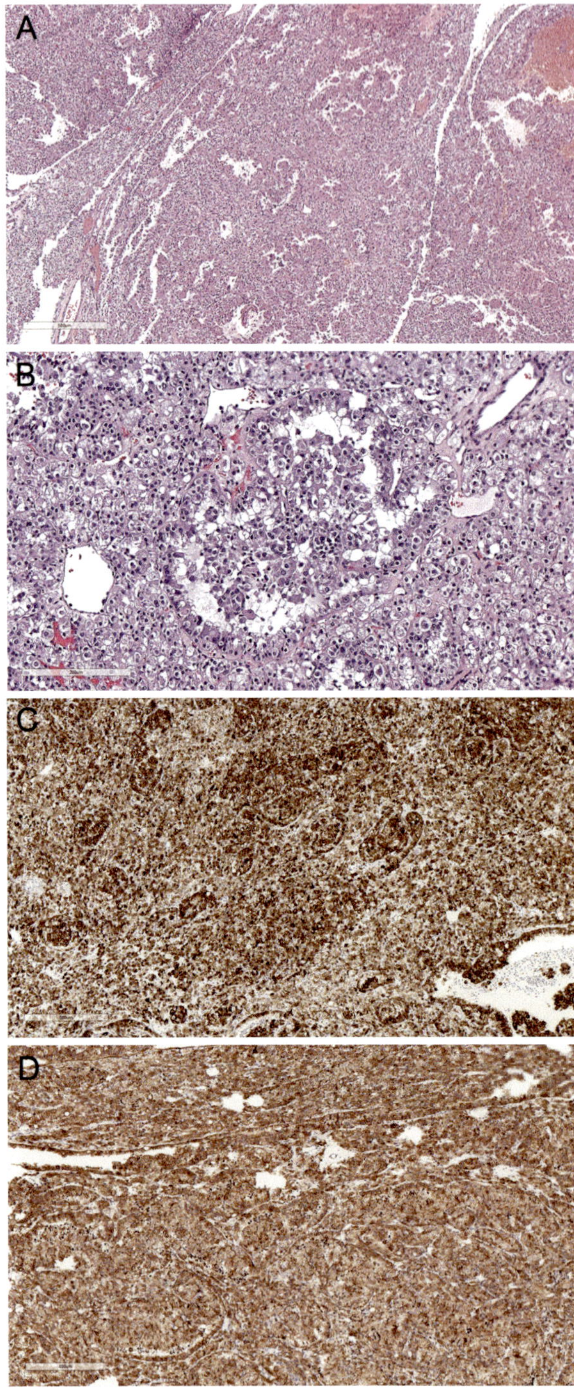

Fig. 6.3 MiT family translocation-associated renal cell carcinoma associated with TFEB gene fusion. (**a**) Tumors show a more solid growth pattern when compared with TFE3 RCCs. (**b**) The tumor often shows a biphasic appearance and shows the presence of "glomeruloid" areas that are composed of smaller cells centrally and are surrounded by larger cells with more voluminous cytoplasm. (**c**) Melan-A stain showing strong staining within the tumor. (**d**) Cathepsin-K typically shows strong and diffuse staining and can be used as a surrogate marker for FISH testing

directed to the C-terminal potion of the TFE3 gene. However, the TFE3 immunohistochemical stain is technically challenging and highly dependent on proper fixation of the tumor. The TFE3 break apart fluorescence in situ hybridization (FISH) assay is less susceptible to the vagaries of tumor fixation and is now widely considered to be the more reliable way to detect a translocation involving the TFE3 gene.

For t(6;11) RCC, the diagnostic immunohistochemical stain is the nuclear expression of TFE-B by immunohistochemistry. These tumors express PAX8, CD10, and low-molecular-weight cytokeratin Cam5.2. A unique finding is the consistent diffuse expression of Melan-A by these tumors which serves to distinguish this tumor type from other subtypes of RCC. Tumors also show patchy labeling for HMB45, but unlike malignant melanoma, they are negative for MiTF and S100 protein. Virtually, all t(6;11) RCCs are also positive for cathepsin K, which can be used as a surrogate maker for TFE-B. However, as with TFE3 RCC, detection of the gene rearrangement by FISH using a break apart probe for the TFEB is considered to be the most specific confirmatory test and is widely regarded to be more sensitive and specific than the immunohistochemical stain [7].

Differential Diagnosis

ccRCC enters the differential diagnosis of Xp11.2 RCC due to the abundant clear cytoplasm. However, presence of extensive papillary architecture, lack of the typical vascular pattern of ccRCC, and the presence of psammoma bodies should raise concern for Xp11.2 RCC. By immunohistochemistry, the diffuse expression of CAIX in ccRCC is usually lacking in MiT family RCCs. The presence of strong cytokeratin 7 expression in a tumor favors the diagnosis of papillary RCC as CK7 is typically negative in both MiT family RCCs and ccRCC. Clear cell papillary RCC may enter the differential diagnosis due to the presence of clear cells and a prominent papillary architecture. However, the latter tend to be small, localized tumors with distinct nuclear features with linear polarization, wherein the nuclei are arranged away from the basement membrane. These tumors, like papillary RCC, also show diffuse expression of CK7, which helps in the separation from MiT family RCC.

The differential diagnostic considerations for t(6;11) RCC, in addition to ccRCC and Xp11.2 RCC, includes epithelioid angiomyolipoma due to expression of melanocytic markers. Both epithelioid angiomyolipoma and t(6;11) RCC show overlapping histology and immunohistochemical findings. These include epithelioid cells without significant atypia or mitosis activity. Both tumors show staining with cathepsin K, HMB45, and Melan A and may be negative for broad-spectrum cytokeratins. However, staining with PAX8 supports the diagnosis of t(6;11) RCC over that of epithelioid angiomyolipoma [4].

As mentioned before, since the MiT translocation RCCs mimic other types of RCC, we generally recommend cytokeratin stain in RCCs arising in children or young adults less than 30 years, regardless of tumor histology. If cytokeratin is diffusely and strongly positive, this is not MiT translocation tumors. When the cytokeratin is negative or weakly positive, we then recommend cathepsin K, TFE3, and TFEB stains with FISH analysis for the diagnosis of MiT translocation tumors.

The prognosis of Xp11.2 RCCs is variable. One large series reported the prognosis of this subtype to be similar to ccRCC, but prognosis is ultimately determined by stage of the tumor [8]. TFEB RCCs tend to follow a more indolent clinical course with some patients reported as developing late metastases, underscoring the need for long-term follow-up.

Clear Cell Papillary Renal Cell Carcinoma

Clear cell papillary renal cell carcinoma (ccpRCC) first received recognition by Tickoo et al., who described 15 tumors with distinctive morphology in patients with end-stage renal disease [9]. Since then ccpRCC has been widely documented in sporadic settings and accounts for approximately 4% of renal tumors, making it the fourth most common renal tumor [10]. The majority of tumors are asymptomatic and are often incidentally detected.

Macroscopic Appearance

Grossly, the majority of ccpRCCs are partially to extensively cystic and small in size. In a study of 36 tumors by Aydin et al., the authors found the mean tumor size to be 2.4 cm and described multifocal tumors in 17% of cases [11].

Histologic Appearance

Histologically, tumors are usually at least partially cystic and demonstrate a partial or circumferential fibrous capsule around the tumor. Tumors show a tubulopapillary appearance with fibrotic intervening stroma. Nuclear features are distinct with low-grade cytology and uniform nuclei that are arranged away from the basement membranes (reversed linear nuclear polarization) (Fig. 6.4).

Tumors with similar morphologic appearance, but with prominent smooth muscle stroma were first reported by Michal et al in 2000. The tumors in their study showed an identical immunohistochemical profile to ccpRCC [12–14]. This variant, now termed renal angiomyoadenomatous tumor (RAT), shows a prominent smooth muscle accompanied by abortive vascular structures and an epithelial component that is identical to that which is seen in ccpRCC (Fig. 6.5) [12].

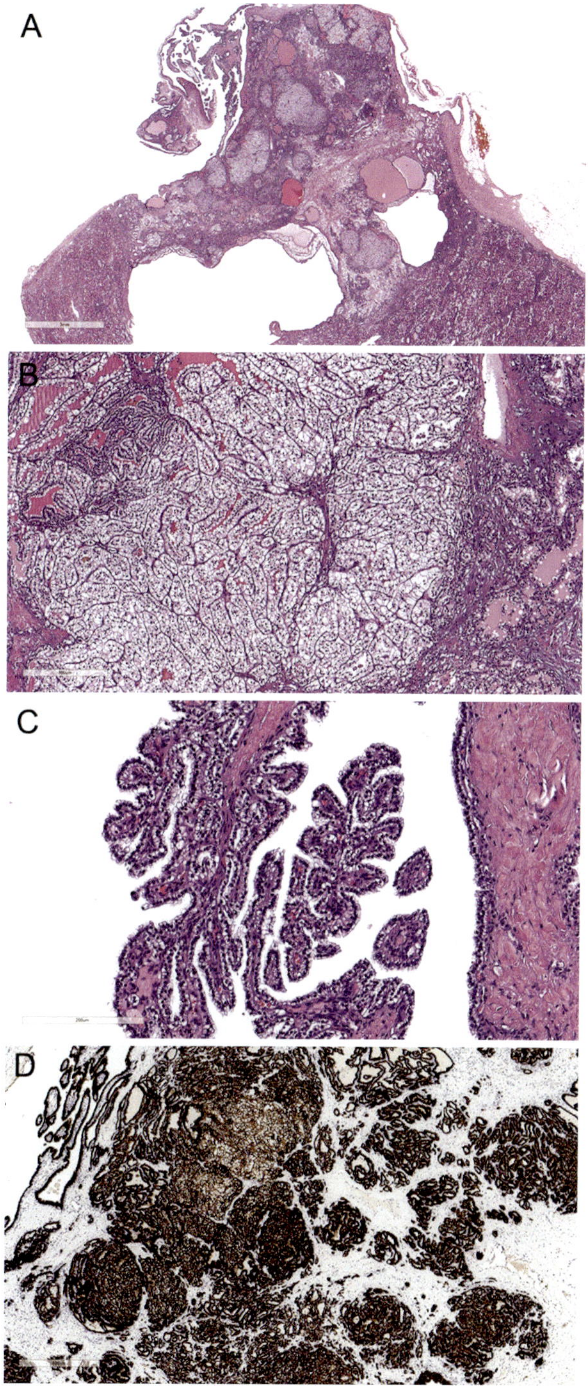

Fig. 6.4 Clear cell papillary renal cell carcinoma. (**a**) The majority of tumors show at least a partially cystic appearance. (**b**) Tumors show a tubulopapillary appearance and lack the typical vascular pattern of clear cell renal cell carcinoma. (**c**) Papillary areas that show delicate branching papillae. Tumor cells are of low nuclear grade and show nuclei with a "picket-fence"-like appearance that line up away from the basement membrane. (**d**) Tumors are diffusely positive for CK7. (**e**) P504S is negative in the tumor. (**f**) CAIX is positive with a "cup-shaped" staining pattern

Fig. 6.4 (continued)

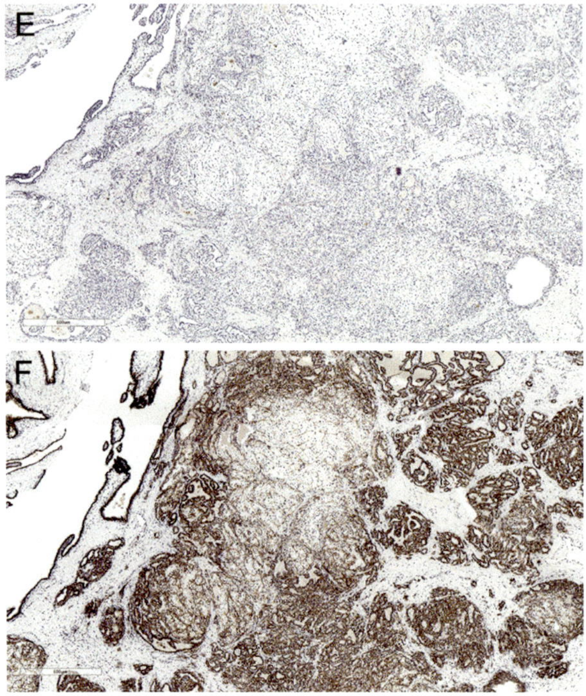

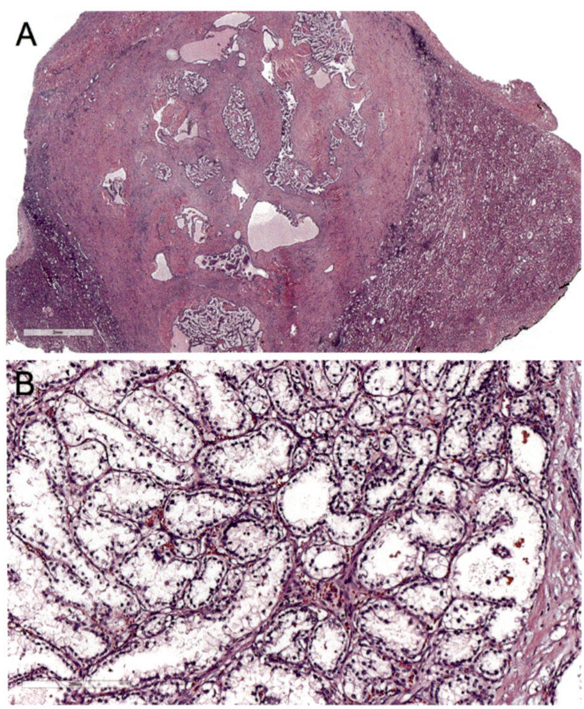

Fig. 6.5 Renal angiomyoadenomatous tumor. (**a**) Renal angiomyoadenomatous tumor (RAT) is widely considered to be within the nosologic spectrum of ccpRCC. Tumors are characterized by prominent smooth muscle stroma with interspersed nests of cells with clear cytoplasm. (**b**) Nuclear features are similar to those of ccpRCC and show clear cells with a low nuclear grade and cells arranged away from the basement membrane

Immunohistochemical Findings

By immunohistochemistry, ccpRCC is diffusely and strongly positive for CK7, which helps in the distinction from ccRCC. Carbonic anhydrase IX is positive in more than 90% of ccpRCCs and shows a "cup-like" pattern of staining. P504S and CD10 are usually negative or only focally positive in ccpRCC, which helps in its distinction from ccRCC and papillary RCC [15].

Distinction from other subtypes of RCC is important, as ccpRCC shows an excellent prognosis with no reported local recurrences or metastasis thus far. Genetically, these tumors do not show any distinct molecular aberrations. These tumors lack 3p deletions, even when they occur in the setting of Von Hippel–Lindau disease (VHL), thus underscoring need for separation from ccRCC [16].

Interestingly, tumors with ccpRCC-like morphology have been described in the setting of VHL disease. Tumors in this clinical setting are often concurrently seen with ccRCC and show a similar histologic appearance to that of ccpRCC, including a tubulopapillary pattern of growth, flattened cysts, and apically arranged nuclei [17]. Unlike ccpRCC, this variant often shows only focal or absent expression of CK7 and CD10 expression in the majority of cases. Tumors in this setting also show 3p deletions classically associated with ccRCC in the setting of VHL disease. Awareness of this histologic variant of ccRCC is important for accurate classification and therapeutic options.

Molecular Findings

ccpRCCs and RATs do not appear to demonstrate any consistent chromosomal abnormalities. These tumors lack the trisomy/polysomy for chromosomes 7 and 17 and do not demonstrate loss of chromosome Y, which are abnormalities typically associated with papillary RCC. A small number of ccpRCC cases have been reported to show mutations in the VHL gene, even in the setting of classic morphology and immunohistochemical findings [18].

Acquired Cystic Disease-Associated Renal Cell Carcinoma

Acquired cystic disease-associated renal cell carcinoma (ACD-RCC) was first recognized in 2006 as a unique tumor that arises specifically in the background of end-stage renal disease (ESRD) [9]. The tumor was formally inducted into the ISUP classification of renal tumors in 2013 as a distinct entity (Fig. 6.6).

Macroscopic Appearance

On gross examination, the background kidneys have the appearance of typical ESRD, including atrophy and diffuse cortical cysts. Tumors may be solitary or multifocal and may be bilateral in about 20% of cases. Size may be variable, and the cut surface ranges from yellow tan to white [19].

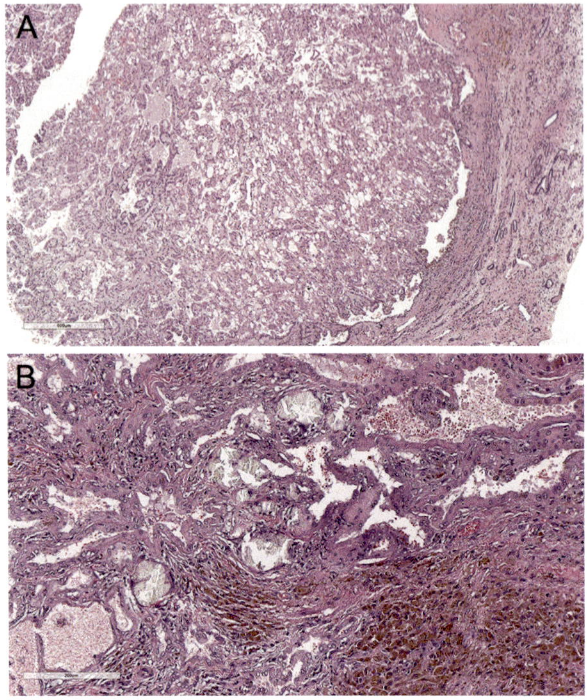

Fig. 6.6 (**a**, **b**) Acquired cystic disease-associated renal cell carcinoma

Histologic Appearance

Histologically, the classic pattern that has been described is that of a cribriform/sieve-like lesion with papillary or tubulopapillary architecture, often arising within a cyst wall. Tumor cells are typically eosinophilic with a high nuclear grade. The pathognomonic feature is the presence of intratumoral polarizable calcium oxalate crystals that are associated with the tumor and the surrounding renal parenchyma.

Immunohistochemical Findings

Immunohistochemistry is typically not required for the diagnosis due to the classic clinical presentation and typical histology. However, tumor cells reportedly express PAX8, CD10, and AMACR and are usually negative or only focally positive for CK7.

Molecular Findings

Multiple chromosomal abnormalities have been reported including gain of chromosomes 1, 2, 3, 6, 7, 16, and Y, however there have been no pathognomonic molecular abnormalities identified. Gains of chromosome 3 have been among the more consistently reported findings [3].

Although most reported cases have shown a good prognosis, this is likely due to early detection of these neoplasms. ACD-RCC is widely recognized as being a high-grade neoplasm with a distinct potential to metastasize, which makes accurate identification of this tumor crucial.

Emerging Entities

Thyroid-Like Follicular Renal Cell Carcinoma

Thyroid-like follicular renal cell carcinoma (TLF-RCC) has been first reported by Jung et al., [20] and provisionally recognized by the ISUP as a distinct neoplasm that resembles well-differentiated follicular carcinoma of the thyroid (Fig. 6.7). The reported age at presentation is wide and there is a slight female preponderance.

Macroscopic Appearance

Macroscopically, tumors are homogeneous, tan brown, well circumscribed, and solid.

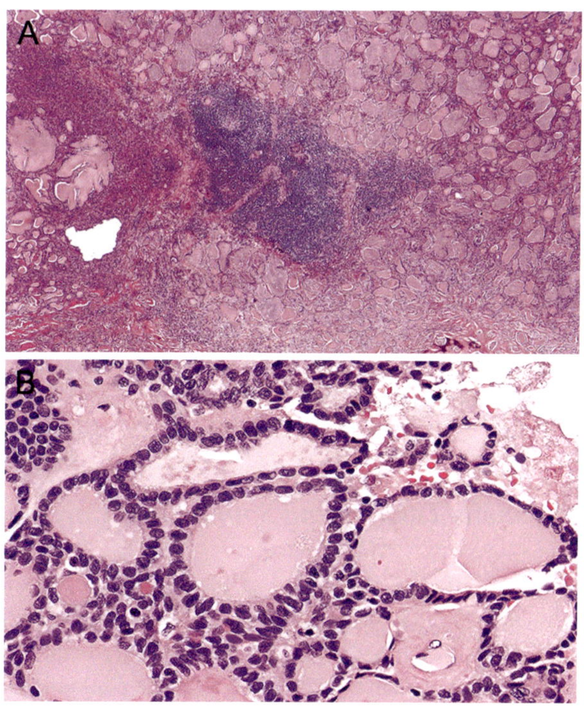

Fig. 6.7 Thyroid-like follicular renal cell carcinoma. (**a**) Tumors show a characteristic appearance resembling that of follicular carcinoma of the thyroid. Inspissated colloid-like material and a prominent lymphocytic infiltrate is a prominent histologic feature. (**b**) Nuclei are round to oval and of a low nuclear grade and histologically similar to papillary renal cell carcinoma

Histologic Appearance

Microscopically, these tumors show a striking follicular architecture with the tumor being composed exclusively of macro- and microfollicles with eosinophilic colloid-like material in the lumen. The follicles are lined by uniform round to cuboidal cells with Fuhrman nuclear grade 2 or 3 nuclei.

Immunohistochemical Findings

By immunohistochemistry, tumor cells are negative for thyroglobulin and TTF1, which helps to distinguish this tumor from metastatic follicular carcinoma of the thyroid. Beyond this, stains are rarely required due to the classic morphology, however, variable staining for CK7, PAX2, and PAX8 are reportedly variable [21]. Although the majority of cases have shown to behave in an indolent manner, there have been cases of lymph node and lung metastasis reported [22].

ALK Translocation RCC

ALK translocation RCC is a rare variant of RCC with gene fusions involving the ALK gene. Cases have been reported in younger patients with sickle cell trait as well as in patients without sickle cell trait. Unlike renal medullary carcinoma (RMC), these tumors do not demonstrate loss of INI-1 staining within the tumor. Tumors in younger patients have shown to harbor a t(2;10)(p23;q22) translocation resulting in a fusion of the gene for the cytoskeletal protein vinculin (VCL) with the anaplastic lymphoma kinase (ALK) gene. In the limited number of reported cases, tumors are composed of polygonal to spindle cells with vesicular nuclei, abundant eosinophilic cytoplasm, and intracytoplasmic lumina. Tumors without VCL as a partner have shown papillary, tubular, or cribriform morphology, but the case numbers are limited [23]. The prognosis of these tumors is less aggressive than that of RMC and the presence of ALK rearrangement presents an opportunity for targeted therapy with ALK inhibitors. ALK expression can be seen by IHC in these tumors, which helps in the diagnosis. Distinction from RMC is crucial in patients with sickle cell trait due to therapeutic and prognostic implications.

Mucinous Tubular and Spindle Cell Carcinoma

Mucinous tubular and spindle cell carcinoma (MTSCC) was first formally recognized as distinct entity in 2004 World Health Organization (WHO) classification of tumors [24]. This tumor usually occurs in adults, with a wide age range at presentation (range 13–81 years; median 60 years) and a female predominance (male to female 1:4) [25].

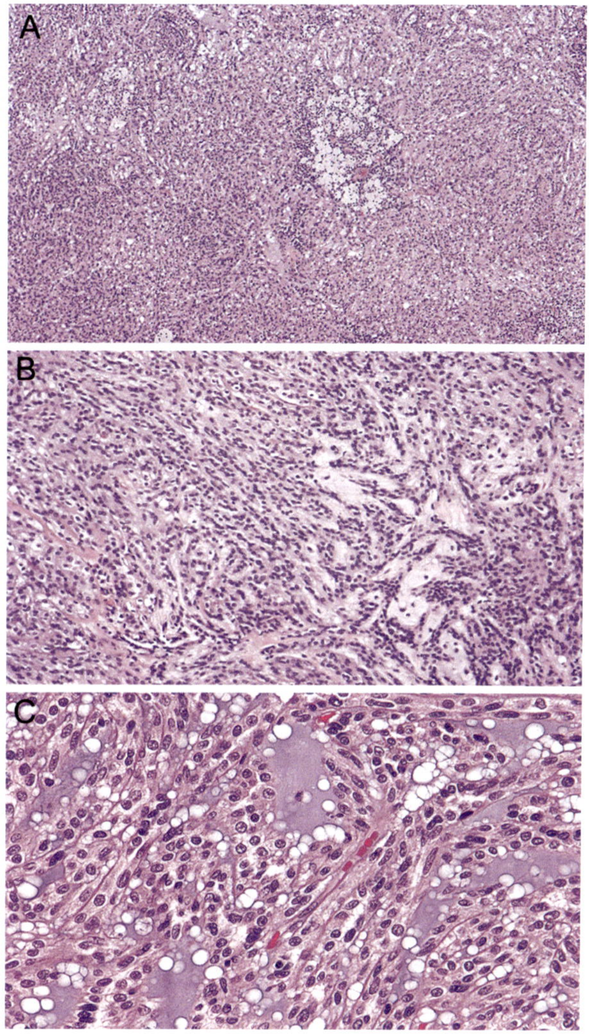

Fig. 6.8 Mucinous tubular and renal cell carcinoma. (**a**) Tumors show a prominent tubular component reminiscent of type 1 papillary RCC. Histiocytic clusters are also commonly identified (**b**) a low-grade spindle cell component and (**c**) extracellular blue mucin–myxoid matrix. The nuclei are typically low grade without any significant mitotic activity and small to intermediate round nucleoli

Macroscopic Appearance

Grossly, tumors are generally well circumscribed with a solid tan cut surface. Necrosis, cystic changes, and hemorrhage are uncommon in MTSCC (Fig. 6.8).

Histologic Appearance

Microscopically, the classic histologic pattern of MTSCC consists of three components, which are (a) a tubular component reminiscent of type 1 papillary RCC, (b) a low-grade spindle cell component, and (c) extracellular blue mucin–myxoid matrix.

The nuclei are typically low grade without any significant mitotic activity and have small to intermediate round nucleoli. The spindle cell component shows histologic features that are identical to the adjacent tubular component and is believed to result from compression of the neoplastic tubules. It is crucial not to confuse the spindle cell areas as sarcomatoid change, especially in needle biopsies where the other components may not be identifiable due to sampling. The indolent nuclear features and lack of mitotic activity should present a clue to the pathologist that the spindle cells are part of a low-grade process rather than true sarcomatoid change, which shows high nuclear grade as well as a high mitotic count and/or necrosis. All three components are not required in order to make the diagnosis, and the presence of any two of the three above-mentioned components is sufficient to establish a diagnosis of MTSCC. True sarcomatoid change, although rare, has been reported in MTSCC and can be identified by the presence of high-grade cytology and mitotic activity within the spindle cell component. In these situations, it is helpful to compare the nuclei in the sarcomatoid component to the adjacent low-grade tubular component, to determine if they are similar, in order to make the diagnosis of sarcomatoid dedifferentiation [26].

The main differential diagnosis is type 1 papillary renal cell carcinoma, which can show identical histology and immunohistochemical features. True papillary structures such as those seen in PRCC are rare in MTSCC, which tends to demonstrate tubular or pseudopapillary features. Additionally, psammomatous calcification, which is frequently seen in papillary renal cell carcinoma, is rare in MTSCC.

Immunohistochemical Findings

The immunohistochemical profile is similar to PRCC, and these tumors are positive for CK7, AE1/AE3, CK19, EMA, and AMACR [25]. Clinically, the majority of tumors are managed surgically and have an excellent prognosis, although rare cases of metastasis have been reported [27].

Molecular Findings

Molecular analysis of MTSCC has shown loss of chromosomes 1, 4, 6, 8, 9, 13, 14, 15, 18, 21, and 22. However, gain of chromosomes 7 and 17 and loss of chromosome Y that is characteristic of papillary renal cell carcinoma are usually not seen in MTSCC [28].

Oncocytic Renal Cell Carcinoma Occurring After Neuroblastoma

Survivors of neuroblastoma have a 329-fold increased lifetime risk of developing renal cell carcinoma [29]. Although several of the common RCC variants, including clear cell RCC and MiTF translocation family-associated RCC, have been described in this clinical setting, the classic postneuroblastoma RCC is described as being oncocytic. The findings were first described by Medeiros et al in 1999 and the entity was formally inducted into the 2004 WHO classification of renal tumors [30]. The typical tumors may show solid, nested, or papillary growth patterns and are characterized by abundant eosinophilic, variably granular cytoplasm with irregular nuclei and mildly enlarged and prominent nucleoli [31]. A major differential diagnostic consideration is succinate dehydrogenase (SDH)-deficient RCC, which shows loss of expression of cytoplasmic SDH protein, in contrast to oncocytic RCC occurring after neuroblastoma, where SDH expression remains intact.

Renal Cell Carcinoma with (Angio) Leiomyomatous Stroma

Renal cell carcinomas (RCCs) with a prominent smooth muscle stroma are rare neoplasms, which were first described in 1993 [32]. Microscopically, these tumors are composed of an admixture of epithelial and stromal components. The epithelial component is typically composed of clear epithelial cells with a low Fuhrman nuclear grade 2. The epithelium is arranged in a nested or tubular pattern and may show prominent papillary morphology. The stromal element is composed of thick smooth muscle bundles associated with a prominent vascular component. While some authors consider RCC with angioleiomyomatous stroma to be a variant of RCC, others have suggested that these may represent a distinct entity due to absence of VHL gene mutations that are typical of ccRCC. Tumors show variable reactivity for CK7 and AMACR. CD10 and CAIX are typically positive in the majority of cases [32–34]. The main differential diagnostic consideration is ccpRCC/RAT, which has been described under the section ccpRCC. These tumors are widely considered to be within the nosolgic spectrum of ccpRCC and show identical immunohistochemical profiles, with the only distinguishing feature being the presence of prominent smooth muscle stroma in RAT.

Eosinophilic Solid Cystic Renal Cell Carcinoma (ESC-RCC)

Eosinophilic solid cystic renal cell carcinoma (ESC-RCC) is a recently described, emerging subtype of RCC that has unique histologic and molecular features. The tumor is rare and accounts for less than 0.5% of all renal tumors. Clinically, these tumors occur overwhelmingly in women with only rare cases reported to occur in men. While the majority of cases occur sporadically, approximately 10% can occur in the setting of tuberous sclerosis. Mean age at diagnosis is in the sixth decade of life [35–37].

These tumors show a solid and cystic gross appearance composed of an admixture of macrocysts and microcysts that are lined by eosinophilic tumor cells with voluminous cytoplasm that show a "hobnail" appearance. By immunohistochemistry, >80% of tumors show at least some staining with CK20 (Fig. 6.9). CK7 is typi-

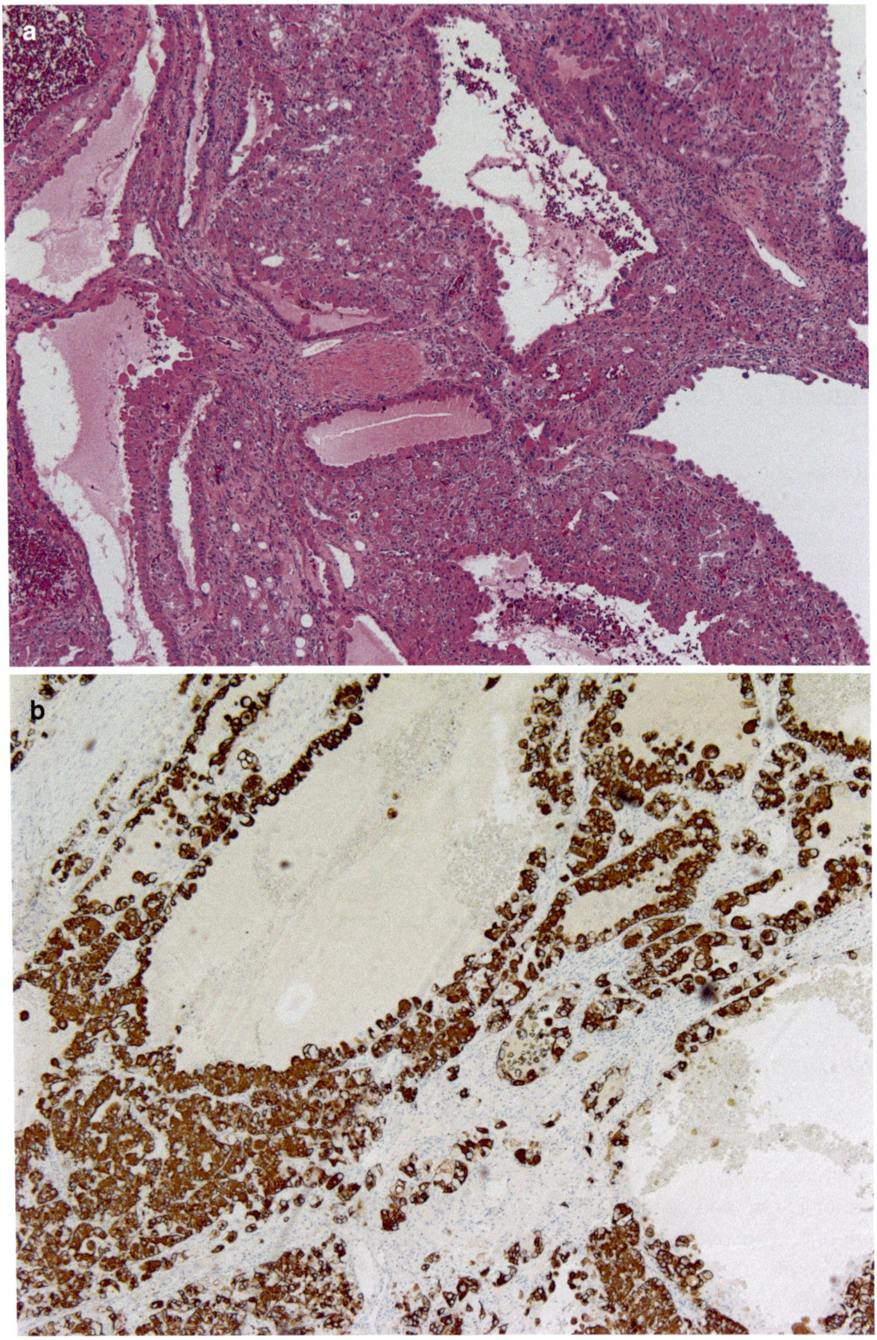

Fig. 6.9 (**a**) ESC-RCC showing solid and cystic areas, with cysts lined by eosinophilic cells with voluminous cytoplasm. (**b**) The hallmark of this tumor is the staining with CK 20, which is seen in >80% of tumors

cally negative or only focally positive and CD117 is typically negative, which helps distinguish this entity from other eosinophilic tumors.

While the majority of these tumors have an indolent clinical course, there have been a few documented cases of metastasis [38]. Recent molecular studies have demonstrated recurrent somatic, biallelic loss or mutations of the TSC gene [39, 40].

Atrophic Kidney-Like RCC

This is a recently described entity with fewer than 10 reported cases in the literature. Tumors have been described as being encapsulated with a homogenous tan brown to white cut surface. Microscopically, the tumors are composed of follicles of varying sizes, similar to that of thyroid-like follicular RCC. The follicles are typically lined by flattened atrophic epithelium in contrast to the more cuboidal or columnar epithelium associated with thyroid-like follicular RCC. The follicles contain dense eosinophilic secretions and frequent associated microcalcifications. Tumors are positive for CK7 and PAX8 and negative for thyroid markers [41, 42].

Clear Cell RCC with Giant Cells and Emperipolesis

There have been rare cases of ccRCC associated with syncytial giant cells and emperipolesis described. These tumors have a male preponderance. Grossly, they are indistinguishable from ccRCC. Histologically, tumors show areas of typical ccRCC admixed with areas with large histiocyte-like tumor cells with multinucleated giant cells that resemble syncytiotrophoblasts. Emperipolesis may be seen in larger voluminous tumor cells and associated areas with rhabdoid morphology also may be seen. The immunohistochemical pattern is similar to that of typical ccRCC with staining for CAIX, vimentin, and PAX8 and lack of staining with CK7, TFE3, and melanocytic markers [43].

Warthin-Like Papillary Renal Cell Carcinoma

This is a recently described variant of papillary renal cell carcinoma that closely resembles Warthin's tumor of the salivary gland. These tumors are characterized by oncocytic tumor cells with a prominent papillary architecture and a dense lymphoid infiltrate within the stroma. By immunohistochemistry, tumor cells are positive for PAX8 and AMACR, with approximately 50% of cases showing staining with CK7. Warthin-like PRCC appears to be a variant of oncocytic PRCC and differed from the latter by the presence of a dense lymphoid infiltrate within the stroma [44].

Renal Cell Carcinoma, Unclassified, with Medullary Phenotype (RCCU-M)

This is an emerging subtype of renal cell carcinoma with fewer than 10 cases reported in the literature. This terminology is reserved for a subset of tumors that show the morphology and immunophenotype of renal medullary carcinoma that occur in patients without evidence of a hemoglobinopathy (sickle cell trait or disease). Tumors present as a high-grade adenocarcinoma with nested, solid, and/or tubulopapillary growth patterns. Sarcomatoid and rhabdoid features have been reported to occur. By immunohistochemistry, all tumors show loss of staining for INI-1 (SMARCB1) and the majority of tumors show expression of OCT4. It is believed that these represent a sporadic variant of renal medullary carcinoma that occurs in patients without sickle cell trait [45, 46].

Low-Grade Oncocytic Renal Tumor

This refers to a subset of tumors with overlapping features of chromophobe renal cell carcinoma and renal oncocytoma. These tumors have a unique immunohistochemical profile and are negative for CD117 and strongly positive for CK7. Tumors present as small organ confined solitary tumors with a tan brown cut surface. By microscopy, tumors lack a capsule and show a solid, nested, papillary, or tubulopapillary architecture. Tumors resemble oncocytoma in which they show prominent edematous stroma separating the nests and low-grade round to oval nuclei without significant nuclear atypia or perinuclear halos. Tumor cells are positive for AE1/AE3, PAX8, E-cadherin, BerEP4, and MOC31 and are negative for CAIX, vimentin, CK20, and melanocytic markers. AMACR is usually negative or only focally positive. The prognosis is good with no reported cases of metastasis [47].

References

1. Amin MB, MacLennan GT, Gupta R, Grignon D, Paraf F, Vieillefond A, et al. Tubulocystic carcinoma of the kidney: clinicopathologic analysis of 31 cases of a distinctive rare subtype of renal cell carcinoma. Am J Surg Pathol. 2009;33(3):384–92.
2. Yang XJ, Zhou M, Hes O, Shen S, Li R, Lopez J, et al. Tubulocystic carcinoma of the kidney: clinicopathologic and molecular characterization. Am J Surg Pathol. 2008;32(2):177–87.
3. Srigley JR, Delahunt B, Eble JN, Egevad L, Epstein JI, Grignon D, et al. The International Society of Urological Pathology (ISUP) Vancouver classification of renal neoplasia. Am J Surg Pathol. 2013;37(10):1469–89.
4. Argani P. MiT family translocation renal cell carcinoma. Semin Diagn Pathol. 2015;32(2):103–13.
5. Komai Y, Fujiwara M, Fujii Y, Mukai H, Yonese J, Kawakami S, et al. Adult Xp11 translocation renal cell carcinoma diagnosed by cytogenetics and immunohistochemistry. Clin Cancer Res. 2009;15(4):1170–6.

6. Zhong M, De Angelo P, Osborne L, Keane-Tarchichi M, Goldfischer M, Edelmann L, et al. Dual-color, break-apart FISH assay on paraffin-embedded tissues as an adjunct to diagnosis of Xp11 translocation renal cell carcinoma and alveolar soft part sarcoma. Am J Surg Pathol. 2010;34(6):757–66.
7. Argani P, Lae M, Hutchinson B, Reuter VE, Collins MH, Perentesis J, et al. Renal carcinomas with the t(6;11)(p21;q12): clinicopathologic features and demonstration of the specific alpha-TFEB gene fusion by immunohistochemistry, RT-PCR, and DNA PCR. Am J Surg Pathol. 2005;29(2):230–40.
8. Sukov WR, Hodge JC, Lohse CM, Leibovich BC, Thompson RH, Pearce KE, et al. TFE3 rearrangements in adult renal cell carcinoma: clinical and pathologic features with outcome in a large series of consecutively treated patients. Am J Surg Pathol. 2012;36(5):663–70.
9. Tickoo SK, de Peralta-Venturina MN, Harik LR, Worcester HD, Salama ME, Young AN, et al. Spectrum of epithelial neoplasms in end-stage renal disease: an experience from 66 tumor-bearing kidneys with emphasis on histologic patterns distinct from those in sporadic adult renal neoplasia. Am J Surg Pathol. 2006;30(2):141–53.
10. Zhou H, Zheng S, Truong LD, Ro JY, Ayala AG, Shen SS. Clear cell papillary renal cell carcinoma is the fourth most common histologic type of renal cell carcinoma in 290 consecutive nephrectomies for renal cell carcinoma. Hum Pathol. 2014;45(1):59–64.
11. Aydin H, Chen L, Cheng L, Vaziri S, He H, Ganapathi R, et al. Clear cell tubulopapillary renal cell carcinoma: a study of 36 distinctive low-grade epithelial tumors of the kidney. Am J Surg Pathol. 2010;34(11):1608–21.
12. Michal M, Hes O, Nemcova J, Sima R, Kuroda N, Bulimbasic S, et al. Renal angiomyoadenomatous tumor: morphologic, immunohistochemical, and molecular genetic study of a distinct entity. Virchows Arch. 2009;454(1):89–99.
13. Petersson F, Grossmann P, Hora M, Sperga M, Montiel DP, Martinek P, et al. Renal cell carcinoma with areas mimicking renal angiomyoadenomatous tumor/clear cell papillary renal cell carcinoma. Hum Pathol. 2013;44(7):1412–20.
14. Michal M, Hes O, Havlicek F. Benign renal angiomyoadenomatous tumor: a previously unreported renal tumor. Ann Diagn Pathol. 2000;4(5):311–5.
15. Williamson SR, Eble JN, Cheng L, Grignon DJ. Clear cell papillary renal cell carcinoma: differential diagnosis and extended immunohistochemical profile. Mod Pathol. 2013;26(5):697–708.
16. Rao P, Monzon F, Jonasch E, Matin SF, Tamboli P. Clear cell papillary renal cell carcinoma in patients with von Hippel-Lindau syndrome – clinicopathological features and comparative genomic analysis of 3 cases. Hum Pathol. 2014;45(9):1966–72.
17. Williamson SR, Zhang S, Eble JN, Grignon DJ, Martignoni G, Brunelli M, et al. Clear cell papillary renal cell carcinoma-like tumors in patients with von Hippel-Lindau disease are unrelated to sporadic clear cell papillary renal cell carcinoma. Am J Surg Pathol. 2013;37(8):1131–9.
18. Aron M, Chang E, Herrera L, Hes O, Hirsch MS, Comperat E, et al. Clear cell-papillary renal cell carcinoma of the kidney not associated with end-stage renal disease: clinicopathologic correlation with expanded immunophenotypic and molecular characterization of a large cohort with emphasis on relationship with renal angiomyoadenomatous tumor. Am J Surg Pathol. 2015;39(7):873–88.
19. Foshat M, Eyzaguirre E. Acquired cystic disease-associated renal cell carcinoma: review of pathogenesis, morphology, ancillary tests, and clinical features. Arch Pathol Lab Med. 2017;141(4):600–6.
20. Jung SJ, Chung JI, Park SH, Ayala AG, Ro JY. Thyroid follicular carcinoma-like tumor of kidney: a case report with morphologic, immunohistochemical, and genetic analysis. Am J Surg Pathol. 2006;30(3):411–5.
21. Amin MB, Gupta R, Ondrej H, McKenney JK, Michal M, Young AN, et al. Primary thyroid-like follicular carcinoma of the kidney: report of 6 cases of a histologically distinctive adult renal epithelial neoplasm. Am J Surg Pathol. 2009;33(3):393–400.

22. Dhillon J, Tannir NM, Matin SF, Tamboli P, Czerniak BA, Guo CC. Thyroid-like follicular carcinoma of the kidney with metastases to the lungs and retroperitoneal lymph nodes. Hum Pathol. 2011;42(1):146–50.
23. Mehra R, Smith SC, Divatia M, Amin MB. Emerging entities in renal neoplasia. Surg Pathol Clin. 2015;8(4):623–56.
24. Lopez-Beltran A, Scarpelli M, Montironi R, Kirkali Z. 2004 WHO classification of the renal tumors of the adults. Eur Urol. 2006;49(5):798–805.
25. Fine SW, Argani P, DeMarzo AM, Delahunt B, Sebo TJ, Reuter VE, et al. Expanding the histologic spectrum of mucinous tubular and spindle cell carcinoma of the kidney. Am J Surg Pathol. 2006;30(12):1554–60.
26. Dhillon J, Amin MB, Selbs E, Turi GK, Paner GP, Reuter VE. Mucinous tubular and spindle cell carcinoma of the kidney with sarcomatoid change. Am J Surg Pathol. 2009;33(1): 44–9.
27. Asghar AM, Uhlman MA, Dahmoush L, Deorah S. Osseous metaplasia in mucinous tubular and spindle cell carcinoma of the kidney: a case of massive, bilateral tumors. Case Rep Urol. 2015;2015:465450.
28. Mehra R, Vats P, Cieslik M, Cao X, Su F, Shukla S, et al. Biallelic alteration and dysregulation of the hippo pathway in mucinous tubular and spindle cell carcinoma of the kidney. Cancer Discov. 2016;6(11):1258–66.
29. Bassal M, Mertens AC, Taylor L, Neglia JP, Greffe BS, Hammond S, et al. Risk of selected subsequent carcinomas in survivors of childhood cancer: a report from the Childhood Cancer Survivor Study. J Clin Oncol. 2006;24(3):476–83.
30. Medeiros LJ, Palmedo G, Krigman HR, Kovacs G, Beckwith JB. Oncocytoid renal cell carcinoma after neuroblastoma: a report of four cases of a distinct clinicopathologic entity. Am J Surg Pathol. 1999;23(7):772–80.
31. Falzarano SM, McKenney JK, Montironi R, Eble JN, Osunkoya AO, Guo J, et al. Renal cell carcinoma occurring in patients with prior neuroblastoma: a heterogenous group of neoplasms. Am J Surg Pathol. 2016;40(7):989–97.
32. Canzonieri V, Volpe R, Gloghini A, Carbone A, Merlo A. Mixed renal tumor with carcinomatous and fibroleiomyomatous components, associated with angiomyolipoma in the same kidney. Pathol Res Pract. 1993;189(8):951–6; discussion 7-9
33. Kuhn E, De Anda J, Manoni S, Netto G, Rosai J. Renal cell carcinoma associated with prominent angioleiomyoma-like proliferation: report of 5 cases and review of the literature. Am J Surg Pathol. 2006;30(11):1372–81.
34. Shannon BA, Cohen RJ, Segal A, Baker EG, Murch AR. Clear cell renal cell carcinoma with smooth muscle stroma. Hum Pathol. 2009;40(3):425–9.
35. Guo J, Tretiakova MS, Troxell ML, Osunkoya AO, Fadare O, Sangoi AR, et al. Tuberous sclerosis-associated renal cell carcinoma: a clinicopathologic study of 57 separate carcinomas in 18 patients. Am J Surg Pathol. 2014;38(11):1457–67.
36. Trpkov K, Abou-Ouf H, Hes O, Lopez JI, Nesi G, Comperat E, et al. Eosinophilic solid and cystic renal cell carcinoma (ESC RCC): further morphologic and molecular characterization of ESC RCC as a distinct entity. Am J Surg Pathol. 2017;41(10):1299–308.
37. Trpkov K, Hes O, Bonert M, Lopez JI, Bonsib SM, Nesi G, et al. Eosinophilic, solid, and cystic renal cell carcinoma: clinicopathologic study of 16 unique, sporadic neoplasms occurring in women. Am J Surg Pathol. 2016;40(1):60–71.
38. McKenney JK, Przybycin CG, Trpkov K, Magi-Galluzzi C. Eosinophilic solid and cystic renal cell carcinomas have metastatic potential. Histopathology. 2018;72(6):1066–7.
39. Mehra R, Vats P, Cao X, Su F, Lee ND, Lonigro R, et al. Somatic bi-allelic loss of TSC genes in eosinophilic solid and cystic renal cell carcinoma. Eur Urol. 2018;74(4): 483–6.
40. Palsgrove DN, Li Y, Pratilas CA, Lin MT, Pallavajjalla A, Gocke C, et al. Eosinophilic solid and cystic (ESC) renal cell carcinomas harbor TSC mutations: molecular analysis supports an expanding clinicopathologic spectrum. Am J Surg Pathol. 2018;42(9):1166–81.

41. Hes O, de Souza TG, Pivovarcikova K, Grossmann P, Martinek P, Kuroda N, et al. Distinctive renal cell tumor simulating atrophic kidney with 2 types of microcalcifications. Report of 3 cases. Ann Diagn Pathol. 2014;18(2):82–8.
42. Oshiro Y, Hida AI, Tamiya S, Toyoshima S, Kuroda N, Hes O, et al. Bilateral atrophic kidney-like tumors. Pathol Int. 2014;64(9):478–80.
43. Williamson SR, Kum JB, Goheen MP, Cheng L, Grignon DJ, Idrees MT. Clear cell renal cell carcinoma with a syncytial-type multinucleated giant tumor cell component: implications for differential diagnosis. Hum Pathol. 2014;45(4):735–44.
44. Skenderi F, Ulamec M, Vanecek T, Martinek P, Alaghehbandan R, Foix MP, et al. Warthin-like papillary renal cell carcinoma: clinicopathologic, morphologic, immunohistochemical and molecular genetic analysis of 11 cases. Ann Diagn Pathol. 2017;27:48–56.
45. Sirohi D, Smith SC, Ohe C, Colombo P, Divatia M, Dragoescu E, et al. Renal cell carcinoma, unclassified with medullary phenotype: poorly differentiated adenocarcinomas overlapping with renal medullary carcinoma. Hum Pathol. 2017;67:134–45.
46. Lai JZ, Lai HH, Cao D. Renal cell carcinoma, unclassified with medullary phenotype and synchronous renal clear cell carcinoma present in a patient with no sickle cell trait/disease: diagnostic and therapeutic challenges. Anticancer Res. 2018;38(6):3757–61.
47. Trpkov K, Hes O. New and emerging renal entities: a perspective post-WHO 2016 classification. Histopathology. 2019;74(1):31–59.

Chapter 7
Renal Mass Biopsy

Kanishka Sircar and Pheroze Tamboli

Evaluation of renal masses is critical for proper patient management. Clinical and radiological evaluations are paramount with the latter indicating whether a renal mass is solid or cystic and the complexity of a radiographically detected cyst using the Bosniak criteria [1]. Historically, virtually all solid or complex cystic renal masses were surgically resected without biopsy confirmation, as it did not alter management and was viewed as introducing unnecessary morbidity. Over the past two decades, clinical thinking has gradually changed to accept the safety and utility of renal mass biopsy for subsets of patients for whom histologic biopsy diagnosis is potentially useful. While the large majority of patients who undergo surgical resection of their renal masses are still not biopsied, many patients with smaller tumors who are candidates for ablation or surveillance or patients with advanced disease are increasingly biopsied in contemporary practice [2, 3]. Accordingly, we will discuss the clinical situations where renal mass biopsy may be indicated, its performance characteristics, as well as the general approach to pathologic evaluation and limitations of renal mass biopsy.

Biopsies are generally performed using coaxial needle biopsies as this technique allows for a greater diagnostic yield without differences in procedure-related morbidity [4]. A variable number of tissue cores are obtained using an 18-gauge needle under computed tomography (CT) or ultrasound guidance (Fig. 7.1a). An 18-gauge needle has been reported to be associated with the best diagnostic accuracy [5],

K. Sircar (✉)
Division of Pathology and Laboratory Medicine, Departments of Pathology and Translational Molecular Pathology, The University of Texas MD Anderson Cancer Center, Houston, TX, USA
e-mail: ksircar@mdanderson.org

P. Tamboli
Division of Pathology and Laboratory Medicine, Department of Pathology, The University of Texas MD Anderson Cancer Center, Houston, TX, USA

M. K. Divatia et al. (eds.), *Kidney Cancer*, https://doi.org/10.1007/978-3-030-28333-9_7

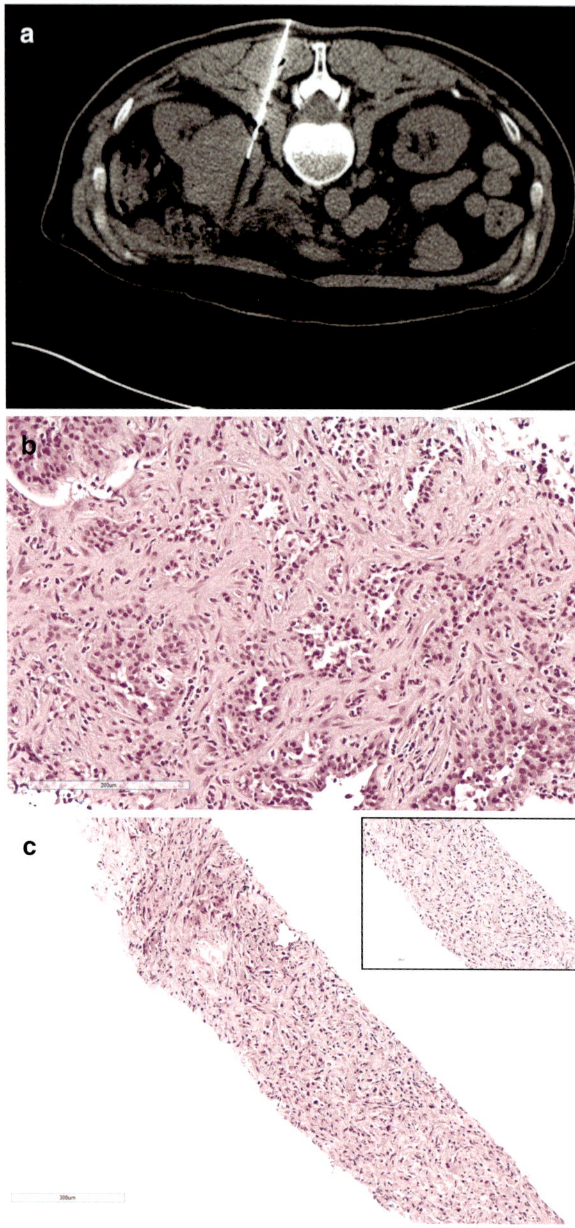

Fig. 7.1 Renal mass biopsy. (**a**) Tissue obtained under computed tomography (CT) guidance; Biopsy showing (**b**) collecting duct RCC and (**c**) sarcomatoid RCC histologies

whereas the choice of using ultrasound or CT depends on various factors, without obvious benefit using either modality in one study [6]. The optimal number of tissue cores taken at biopsy is not established; however, the diagnostic accuracy of renal mass biopsy using a one-, two-, or three-core strategy was directly proportional to the number of cores sampled [7].

Clinical Scenarios Where Renal Masses Are Biopsied

Indications for renal mass biopsy have evolved over time and may be individualized to the patient. In general, renal mass biopsies (RMB) may be performed in the following scenarios.

Patient with Another Nonrenal Primary Tumor

Biopsy is used to determine whether the renal mass represents a primary renal tumor or metastatic involvement of the kidney from the patient's extrarenal primary neoplasm. If the renal tumor is a second primary, it may be further characterized as to its malignant potential.

The therapeutic strategy will differ significantly depending on the outcome of the biopsy. Metastatic tumor will likely be treated using systemic therapies whereas a primary renal tumor will generally be managed with local extirpation according to the malignant potential of the tumor and patient-related factors.

Patient with an Unresectable Renal Mass

This scenario involves an advanced, surgically unresectable renal mass. Biopsy of the renal mass is used to document the tumor's histologic type prior to initiation of systemic therapy. The precise histologic subtype will aid in guiding therapy. For example, a biopsy diagnosis of urothelial or collecting duct carcinoma (Fig. 7.1b) will trigger different treatment modalities, usually MVAC-based chemotherapies, versus a renal cortical carcinoma of proximal nephron origin. Further, a clear cell renal cell carcinoma (RCC) subtype may be treated differently than non-clear cell RCC, with greater utility of antiangiogenic drugs.

Patient with a Renal Mass and Clinical Metastasis

These patients will require histologic subtyping of their tumor to direct the appropriate sequence of therapies. In addition to different approaches for urothelial and collecting duct carcinomas and rarer lymphomas, sarcomas, or neuroendocrine tumors, patients with the more common RCC are also managed in a subtype specific manner. Hence, a patient with renal cell carcinoma of clear cell subtype will generally be treated with antiangiogenic drugs and cytoreductive nephrectomy whereas non-clear cell RCC will proceed directly to nephrectomy followed by systemic therapy. If sarcomatoid features are detected (Fig. 7.1c), patients will forgo nephrectomy and proceed to upfront systemic therapy as sarcomatoid tumors usually grow too quickly to allow for convalescence from surgery.

Clear RCC Neoadjuvant Clinical Trials

There are clinical trials designed for specific RCC subtypes in the neoadjuvant setting. In these cases, a biopsy is needed for confirmation of histologic subtype. Most commonly, these trials are applicable to clear cell RCC and where non-clear cell RCC histology is an exclusion criterion.

Patient with a Renal Mass That May Be Non-neoplastic

Renal mass lesions that are suspected to be infectious in etiology, such as pyelonephritis, require biopsy for confirmation. These lesions may be treated nonsurgically.

Therapy with Ablative Techniques

Newer nephron sparing approaches include radiofrequency ablation (RFA), cryoablation, microwave ablation, and high-intensity focused ultrasound (HIFU), wherein the tumor is ablated using thermal (extreme heat or cold) and nonthermal energy, but not surgically resected [8]. The aim of these modalities is to destroy lesional tumor tissue while preserving a rim of viable renal parenchyma. Optimal candidates for ablative therapy include patients with small renal masses who are not good candidates for partial nephrectomy such as individuals who have significant comorbidities, who are elderly, or who have medical renal disease [9, 10]. Although selection of ablation versus partial nephrectomy depends on a host of patient and tumor-related factors, it is generally true that ablation (RFA) shows maximal efficacy in very small (< 3 cm in diameter) and peripherally located renal tumors where tumor necrosis can be achieved in a single ablation rather than multiple ablation sessions [11, 12]. Cryoablation also showed decreased efficacy with larger tumors in that tumor recurrence was significantly higher for cryoablated versus surgically resected tumors in the 4–7 cm diameter range [13].

The renal biopsy taken prior to the procedure is the only specimen available for rendering a tissue diagnosis and subtyping the tumor. This is important for recording clinical follow-up data given that RFA has shown greater efficacy in treatment of specific subtypes, for example, papillary RCC showing superior response compared to clear cell RCC [14]; and to potentially spare unnecessary treatment of benign masses. Although biopsy sampling is considered standard of care in this setting, the majority of patients get biopsied during the ablation session and many get inadequate or suboptimal tumor sampling [8, 15]. The effectiveness of ablation is generally measured based on radiographic parameters of tumor involution with a post ablation biopsy occasionally performed when the tumor does not involute radiographically as expected. Radiology is imperfect in measuring tumor viability, however, as one study, involving multisite biopsies taken approximately 24 months after RFA in a subset of patients with non-enhancing and non-involuting tumors, showed a 7.9% rate of viable tumor cells [16]. The pathologist is tasked with identifying viable tumor based mainly on the hematoxylin and eosin (H&E) stain. A nicotinamide adenine dinucleotide (NaDH) stain for viability requires frozen tissue, has to be freshly prepared, and is capricious, limiting its utility in a clinical setting.

Risk Stratification of Kidney Tumors

With advances in imaging of renal masses over the past two decades, there are significantly more cases of RCC that are detected. That increased detection has not translated into a corresponding decrease in RCC cancer mortality, suggesting that many smaller and incidentally detected tumors are not biologically aggressive [17]. Tumors that behave indolently include those showing benign histology and those with malignant histology but lacking high-grade and high-stage pathological features. Histologically benign tumors encompassing, in descending frequency, oncocytoma, angiomyolipoma, papillary adenoma, and metanephric adenoma, represent approximately 20% of all excised renal masses. The proportion of tumors that are histologically benign is reported to be inversely proportional to the tumor size, as 30% of tumors measuring <2 cm in diameter showed benign histology versus approximately 6% benign histology for tumors with a diameter of >7 cm [18]. The histologic type of renal masses also differs according to tumor size, with the fraction of clear cell renal carcinoma and papillary renal cell carcinoma showing a direct and inverse correlation with tumor diameter, respectively [18].

Smaller renal masses harboring malignant histology are generally not biologically aggressive given their tendency to demonstrate lower pathologic grade and stage [18, 19]. However, small renal masses, defined as tumors ≤4 cm in diameter [20], are not uniformly innocuous with up to one-quarter of cases showing high-grade histology and up to one-third of cases showing locally advanced disease [21, 22]. Surveillance, Epidemiology and End Results (SEER) data indicate metastasis and cancer-specific mortality rates of 7.4% and 5.3%, respectively for tumors measuring 3.1–4.0 cm in diameter [23]. Further, multi-institutional data reveal that patients with localized small renal masses show a low but definite cancer-specific mortality of approximately 3% [24]. In view of the uncertainty of predicting the biological aggressiveness of small renal masses by clinical or radiological parameters, renal mass biopsy may be used for risk stratification of kidney tumors [19]. This applies to small renal masses that may be benign or of low malignant potential and potentially manageable with surveillance approaches, particularly in patients who are poor surgical candidates.

Performance Characteristics of Renal Mass Biopsy Sampling

The performance characteristics of renal mass biopsies, summarized in Table 7.1, are important since risk-adapted treatment of small renal masses involves a trade-off between risks and benefits. Importantly, renal mass biopsies are an established diagnostic modality mainly for solid masses with significantly less applicability for cystic lesions of the kidney [25, 26].

The risks associated with RMB are minimal and include most commonly post biopsy hematoma (5%) as well as pain, hematuria and pneumothorax, occurring in <1% of patients, and all of which are easily manageable [27]. Needle biopsy tract seeding of carcinoma has been described historically, but only twice in the contemporary literature [28, 29]. With respect to furnishing adequate diagnostic tissue, renal biopsy shows a technical failure rate of around 15% [27], with higher failure rates associated with smaller tumors, greater distance between skin and tumor, and cystic tumors [28, 30]. Inadequate diagnostic tissue may be due to under-sampled tumor or to missing the tumor entirely with pathologic evaluation showing only renal parenchyma, connective tissue, or hemorrhage/necrosis. Repeat biopsy after initial nondiagnostic biopsy sampling is successful in rendering a diagnosis in approximately 80% of cases [28, 30–34]. These subsequent biopsies frequently show malignant tumor [28, 32, 35–38]; therefore, a nondiagnostic initial biopsy is not tantamount to an indolent tumor.

Once adequate diagnostic tissue has been procured, the reliability of biopsy is measured by its ability to diagnose malignancy, tumor type, and tumor grade. Though renal biopsy is used in conjunction with patient-related factors to decide the appropriate therapeutic approach, pathological diagnosis by itself has significance beyond clinical and radiological parameters [39–42]. In a large single institution series, active surveillance of renal masses was instituted for 77% of benign or low

Table 7.1 Performance characteristics of renal mass biopsy

Safe procedure
Serious morbidity is negligible
Applicable mainly to solid masses
Inadequate tissue procured (~15%)
Repeat biopsy diagnostic in ~80%
Frequently positive for malignancy
Excellent positive predictive value for malignant diagnosis (> 99%)
High concordance for histologic subtype (>95%)
Ancillary immunohistochemical tests improve accuracy
Poor concordance for histologic grade (50–75%) and sarcomatoid features
Histological upgrading at resection
Moderate negative predictive value for malignant diagnosis (~70%)
Pathologic heterogeneity of renal oncocytic neoplasms

malignant potential tumors versus an active surveillance rate of only 17% for clear cell renal carcinomas [35]. The exact proportion of tumor subtypes diagnosed by biopsy of renal masses is variable, depending on the cohort and indications for biopsy. Clear cell RCC is the most common subtype diagnosed (45–52%) across cohorts where indications for biopsy included indeterminate mass [41], asymptomatic small renal mass [32], patients treated with RFA [16], and consecutive biopsies performed for different indications [35]. Renal oncocytic neoplasm was the second most frequent biopsy diagnosis (13–23%) followed by papillary RCC (4–14%), and chromophobe RCC (1–14%). Historical data overestimate papillary RCC incidence due to inclusion of mimics such as clear cell papillary RCC and MiTF translocation RCC whereas renal oncocytic neoplasms encompass oncocytoma, hybrid oncocytic chromophobe tumors, and some chromophobe RCC. Angiomyolipoma is the second most frequent benign diagnosis, after oncocytoma, ranging from 1% to 7%.

In the case of a biopsy that is diagnostic and positive for malignancy, the positive predictive value (PPV) is very high (>99%) when assessed against the pathology reading from the surgically resected specimen [27]. Contemporary series comparing biopsy with nephrectomy pathology also show high concordance in terms of histological RCC subtype, ranging from 95% to 100% [38, 43–45], and encompassing clear and non-clear cell RCC. Improved diagnostic accuracy is partly related to the use of reliable ancillary immunohistochemical tests and increased pathologist experience in interpreting renal biopsies [46]. Renal biopsy performed less well in determining the final histologic grade, with concordance reported in the 50–75% range [45, 47]. This is not surprising, given the inherent grade heterogeneity of RCC and that the final assigned grade is based on the highest-grade focus, which may span only a few microscopic fields. Thus, RCC tumors are prone to upgrading at resection [27]. Accordingly, renal biopsy performs poorly in identifying sarcomatoid features [48], although given the very low incidence of sarcomatoid histology in small, low-stage tumors [49], this issue is less relevant than with larger tumors.

Interestingly, approximately 37% of biopsies that are read as showing benign histology are subsequently found to be malignant on the resected specimen [27]. While only a minority of benign biopsies are resected, potentially introducing bias, an analysis of data that is potentially less confounded by bias still showed a negative predictive value of renal mass biopsy of 73% [15, 45, 47, 50]. While benign diagnoses of angiomyolipoma and metanephric adenoma may be confidently rendered on biopsy specimens from small renal masses [32], oncocytic renal neoplasms, which constitute the large majority of benign pathologic diagnoses rendered on biopsy, show relatively poor concordance between biopsy and final pathology on the resected specimen. In a meta-analysis of over 200 oncocytic neoplasms diagnosed on biopsy and 22% with available final pathology, the positive predictive value for oncocytoma was 67%; 25% of cases showed RCC on the resected specimen, with 6% showing a hybrid oncocytic/chromophobe tumor [51]. Examination of renal oncocytic tumors by dedicated genitourinary pathologists at a single academic center employing the latest ancillary tests showed a degree of diagnostic uncertainly. Approximately, two-thirds of oncocytic tumors were placed in the "favor oncocytoma" category with a PPV of 83%; the "cannot exclude RCC" and "favor RCC" groups showed PPVs of 90% and 100%, respectively [52].

Approach to Handling and Pathologic Reporting of Renal Mass Biopsies

The approach to handling renal mass biopsies at our institution is to cut at eight consecutive levels: The first and eighth levels are stained with H&E, with the intervening six levels cut as unstained sections on charged slides for potential immunohistochemical studies (Fig. 7.2). We examine the H&E stained section for specimen adequacy in terms of whether there is sufficient lesional tissue. If diagnostic tumor tissue is not seen, we cut deeper into the block in the hopes of identifying the lesion; otherwise, it is considered as a nondiagnostic biopsy. In all cases, we correlate our pathology findings with those obtained by fine-needle aspiration cytology.

The approach to reporting renal mass biopsies is similar to that used for resected kidneys with the caveat that only a limited tissue sampling is possible with biopsies. We report on the adequacy of the biopsy, whether there is a neoplastic or nonneoplastic process present, and if neoplastic, we then refine our diagnosis, often with the aid of immunohistochemical studies. The first categorization for renal neoplasms is whether they represent a benign or malignant tumor. Angiomyolipoma and metanephric adenoma are benign diagnoses that can be rendered on biopsy with appropriate ancillary studies as illustrated in Fig. 7.3a–e. Papillary adenoma, by contrast, should generally not be diagnosed at biopsy since focal sampling cannot guarantee the absence of a capsule or of higher-grade foci, which would preclude this diagnosis. We would typically report a papillary renal epithelial tumor (Fig. 7.3f) with ISUP grade 1–2 nuclear features as presenting a differential diagnosis of papillary adenoma versus type 1 papillary RCC depending on whether the tumor measures ≤1.5 cm in diameter, possesses a capsule, or ISUP grade 3–4 foci. Diagnosing renal oncocytoma is also problematic on biopsy because "oncocytoma-like" areas have been reported in chromophobe renal cell carcinoma resections [53]. These tumors likely represent the so-called hybrid renal oncocytic neoplasm, which may show either distinct oncocytoma-like and chromophobe RCC-like zones, or, ambiguous morphology [54, 55]. Given the

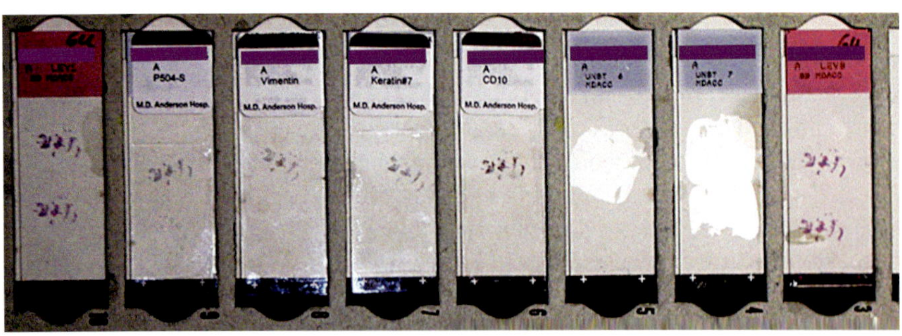

Fig. 7.2 Renal mass biopsy processing. Eight consecutive levels are cut, with the first and eighth levels stained with H&E and the intervening six levels cut as unstained sections on charged slides for potential immunohistochemical studies

focal nature of these morphologic changes and the low malignant potential of hybrid tumors [53, 56], it is risky to guarantee a diagnosis of oncocytoma on biopsy.

Malignant diagnoses rendered on biopsy are reliable and highly concordant with final pathology in terms of malignancy and RCC subtype, and less so for grade, as previously mentioned. However, ancillary studies are often required for an accurate

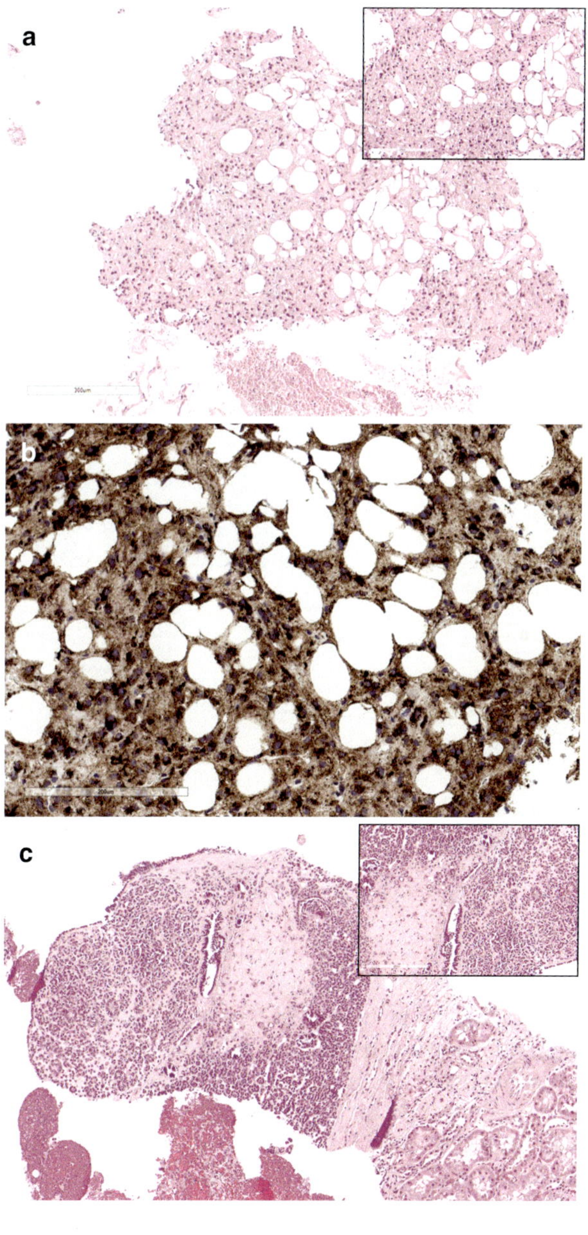

Fig. 7.3 Benign diagnoses reportable on biopsy include (**a**) angiomyolipoma showing immunoreactivity for Cathepsin K (**b**); and (**c**) metanephric adenoma showing immunoreactivity for (**d**) CD57 and (**e**) WT1. (**f**) Papillary adenoma may show similar histologic features as type 1 papillary RCC and cannot be reliably distinguished from the latter on biopsy

Fig. 7.3 (continued)

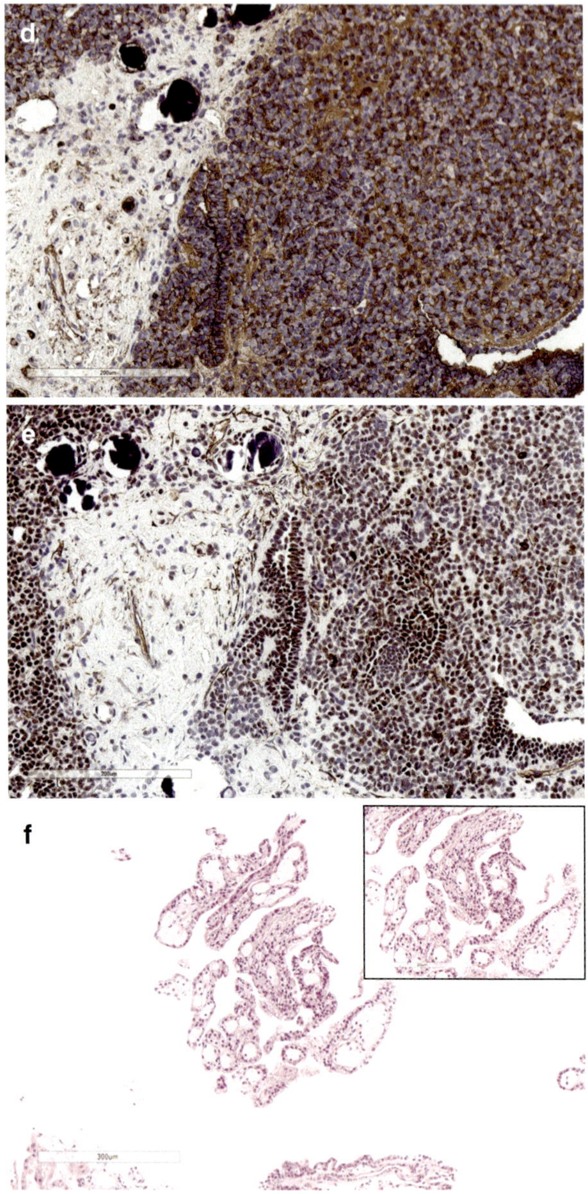

diagnosis given the mixed architectural features that characterize some RCC subtypes and based on the clinical scenario. For example, it is prudent to use a battery of immunohistochemical markers in a biopsy sampling of a renal cell carcinoma from a younger patient with clear cell features that can resolve the differential diagnosis between: clear cell RCC, clear cell papillary RCC, papillary RCC with clear cells, and MiT family translocation RCC as illustrated in Fig. 7.4a–e. Similarly, tumors with oncocytic cytoplasm have a broad differential diagnosis that spans benign (oncocytoma) and malignant (papillary RCC, chromophobe RCC) entities. While it may not be possible to guarantee a benign diagnosis of oncocytoma, immunohistochemistry is helpful in ruling in the malignant diagnoses of papillary and chromophobe RCC, as illustrated in Fig. 7.5a–e.

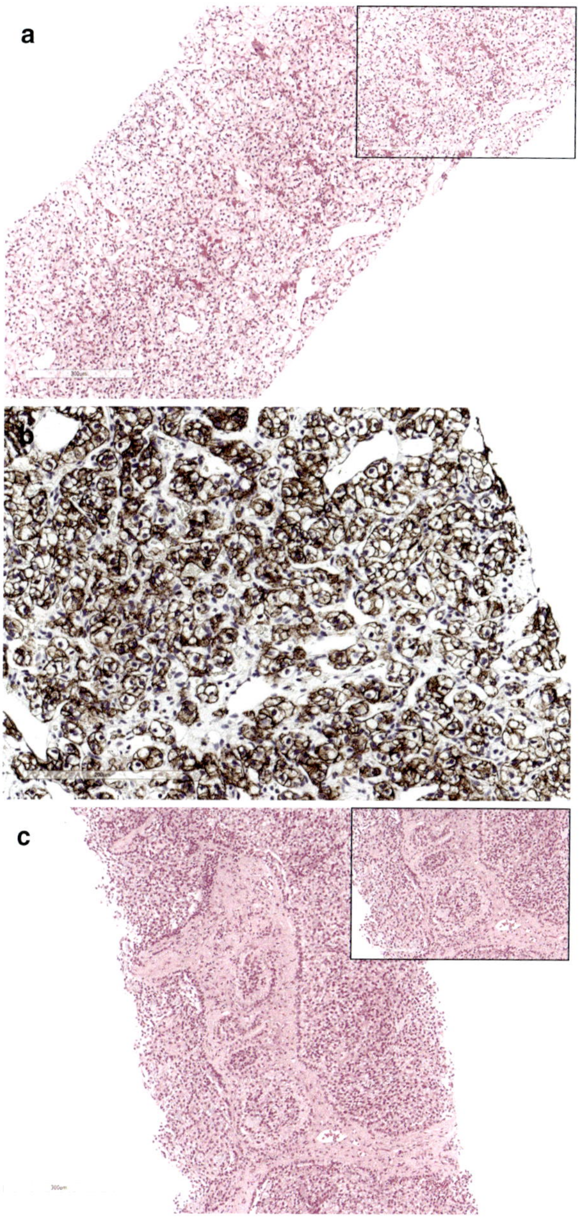

Fig. 7.4 Malignant diagnoses may require ancillary tests given the mixed architectural features of RCC subtypes and the limited biopsy sampling of the tumor. Renal cell carcinoma subtypes with clear cytoplasm include (**a**) clear cell RCC with labeling for CAIX (**b**); (**c**) papillary RCC with labeling for CK7 (**d**); and (**e**) MiTF translocation RCC

Fig. 7.4 (continued)

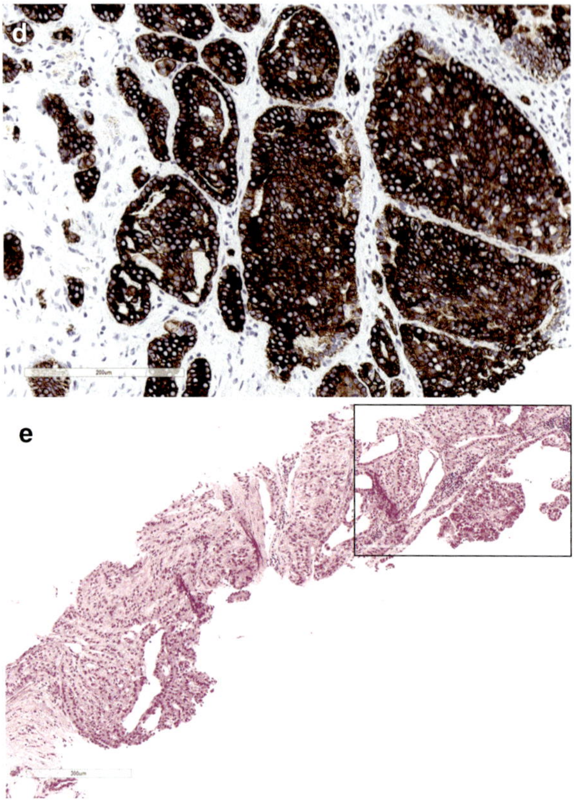

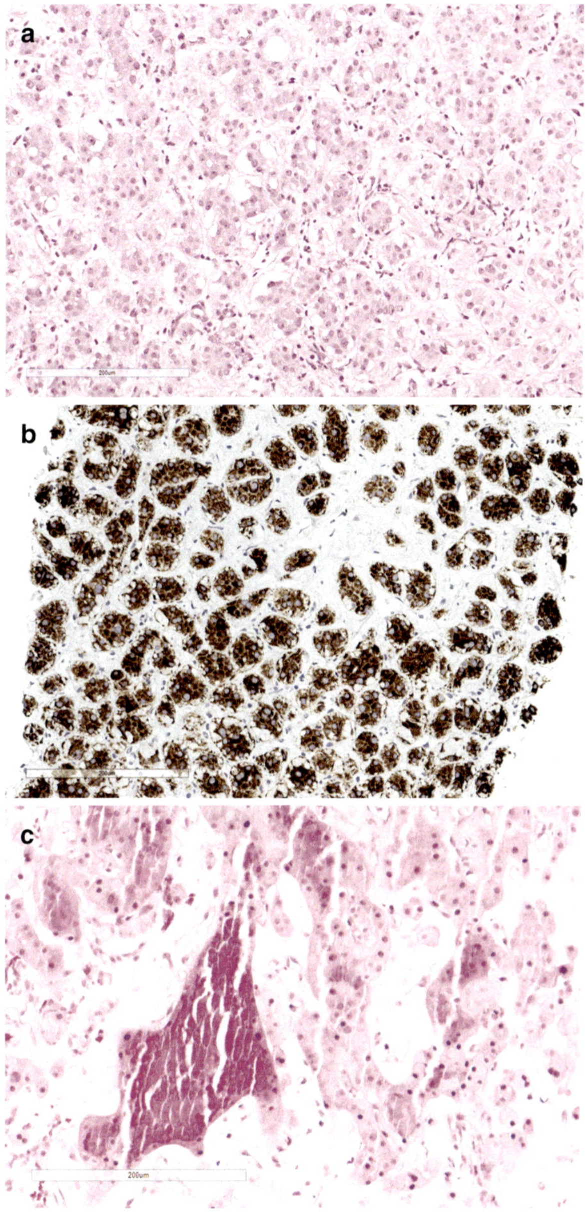

Fig. 7.5 Renal oncocytic tumors present a differential diagnosis including (**a**) papillary type 2 RCC that labels for P504s (**b**). Renal biopsy may be suggestive of renal oncocytoma (**c**) or chromophobe RCC (**d**) with immunohistochemical expression of CK7 (**e**). However, the existence of hybrid renal oncocytoma-like and chromophobe RCC-like areas in occasional tumors limits a biopsy diagnosis

Fig. 7.5 (continued)

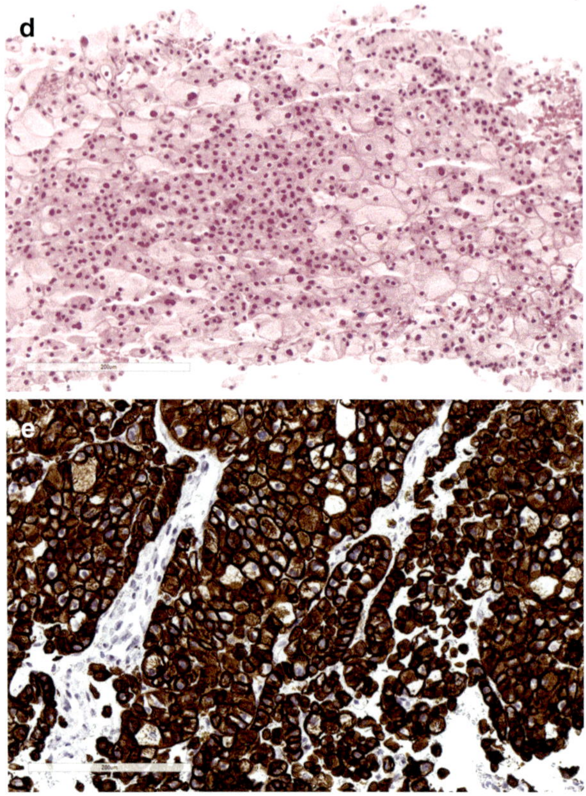

References

1. Bosniak MA. The Bosniak renal cyst classification: 25 years later. Radiology. 2012;262:781–5.
2. Kunkle DA, Egleston BL, Uzzo RG. Excise, ablate or observe: the small renal mass dilemma--a meta-analysis and review. J Urol. 2008;179:1227–33; discussion 33–4.
3. Leppert JT, Hanley J, Wagner TH, Chung BI, Srinivas S, Chertow GM, Brooks JD, Saigal CS, Urologic Diseases in America P. Utilization of renal mass biopsy in patients with renal cell carcinoma. Urology. 2014;83:774–9.
4. Appelbaum AH, Kamba TT, Cohen AS, Qaisi WG, Amirkhan RH. Effectiveness and safety of image-directed biopsies: coaxial technique versus conventional fine-needle aspiration. South Med J. 2002;95:212–7.
5. Breda A, Treat EG, Haft-Candell L, Leppert JT, Harper JD, Said J, Raman S, Smith RB, Belldegrun AS, Schulam PG. Comparison of accuracy of 14-, 18- and 20-G needles in ex-vivo renal mass biopsy: a prospective, blinded study. BJU Int. 2010;105:940–5.
6. Rybicki FJ, Shu KM, Cibas ES, Fielding JR, van Sonnenberg E, Silverman SG. Percutaneous biopsy of renal masses: sensitivity and negative predictive value stratified by clinical setting and size of masses. AJR Am J Roentgenol. 2003;180:1281–7.
7. Hobbs DJ, Zhou M, Campbell SC, Aydin H, Weight CJ, Lane BR. The impact of location and number of cores on the diagnostic accuracy of renal mass biopsy: an ex vivo study. World J Urol. 2013;31:1159–64.

8. Ginzburg S, Tomaszewski JJ, Kutikov A. Focal ablation therapy for renal cancer in the era of active surveillance and minimally invasive partial nephrectomy. Nat Rev Urol. 2017;14:669–82.
9. Woldrich JM, Palazzi K, Stroup SP, Sur RL, Parsons JK, Chang D, Derweesh IH. Trends in the surgical management of localized renal masses: thermal ablation, partial and radical nephrectomy in the USA, 1998-2008. BJU Int. 2013;111:1261–8.
10. Ljungberg B, Bensalah K, Canfield S, Dabestani S, Hofmann F, Hora M, Kuczyk MA, Lam T, Marconi L, Merseburger AS, Mulders P, Powles T, Staehler M, Volpe A, Bex A. EAU guidelines on renal cell carcinoma: 2014 update. Eur Urol. 2015;67:913–24.
11. Gervais DA, McGovern FJ, Arellano RS, McDougal WS, Mueller PR. Radiofrequency ablation of renal cell carcinoma: part 1, indications, results, and role in patient management over a 6-year period and ablation of 100 tumors. AJR Am J Roentgenol. 2005;185:64–71.
12. Breen DJ, Rutherford EE, Stedman B, Roy-Choudhury SH, Cast JE, Hayes MC, Smart CJ. Management of renal tumors by image-guided radiofrequency ablation: experience in 105 tumors. Cardiovasc Intervent Radiol. 2007;30:936–42.
13. Caputo PA, Zargar H, Ramirez D, Andrade HS, Akca O, Gao T, Kaouk JH. Cryoablation versus partial nephrectomy for clinical T1b renal tumors: a matched group comparative analysis. Eur Urol. 2017;71:111–7.
14. Lay AH, Faddegon S, Olweny EO, Morgan M, Lorber G, Trimmer C, Leveillee R, Cadeddu JA, Gahan JC. Oncologic efficacy of radio frequency ablation for small renal masses: clear cell vs papillary subtype. J Urol. 2015;194:653–7.
15. Halverson SJ, Kunju LP, Bhalla R, Gadzinski AJ, Alderman M, Miller DC, Montgomery JS, Weizer AZ, Wu A, Hafez KS, Wolf JS Jr. Accuracy of determining small renal mass management with risk stratified biopsies: confirmation by final pathology. J Urol. 2013;189:441–6.
16. Karam JA, Ahrar K, Vikram R, Romero CA, Jonasch E, Tannir NM, Rao P, Wood CG, Matin SF. Radiofrequency ablation of renal tumours with clinical, radiographical and pathological results. BJU Int. 2013;111:997–1005.
17. Hollingsworth JM, Miller DC, Daignault S, Hollenbeck BK. Rising incidence of small renal masses: a need to reassess treatment effect. J Natl Cancer Inst. 2006;98:1331–4.
18. Frank I, Blute ML, Cheville JC, Lohse CM, Weaver AL, Zincke H. Solid renal tumors: an analysis of pathological features related to tumor size. J Urol. 2003;170:2217–20.
19. Lane BR, Babineau D, Kattan MW, Novick AC, Gill IS, Zhou M, Weight CJ, Campbell SC. A preoperative prognostic nomogram for solid enhancing renal tumors 7 cm or less amenable to partial nephrectomy. J Urol. 2007;178:429–34.
20. Gill IS, Aron M, Gervais DA, Jewett MA. Clinical practice. Small renal mass. N Engl J Med. 2010;362:624–34.
21. Remzi M, Ozsoy M, Klingler HC, Susani M, Waldert M, Seitz C, Schmidbauer J, Marberger M. Are small renal tumors harmless? Analysis of histopathological features according to tumors 4 cm or less in diameter. J Urol. 2006;176:896–9.
22. Pahernik S, Ziegler S, Roos F, Melchior SW, Thuroff JW. Small renal tumors: correlation of clinical and pathological features with tumor size. J Urol. 2007;178:414–7; discussion 6–7.
23. Nguyen MM, Gill IS. Effect of renal cancer size on the prevalence of metastasis at diagnosis and mortality. J Urol. 2009;181:1020–7; discussion 7.
24. Klatte T, Patard JJ, de Martino M, Bensalah K, Verhoest G, de la Taille A, Abbou CC, Allhoff EP, Carrieri G, Riggs SB, Kabbinavar FF, Belldegrun AS, Pantuck AJ. Tumor size does not predict risk of metastatic disease or prognosis of small renal cell carcinomas. J Urol. 2008;179:1719–26.
25. Silverman SG, Gan YU, Mortele KJ, Tuncali K, Cibas ES. Renal masses in the adult patient: the role of percutaneous biopsy. Radiology. 2006;240:6–22.
26. Caoili EM, Davenport MS. Role of percutaneous needle biopsy for renal masses. Semin Intervent Radiol. 2014;31:20–6.
27. Patel HD, Johnson MH, Pierorazio PM, Sozio SM, Sharma R, Iyoha E, Bass EB, Allaf ME. Diagnostic accuracy and risks of biopsy in the diagnosis of a renal mass suspicious for localized renal cell carcinoma: systematic review of the literature. J Urol. 2016;195:1340–7.

28. Leveridge MJ, Finelli A, Kachura JR, Evans A, Chung H, Shiff DA, Fernandes K, Jewett MA. Outcomes of small renal mass needle core biopsy, nondiagnostic percutaneous biopsy, and the role of repeat biopsy. Eur Urol. 2011;60:578–84.
29. Mullins JK, Rodriguez R. Renal cell carcinoma seeding of a percutaneous biopsy tract. Can Urol Assoc J. 2013;7:E176–9.
30. Prince J, Bultman E, Hinshaw L, Drewry A, Blute M, Best S, Lee FT Jr, Ziemlewicz T, Lubner M, Shi F, Nakada SY, Abel EJ. Patient and tumor characteristics can predict nondiagnostic renal mass biopsy findings. J Urol. 2015;193:1899–904.
31. Park SY, Park BK, Kim CK, Kwon GY. Ultrasound-guided core biopsy of small renal masses: diagnostic rate and limitations. J Vasc Interv Radiol. 2013;24:90–6.
32. Shannon BA, Cohen RJ, de Bruto H, Davies RJ. The value of preoperative needle core biopsy for diagnosing benign lesions among small, incidentally detected renal masses. J Urol. 2008;180:1257–61; discussion 61.
33. Salem S, Ponsky LE, Abouassaly R, Cherullo EE, Isariyawongse JP, Maclennan GT, Nakamoto D, Haaga JR. Image-guided biopsy of small renal masses in the era of ablative therapies. Int J Urol. 2013;20:580–4.
34. Richard PO, Jewett MA, Bhatt JR, Kachura JR, Evans AJ, Zlotta AR, Hermanns T, Juvet T, Finelli A. Renal tumor biopsy for small renal masses: a single-center 13-year experience. Eur Urol. 2015;68:1007–13.
35. Gellert LL, Mehra R, Chen YB, Gopalan A, Fine SW, Al-Ahmadie H, Reuter VE, Tickoo SK. The diagnostic accuracy of percutaneous renal needle core biopsy and its potential impact on the clinical management of renal cortical neoplasms. Arch Pathol Lab Med. 2014;138:1673–9.
36. Somani BK, Nabi G, Thorpe P, N'Dow J, Swami S, McClinton S, Aberdeen A, Clinical Urological Surgeons G. Image-guided biopsy-diagnosed renal cell carcinoma: critical appraisal of technique and long-term follow-up. Eur Urol. 2007;51:1289–95; discussion 96–7.
37. Lebret T, Poulain JE, Molinie V, Herve JM, Denoux Y, Guth A, Scherrer A, Botto H. Percutaneous core biopsy for renal masses: indications, accuracy and results. J Urol. 2007;178:1184–8; discussion 8.
38. Wang R, Wolf JS Jr, Wood DP Jr, Higgins EJ, Hafez KS. Accuracy of percutaneous core biopsy in management of small renal masses. Urology. 2009;73:586–90; discussion 90–1.
39. Lhermitte B, de Leval L. Interpretation of needle biopsies of the kidney for investigation of renal masses. Virchows Arch. 2012;461:13–26.
40. Maturen KE, Nghiem HV, Caoili EM, Higgins EG, Wolf JS Jr, Wood DP Jr. Renal mass core biopsy: accuracy and impact on clinical management. AJR Am J Roentgenol. 2007;188:563–70.
41. Shah RB, Bakshi N, Hafez KS, Wood DP Jr, Kunju LP. Image-guided biopsy in the evaluation of renal mass lesions in contemporary urological practice: indications, adequacy, clinical impact, and limitations of the pathological diagnosis. Hum Pathol. 2005;36:1309–15.
42. Menogue SR, O'Brien BA, Brown AL, Cohen RJ. Percutaneous core biopsy of small renal mass lesions: a diagnostic tool to better stratify patients for surgical intervention. BJU Int. 2013;111:E146–51.
43. Millet I, Curros F, Serre I, Taourel P, Thuret R. Can renal biopsy accurately predict histological subtype and Fuhrman grade of renal cell carcinoma? J Urol. 2012;188:1690–4.
44. Volpe A, Mattar K, Finelli A, Kachura JR, Evans AJ, Geddie WR, Jewett MA. Contemporary results of percutaneous biopsy of 100 small renal masses: a single center experience. J Urol. 2008;180:2333–7.
45. Schmidbauer J, Remzi M, Memarsadeghi M, Haitel A, Klingler HC, Katzenbeisser D, Wiener H, Marberger M. Diagnostic accuracy of computed tomography-guided percutaneous biopsy of renal masses. Eur Urol. 2008;53:1003–11.
46. Al-Ahmadie HA, Alden D, Fine SW, Gopalan A, Touijer KA, Russo P, Reuter VE, Tickoo SK. Role of immunohistochemistry in the evaluation of needle core biopsies in adult renal cortical tumors: an ex vivo study. Am J Surg Pathol. 2011;35:949–61.

47. Sofikerim M, Tatlisen A, Canoz O, Tokat F, Demirtas A, Mavili E. What is the role of percutaneous needle core biopsy in diagnosis of renal masses? Urology. 2010;76:614–8.
48. Abel EJ, Culp SH, Matin SF, Tamboli P, Wallace MJ, Jonasch E, Tannir NM, Wood CG. Percutaneous biopsy of primary tumor in metastatic renal cell carcinoma to predict high risk pathological features: comparison with nephrectomy assessment. J Urol. 2010;184:1877–81.
49. Abel EJ, Culp SH, Meissner M, Matin SF, Tamboli P, Wood CG. Identifying the risk of disease progression after surgery for localized renal cell carcinoma. BJU Int. 2010;106:1277–83.
50. Reichelt O, Gajda M, Chyhrai A, Wunderlich H, Junker K, Schubert J. Ultrasound-guided biopsy of homogenous solid renal masses. Eur Urol. 2007;52:1421–6.
51. Patel HD, Druskin SC, Rowe SP, Pierorazio PM, Gorin MA, Allaf ME. Surgical histopathology for suspected oncocytoma on renal mass biopsy: a systematic review and meta-analysis. BJU Int. 2017;119:661–6.
52. Alderman MA, Daignault S, Wolf JS Jr, Palapattu GS, Weizer AZ, Hafez KS, Kunju LP, Wu AJ. Categorizing renal oncocytic neoplasms on core needle biopsy: a morphologic and immunophenotypic study of 144 cases with clinical follow-up. Hum Pathol. 2016;55:1–10.
53. Amin MB, Paner GP, Alvarado-Cabrero I, Young AN, Stricker HJ, Lyles RH, Moch H. Chromophobe renal cell carcinoma: histomorphologic characteristics and evaluation of conventional pathologic prognostic parameters in 145 cases. Am J Surg Pathol. 2008;32:1822–34.
54. Petersson F, Gatalica Z, Grossmann P, Perez Montiel MD, Alvarado Cabrero I, Bulimbasic S, Swatek A, Straka L, Tichy T, Hora M, Kuroda N, Legendre B, Michal M, Hes O. Sporadic hybrid oncocytic/chromophobe tumor of the kidney: a clinicopathologic, histomorphologic, immunohistochemical, ultrastructural, and molecular cytogenetic study of 14 cases. Virchows Arch. 2010;456:355–65.
55. Pote N, Vieillefond A, Couturier J, Arrufat S, Metzger I, Delongchamps NB, Camparo P, Mege-Lechevallier F, Molinie V, Sibony M. Hybrid oncocytic/chromophobe renal cell tumours do not display genomic features of chromophobe renal cell carcinomas. Virchows Arch. 2013;462:633–8.
56. Aslam MI, Spencer L, Garcea G, Pollard C, Metcalfe MS, Harrison RF, Dennison AR. A case of liver metastasis from an oncocytoma with a focal area of chromophobe renal cell carcinoma: a wolf in sheep's clothing. Int J Surg Pathol. 2009;17:158–62.

Chapter 8
Mesenchymal Kidney Tumors

Andres Matoso, Evgeny Yakirevich, and Shamlal Mangray

Mesenchymal tumors involving the kidney include a wide range of benign and malignant tumors and are relatively rare compared to epithelial neoplasms. Within the last two decades, there have been major discoveries in the underlying genomic alterations that drive the neoplastic process in mesenchymal lesions of the kidney. Specifically, a variety of translocation-associated sarcomas have been described arising from the kidney, significantly expanding the differential diagnosis of mesenchymal tumors primary to the kidney. This chapter is devoted to the clinical, morphologic, immunohistochemical, and genomic alterations of mesenchymal tumors that primarily occur in adults, with discussion of the differential diagnosis of specific entities. In contrast to the childhood lesions, most of these entities occur primarily in somatic soft tissue sites, but are also described in the kidney, and constitute an ever-increasing list that appear to have a predilection for this location. It must be recognized that many of the neoplasms reviewed also occur in children.

Sarcomas with "Small Round and/or Spindle Cell" Morphology

This group of tumor is composed by primitive sarcomas in which the cells are generally round or oval with spindle nuclei and scant cytoplasm. The designation of "small" has traditionally been appended to these tumors which can be misleading to the novice

A. Matoso (✉)
Department of Pathology, Urology, and Oncology, Johns Hopkins Medical Institutions, Baltimore, MD, USA
e-mail: amatoso1@jhmi.edu

E. Yakirevich · S. Mangray
Department of Pathology, Lifespan Academic Medical Center and Brown University, Providence, RI, USA

M. K. Divatia et al. (eds.), *Kidney Cancer*, https://doi.org/10.1007/978-3-030-28333-9_8

since the neoplastic cells are usually multiple orders of the size of small lymphocytes or red blood cells, but the scant cytoplasm has been responsible for the use of this adjective akin to small cell carcinoma of the lung. They have significant morphologic and immunophenotypic overlap, making the differential diagnosis challenging. Many of these neoplasms have characteristic translocations, and demonstration of these genomic alterations is key to confirmation of the diagnosis. The tumors of this group include Ewing sarcoma/primitive neuroectodermal tumor (EWS/PNET), Ewing-like sarcomas with *CIC* gene rearrangement and *BCOR-CCNB3* fusion, synovial sarcoma, desmoplastic small round cell tumor (DSRCT), and rhabdomyosarcoma (RMS).

Ewing Sarcoma/Primitive Neuroectodermal Tumor (EWS/PNET)

EWS/PNET are small round cell sarcomas that harbor the characteristic somatic reciprocal translocation t(11;22) that fuses *EWSR1* and *FLI1* to generate the EWSR1–FLI1 oncoprotein in the vast majority of cases. A literature review paper published in 2013 included 116 cases reported between 1975 and 2012 [1]. A recently published series of 23 cases included patients from 8 to 70 years old with a similar male: female distribution [2]. In this series, all cases were unilateral and presented as large masses with an average size of 12 cm with frequent extrarenal extension.

The gross appearance is of a fleshy tan tumor with hemorrhage, necrosis, and cystic change. Microscopically, most tumors are composed of uniform small round cells with round nuclei with fine chromatin and scant clear cytoplasm (Fig. 8.1). Neuroectodermal differentiation is variable with cells arranged in pseudorosettes. The growth pattern is solid in the majority of cases, but some may show focal papillary formation or alveolar pattern. Mitotic activity is brisk and necrosis and vascular invasion are common.

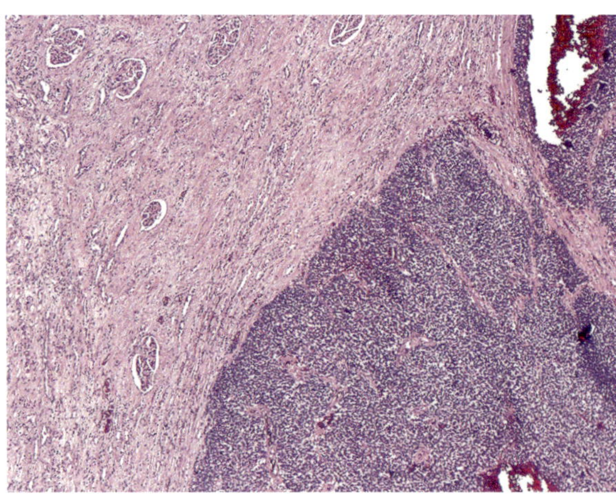

Fig. 8.1 Primitive neuroectodermal tumor/Ewing sarcoma of the kidney. Low power view shows a tumor composed of small blue cells with scant cytoplasm

By immunohistochemistry, tumor cells are usually positive for CD99, vimentin, and neuron-specific enolase and a subset of tumors can be positive for synaptophysin, or CD56. Although diffuse membranous CD99 positivity tends to be characteristic of EWS/PNET, studies on extrarenal EWS/PNETs have shown that such CD99 positivity can also be seen in other round cell tumors frequently considered in the differential diagnosis, including lymphoblastic lymphoma [3, 4], Merkel cell carcinoma [5], small cell carcinoma [6], rhabdomyosarcoma [7], desmoplastic small round cell tumor [8], small cell osteosarcoma [9], and mesenchymal chondrosarcoma [10]. While cytokeratins are usually negative, focal staining has been reported in up to 30% of kidney PNET/EWS cases [11]. Most recently, the transcription factor NKX2.2 has shown high sensitivity and relatively high specificity for EWS/PNET [12]. Still, a subset of tumors that enter in the differential diagnosis can be positive, including small cell carcinoma, myoepithelial carcinoma, desmoplastic small round cell tumor, and a high proportion of mesenchymal chondrosarcoma [13]. Molecular testing for the t(11;22) is usually used to confirm the diagnosis. This translocation is present in 85% of PNET/EWS. Other translocations found include *EWSR1–ERG, EWSR1–ETV1, EWSR1–ETV4, EWSR1–FEV, FUS–ERG, FUS–FEV* [14, 15]. Alternatively, fluorescence in situ hybridization (FISH) for demonstration of *EWSR1* rearrangement is used, but it has to be taken in the context of the immunophenotype of the neoplasm since other tumors in the differential diagnosis (e.g., DSRCT) share this rearrangement but have a different immunophenotype (see below).

Ewing-Like Sarcomas

This group of sarcomas are morphologically similar to PNET/EWS but lack rearrangements in the *EWSR1* gene. These tumors were initially termed Ewing-like sarcomas, and some studies found that approximately 70% of *EWSR1*-negative tumors harbor a *CIC–DUX4* or *CIC–FOXO4* rearrangement [16, 17]. Recently, primary renal *CIC*-rearranged tumors have been reported in both children and adults as individual case reports, small case series [18, 19] or within larger series of cases from all sites [20]. The first reported case was in a 9-year-old boy previously treated with chemotherapy, radiation, and stem cell transplantation for neuroblastoma [18]. Reported cases were large masses measuring between 7.8 and 18 cm. On cut surface, the tumors were solid with areas of necrosis and hemorrhage. Histologically, the tumors were composed of spindle and round cells with nuclei with coarse chromatin and areas with prominent nucleoli (Fig. 8.2). The cytoplasm was scant although one case showed focal rhabdoid morphology. The background was myxoid. Mitotic activity was high (>20/10 high-power fields). By immunohistochemistry, tumor cells showed variable membranous CD99, and one case had diffuse staining for bcl-2 and focal cytokeratin staining. One case was also positive for CD10. Reported cases were usually positive for WT1, either nuclear or cytoplasmic, as first described by Specht et al. in extrarenal tumors [21]. The first

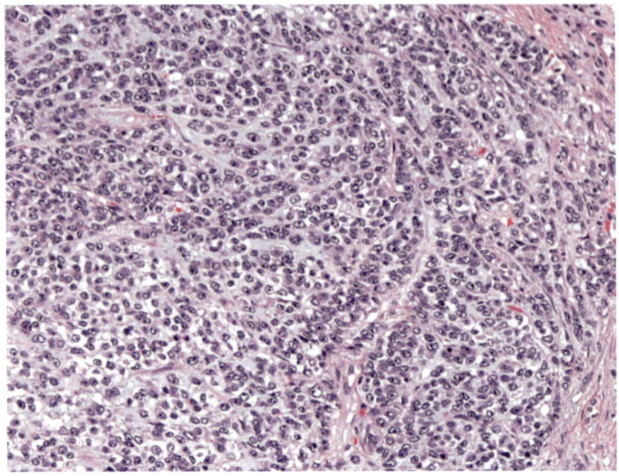

Fig. 8.2 Ewing-like sarcoma of the kidney with *CIC* gene rearrangement. The tumor is characterized by a population of small cells with scant cytoplasm and some myxoid background. Note nuclei with prominent nucleoli

case with nuclear staining for WT1 had been erroneously diagnosed as Wilms tumor prior to *CIC*-rearranged sarcomas becoming a well-established entity and was retrospectively diagnosed after recognition. Cases were diagnosed by FISH or RT-PCR, and further delineation of the fusions by next generation sequencing (NGS) was performed in a subset of cases [22]. Patients have responded poorly to therapy with the development of metastatic disease to lungs and brain, but treatment has varied results in reported cases. From available survival data in six reported cases, five patients died of disease or complications of treatment within 18 months of diagnosis, with only one child alive and free of disease at 24 months follow-up [22].

In addition to *CIC–DUX4* rearrangements, some "Ewing-like" sarcomas harbor fusion of *BCOR–CCNB3*, resulting in overexpression of BCOR and CCNB3 [23]. Recently, two primary renal sarcomas harboring BCOR–CCNB3 fusion were reported in 11-year-old and 12-year-old boys [24]. Both of these cases consisted of large tumors (13 and 27 cm) with solid areas but extensively cystic. Similar to other stromal tumors discussed here, the cystic spaces were lined by nonneoplastic entrapped renal tubules (Fig. 8.3). Beneath these cystic spaces, the neoplastic cells were spindled, monomorphic, and relatively bland. Areas with more epithelioid morphology were also described. By immunohistochemistry, both cases were diffusely positive for BCOR, Bcl2, and CD56. SATB2, cyclin D1, TLE1, Desmin, S100, cytokeratin AE1/AE3, CD34, and PAX8 were negative in both cases. FISH demonstrated the BCOR–CCNB3 fusion in both cases.

Synovial Sarcoma

Synovial sarcomas of the kidney are also rare and can affect both men and women with a wide age range [25–27]. The clinical presentation is that of any kidney mass including pain, hematuria, or incidental finding on imaging studies. The gross

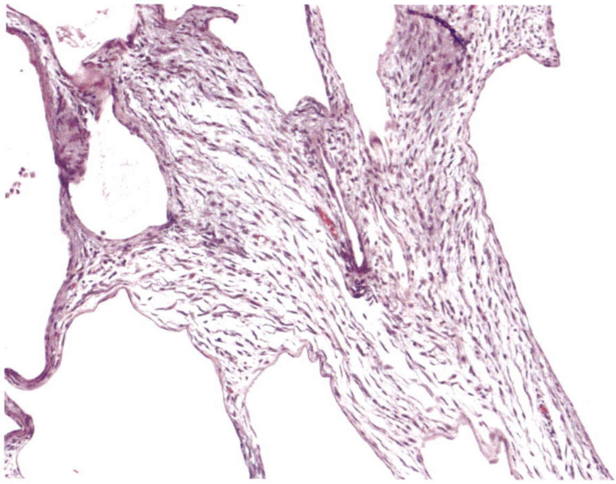

Fig. 8.3 Ewing-like sarcoma of the kidney with BCOR–CCNB3 rearrangement. The tumor shows solid areas but is extensively cystic. The cystic spaces are lined by nonneoplastic entrapped renal tubules. The neoplastic cells are spindled, monomorphic, and relatively bland

appearance is of a well-demarcated tumor with a soft gray cut surface. Some tumors have foci of hemorrhage and necrosis or smooth wall cysts. In the majority of the reported cases, these cysts were different from pseudocysts formed as a result of degenerative changes. They are typically not surrounded by fibrous pseudocapsule. Approximately, two-thirds of the reported cases are monophasic, with the remaining being either poorly differentiated synovial sarcoma with clusters of epithelioid cells with rhabdoid features or glandular formation [28–30]. Histologically, the tumor is composed of monomorphic plump spindle cells with scant cytoplasm and indistinct cell borders forming intersecting fascicles (Fig. 8.4). Nuclear anaplasia or prominent nucleoli are not seen. Mitotic activity is easily identifiable in all cases. In cases with cyst formation, cells having abundant eosinophilic cytoplasm with luminal snouts (hobnail appearance) line the cysts (Fig. 8.5). By immunohistochemistry, tumor cells are variably positive for pancytokeratin and EMA and negative for CK7, CK20, and WT1. The spindle cells can also be positive for vimentin, and variably BCL2. The epithelial cysts are positive for cytokeratin, PAX2, and PAX8, consistent with entrapped renal tubules [31]. The diagnosis can be confirmed by real-time PCR to detect SYT-SSX1 or SYT-SSX2 fusion transcript products of t(X;18). The main differential diagnosis is with sarcomatoid renal cell carcinoma or urothelial carcinoma for which the identification of a carcinomatous component is helpful. Immunohistochemistry for cytokeratin is not helpful in this situation as both tumors can be focally positive for various cytokeratin stains; however, the spindle cell component of a sarcomatoid carcinoma is usually more pleomorphic.

Desmoplastic Small Round Cell Tumor

It is a rare neoplasm that affects children and young adults, with approximately 10 cases reported in the kidney [32–38]. Tumors are solid with areas of necrosis and hemorrhage. As the name indicates, tumors are composed of small round cells with

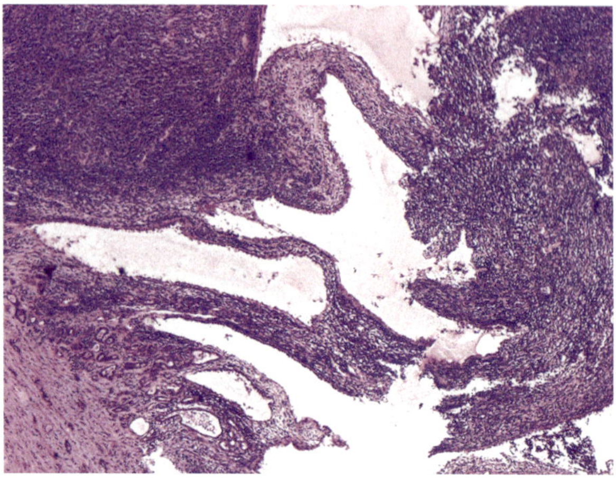

Fig. 8.4 Synovial sarcoma of the kidney. The tumor is hypercellular composed of a monomorphic population of spindle cells with scant cytoplasm. Note entrapped renal tubules forming cystic spaces

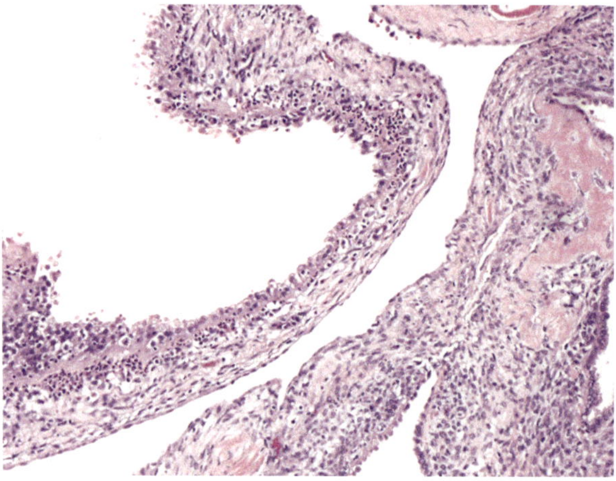

Fig. 8.5 Synovial sarcoma of the kidney mimicking mixed epithelial and stromal tumor (MEST). Extensive cystic change can distract the attention to the stromal component and lead to a misdiagnosis of MEST

scant cytoplasm and hyperchromatic nuclei. Mitotic activity is usually high. By immunohistochemistry, tumor cells are positive for vimentin, pancytokeratin, cytokeratin CAM5.2, EMA, smooth muscle actin, muscle-specific actin, desmin, FLI1, WT1 (the antibody to the C-terminal), and CD56. Perinuclear dot-like staining of desmin is a helpful feature in the differential diagnosis. The tumor harbors a t [11, 22] gene fusion between EWS and WT1, which is also helpful in the differential diagnosis with other small round cell tumors including Wilms.

Rhabdomyosarcoma

Primary rhabdomyosarcoma of the kidney is more frequent in children and young adults but has been reported at any age. While the genitourinary system is one of the most commonly systems involved by rhabdomyosarcoma, primary tumors of the

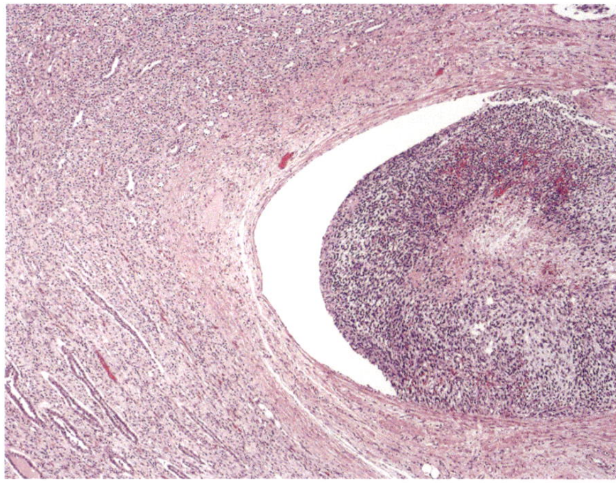

Fig. 8.6 Embryonal rhabdomyosarcoma arising in the renal pelvis. The tumor is composed of small blue cells underlying the urothelium of the renal pelvis

kidney are rare with only case reports published in the literature [39, 40]. Most tumors are embryonal type and botryoid type arising in the renal pelvis [41, 42]. Rhabdomyosarcomas are usually large with a soft grayish cut surface. Histologically, since most of these tumors are embryonal type, they are characterized by the following features (Fig. 8.6): (1) variable degrees of cellularity; (2) composed of small round cells with hyperchromatic nuclei and scant cytoplasm and cells with granular eosinophilic cytoplasm characteristic of rhabdomyoblasts; (3) more differentiated tumors show areas of spindle cells with occasional cross-striations; and (4) varying amount of myxoid background. Immunohistochemistry is essential to arrive at the diagnosis in most cases. The most commonly used markers include desmin and myogenin, which are positive in approximately 90% of rhabdomyosarcomas while negative in entities most frequently considered in the differential diagnosis, including Ewing family tumors and neuroblastomas. Alveolar rhabdomyosarcomas can show positive staining for cytokeratins and neuroendocrine markers, leading to confusions with other entities, especially Ewing family tumors [11]. PAX5 is also positive in alveolar rhabdomyosarcoma, particularly those harboring t(2;13) or (1;13). PCR or FISH techniques targeting these translocations can help in the differential diagnosis, but these are characteristic of the alveolar subtype and not the embryonal. The differential diagnosis should also include lymphoma, synovial sarcoma, desmoplastic small round cell tumor, and poorly differentiated angiosarcoma.

Smooth Muscle Tumors

Leiomyoma and Leiomyosarcoma

Benign and malignant tumors with smooth muscle differentiation constitute less than 1% of resected kidney tumors and are more frequent in women. They are more commonly located in the capsular/subcapsular area and around renal pelvis and renal vessels [43, 44]. Both leiomyomas and leiomyosarcomas in the kidney are morphologically identical to those found elsewhere. The characteristic morphology of bundles of smooth muscle cells without nuclear atypia arranged in nodules of varying sizes separated by stroma with thick wall vessels. Hyalinization can be pronounced. The presence of mitoses, hypercellularity, and nuclear atypia should raise consideration of leiomyosarcoma. The most recently published series of leiomyomas of the kidney included nine cases occurring in females. The majority of them (7/9) were asymptomatic, one patient presented with gross hematuria and one with abdominal pain. Five tumors were located in the renal capsule, two in the subcapsular area, and one originated in the large vessel in the renal sinus. The sizes varied from less than 1 to 7 cm [45].

The largest study of primary renal leiomyosarcomas was by Miller et al., who reviewed 27 cases from three institutions over a 23-year period in patients 22–83 years (mean 58.5) of age. The average size of tumors was 13.4 cm (range 4–26). The average mitotic rate was 11 per 10 high-power fields (HPFs; range 0–50) and the average extent of necrosis was 21% (range 0–50). Nuclear pleomorphism ranged from focal to extensive. Follow-up data were available in 20 cases and averaged 2.8 years (range 0.25–9), distant metastases found in 90% of these patients, and 75% eventually died of tumor burden [46].

By immunohistochemistry, smooth muscle tumors label with smooth muscle actin, desmin, heavy chain caldesmon, and calponin and are negative for markers of angiomyolipomas, including HMB45, Melan-A, and cathepsin-K. By and large, the tumors are negative with antibodies to cytokeratin, EMA, CD34, and S100, but focal aberrant expression may be seen. Estrogen and progesterone receptor are positive in the majority of renal leiomyomas [45].

Adipocytic Tumors

Lipoma and Liposarcoma

Lipomas are extremely rare in the kidney and an undersampled angiomyolipoma should be suspected. Well-differentiated/dedifferentiated liposarcoma could represent invasion from a retroperitoneal tumor. Immunohistochemistry markers for angiomyolipomas (HMB-45, melan-A, cathepsin-K, smooth muscle actin, and estrogen receptor) should be negative before diagnosing a fatty tumor in the kidney as lipoma. The differential diagnosis should also include idiopathic renal lipomatosis and fatty expansion of the renal sinus [47]. Two cases have been reported of liposarcomatous differentiation in chromophobe renal cell carcinoma [48, 49].

Nerve Sheath Tumors

Schwannoma This tumor is rare in the kidney with the majority of the reports being isolated cases or small series [50–52]. They are more common in women and can be located anywhere in the kidney but more frequently near the renal hilum. Tumors are usually well circumscribed and encapsulated, but multinodular cases and cystic change have also been reported [50]. The microscopic features are the same as schwannomas in other sites. A proportion of the cases can be classified as cellular characterized by entirely Antoni A pattern and absence of Verocay bodies. Additionally, bizarre nuclear atypia, also known as ancient change, is clinically important to recognize and to avoid overdiagnosing the lesion as malignant or sarcomatoid carcinoma, especially in needle biopsy specimens. In addition to sarcomatoid carcinoma, the differential diagnoses include malignant peripheral nerve sheath tumor, angiomyolipoma, synovial sarcoma, solitary fibrous tumor, leiomyoma, rhabdomyosarcoma, and angiosarcoma.

Vascular Tumors

Angiomyolipoma Renal angiomyolipomas (AMLs) are tumors formed of variable amounts of three components: adipose tissue, tortuous thick-walled vessels, and cells with smooth muscle differentiation (Fig. 8.7). There is evidence that the AMLs belong to the family of perivascular epithelioid cell tumors (PEComas) [53]. It can be associated with tuberous sclerosis but they are most frequently sporadic [54]. Sporadic AMLs are four times more frequent in women. The clinical presentation is similar to other renal masses: incidental finding, abdominal pain, and/or hematuria. A minority of patients may present with rupture and intraabdominal bleeding. Grossly, AMLs are typically well circumscribed, sometimes with infiltrating edges. It may involve the perirenal soft tissue and even lymph nodes (Fig. 8.8), but these features are not associated with malignancy. Histologically, AMLs show vessels with thick wall and spindle cells radiating off the wall. The spindle cells have an appearance similar to smooth muscle cells with blunt end elongated nuclei and eosinophilic cytoplasm. Variants of AMLs include fat poor, epithelioid [55], epithelioid AML with atypia [56], and angiomyolipoma with epithelial cysts [57]. Fat poor-AMLs are more common in needle biopsy specimens because they are difficult to distinguish from renal cell carcinoma on image studies, and therefore, undergo more frequent biopsy [58]. The epithelioid variant is characterized by round cells with variable amount of eosinophilic or clear cytoplasm and sometimes bizarre nuclear atypia (atypical epithelioid AMLs). Rarely, epithelioid AMLs can have a malignant behavior. Malignancy in AMLs has been associated with the presence of at least three of the following findings: (1) >70% atypical epithelioid cells,

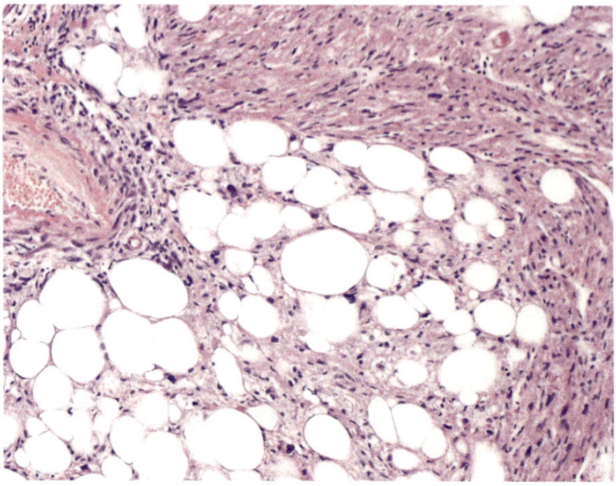

Fig. 8.7 Angiomyolipoma (AML) composed of its three elements: blood vessels, adipose tissue, and spindle cells with smooth muscle differentiation. Note scattered nuclear enlargement and irregular nuclear membranes occasionally seen in AMLs, a feature not associated with poor clinical outcome

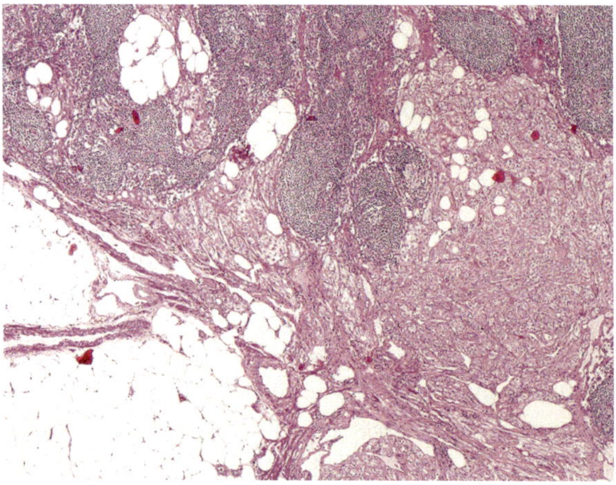

Fig. 8.8 Angiomyolipoma (AML) involving a perirenal lymph node. This finding is not associated with aggressive clinical course

(2) two or more mitotic figures per 10 HPFs, (3) atypical mitotic figures, or (4) necrosis [56]. By immunohistochemistry, AMLs are positive for melanocytic markers HMB45, Melan-A, and tyrosinase. These are often focally positive and therefore a panel of markers is recommended. Other positive markers include cathepsin-K and smooth muscle actin. PAX-8 and keratin stains are frequently negative and might be helpful in the distinction of epithelioid AMLs and renal cell carcinoma.

Hemangioma and Anastomosing Hemangioma

This rare benign vascular proliferation can be seen in patients with Klippel–Trenaunay and Sturge–Weber syndromes, end-stage renal disease, or sporadically. Hemangiomas are usually solitary, unilateral, and do not have a sex predilection. A study of 76 surgical and autopsy specimens revealed that the lesions are most

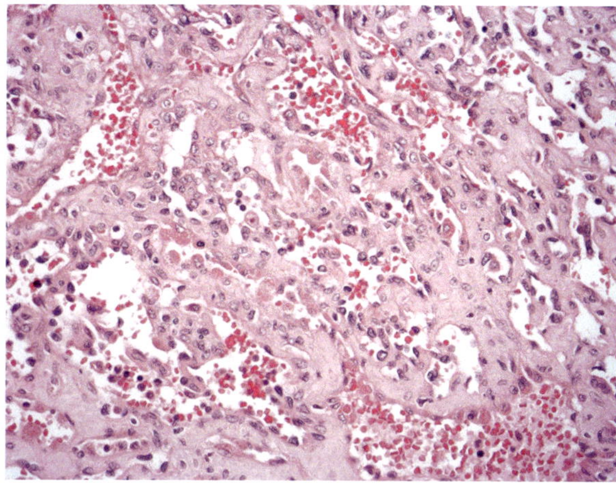

Fig. 8.9 Anastomosing hemangioma of the kidney. The tumor is composed of anastomosing sinusoidal capillary-size blood vessels with focal hobnail nuclei but without nuclear stratification or significant nuclear atypia

commonly located in the mucosa or submucosa of the renal pelvis, pyramids, and cortex [59]. They can cause intraparenchymal bleeding. Anastomosing hemangiomas have also been reported in the kidney with the caveat that they have to be differentiated from angiosarcoma [60]. Grossly, these tumors were located near the renal hilum, measured up to 1.7 cm and had a hemorrhagic and mahogany spongy cut surface. In three of four cases in this series, the tumor showed minor extension into the perirenal adipose tissue. On histologic examination, the tumors were composed of anastomosing sinusoidal capillary-size blood vessels with focal hobnail nuclei but without nuclear stratification or significant nuclear atypia (Fig. 8.9). Mitoses were absent or rare. Extramedullary hematopoiesis was identified in a minority of cases. The anastomosing pattern can raise concern for angiosarcoma; however, the small size, well-defined borders, lack of significant atypia, and infrequent mitoses should be deterrent of a malignant diagnosis. Additionally, vascular lesions of the kidney should be examined carefully to exclude a renal cell carcinoma with prominent vasculature, recently reported as hemangioma-like renal cell carcinoma [61].

Hemangioblastoma

Renal hemangioblastomas are extremely rare and consist of a network of capillary-sized and thin blood vessels and interstitial microvacuolated stromal cells. Hemangioblastomas are one of the manifestations of von Hippel–Lindau disease caused by germline mutation of the *VHL* tumor suppressor gene. There was no association with von Hippel–Lindau in any of the renal cases reported in the literature [62–64]. The clinical presentation is that of any kidney mass and they can vary in size from 2 to more than 10 cm. Grossly, these tumors show a gray cut surface with focal cystic change. On light microscopy, the tumor is composed by a network of small vessels surrounded by cells with large pale eosinophilic cytoplasm and

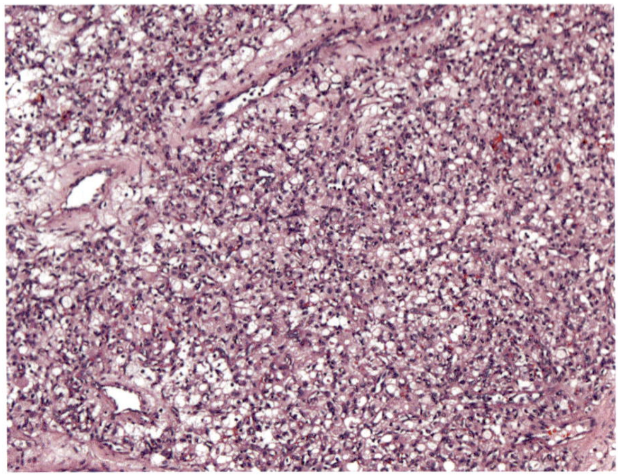

Fig. 8.10 Renal hemangioblastoma. The tumor is composed of a network of small vessels surrounded by cells with large pale eosinophilic cytoplasm and round to oval nuclei

round to oval nuclei (Fig. 8.10). These large cells can be morphologically confused with clear cell renal cell carcinoma, histiocytes, or lipoblasts. By immunohistochemistry, hemangioblastomas are positive for inhibin, neuron-specific enolase, and S-100. PAX8 can be positive, adding confusion with clear cell renal cell carcinoma. Recurrence or metastasis has not been reported after resection.

Lymphangioma

Renal lymphangiomas are rare and can occur in children and adults and anywhere in the kidney parenchyma [65–69]. Clinically, they can cause mass-related symptoms including urinary obstruction [70]. Due to its multicystic appearance, it can be confused with a cystic nephroma. Vascular markers CD31, Factor VIII, and D2-40 would be positive in lymphangiomas and not in cystic nephromas. Lymphangiomas are benign lesions and excision should be curative.

Angiosarcoma

Primary renal angiosarcomas are more frequent in the sixth and seventh decades and have a clear predilection for males [71]. Renal angiosarcomas are infiltrative lesions with extensive parenchymal destruction and are more commonly composed of highly atypical spindle and epithelioid cells (Figs. 8.11 and 8.12). The main differential diagnosis is with sarcomatoid carcinoma and the diagnosis is supported by positive immunohistochemistry for CD31, CD34, or FLI-1. Renal angiosarcomas have a poor prognosis and most patients die within months to 1 year after the initial diagnosis [72].

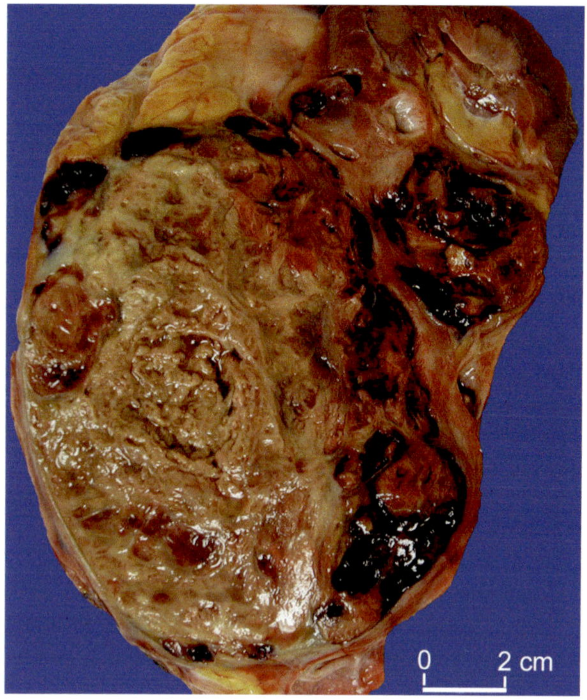

Fig. 8.11 Gross image of a large renal angiosarcoma

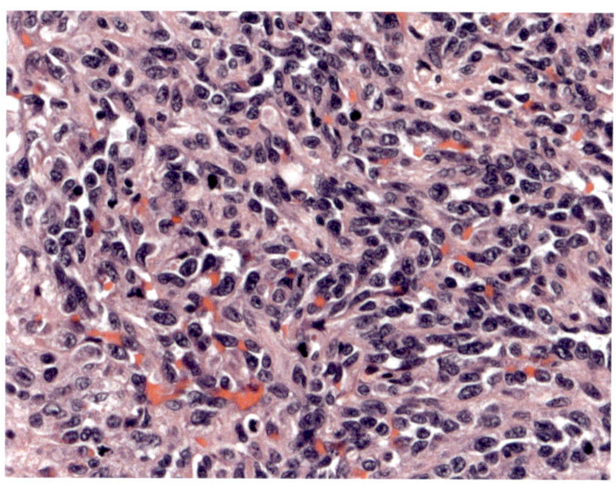

Fig. 8.12 Angiosarcoma composed of highly atypical spindle cells with intercalated red blood cells and red blood cell fragments. Note brisk mitotic activity

Other Vascular Tumors

Glomus tumor [73, 74], glomangiomyomas [75], and myopericytomas [76–78] involving the kidney have also been reported in the literature. They have similar morphologic features as those in other sites. By immunohistochemistry, tumor cells are positive for smooth muscle actin and CD34 highlights the endothelial cells surrounded by the tumor cells, consistent with their perivascular origin. In general, these tumors are benign, although a case of malignant glomus tumor of the kidney has been reported in the literature [79].

Fibrous Tumors

Medullary Fibroma

Also called renomedullary interstitial cell tumor, medullary fibroma is a common tumor usually found incidentally or in autopsy. There is a female predominance. The tumor originates from interstitial cells of the medulla. The majority of these tumors are asymptomatic, but there are rare reports of urinary obstruction due to protrusion into the renal pelvis [80].

Grossly, medullary fibromas are solid white and well circumscribed usually subcentimeter in size. Histologically, tumor cells are spindle with bland ovoid nuclei and can entrap renal tubules (Fig. 8.13). By immunohistochemistry, tumor cells are usually positive for CD35 and smooth muscle actin, although these are rarely required to arrive at the diagnosis. These are benign tumors and do not require treatment except for the rare situation of renal outflow obstruction [81].

Sclerosing Epithelioid Fibrosarcoma

Primary sclerosing fibrosarcomas of the kidney were recently described by Argani et al. with only two cases reported [82]. The gross appearance of these tumors is described as firm and white with protrusion of the renal capsule or renal pelvis.

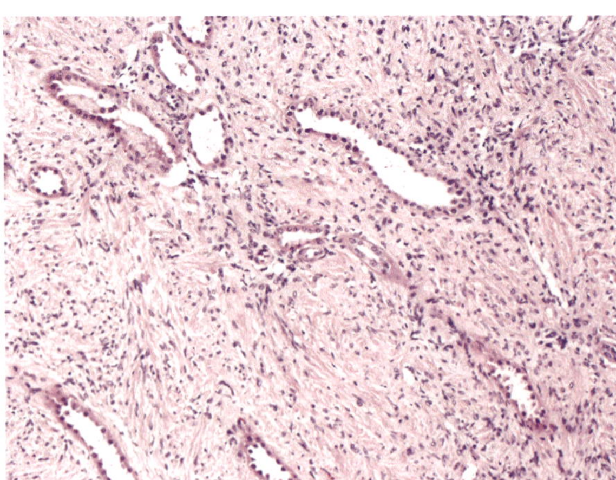

Fig. 8.13 Medullary fibroma. Tumor cells are spindle with bland ovoid nuclei and can entrap renal tubules

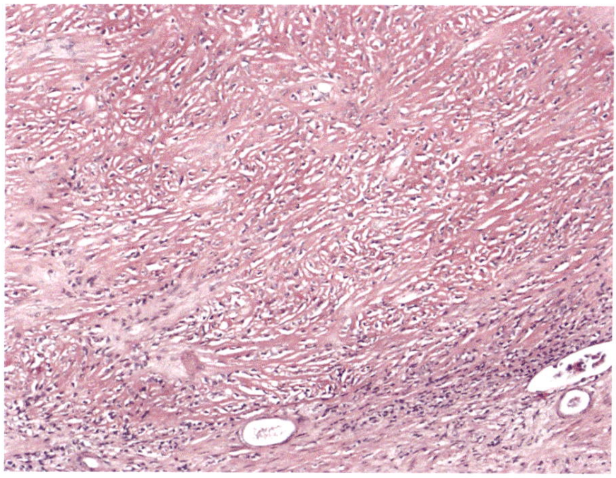

Fig. 8.14 Sclerosing epithelioid fibrosarcoma. Tumor cells have an epithelioid appearance with small angulated nuclei and clear cytoplasm arranged in cords in a background of hyaline sclerosis

Histologically, tumor cells have an epithelioid appearance with small angulated nuclei and clear cytoplasm arranged in cords in a background of hyaline sclerosis (Fig. 8.14). Cellularity is variable. One of the cases reported showed entrapped renal tubules with tubulopapillary hyperplasia, resembling a biphasic neoplasm. One case also demonstrated an area of myxoid background with bland spindle cells in a swirling pattern, closely resembling low-grade fibromyxoid sarcoma. Clinically, one case showed liver and the epidural metastases. By immunohistochemistry, both cases were diffusely positive for MUC4, bcl2, and vimentin. Negative stains include cytokeratin AE1/AE3, desmin, and S100 protein. By FISH, both neoplasm demonstrated the presence of *EWSR1–CREB3L1* rearrangement.

Solitary Fibrous Tumor

Solitary fibrous tumor (SFT) of the kidney is rare with the first case described in 1996 [83]. Since then many other reports have added to the literature and currently there are more than 40 cases have been reported [84]. The clinical presentation is that of any kidney mass, either discovered incidentally or causing symptoms including pain, hematuria, or palpable mass [85]. The paraneoplastic syndrome of hypoglycemia due to secretion of insulin-like growth factor has not been reported so far in primary kidney SFTs. Grossly, kidney SFTs vary in size and there are reported cases of up to 25 cm. They are most commonly well-demarcated tumors with a tan-white cut surface. Malignant cases may show cystic changes, necrosis, and hemorrhage. Histologically, SFTs are characterized by variable patterns both within the same tumor and among different cases. Tumor cells are spindle with bland nuclei and arranged in several different patterns including whorled, short fascicular, or storiform neurofibroma-like pattern [86]. The background usually shows areas of dense hyaline collagen intercalated with more cellular regions and foci of myxoid change. The tumor shows a characteristic vasculature composed of elongated thin-walled vessels with branching often referred to as "staghorn vessels" or "hemangiopericytoma-like vessels." SFTs are typically immunoreactive to CD34, CD99, bcl2, and STAT6, and negative for S100, desmin, smooth muscle actin, and cytokeratins [87, 88].

Miscellaneous

Renal myxoma Renal myxomas are extremely rare and have been reported to arise from the renal parenchyma or the renal capsule [89–91]. This tumor is usually well circumscribed with a gelatinous cut surface. Histologically, the tumor is hypocellular, hypovascular, and composed of small angulated cells with hyperchromatic nuclei and elongated cytoplasm, sometimes with stellate appearance. The background is myxoid with a loose meshwork of thin reticulin fibers. There is minimal nuclear pleomorphism and multinucleated cells are not seen. The differential diagnosis includes any other tumor with a myxoid background but the hypocellular nature, the bland appearance of the tumor cells, lack of pleomorphism, and absence of mitoses should provide enough diagnostic clues. The intramuscular myxomas can show areas of hypercellularity and hypervascularity, but tumor cells preserve the nuclear characteristics of benign myxomas [92]. Myxomas are benign and resection should be curative.

Juxtaglomerular Cell Tumor (JGCT)

JGCT is a rare renin-secreting tumor that typically occurs in young adults and more commonly occurs in females (M:F = 1:2). Patients present with features of uncontrolled hypertension and on imaging workup, a unilateral peripherally located solitary renal mass is identified accompanied by laboratory features of hyperaldosteronism and hypokalemia [93].

Most tumors are between 3 and 5 cm circumscribed yellow-tan mass, but subcentimeter examples as well as lesions as large as 15 cm have been reported. Histologically, lesional cells are polygonal or spindled with indistinct cell borders, and round or oval nuclei. Vascular structures are prominent with both thin-walled and thick-walled vessels and a hemangiopericytoma-like pattern may be encountered. Rarely, these tumors can have a papillary configuration or nuclear pleomorphism [94, 95]. In the cases with a papillary configuration, a mixed epithelial and stromal tumor (MEST) or metanephric adenofibroma (MAF) will be in the differential diagnosis especially since juxtaglomerular cell hyperplasia can be seen in the stromal component of MAF (Fig. 8.15). The presence of hypertension is helpful in making the distinction, but MAF may also have hypertension. The neoplastic cells of JGCT express SMA, muscle-specific actin, CD34, CD117, vimentin, and renin [95]. Desmin, S-100, HMB45, chromogranin, and synaptophysin are negative. Cytokeratin is negative, but the entrapped renal tubular epithelium is highlighted

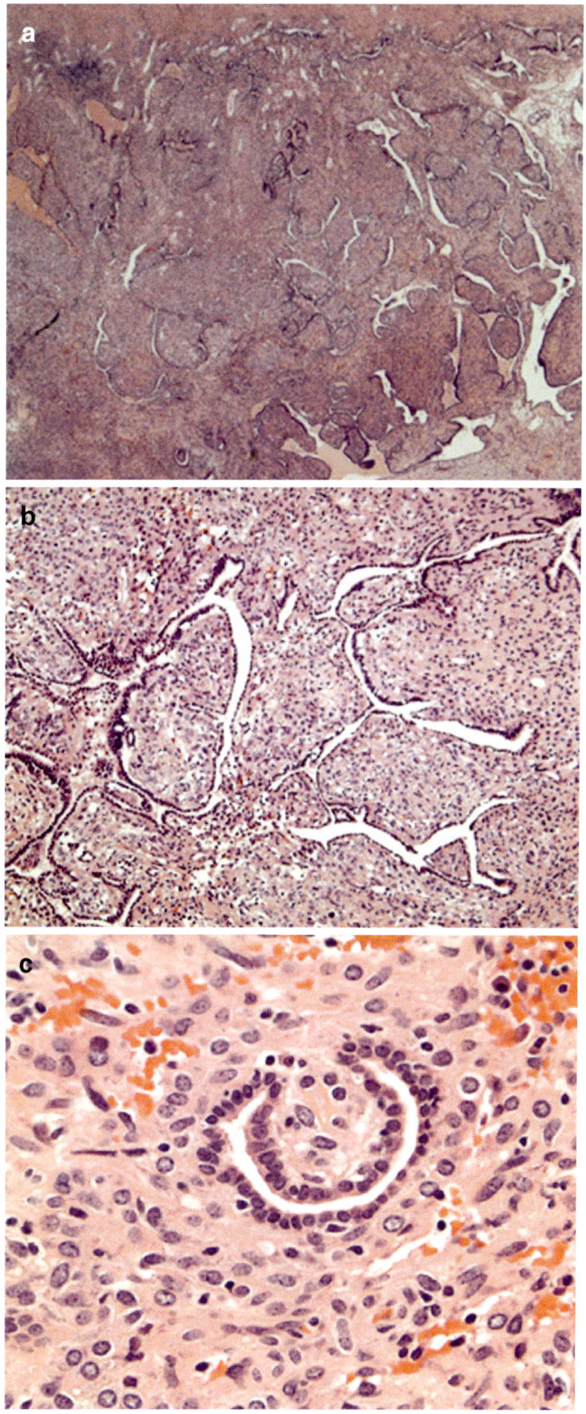

Fig. 8.15 Juxtaglomerular cell tumor (JGCT). (**a**) Low power H&E image demonstrates a papillary configuration. (**b**) Medium power H&E image demonstrates the entrapped renal tubular epithelium lining the papillary processes. (**c**) High power demonstrates eosinophilic lesional cells with indistinct cytoplasmic borders and entrapped epithelium with a glomeruloid configuration. (**d**) Thick-walled arteries (arrowheads) are present in this JGCT. (**e**) Cytokeratin highlights the entrapped epithelium. (**f**) A CD34 stain is positive in the neoplastic cells

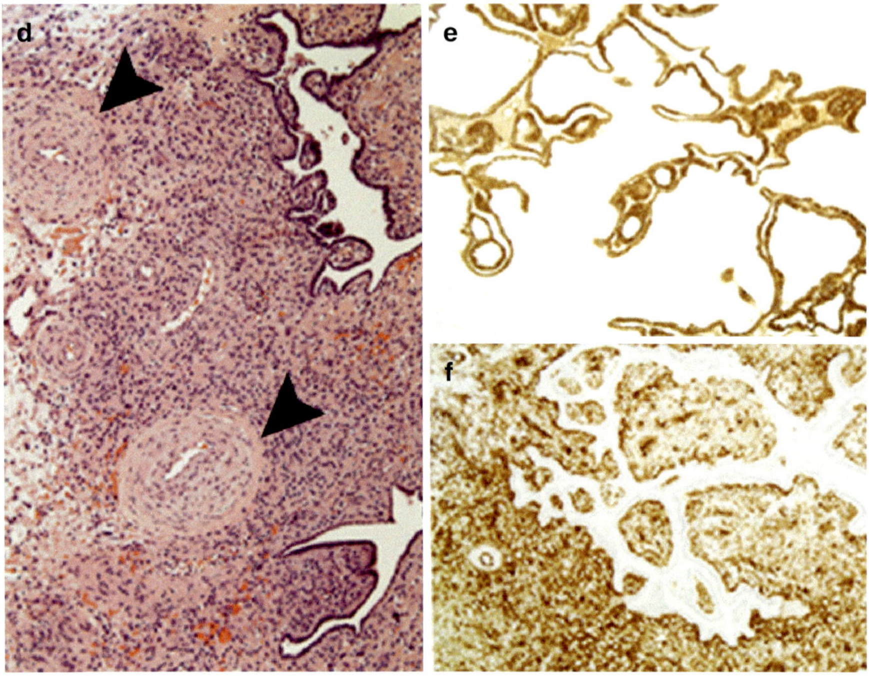

Fig. 8.15 (continued)

and is profuse in examples with a papillary configuration (Fig. 8.15). Cytogenetic studies have revealed gains of chromosome 4 and 10, loss of chromosome 9 and 11, and aneusomy as well as upregulation and downregulation of multiple genes involved in neoplasia [95]. The vast majority of JGCT are benign and there is usually resolution of hypertension after excision, rare examples of malignant cases with metastatic disease are reported [96].

References

1. Risi E, Iacovelli R, Altavilla A, et al. Clinical and pathological features of primary neuroectodermal tumor/Ewing sarcoma of the kidney. Urology. 2013;82:382–6.
2. Murugan P, Rao P, Tamboli P, et al. Primary Ewing sarcoma / primitive neuroectodermal tumor of the kidney: a clinicopathologic study of 23 cases. Pathol Oncol Res. 2018;24(1):153–9.
3. Ozdemirli M, Fanburg-Smith JC, Hartmann DP, et al. Precursor B-lymphoblastic lymphoma presenting as a solitary bone tumor and mimicking Ewing's sarcoma: a report of four cases and review of the literature. Am J Surg Pathol. 1998;22:795–804.
4. Ozdemirli M, Fanburg-Smith JC, Hartmann DP, et al. Differentiating lymphoblastic lymphoma and Ewing's sarcoma: lymphocyte markers and gene rearrangement. Mod Pathol. 2001;14:1175–82.
5. Perlman EJ, Lumadue JA, Hawkins AL, et al. Primary cutaneous neuroendocrine tumors. Diagnostic use of cytogenetic and MIC2 analysis. Cancer Genet Cytogenet. 1995;82:30–4.

6. Lumadue JA, Askin FB, Perlman EJ. MIC2 analysis of small cell carcinoma. Am J Clin Pathol. 1994;102:692–4.
7. Folpe AL, Hill CE, Parham DM, et al. Immunohistochemical detection of FLI-1 protein expression: a study of 132 round cell tumors with emphasis on CD99-positive mimics of Ewing's sarcoma/primitive neuroectodermal tumor. Am J Surg Pathol. 2000;24:1657–62.
8. Gerald WL, Ladanyi M, De Alava E, et al. Clinical, pathologic, and molecular spectrum of tumors associated with T(11;22)(P13;Q12): desmoplastic small round-cell tumor and its variants. J Clin Oncol. 1998;16:3028–36.
9. Devaney K, Abbondanzo SL, Shekitka KM, et al. MIC2 detection in tumors of bone and adjacent soft tissues. Clin Orthop Relat Res. 1995:176–87.
10. Granter SR, Renshaw AA, Fletcher CD, et al. CD99 reactivity in mesenchymal chondrosarcoma. Hum Pathol. 1996;27:1273–6.
11. Folpe AL, Goldblum JR, Rubin BP, et al. Morphologic and immunophenotypic diversity in Ewing family tumors: a study of 66 genetically confirmed cases. Am J Surg Pathol. 2005;29:1025–33.
12. Yoshida A, Sekine S, Tsuta K, et al. NKX2.2 is a useful immunohistochemical marker for Ewing sarcoma. Am J Surg Pathol. 2012;36:993–9.
13. Hung YP, Fletcher CD, Hornick JL. Evaluation of NKX2-2 expression in round cell sarcomas and other tumors with EWSR1 rearrangement: imperfect specificity for Ewing sarcoma. Mod Pathol. 2016;29:370–80.
14. Ng TL, O'sullivan MJ, Pallen CJ, et al. Ewing sarcoma with novel translocation T(2;16) producing an in-frame fusion of FUS and FEV. J Mol Diagn. 2007;9:459–63.
15. Shing DC, Mcmullan DJ, Roberts P, et al. FUS/ERG gene fusions in Ewing's tumors. Cancer Res. 2003;63:4568–76.
16. Graham C, Chilton-Macneill S, Zielenska M, et al. The CIC-DUX4 fusion transcript is present in a subgroup of pediatric primitive round cell sarcomas. Hum Pathol. 2012;43:180–9.
17. Italiano A, Sung YS, Zhang L, et al. High prevalence of cic fusion with double-homeobox (DUX4) transcription factors in EWSR1-negative undifferentiated small blue round cell sarcomas. Genes Chromosomes Cancer. 2012;51:207–18.
18. Mangray S, Somers GR, He J, et al. Primary undifferentiated sarcoma of the kidney harboring a novel variant of CIC-DUX4 gene fusion. Am J Surg Pathol. 2016;40:1298–301.
19. Bergerat S, Barthelemy P, Mouracade P, et al. Primary CIC-DUX4 round cell sarcoma of the kidney: a treatment-refractory tumor with poor outcome. Pathol Res Pract. 2017;213:154–60.
20. Antonescu CR, Owosho AA, Zhang L, et al. Sarcomas with CIC-rearrangements are a distinct pathologic entity with aggressive outcome: a clinicopathologic and molecular study of 115 cases. Am J Surg Pathol. 2017;41:941–9.
21. Specht K, Sung YS, Zhang L, et al. Distinct transcriptional signature and immunoprofile of CIC-DUX4 fusion-positive round cell tumors compared to EWSR1-rearranged Ewing sarcomas: further evidence toward distinct pathologic entities. Genes Chromosomes Cancer. 2014;53:622–33.
22. Mangray S, Kelly D, Leguellec S, et al. Clinical, morphologic, immunohistochemical and molecular features of a series of primary renal CIC-rearranged sarcomas. Am J Surg Pathol. 2018;42(10):1360–9.
23. Pierron G, Tirode F, Lucchesi C, et al. A new subtype of bone sarcoma defined by BCOR-CCNB3 gene fusion. Nat Genet. 2012;44:461–6.
24. Argani P, Kao YC, Zhang L, et al. Primary renal sarcomas with BCOR-CCNB3 gene fusion: a report of 2 cases showing histologic overlap with clear cell sarcoma of kidney, suggesting further link between BCOR-related sarcomas of the kidney and soft tissues. Am J Surg Pathol. 2017;41:1702–12.
25. Mirza M, Zamilpa I, Bunning J. Primary renal synovial sarcoma. Urology. 2008;72:716.. E711-712
26. Shannon BA, Murch A, Cohen RJ. Primary renal synovial sarcoma confirmed by cytogenetic analysis: a lesion distinct from sarcomatoid renal cell carcinoma. Arch Pathol Lab Med. 2005;129:238–40.

27. Argani P, Faria PA, Epstein JI, et al. Primary renal synovial sarcoma: molecular and morphologic delineation of an entity previously included among embryonal sarcomas of the kidney. Am J Surg Pathol. 2000;24:1087–96.
28. Palau LM, Thu Pham T, Barnard N, et al. Primary synovial sarcoma of the kidney with rhabdoid features. Int J Surg Pathol. 2007;15:421–8.
29. Chen PC, Chang YH, Yen CC, et al. Primary renal synovial sarcoma with inferior vena cava and right atrium invasion. Int J Urol. 2003;10:657–60.
30. Vesoulis Z, Rahmeh T, Nelson R, et al. Fine needle aspiration biopsy of primary renal synovial sarcoma. A case report. Acta Cytol. 2003;47:668–72.
31. Karafin M, Parwani AV, Netto GJ, et al. Diffuse expression of Pax2 and Pax8 in the cystic epithelium of mixed epithelial stromal tumor, angiomyolipoma with epithelial cysts, and primary renal synovial sarcoma: evidence supporting renal tubular differentiation. Am J Surg Pathol. 2011;35:1264–73.
32. Eklund MJ, Cundiff C, Shehata BM, et al. Desmoplastic small round cell tumor of the kidney with unusual imaging features. Clin Imaging. 2015;39:904–7.
33. Egloff AM, Lee EY, Dillon JE, et al. Desmoplastic small round cell tumor of the kidney in a pediatric patient: sonographic and multiphase CT findings. AJR Am J Roentgenol. 2005;185:1347–9.
34. Eaton SH, Cendron MA. Primary desmoplastic small round cell tumor of the kidney in a 7-year-old girl. J Pediatr Urol. 2006;2:52–4.
35. Wang LL, Perlman EJ, Vujanic GM, et al. Desmoplastic small round cell tumor of the kidney in childhood. Am J Surg Pathol. 2007;31:576–84.
36. Walton WJ, Flores RR. Desmoplastic small round cell tumor of the kidney: AIRP best cases in radiologic-pathologic correlation. Radiographics. 2016;36:1533–8.
37. Su MC, Jeng YM, Chu YC. Desmoplastic small round cell tumor of the kidney. Am J Surg Pathol. 2004;28:1379–83.
38. Janssens E, Desprechins B, Ernst C, et al. Desmoplastic small round cell tumor of the kidney. JBR-BTR. 2009;92:60.
39. Parvin S, Ghosh R, Das RN, et al. Primary renal rhabdomyosarcoma: an unusual bone metastasizing tumor of kidney. Fetal Pediatr Pathol. 2016;35:251–9.
40. Lin WC, Chen JH, Westphalen A, et al. Primary renal rhabdomyosarcoma in an adolescent with tumor thrombosis in the inferior vena cava and right atrium: a case report and review of the literature. Medicine (Baltimore). 2016;95:e3771.
41. Kren L, Goncharuk VN, Votava M, et al. Botryoid-type of embryonal rhabdomyosarcoma of renal pelvis in an adult. A case report and review of the literature. Cesk Patol. 2003;39:31–5.
42. Kaabneh A, Lang C, Eichel R, et al. Botryoid-type of embryonal rhabdomyosarcoma of renal pelvis in a young woman. Urol Ann. 2014;6:81–4.
43. Kuroda N, Inoue Y, Taguchi T, et al. Renal leiomyoma: an immunohistochemical, ultrastructural and comparative genomic hybridization study. Histol Histopathol. 2007;22:883–8.
44. Lee S, Hsu H, Chang C, et al. Renal capsular leiomyoma--imaging features on computed tomography and angiography. Nephrol Dial Transplant. 2006;21:228–9.
45. Patil PA, Mckenney JK, Trpkov K, et al. Renal leiomyoma: a contemporary multi-institution study of an infrequent and frequently misclassified neoplasm. Am J Surg Pathol. 2015;39:349–56.
46. Miller JS, Zhou M, Brimo F, et al. Primary leiomyosarcoma of the kidney: a clinicopathologic study of 27 cases. Am J Surg Pathol. 2010;34:238–42.
47. Shah VB, Rupani AB, Deokar MS, et al. Idiopathic renal replacement lipomatosis: a case report and review of literature. Indian J Pathol Microbiol. 2009;52:552–3.
48. Petersson F, Michal M, Franco M, et al. Chromophobe renal cell carcinoma with liposarcomatous dedifferentiation – report of a unique case. Int J Clin Exp Pathol. 2010;3:534–40.
49. Anila KR, Mathew AP, Somanathan T, et al. Chromophobe renal cell carcinoma with heterologous (liposarcomatous) differentiation: a case report. Int J Surg Pathol. 2012;20:416–9.

50. Alvarado-Cabrero I, Folpe AL, Srigley JR, et al. Intrarenal schwannoma: a report of four cases including three cellular variants. Mod Pathol. 2000;13:851–6.
51. Kelley J, Collins R, Allam C. Robot-assisted laparoscopic renal schwannoma excision. J Endourol Case Rep. 2016;2:221–3.
52. Gobbo S, Eble JN, Huang J, et al. Schwannoma of the kidney. Mod Pathol. 2008;21:779–83.
53. Eble JN. Angiomyolipoma of kidney. Semin Diagn Pathol. 1998;15:21–40.
54. Lin C, Jin L, Yang Y, et al. Tuberous sclerosis-associated renal angiomyolipoma: a report of two cases and review of the literature. Mol Clin Oncol. 2017;7:706–8.
55. Nese N, Martignoni G, Fletcher CD, et al. Pure epithelioid pecomas (so-called epithelioid angiomyolipoma) of the kidney: a clinicopathologic study of 41 cases: detailed assessment of morphology and risk stratification. Am J Surg Pathol. 2011;35:161–76.
56. Brimo F, Robinson B, Guo C, et al. Renal epithelioid angiomyolipoma with atypia: a series of 40 cases with emphasis on clinicopathologic prognostic indicators of malignancy. Am J Surg Pathol. 2010;34:715–22.
57. Fine SW, Reuter VE, Epstein JI, et al. Angiomyolipoma with epithelial cysts (AMLEC): a distinct cystic variant of angiomyolipoma. Am J Surg Pathol. 2006;30:593–9.
58. Park BK. Renal angiomyolipoma: radiologic classification and imaging features according to the amount of fat. AJR Am J Roentgenol. 2017;209:826–35.
59. Jahn H, Nissen HM. Haemangioma of the urinary tract: review of the literature. Br J Urol. 1991;68:113–7.
60. Montgomery E, Epstein JI. Anastomosing hemangioma of the genitourinary tract: a lesion mimicking angiosarcoma. Am J Surg Pathol. 2009;33:1364–9.
61. Taneja K, Arora S, Rogers CG, et al. Unclassified hemangioma-like renal cell carcinoma: a potential diagnostic pitfall. Hum Pathol. 2018;75:132–6.
62. Ip YT, Yuan JQ, Cheung H, et al. Sporadic hemangioblastoma of the kidney: an underrecognized pseudomalignant tumor? Am J Surg Pathol. 2010;34:1695–700.
63. Liu Y, Qiu XS, Wang EH. Sporadic hemangioblastoma of the kidney: a rare renal tumor. Diagn Pathol. 2012;7:49.
64. Doyle LA, Fletcher CD. Peripheral hemangioblastoma: clinicopathologic characterization in a series of 22 cases. Am J Surg Pathol. 2014;38:119–27.
65. Chaabouni A, Rebai N, Fourati M, et al. Cystic lymphangioma of the kidney: diagnosis and management. Int J Surg Case Rep. 2012;3:587–9.
66. Caduff RF, Schwobel MG, Willi UV, et al. Lymphangioma of the right kidney in an infant boy. Pediatr Pathol Lab Med. 1997;17:631–7.
67. Zapzalka DM, Krishnamurti L, Manivel JC, et al. Lymphangioma of the renal capsule. J Urol. 2002;168:220.
68. Nakai Y, Namba Y, Sugao H. Renal lymphangioma. J Urol. 1999;162:484–5.
69. Honma I, Takagi Y, Shigyo M, et al. Lymphangioma of the kidney. Int J Urol. 2002;9:178–82.
70. Topaloglu H, Karakoyunlu N, Ozok U, et al. Lymphangioma of pyeloureteral junction: an extremely rare case. Urol Int. 2013;90:243–5.
71. Omiyale AO. Clinicopathological features of primary angiosarcoma of the kidney: a review of 62 cases. Transl Androl Urol. 2015;4:464–73.
72. Brown JG, Folpe AL, Rao P, et al. Primary vascular tumors and tumor-like lesions of the kidney: a clinicopathologic analysis of 25 cases. Am J Surg Pathol. 2010;34:942–9.
73. Al-Ahmadie HA, Yilmaz A, Olgac S, et al. Glomus tumor of the kidney: a report of 3 cases involving renal parenchyma and review of the literature. Am J Surg Pathol. 2007;31:585–91.
74. Herawi M, Parwani AV, Edlow D, et al. Glomus tumor of renal pelvis: a case report and review of the literature. Hum Pathol. 2005;36:299–302.
75. Siddiqui N, Rogalska A, Basil IS. Glomangiomyoma (glomus tumor) of the kidney. Arch Pathol Lab Med. 2005;129:1172–4.
76. Lau SK, Klein R, Jiang Z, et al. Myopericytoma of the kidney. Hum Pathol. 2010;41:1500–4.
77. Dhingra S, Ayala A, Chai H, et al. Renal myopericytoma: case report and review of literature. Arch Pathol Lab Med. 2012;136:563–6.

78. Zhang Z, Yu D, Shi H, et al. Renal myopericytoma: a case report with a literature review. Oncol Lett. 2014;7:285–7.
79. Lamba G, Rafiyath SM, Kaur H, et al. Malignant glomus tumor of kidney: the first reported case and review of literature. Hum Pathol. 2011;42:1200–3.
80. Mai K. Giant renomedullary interstitial cell tumor. J Urol. 1994;151:986–8.
81. Kuroda N, Toi M, Miyazaki E, et al. Participation of alpha-smooth muscle actin-positive cells in renomedullary interstitial cell tumors. Oncol Rep. 2002;9:745–50.
82. Argani P, Lewin JR, Edmonds P, et al. Primary renal sclerosing epithelioid fibrosarcoma: report of 2 cases with EWSR1-CREB3L1 gene fusion. Am J Surg Pathol. 2015;39:365–73.
83. Gelb AB, Simmons M, Weidner N. Solitary fibrous tumor involving the renal capsule. Am J Surg Pathol. 1996;20:1288–95.
84. Khater N, Khauli R, Shahait M, et al. Solitary fibrous tumors of the kidneys: presentation, evaluation, and treatment. Urol Int. 2013;91:373–83.
85. Wang J, Arber DA, Frankel K, et al. Large solitary fibrous tumor of the kidney: report of two cases and review of the literature. Am J Surg Pathol. 2001;25:1194–9.
86. Hasegawa T, Matsuno Y, Shimoda T, et al. Extrathoracic solitary fibrous tumors: their histological variability and potentially aggressive behavior. Hum Pathol. 1999;30:1464–73.
87. Doyle LA, Vivero M, Fletcher CD, et al. Nuclear expression of STAT6 distinguishes solitary fibrous tumor from histologic mimics. Mod Pathol. 2014;27:390–5.
88. Hasegawa T, Hirose T, Seki K, et al. Solitary fibrous tumor of the soft tissue. An immunohistochemical and ultrastructural study. Am J Clin Pathol. 1996;106:325–31.
89. Nishimoto K, Sumitomo M, Kakoi N, et al. Case of renal myxoma. Int J Urol. 2007;14:242–4.
90. Thakker P, Ramsey T, Navarro F. Renal myxoma, an incidental finding. Urol Case Rep. 2017;13:131–2.
91. Suthar KS, Vanikar AV, Patel RD, et al. Renal myxoma- a rare variety of benign genitourinary tumour. J Clin Diagn Res. 2015;9:ED11–2.
92. Nielsen GP, O'connell JX, Rosenberg AE. Intramuscular myxoma: a clinicopathologic study of 51 cases with emphasis on hypercellular and hypervascular variants. Am J Surg Pathol. 1998;22:1222–7.
93. Wu T, Gu JQ, Duan X, et al. Hypertension due to juxtaglomerular cell tumor of the kidney. Kaohsiung J Med Sci. 2016;32:276–7.
94. Soni A, Gordetsky JB. Adult pleomorphic juxtaglomerular cell tumor. Urology. 2016;87:E5–7.
95. Kuroda N, Maris S, Monzon FA, et al. Juxtaglomerular cell tumor: a morphological, immunohistochemical and genetic study of six cases. Hum Pathol. 2013;44:47–54.
96. Duan X, Bruneval P, Hammadeh R, et al. Metastatic juxtaglomerular cell tumor in a 52-year-old man. Am J Surg Pathol. 2004;28:1098–102.

Chapter 9
Pediatric Renal Tumors: Diagnostic Updates

Maren Y. Fuller

Pediatric solid tumors are rare, and only approximately 6–7% of them are from the kidney [1]. As in many pediatric malignancies, age of the patient is an important consideration. For example, Wilms tumor, the most common pediatric kidney tumor, is most common in children ages 2–5 years old, and is rare in infants and in adults. In contrast, mesoblastic nephroma is the most common kidney tumor in neonates, and is rare in children older than 1 year. Renal cell carcinoma is very rare in children, but may be seen, especially in older children and young adults. An additional consideration in pediatric tumors is retaining sufficient material for ancillary testing, including fluorescent in situ hybridization (FISH), molecular testing, cytogenetics, and for centralized studies. These findings are necessary for diagnosis (such as specific translocations in mesoblastic nephroma and clear cell sarcoma of the kidney) and for prognosis (loss of heterozygosity in Wilms tumor). Some pediatric kidney tumors also have associations with specific genetic alterations and syndromes.

General Principles

There are a few general principles that apply to most pediatric kidney tumor specimens. As with many pediatric tumors, age is an important variable, and may guide your diagnostic considerations. This is especially true in renal tumors, as tumors may characteristically occur only in infants, children between 2 and 5 years old, or older children/young adults (Table 9.1). In general, intraoperative frozen sections should be avoided, due to the potential for diagnostic error. The only exception would be to confirm the presence of viable tumor. When grossing, the intact nephrectomy specimen should be photographed and weighed, and the surface

M. Y. Fuller (✉)
Texas Children's Hospital/Baylor College of Medicine, Houston, TX, USA

M. K. Divatia et al. (eds.), *Kidney Cancer*, https://doi.org/10.1007/978-3-030-28333-9_9

Table 9.1 Characteristics of pediatric renal tumors

Tumor	Average age at presentation	Diagnostic genetic alterations	Prognosis
Mesoblastic nephroma	0–3 months	t(12;15) *ETV6-NTRK3* (cellular variant only)	Very good
Rhabdoid tumor	1–2 years	Mutations or deletions of *SMARCB1*	Poor
Wilms tumor	2–4 years	n/a	Good
Clear cell sarcoma	2–3 years	BCOR internal tandem duplication repeats OR *YWHAE* and *NUTM2B/NUTM2E* fusions	Improved with multimodality therapy
Cystic nephroma	0–4 years	*DICER1* mutations	Very good, rare sarcomatous transformation
Anaplastic sarcoma	5 years	*DICER1* mutations	Unknown
Renal cell carcinoma	10–11 years	*MiT*-translocation (translocation RCC); *SMARCB1* alterations (medullary carcinoma)	Variable

should be inked before the kidney is bi-valved. The nephrectomy weight is of particular importance, as this data point may guide therapy and may be required for entry into clinical trials. If any areas of possible tumor rupture are noted grossly, it is recommended to ink the suspicious area in a different color and sample it for histology. The capsule should never be stripped, as capsule invasion changes the tumor stage. The renal vein should be examined for gross evidence of tumor thrombus. Ideally, fresh tumor and non-neoplastic kidney should be snap-frozen for possible future studies, and unstained tumor touch imprints may be performed for possible FISH studies.

It is also important to consider differences in staging between classically pediatric renal tumors and renal cell carcinomas. Pediatric renal tumors, including Wilms tumor, congenital mesoblastic nephroma, clear cell sarcoma, and rhabdoid tumor, are staged via the Children's Oncology Group (COG) protocol. Renal cell carcinomas, including those in the pediatric age group are staged via the TNM classification, American Joint Committee on Cancer (AJCC) protocol. Although many elements in the two staging protocols are similar, there are also relevant differences (Table 9.2).

Wilms Tumor

Wilms tumor (nephroblastoma) is the most common pediatric renal tumor. It is generally a tumor of young children, with an average age at presentation of 2–5 years old. It is uncommon in neonates and infants, and is only rarely reported in adults. Wilms tumors are often asymptomatic, and the classic presentation is of an

Table 9.2 Differences between COG and pTNM AJCC staging of kidney tumors

	Children's Oncology Group (COG)		pTNM, American Joint Committee on Cancer (AJCC)	
Tumor types	Wilms tumor, congenital mesoblastic nephroma, clear cell sarcoma, rhabdoid tumor		Renal cell carcinoma (including renal medullary carcinoma and translocation renal cell carcinomas)	
Stage	I	Tumor limited to kidney and completely resected	pT1	Tumor ≤7 cm, limited to the kidney
	II	Tumor extends beyond kidney (including through renal capsule, extrarenal/renal sinus lymph-vascular spaces, renal vein, and/or renal sinus soft tissue), but is completely resected with negative lymph nodes	pT2	Tumor >7 cm, limited to the kidney
	III	Residual tumor (present at margin, tumor rupture/spill, piecemeal excision, prior biopsy, and/or regional lymph node involvement)	pT3	Tumor extends into major veins or perinephric tissues (pelvicaliceal system, perirenal fat, and/or renal sinus fat)
	IV	Hematogenous or lymph node metastases beyond abdomino-pelvic region	pT4	Tumor extends beyond Gerota's fascia (e.g., invasion into adrenal gland)
	V	Bilateral renal tumors at diagnosis (also stage each side separately)		

abdominal mass palpated by a caregiver when bathing the child. Other presentations include hypertension, hematuria, and abdominal pain. Importantly, about 10% of these tumors have an associated syndrome, including WAGR syndrome, Denys–Drash, Beckwith–Wiedemann, Li–Fraumeni, and others. Approximately, 4% of Wilms tumors are bilateral.

Treatment approaches vary based on the clinical stage at presentation, as well as the presence or absence "unfavorable histology," defined as diffuse anaplasia. In the United States, Children's Oncology Group (COG) recommends primary resection, then further therapy depending on the stage and unfavorable histology. In Europe, Société Internationale d'Oncologie Pédiatrique (SIOP) recommends neoadjuvant therapy, then surgical resection. Nevertheless, both approaches have a similarly good prognosis, with an overall survival of over 90% [2, 3].

Grossly, most tumors are solitary and well circumscribed with a fibrous pseudocapsule. The cut surface is soft and usually uniformly tan-pink. Hemorrhage, necrosis, and cystic changes are common. Important considerations at grossing include recording the weight of the nephrectomy specimen, evaluation of any areas of suspected tumor rupture, and extensive sampling of the renal sinus. The kidney weight is an essential element, as stage I tumors with kidney weights <550 g may not require further therapy. Evaluation of tumor rupture as well as renal vein and sinus invasion are essential for staging, as either of these findings correlate to stage

III. Furthermore, a tumor "map" of where each section is taken is strongly recommended, as this is often critical for staging as well as identifying diffuse versus focal anaplasia. Sampling of the uninvolved kidney parenchyma is also critical for evaluation of nephrogenic rests.

Wilms tumor histology is triphasic, including blastemal, epithelial, and stromal elements (Fig. 9.1). However, it is not necessary to see all three components for a diagnosis of Wilms tumor. The blastemal component is composed of densely packed small cells with scant cytoplasm, nuclear overlapping, coarse chromatin, and many mitoses. The epithelial component often resembles primitive tubules and glomerular structures, and can also include maturing to mature tubules. Variable differentiation, including squamous, mucinous, neuroendocrine, and neuroepithelial can be seen. The stromal component is often bland spindled to loose myxoid, and can include heterologous differentiation such as cartilage, bone, skeletal muscle, or fat. Wilms tumors with extensive mature epithelial and stromal heterologous differentiation have been termed "teratoid Wilms tumor." As opposed to immature teratomas of the kidney, teratoid Wilms tumors are more disorganized and have blastemal or nephrogenic epithelial elements.

Presence of anaplasia is the only marker of "unfavorable histology" in Wilms Tumors, and is only present in approximately 5% of tumors. Although rare, it is the most important prognostic marker [4]. Anaplasia is defined as large hyperchromatic nuclei greater than three times larger than neighboring nuclei (Fig. 9.2), as well as large atypical/multipolar mitotic figures. It is also considered a marker of *TP53* mutations and resistance to chemotherapy. Focal anaplasia is limited to 1 to "few" discrete areas, surrounded by nonanaplastic tissue, and the remaining tumor cannot show severe nuclear unrest. Severe nuclear unrest is defined as nuclear pleomorphism or atypia that does not quite reach the threshold of anaplasia. Diffuse anaplasia is defined as any of the following: Anaplasia in any extrarenal site, anaplasia in a random biopsy, or anaplasia that is more than the criteria set as focal anaplasia [5]. Chemotherapy and radiation therapy are not considered to result in tumor anaplasia, thus, these criteria can be applied to both primary resection and posttherapy resection tumors. It is also

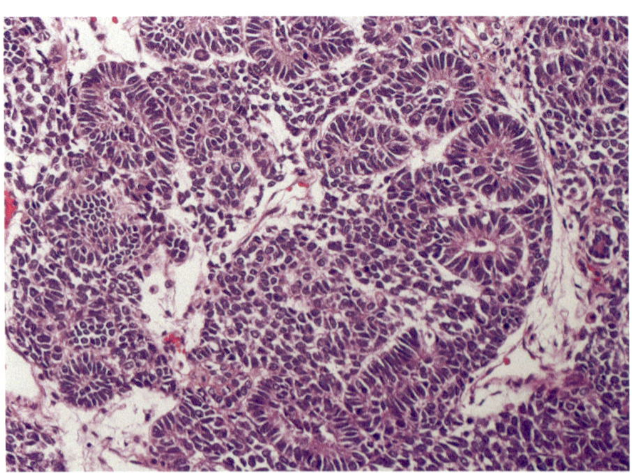

Fig. 9.1 Triphasic Wilms tumor histology, including epithelial, blastema, and stromal components

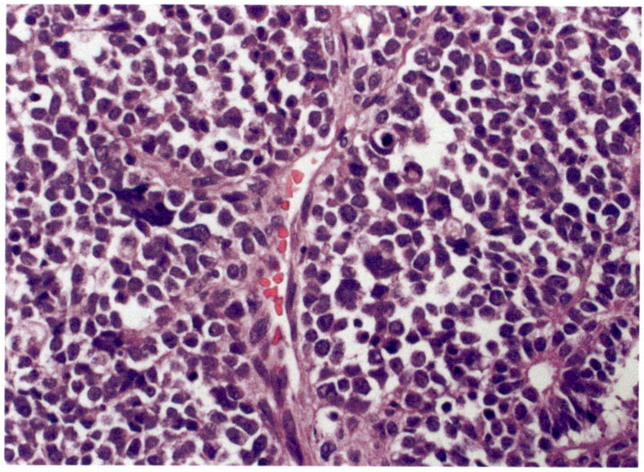

Fig. 9.2 Wilms tumor with anaplasia, characterized by 3x enlarged, hyperchromatic nuclei

important to examine the uninvolved kidney parenchyma for nephrogenic rests, as their presence is a marker for increased risk of bilateral Wilms tumors.

Although immunohistochemistry is not often necessary to make a diagnosis of Wilms tumor in a resection specimen, it is invaluable in blastemal–predominant biopsies. The blastemal and epithelial components usually stain strongly and diffusely with immunohistochemistry for WT1, but the stromal component will be negative. Desmin may be positive in blastema, but myogenin, MyoD1, actin, and other muscle markers should be negative [6]. Although strong nuclear staining of p53 correlates with unfavorable/anaplastic histology, it is not currently part of the COG risk-stratification system.

Molecular testing for loss of heterozygosity (LOH) at chromosomes 1p and 16q is under active investigation for risk stratification of Wilms tumors, and as such, performing this testing may be warranted in many Wilms tumor specimens [2–4]. A wide variety of genetic changes have been described in Wilms tumor, including changes in *WT1* and *TP53*. Recent research has uncovered more of the genetic landscape of these tumors, providing insight into Wilms tumor development as well as future therapies [4, 7, 8].

In most cases of Wilms tumor, the triphasic histology is diagnostic. However, in small biopsies or blastema-predominant tumors, the differential diagnosis includes other small round blue cell tumors such as neuroblastoma and rhabdomyosarcoma. Epithelial-predominant Wilms tumors must be differentiated from metanephric adenoma and papillary renal cell carcinoma.

Mesoblastic Nephroma

Congenital mesoblastic nephroma is a spindle cell myofibroblastic neoplasm of the kidney, which occurs most commonly in the first year of life, and may be congenital. Most patients are cured with complete surgical excision, but incompletely

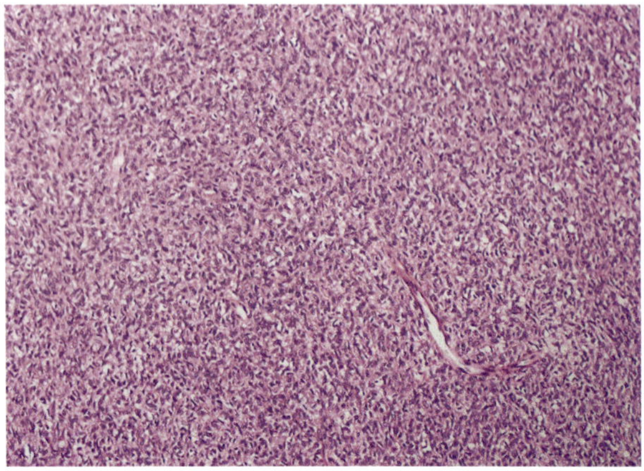

Fig. 9.3 Cellular variant of mesoblastic nephroma with many spindled cells and mitoses

excised tumors may recur. Due to the often infiltrative and indistinct tumor borders, complete nephrectomy is often the treatment of choice. There are two main subtypes: the classic type, with whorled cut surfaces and indistinct separation from the nonneoplastic kidney, and the cellular type, which is more fleshy and well circumscribed. Both may arise centrally and involve the renal sinus.

The classic variant is less common, and represents approximately one-fourth of cases. Histologically, it is composed of bundles of spindle cells with minimal atypia and inconspicuous mitoses. The tumor edges show extensive infiltration into the adjacent renal parenchyma as well as entrapped nonneoplastic tubules. Associated islands of cartilage are also often seen. The cellular variant is composed of a more densely cellular lesion with pushing borders, more frequent mitoses, and more sarcomatous areas (Fig. 9.3). Approximately, 10–20% of cases show mixed classic and cellular histology. All histologic patterns show variable positivity for vimentin, SMA, and desmin immunohistochemistry [6]. The cellular variant of mesoblastic nephroma is characterized by t(12;15)(p13;q25) *ETV6–NTRK3* gene fusion, the same fusion as found in infantile fibrosarcoma [9, 10]. Variant *NTRK1* and *NTRK2* translocations have also been described. Pan-Trk immunohistochemistry shows promise as a sensitive and specific surrogate marker for *NTRK* rearrangements [11]. The classic variant does not have a consistently identified genetic abnormality.

The differential diagnosis includes metanephric fibroma, clear cell sarcoma of kidney, blastema-predominant Wilms tumor, and rhabdoid tumor of kidney.

Clear Cell Sarcoma

Clear cell sarcoma of the kidney is a very rare tumor, but is clinically important to consider due to its aggressive clinical course and proclivity for metastasis, including to the bone. It presents in a similar age group to Wilms tumor (peak at 2–3 years old) as a large renal mass. There may be associated hematuria,

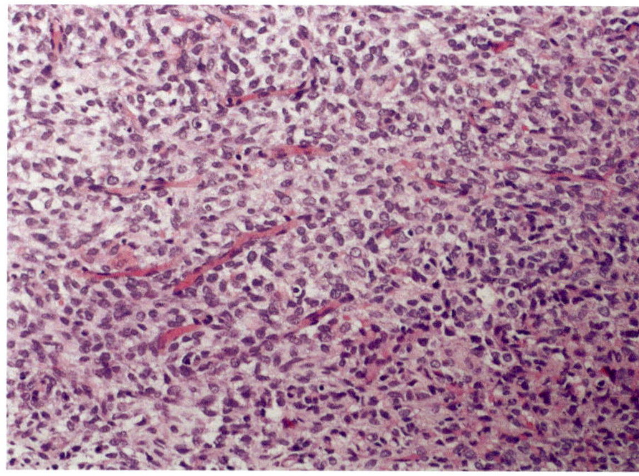

Fig. 9.4 The characteristic delicate, "chicken-wire" vasculature may be the only morphologic clue to clear cell sarcoma

hypertension, as well as possible lymph node metastases at diagnosis. The prognosis has improved with intensive multimodality therapy [12].

Grossly, they are a large well-circumscribed renal mass with a tan-white, mucoid cyst surface, with frequent hemorrhage, necrosis, and cystic change. The classic microscopic features are a relatively homogeneous tumor composed of plump ovoid cells with cytoplasmic clearing in a typical background of thin, "chicken-wire" vasculature (Fig. 9.4). The nuclei are round with fine chromatin and inconspicuous nucleoli. However, not all clear cell sarcomas are clear. They may have myriad appearances, including myxoid, sclerosing, spindle cell, epithelioid, palisading, and others. In most cases, the classic histology can be found, at least focally.

Immunohistochemistry is of limited use. If present, diffuse strong nuclear positivity for BCOR is sensitive and specific for clear cell sarcoma of kidney. Recent reports have described strong, diffuse cyclinD1 immunohistochemistry in clear cell sarcoma, which may have utility in distinction from Wilms tumor and rhabdoid tumor [13]. Vimentin is positive in the tumor cells, and vascular markers highlight the delicate vascular network. These tumors have been recently described to commonly have BCOR internal tandem duplication repeats or less commonly, *YWHAE* and *NUTM2B/NUTM2E* fusions [14–19]. Rare cases with *BCOR–CCNB3* fusion have also been described [20, 21].

The differential diagnosis includes but is not limited to blastema-predominant Wilms tumor and congenital mesoblastic nephroma.

Rhabdoid Tumor

Rhabdoid tumor of the kidney is a very rare, aggressive tumor that occurs most commonly in the first 3 years of life. Originally described as a variant of Wilms Tumor [22], it is now understood to be a separate entity. Other tumors with similar features in different anatomical locations include extrarenal malignant rhabdoid

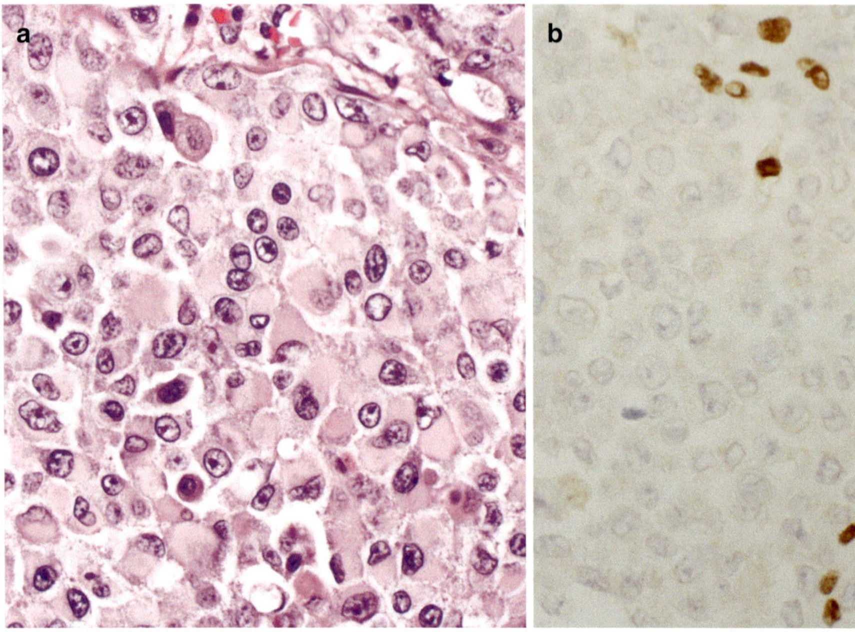

Fig. 9.5 (**a**, **b**) The characteristic eosinophilic inclusions with eccentrically placed nuclei are usually at least focally present in rhabdoid tumor. Nuclear loss of INI1 immunohistochemistry (**b**) is characteristic

tumors and atypical/teratoid rhabdoid tumors [23]. Grossly, they are infiltrative tumors, often with prominent hilar and vascular invasion. The microscopic appearance is somewhat homogeneous, composed of sheets of loosely cohesive cells with large vesicular nuclei with nucleoli. The histologic hallmark is the so-called "rhabdoid" cells with densely eosinophilic cytoplasmic inclusions and an eccentric nucleus (Fig. 9.5). These cells may not be prominent, but are almost always present with careful examination and sufficient tumor sampling. Recently, rhabdoid tumors have been described to have inactivating mutations or deletions in *SMARCB1*, both somatic and germline [23]. The corresponding immunohistochemical finding is loss of nuclear staining of INI1 [24]. The immunohistochemical profile is otherwise nonspecific. Some patients with rhabdoid tumor have *SMARCB1* germline inactivating mutations. Although most of these are de novo mutations, some may be familial and are considered part of rhabdoid tumor predisposing syndrome. These patients often present at a younger age and may have multiple rhabdoid tumors [25]. Although very rare, this syndrome is important to consider so appropriate referral to genetic counseling can be made. Overall, rhabdoid tumor outcomes are very poor, with a median survival of less than 1 year [25].

Translocation Renal Cell Carcinoma

Renal cell carcinoma (RCC) is very rare in children, comprising only about 4% of all pediatric renal cancers [26]. In contrast to adult RCC, pediatric RCC is often associated with unique genetic alterations. Most commonly seen are translocations involving microphthalmia transcription factor (MiT), the so-called "translocation RCCs" [27]. These tumors often are well circumscribed, and are composed of epithelial cells arranged in nests and papillary configurations. The cells often have voluminous clear cytoplasm, distinct cytoplasmic borders, and high nuclear grade with prominent nucleoli (Fig. 9.6). Immunohistochemistry for TFE3 shows strong nuclear positivity, and is a surrogate marker for *TFE3* rearrangements. They often show only minimal positive staining for epithelial membrane antigen (EMA) and cytokeratin 7, and are positive for AMACAR and CD10 [28]. Due to their rarity and fairly recent recognition, the clinical prognosis is still somewhat unclear [26].

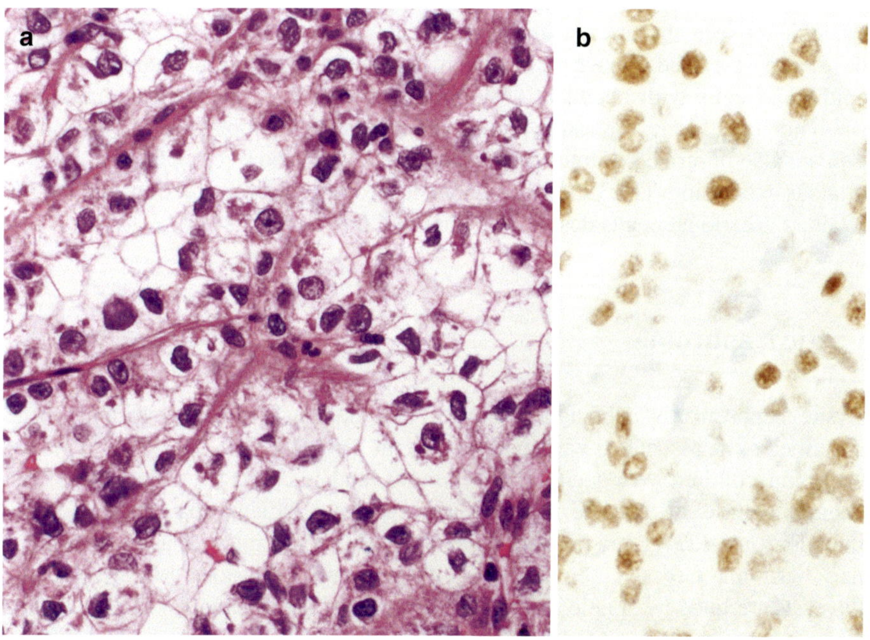

Fig. 9.6 (**a**, **b**) Translocation renal cell carcinomas often have characteristic voluminous, eosinophilic to clear cytoplasm, with high nuclear grade. Immunohistochemistry for TFE3 (**b**) is a surrogate marker for *TFE3* rearrangements

Renal Medullary Carcinoma

Another very rare carcinoma of the pediatric age group is renal medullary carcinoma. It is almost always seen in young patients that carry sickle cell trait, and has an aggressive clinical course [29]. The tumors are often centered on the renal medulla with an infiltrative pattern. Histologically, they are similar to renal collecting duct carcinoma and show a variety of histologic patterns. The tumor cells are large, with eosinophilic cytoplasm and prominent nucleoli. Sickled erythrocytes may be seen within the tumor. Rarely, urine cytology may show tumor cells. These tumors are characterized by loss of INI1 by immunohistochemistry, corresponding to *SMARCB1* loss [30–32]. Prognosis is poor.

ALK-Rearranged Renal Cell Carcinoma

Many pediatric renal cell carcinomas remain in the unclassified category, although recent research has identified additional molecular changes in a subset of these tumors. This includes the recently described group of RCC with *ALK* gene rearrangements seen in patients with sickle-cell trait/disease [33–35]. These tumors have been described to have distinctive histology, including solid architecture with epithelioid cells with abundant eosinophilic cytoplasm, high nuclear grade, and small nucleoli. Intracytoplasmic lumina and variable lymphoplasmacytic inflammation are also described. Immunohistochemically, ALK shows cytoplasmic to membranous expression, TFE3 shows moderate to strong nuclear expression, and INI1 is retained. Rearrangements described include *VCL-ALK* or *TPM3-ALK* [36].

Cystic Nephroma

Cystic nephroma is a benign pediatric renal neoplasm that has recently been described to be associated with mutations in the *DICER1* gene [37–39]. It typically occurs in children younger than 4 years old, and is cured by surgical excision. Genetic counseling may be recommended, as these patients may have germline mutations in *DICER1* and may be at risk for other neoplasms such as pleuropulmonary blastoma. Grossly, they are cystic, well-demarcated lesions. Microscopically, the cysts are lined by simple epithelium that may be flat to cuboidal (Fig. 9.7). The fibrous septae can have a range of cellularity, and may have associated inflammation. No immature nephroblastic elements are present, and if seen, this raises the diagnostic consideration of cystic partially differentiated nephroblastoma. Rarely, there are associated foci of sarcomatous transformation and anaplastic sarcoma [37, 40].

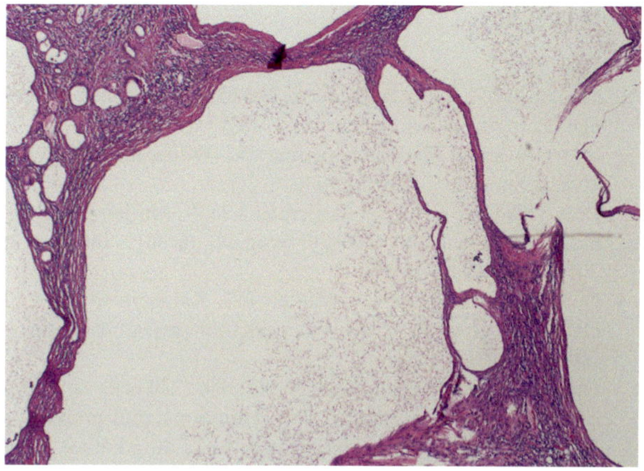

Fig. 9.7 Cystic nephroma is characterized by cysts lined by simple attenuated to low cuboidal epithelium and may have associated inflammation

Anaplastic Sarcoma of the Kidney

A recently described, very rare malignant pediatric kidney tumor, also associated with *DICER1*, is anaplastic sarcoma [41]. It has been described in patients from ages 10 months to 41 years, and the median age at presentation is 5 years [42]. Grossly, it is cystic with a spindle cell component with marked anaplasia. Characteristically, it also has islands of chondroid differentiation or benign and/or malignant cartilage. Typically, the cysts are surrounded by the sarcomatoid component. Rhabdomyoblastic differentiation may also be found. These sarcomas are also characterized by *DICER1* mutations, and are considered to be part of the DICER1 syndrome [43]. Mutations in *TP53* may also be found in many anaplastic sarcomas of the kidney [43].

Ossifying Renal Tumor of Infancy

Ossifying renal tumor of infancy is a very rare, benign kidney tumor seen almost exclusively in infants, first described in 1980 [44]. The average age at diagnosis is 6 months, and most tumors occur in the first year of life. The typical clinical presentation is gross hematuria [45]. The tumors are frequently, but not always, calcified. Histologically, there are three elements: spindle cells, osteoblast-like cells, and an osteoid core. Prognosis is very good; the vast majority of patients are cured with surgical resection. No characteristic genetic alterations have been described to date [46].

References

1. Malkan AD, Loh A, Bahrami A, Navid F, Coleman J, Green DM, et al. An approach to renal masses in pediatrics. Pediatrics. 2015;135(1):142–58.
2. Irtan S, Ehrlich PF, Pritchard-Jones K. Wilms tumor: "State-of-the-art" update, 2016. Semin Pediatr Surg. 2016;25(5):250–6.
3. Dome JS, Graf N, Geller JI, Fernandez CV, Mullen EA, Spreafico F, et al. Advances in wilms tumor treatment and biology: progress through international collaboration. J Clin Oncol. 2015;33(27):2999–3007.
4. Dome JS, Fernandez CV, Mullen EA, Kalapurakal JA, Geller JI, Huff V, et al. Children's Oncology Group's 2013 blueprint for research: renal tumors. Pediatr Blood Cancer. 2013;60(6):994–1000.
5. Faria P, Beckwith JB, Mishra K, Zuppan C, Weeks D, Breslow N, et al. Focal versus diffuse anaplasia in Wilms tumor – new definitions with prognostic significance: a report from the National Wilms Tumor Study Group. Am J Surg Pathol. 1996;20(8):909–20.
6. Picarsic J, Reyes-Múgica M. Phenotype and immunophenotype of the most common pediatric tumors. Appl Immunohistochem Mol Morphol. 2015;23(5):313–26.
7. Gadd S, Huff V, Walz AL, Ooms AHAG, Armstrong AE, Gerhard DS, et al. A Children's Oncology Group and TARGET initiative exploring the genetic landscape of Wilms tumor. Nat Genet. 2017;49(10):1487–94.
8. Treger TD, Chowdhury T, Pritchard-Jones K, Behjati S. The genetic changes of Wilms tumour. Nat Rev Nephrol. 2019;15(4):240–51.
9. Knezevich SR, Garnett MJ, Pysher TJ, Beckwith JB, Grundy PE, Sorensen PHB. ETV6-NTRK3 gene fusions and trisomy 11 establish a histogenetic link between mesoblastic nephroma and congenital fibrosarcoma. Cancer Res. 1998;58(22):5046–8.
10. Rubin BP, Chen CJ, Morgan TW, Xiao S, Grier HE, Kozakewich HP, et al. Congenital mesoblastic nephroma t(12;15) is associated with ETV6-NTRK3 gene fusion: cytogenetic and molecular relationship to congenital (infantile) fibrosarcoma. Am J Pathol. 1998;153(5):1451–8.
11. Rudzinski ER, Lockwood CM, Stohr BA, Vargas SO, Sheridan R, Black JO, et al. Pan-Trk immunohistochemistry identifies NTRK rearrangements in pediatric mesenchymal tumors. Am J Surg Pathol. 2018;42(7):927–35.
12. Gooskens SLM, Furtwängler R, Vujanic GM, Dome JS, Graf N, van den Heuvel-Eibrink MM. Clear cell sarcoma of the kidney: a review. Eur J Cancer. 2012;48(14):2219–26.
13. Mirkovic J, Calicchio M, Fletcher CD, Perez-Atayde AR. Diffuse and strong cyclin D1 immunoreactivity in clear cell sarcoma of the kidney. Histopathology. 2015;67(3):306–12.
14. Ueno-Yokohata H, Okita H, Nakasato K, Akimoto S, Hata JI, Koshinaga T, et al. Consistent in-frame internal tandem duplications of BCOR characterize clear cell sarcoma of the kidney. Nat Genet. 2015;47(8):861–3.
15. Kenny C, Bausenwein S, Lazaro A, Furtwängler R, Gooskens SLM, Van Den Heuvel Eibrink M, et al. Mutually exclusive BCOR internal tandem duplications and YWHAE-NUTM2 fusions in clear cell sarcoma of kidney: not the full story. J Pathol. 2016;238(5):617–20.
16. Kao Y-C, Sung Y-S, Zhang L, Huang S-C, Argani P, Chung CT, et al. Recurrent BCOR internatl tandem duplication and YWHAE-NUTM2B fusions in soft tissue undifferentiated round cell sarcoma of infancy – overlapping genetic features with clear cell sarcoma of kidney. Am J Surg Pathol. 2016;40(8):1009–20.
17. Roy A, Kumar V, Zorman B, Fang E, Haines K, Doddapaneni H, et al. Recurrent internal tandem duplications of BCOR in clear cell sarcoma of the kidney. Nat Commun. 2015;6:8891.
18. O'Meara E, Stack D, Lee CH, Garvin AJ, Morris T, Argani P, et al. Characterization of the chromosomal translocation t(10;17)(q22;p13) in clear cell sarcoma of kidney. J Pathol. 2012;227(1):72–80.
19. Karlsson J, Valid A, Gisselsson D. BCOR internal tandem duplication and YWHAE-NUTM2B/E fusion are mutually exclusive events in clear cell sarcoma of the kidney. Genes Chromosomes Cancer. 2016;55:120–3.

20. Wong MK, Ng CCY, Kuick CH, Aw SJ, Rajasegaran V, Lim JQ, et al. Clear cell sarcomas of the kidney are characterised by *BCOR* gene abnormalities, including exon 15 internal tandem duplications and *BCOR-CCNB3* gene fusion. Histopathology. 2018;72(2):320–9.
21. Argani P, Kao Y-C, Zhang L, Bacchi C, Matoso A, Alaggio R, et al. Primary renal sarcomas with BCOR-CCNB3 gene fusion. Am J Surg Pathol. 2017;41(12):1702–12.
22. Beckwith JB, Palmer NF. Histopathology and prognosis of Wilms tumors: results from the First National Wilms' Tumor Study. Cancer. 1978;41(5):1937–48.
23. Bourdeaut F, Lequin D, Brugières L, Reynaud S, Dufour C, Doz F, et al. Frequent hSNF5/INI1 germline mutations in patients with rhabdoid tumor. Clin Cancer Res. 2011;17(1):31–8.
24. Sigauke E, Rakheja D, Maddox DL, Hladik CL, White CL, Timmons CF, et al. Absence of expression of SMARCB1/INI1 in malignant rhabdoid tumors of the central nervous system, kidneys and soft tissue: an immunohistochemical study with implications for diagnosis. Mod Pathol. 2006;19(5):717–25.
25. Sredni ST, Tomita T. Rhabdoid tumor predisposition syndrome. Pediatr Dev Pathol. 2015;18(1):49–58.
26. Geller JI, Ehrlich PF, Cost NG, Khanna G, Mullen EA, Gratias EJ, et al. Characterization of adolescent and pediatric renal cell carcinoma: a report from the Children's Oncology Group study AREN03B2. Cancer. 2015;121(14):2457–64.
27. Cajaiba MM, Dyer LM, Geller JI, Jennings LJ, George D, Kirschmann D, et al. The classification of pediatric and young adult renal cell carcinomas registered on the children's oncology group (COG) protocol AREN03B2 after focused genetic testing. Cancer. 2018;124(16):3381–9.
28. Perlman EJ. Pediatric renal cell carcinoma. Surg Pathol Clin. 2010;3(3):641–51.
29. Davis CJ, Mostofi FK, Sesterhenn IA. Renal medullary carcinoma. The seventh sickle cell nephropathy. Am J Surg Pathol. 1995;19(1):1–11.
30. Cheng JX, Tretiakova M, Gong C, Mandal S, Krausz T, Taxy JB. Renal medullary carcinoma: rhabdoid features and the absence of INI1 expression as markers of aggressive behavior. Mod Pathol. 2008;21(6):647–52.
31. Liu Q, Galli S, Srinivasan R, Linehan WM, Tsokos M, Merino MJ. Renal medullary carcinoma: molecular, immunohistochemistry, and morphologic correlation. Am J Surg Pathol. 2013;37(3):368–74.
32. Carlo MI, Chaim J, Patil S, Kemel Y, Schram AM, Woo K, et al. Genomic characterization of renal medullary carcinoma and treatment outcomes. Clin Genitourin Cancer. 2017;15(6):e987–94.
33. Debelenko LV, Raimondi SC, Daw N, Shivakumar BR, Huang D, Nelson M, et al. Renal cell carcinoma with novel VCL-ALK fusion: new representative of ALK-associated tumor spectrum. Mod Pathol. 2011;24(3):430–42.
34. Smith N, Deyrup AT, Fletcher JA, Bridge JA, Illei PB, Netto GJ, et al. VCL-ALK renal cell carcinoma in children with sickle-cell trait: the eighth sickle-cell nephropathy? Am J Surg Pathol. 2014;38(6):858–63.
35. Mariño-Enríquez A, Ou W-B, Weldon CB, Fletcher JA, Pérez-Atayde AR. ALK rearrangement in sickle cell trait-associated renal medullary carcinoma. Genes Chromosom Cancer. 2011;50(3):146–53.
36. Cajaiba MM, Jennings LJ, Rohan SM, Perez-Atayde AR, Marino-Enriquez A, Fletcher JA, et al. ALK rearranged renal cell carcinomas in children. Genes Chromosom Cancer. 2016;55(5):442–51.
37. Doros LA, Rossi CT, Yang J, Field A, Williams GM, Messinger Y, et al. DICER1 mutations in childhood cystic nephroma and its relationship to DICER1-renal sarcoma. Mod Pathol. 2014;27(9):1267–80.
38. Cajaiba MM, Khanna G, Smith EA, Gellert L, Chi YY, Mullen EA, et al. Pediatric cystic nephromas: distinctive features and frequent DICER1 mutations. Hum Pathol. 2016;48:81–7.
39. Li Y, Pawel BR, Hill DA, Epstein JI, Argani P. Pediatric cystic nephroma is morphologically, immunohistochemically, and genetically distinct from adult cystic nephroma. Am J Surg Pathol. 2017;41(4):472–81.

40. Wu MK, Cotter MB, Pears J, McDermott MB, Fabian MR, Foulkes WD, et al. Tumor progression in DICER1-mutated cystic nephroma – witnessing the genesis of anaplastic sarcoma of the kidney. Hum Pathol. 2016;53:114–20.
41. Vujanić GM, Kelsey A, Perlman EJ, Sandstedt B, Beckwith JB. Anaplastic sarcoma of the kidney: a clinicopathologic study of 20 cases of a new entity with polyphenotypic features. Am J Surg Pathol. 2007;31(10):1459–68.
42. Sebire NJ, Vujanic GM. Paediatric renal tumours: recent developments, new entities and pathological features. Histopathology. 2009;54(5):516–28.
43. Wu MK, Vujanic GM, Fahiminiya S, Watanabe N, Thorner PS, O'Sullivan MJ, et al. Anaplastic sarcomas of the kidney are characterized by DICER1 mutations. Mod Pathol. 2018;31(1):169–78.
44. Chatten J, Cromie WJ, Duckett JW. Ossifying tumor of infantile kidney: report of two cases. Cancer. 1980;45(3):609–12.
45. Hu J, Wu Y, Qi J, Zhang C, Lv F. Ossifying renal tumor of infancy (ORTI): a case report and review of the literature. J Pediatr Surg. 2013;48(2):e37–40.
46. Guan W, Yan Y, He W, Qiao M, Liu Y, Wang Y, et al. Ossifying renal tumor of infancy (ORIT): the clinicopathological and cytogenetic feature of two cases and literature review. Pathol Res Pract. 2016;212(11):1004–9.

Chapter 10
Neuroendocrine Kidney Tumors

Miao Zhang and Charles C. Guo

Carcinoid Tumor

Carcinoid tumor was first reported as a primary neoplasm of the kidney in 1966. It is a very rare tumor in the kidney with fewer than 100 cases reported in the literature.

Etiology

The histogenesis of carcinoid tumor in the kidney is unclear. Occasionally, carcinoid tumors may arise from renal teratomas [1], which is exceedingly rare. About 20% of cases have been reported to be associated with horseshoe kidney [2, 3]; however, no neuroendocrine cells have been identified in the normal kidney parenchyma.

Clinical Presentation

Clinically, patients present with nonspecific symptoms, such as flank pain, hematuria, or abdominal mass. Very rarely, patients can present with carcinoid syndrome [4]. The average age of diagnosis is 52 years (range 27–78 years) with no significant gender predilection [5].

M. Zhang · C. C. Guo (✉)
Department of Pathology, The University of Texas MD Anderson Cancer Center, Houston, TX, USA
e-mail: ccguo@mdanderson.org

M. K. Divatia et al. (eds.), *Kidney Cancer*, https://doi.org/10.1007/978-3-030-28333-9_10

Gross Pathology

Tumors vary in size with an average of 6.4 cm (range 2–17 cm) [5]. Most tumors are well circumscribed with a distinct interface with nonneoplastic kidney. Cut surface is solid homogenous, yellow tan, or red-brown; focal hemorrhage, calcification, or cystic change can be seen; however, necrosis is rarely seen.

Histology

The most common growth pattern is cords and trabeculae with ribbon-like appearance in scarce, dense and sclerotic stroma (Fig. 10.1a); solid sheet, nests, or gland-like lumina can be seen. Tumor cells are quite uniform with round nuclei and moderate amount of cytoplasm (Fig. 10.1b, c); mild-to-moderate nuclear pleomorphism can be seen. Tumor nuclei show granular and fine chromatin (salt and pepper) with inconspicuous nucleoli (Fig. 10.2). Most cases show <2 mitosis/10 high-power field (HPF); however, mitotic rate of 3–4 mitoses/10 HPF has been reported; Ki-67 proliferation index is mostly less than 5% and sometimes 5–10% (Fig. 10.1d). About 24% of cases are associated with calcification. Extrarenal extension into perinephric adipose tissue has been reported in about 40% of cases [5].

Immunohistochemical Feature

Over 90% of tumors are positive for synaptophysin and cam5.2, while chromogranin is positive in 65% of cases. Interestingly, immunoreactivity for prostatic acid phosphatase (PAP) has been documented [6, 7].

Treatment and Prognosis

Surgical resection is the primary treatment of choice. The clinical outcome is difficult to predict; however, even patients with metastatic disease may suvive for a long time.

High-Grade Neuroendocrine Carcinoma

High-grade neuroendocrine carcinoma of the kidney is a poorly differentiated carcinoma with neuroendocrine differentiation. It is an extremely rare primary tumor of the kidney with fewer than 50 cases reported [8].

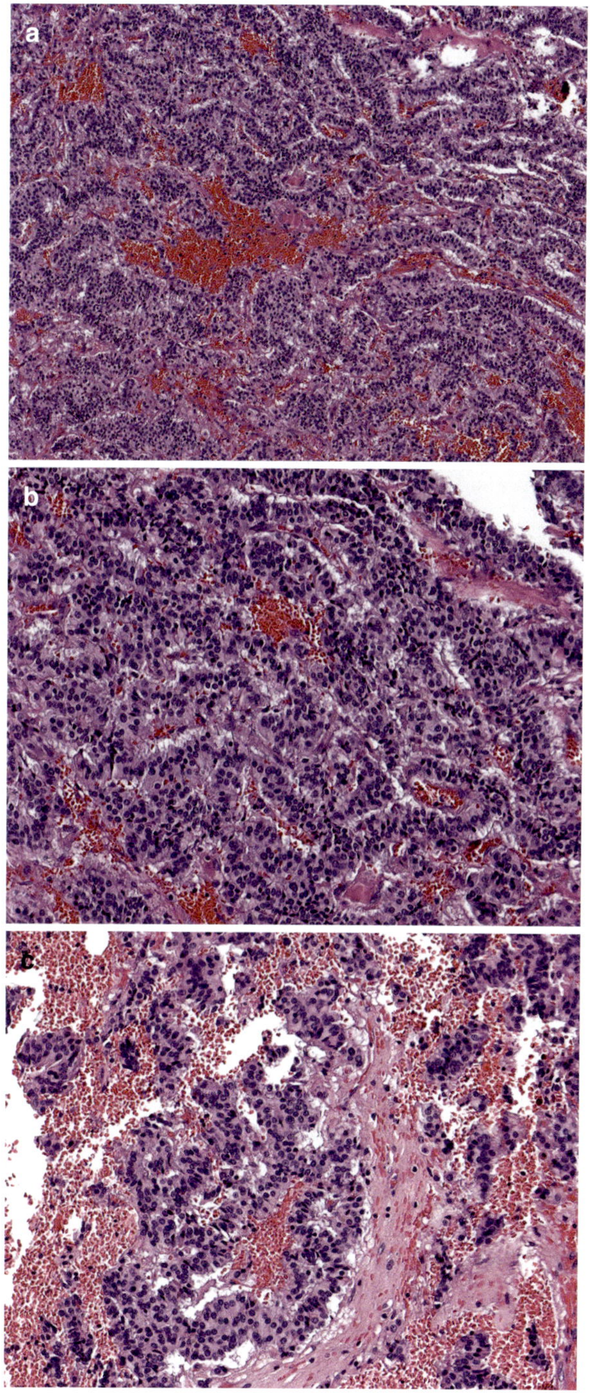

Fig. 10.1 Carcinoid tumor of the kidney. (**a**) Tumor cells show ribbon-like growth; (**b**, **c**) tumor cells are uniform with abundant pink cytoplasm, salt and pepper chromatin; (**d**) Ki-67 proliferation index is less than 5% in most cases

Fig. 10.1 (continued)

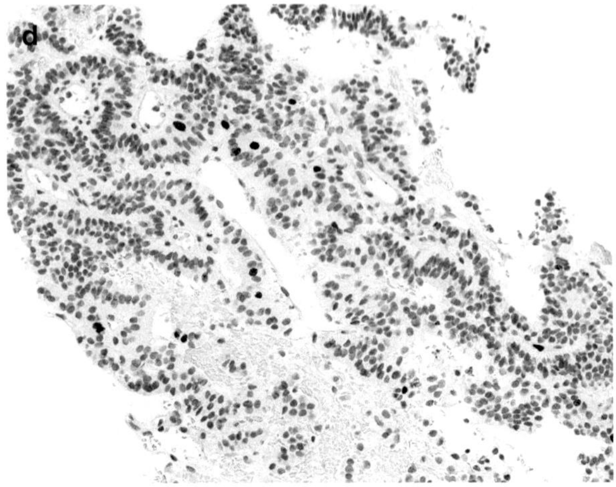

Clinical Presentation

Nausea, abdominal or flank pain, and gross hematuria are common clinical symptoms [9, 10].

Gross Pathology

On gross examination, tumor is lobulated and mostly located at the renal pelvis. Cut surface is white-gray and often associated with necrosis. The reported size ranges from 2.5 to 23 cm (median 8 cm).

Histology

The tumor may be comosed of small cell neuroendocrine carcinoma or large cell neuroendocirne carcinoma. It usually shows sheets and nests of cells infiltrating the kidney parenchyma. It is frequently associated with necrosis (Fig. 10.2a). Tumor cells are small to intermediate in size and show markedly hyperchromatic round to oval nuclei, inconspicuous nucleoli, scan cytoplasm, and poorly defined cytoplasmic borders (Fig. 10.2b–c). Mitotic activity is high (>10 mitoses/10 HPF) (Fig. 10.2c) [9]. Metastasis to regional lymph nodes is frequently seen (Fig. 10.2d).

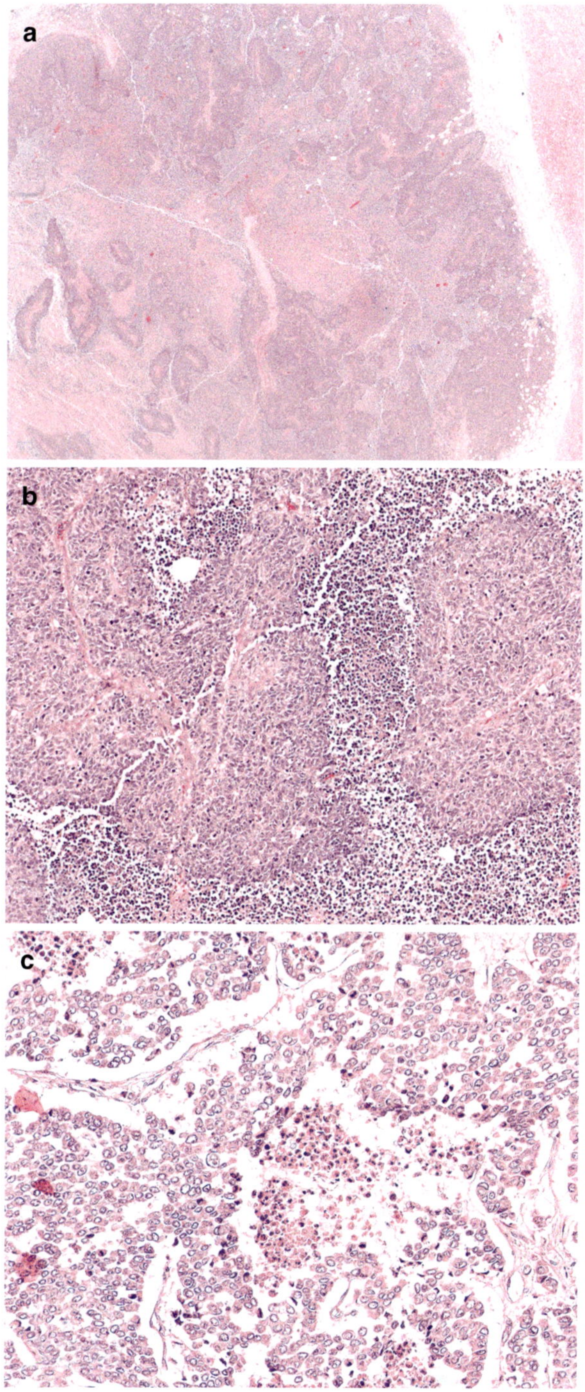

Fig. 10.2 Neuroendocrine carcinoma of the kidney. (**a**) Low power, tumor is composed of a sheet of cells associated with necrosis; (**b**) tumor shows high mitotic counts and necrosis; (**c**, **d**) tumor cells are markedly hyperchromatic with inconspicuous nucleoli; (**e**) neuroendocrine carcinoma of kidney metastasis to hilar lymph node

Fig. 10.2 (continued)

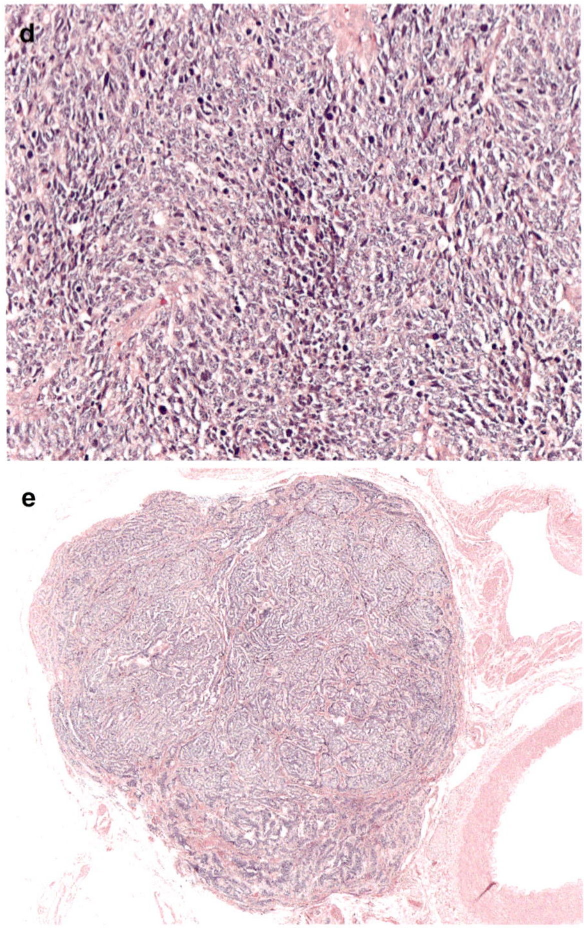

Immunohistochemical Features

Tumor cells show dot-like cytoplasmic staining with cytokeratins and variable positivities for neuroendocrine markers, such as synaptophysin, chromogranin, CD56, and NSE (neuron-specific enolase).

Treatment and Prognosis

Most patients presented with locally advanced tumors that are large in size with invasion of vascular and retroperitoneal structures. Regional lymph node and distant metastases are common. Surgical resection and aggressive chemotherapy are commonly used; however, over 50% of patients died within 1 year [9].

Primitive Neuroectodermal Tumor (PNET)

PNET is a very uncommon entity in the kidney, with approximately 120 cases reported in the literature.

Clinical Presentation

Average age is 23–27 years, but age ranges from the first to eighth decades. Abdominal pain and gross hematuria are common presenting symptoms. About 10% of patients presented with lung, hepatic, and bone metastasis [11].

Gross Pathology

On gross examination, tumor shows a tan, yellow to white lobulated cut surface; tumors are large in size (average 16 cm, range 7–21 cm) and often extensively replace the kidney parenchyma [12].

Histology

Histological features are not different from those in its soft-tissue counterpart with primitive appearing round cells and high nuclear to cytoplasmic ratio. When clear cytoplasm is present, it is frequently associated with the presence of glycogen (diastase-sensitive PAS positivity) [12]. Mitosis and necrosis are easily identified. Homer Wright rosettes are seen in some case.

Immunohistochemical Features

Tumor cells are strongly and diffusely positive for CD99 (membranous pattern). Some show nuclear positivity for FLI-1. Approximately 20% of cases are positive for cytokeratin. It should be noted that all tumor cells are negative for WT-1 and muscle markers, which may help to distinguish from other small round blue cell tumors in the kidney, such as Wilms' tumor and rhabdomyosarcoma. Like its soft-tissue counterpart, the characteristic translocation t (11; 22)(q24;q12) leading to the EWS-FLI1 fusion gene is the most frequent genetic alteration.

Treatment and Prognosis

Pathological stage is the main determinant in the prognosis. Generally, PNET is an aggressive tumor with poor clinical outcome. Recently, the utilization of multidisciplinary therapy includes surgery, chemotherapy, and radiation has improved the median survival significantly [13, 14].

Neuroblastoma

A true neuroblastoma originated from the kidney is exceedingly rare, and only a handful of cases have been registered at the National Wilms' Tumor Study Group Pathology Center [15]. Involvement of the renal tissue by adrenal neuroblastomas is a much more common occurrence. Renal neuroblastomas show similar features as its adrenal counterpart, with primitive neural tissue, Homer Wright rosettes, neurofibrillary stroma, and embryonal cell with round nuclei containing granular, fine (salt and pepper) chromatin. The tumor cells are positive for neuroendocrine markers, such as synaptophysin, chromogranin, and S100.

Paraganglioma/Pheochromocytoma

Paraganglioma is a rare entity in the kidney with only few cases described in the literature [16]. Most tumors are small in size. The gross and histological appearance is identical to paraganglioma/pheochromocytoma of other organs. Grossly, tumor is tan gray and well circumscribed. Microscopically, tumor cells show "zellballen" with distinctive collagenous septa. The nuclei show inconspicuous nucleoli. Mitosis is infrequent. Immunohistochemically, tumor cells are positive for chromogranin, synaptophysin, GATA-3, and CD56. S100 labels the sustentacular cells.

Juxtaglomerular Cell Tumor

Juxtaglomerular cell tumor (JGCT) was first described in 1967 [17]. It is a rare tumor that differentiates toward smooth muscle cells in the afferent arteriole of glomeruli. It is associated with abundant renin production. JGCT usually occurs in younger individuals (mean age: 23 years). It is slightly female predominant (female to male ratio: 2:1) [18].

Clinical Presentation

Patients typically present with hypertension, hypokalemia, and hyperaldosteronism owing to excessive renin production. There was one reported case in which patient presented with normal blood pressure [19].

Gross Pathology

Tumors are usuallly small (less than 3 cm, ranging from 2 mm to 9 cm), well circumscribed with yellow to tan cut surface [20], and necrosis is rarely seen.

Histology

Tumor usually shows a hemangiopericytic growth pattern (Fig. 10.3a). Other growth patterns include trabecular, insular, solid, papillary, cystic, and tubular. Tumor is composed of uniform population of round, polygonal, or spindled cells with granular and eosinophilic cytoplasm (Fig. 10.3b). Tumor cells have distinctive cell borders. Myxoid stroma with prominent vasculature and mast cells are frequently seen (Fig. 10.3c).

Immunohistochemical Features

The cytoplasmic granules are positive for PAS. Immunohistochemically, tumor cells are positive for renin, actin, vimentin, and CD34 (Fig. 10.3d) [18].

Treatment and Prognosis

Surgery is the primary treatment of choice. All clinical symptoms resolve after surgical intervention. There has been no reported case with metastasis or recurrence in literature after long follow-up [21, 22].

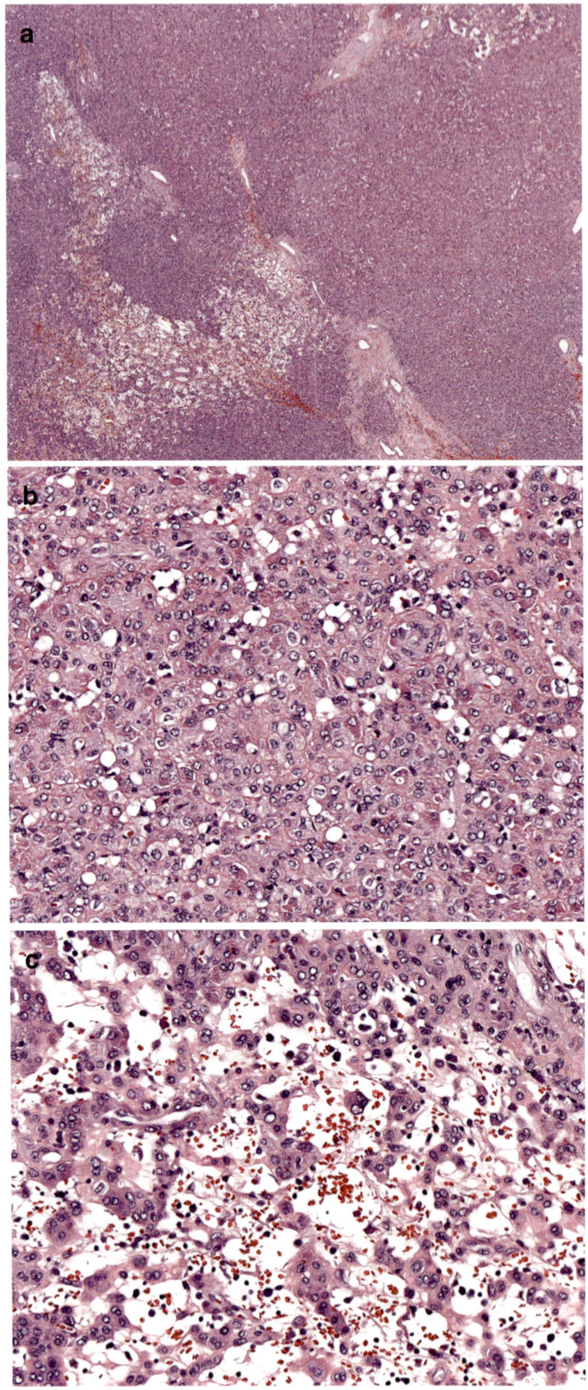

Fig. 10.3 Juxtaglomerular cell tumor of the kidney. (**a**) tumor shows a hemangiopericytic growth pattern; (**b**) tumor is composed of uniform population of round or polygonal cells with eosinophilic cytoplasm; (**c**) tumor shows prominent vasculature with mast cells; (**d**) tumor cells are diffusely positive for CD34

Fig. 10.3 (continued)

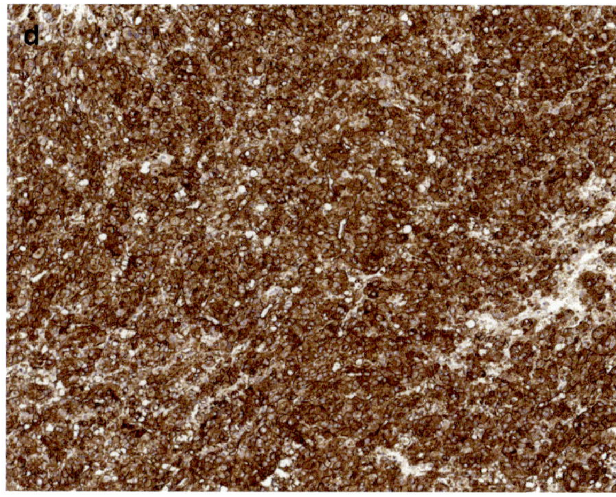

Germ Cell Tumor

Metastasis from gonadal germ cell tumor needs to be excluded before a primary germ cell tumor of the kidney is considered. Primary renal pelvic choriocarcinomas have been reported in the literature and are difficult to distinguish from high-grade urothelial carcinoma due to the overlapping histological and immunohistochemical features [23]. However, treatment regimens utilized for choriocarcinoma of the testis seem to prolong remission of the renal choriocarcinomas, suggesting a similar pathogenetic pathway. Other germ cell tumors, such as teratomas, have also been reported in the kidney [24].

Tumor Metastatic to the Kidney

Involvement of the kidney by secondary malignancies is uncommon, accounting for less than 5% of all renal malignancies [25]. A recent published study shows that the most common solid tumor metastatic to the kidney is of lung primary. Clinical features, such as imaging studies, are almost indistinguishable from primary kidney tumors. Major differential diagnosis includes collecting duct carcinoma, medullary carcinoma, and urothelial carcinoma of the kidney. Clinical, radiological, and pathological correlations are essential for the accurate diagnosis.

References

1. Yoo J, Park S, Jung Lee H, Jin Kang S, Kee Kim B. Primary carcinoid tumor arising in a mature teratoma of the kidney: a case report and review of the literature. Arch Pathol Lab Med. 2002;126(8):979–81.
2. Rodriguez-Covarrubias F, Gomez X, Valerio JC, Lome-Maldonado C, Gabilondo F. Carcinoid tumor arising in a horseshoe kidney. Int Urol Nephrol. 2007;39(2):373–6.
3. Krishnan B, Truong LD, Saleh G, Sirbasku DM, Slawin KM. Horseshoe kidney is associated with an increased relative risk of primary renal carcinoid tumor. J Urol. 1997;157(6):2059–66.
4. McCaffrey JA, Reuter VV, Herr HW, Macapinlac HA, Russo P, Motzer RJ. Carcinoid tumor of the kidney. The use of somatostatin receptor scintigraphy in diagnosis and management. Urol Oncol. 2000;5(3):108–11.
5. Hansel DE, Epstein JI, Berbescu E, Fine SW, Young RH, Cheville JC. Renal carcinoid tumor: a clinicopathologic study of 21 cases. Am J Surg Pathol. 2007;31(10):1539–44.
6. el-Naggar AK, Troncoso P, Ordonez NG. Primary renal carcinoid tumor with molecular abnormality characteristic of conventional renal cell neoplasms. Diagn Mol Pathol. 1995;4(1):48–53.
7. Goldblum JR, Lloyd RV. Primary renal carcinoid. Case report and literature review. Arch Pathol Lab Med. 1993;117(8):855–8.
8. La Rosa S, Bernasconi B, Micello D, Finzi G, Capella C. Primary small cell neuroendocrine carcinoma of the kidney: morphological, immunohistochemical, ultrastructural, and cytogenetic study of a case and review of the literature. Endocr Pathol. 2009;20(1):24–34.
9. Tetu B, Ro JY, Ayala AG, Ordonez NG, Johnson DE. Small cell carcinoma of the kidney. A clinicopathologic, immunohistochemical, and ultrastructural study. Cancer. 1987;60(8):1809–14.
10. Capella C, Eusebi V, Rosai J. Primary oat cell carcinoma of the kidney. Am J Surg Pathol. 1984;8(11):855–61.
11. Casella R, Moch H, Rochlitz C, Meier V, Seifert B, Mihatsch MJ, et al. Metastatic primitive neuroectodermal tumor of the kidney in adults. Eur Urol. 2001;39(5):613–7.
12. Jimenez RE, Folpe AL, Lapham RL, Ro JY, O'Shea PA, Weiss SW, et al. Primary Ewing's sarcoma/primitive neuroectodermal tumor of the kidney: a clinicopathologic and immunohistochemical analysis of 11 cases. Am J Surg Pathol. 2002;26(3):320–7.
13. Cuesta Alcala JA, Solchaga Martinez A, Caballero Martinez MC, Gomez Dorronsoro M, Pascual Piedrola I, Ripa Saldias L, et al. Primary neuroectodermal tumor (PNET) of the kidney: 26 cases. Current status of its diagnosis and treatment. Arch Esp Urol. 2001;54(10):1081–93.
14. Thyavihally YB, Tongaonkar HB, Gupta S, Kurkure PA, Amare P, Muckaden MA, et al. Primitive neuroectodermal tumor of the kidney: a single institute series of 16 patients. Urology. 2008;71(2):292–6.
15. Parham DM, Roloson GJ, Feely M, Green DM, Bridge JA, Beckwith JB. Primary malignant neuroepithelial tumors of the kidney: a clinicopathologic analysis of 146 adult and pediatric cases from the National Wilms' Tumor Study Group Pathology Center. Am J Surg Pathol. 2001;25(2):133–46.
16. Lagace R, Tremblay M. Non-chromaffin paraganglioma of the kidney with distant metastases. Can Med Assoc J. 1968;99(22):1095–8.
17. Robertson PW, Klidjian A, Harding LK, Walters G, Lee MR, Robb-Smith AH. Hypertension due to a renin-secreting renal tumour. Am J Med. 1967;43(6):963–76.
18. Martin SA, Mynderse LA, Lager DJ, Cheville JC. Juxtaglomerular cell tumor: a clinicopathologic study of four cases and review of the literature. Am J Clin Pathol. 2001;116(6):854–63.
19. Hayami S, Sasagawa I, Suzuki H, Kubota Y, Nakada T, Endo Y. Juxtaglomerular cell tumor without hypertension. Scand J Urol Nephrol. 1998;32(3):231–3.
20. Kuroda N, Moriki T, Komatsu F, Miyazaki E, Hayashi Y, Naruse K, et al. Adult-onset giant juxtaglomerular cell tumor of the kidney. Pathol Int. 2000;50(3):249–54.
21. Moss AH, Peterson LJ, Scott CW, Winter K, Olin DB, Garber RL. Delayed diagnosis of juxtaglomerular cell tumor hypertension. N C Med J. 1982;43(10):705–7.

22. Haab F, Duclos JM, Guyenne T, Plouin PF, Corvol P. Renin secreting tumors: diagnosis, conservative surgical approach and long-term results. J Urol. 1995;153(6):1781–4.
23. Msaouel P, Zhang M, Tu SM. Prolonged remission of upper urinary tract urothelial carcinoma with prominent choriocarcinomatous differentiation: a case report. Clin Genitourin Cancer. 2017;15(1):e73–e7.
24. Govender D, Nteene LM, Chetty R, Hadley GP. Mature renal teratoma and a synchronous malignant neuroepithelial tumour of the ipsilateral adrenal gland. J Clin Pathol. 2001;54(3):253–4.
25. Huang H, Tamboli P, Karam JA, Vikram R, Zhang M. Secondary malignancies diagnosed using kidney needle core biopsies: a clinical and pathological study of 75 cases. Hum Pathol. 2016;52:55–60.

Chapter 11
Hereditary Syndromes Associated with Kidney Tumors

Ayhan Ozcan, Seyda Erdogan, and Luan D. Truong

Hereditary renal cell carcinomas (HRCCs) account for about 2–4% of all RCCs [1–7]. However, the actual incidence may be higher due to insufficient family history, clinical evaluation, and limitations in current understanding of genetically linked cancer syndromes [2]. The patients with hereditary renal cell carcinoma (HRCC) syndromes are an important group requiring early screening and careful follow-up, and their relatives should be informed about disease-related morbidity and survival [2]. HRCC syndromes may occur in more than one first (parents, full siblings, or children) – or second (grandparents, grandchildren, aunts, uncles, nephews, nieces, or half-siblings) – degree family members that may be passed on through germ-line mutations.

Ten HRCC syndromes are currently recognized (Table 11.1), and they all show an autosomal dominant inheritance pattern. More common and well-known HRCC syndromes are von Hippel–Lindau (VHL), hereditary papillary RCC, Birt–Hogg–Dubé (BHD), hereditary leiomyomatosis RCC (HLRCC), and tuberous sclerosis. The International Society of Urological Pathology (ISUP) consensus conference on renal neoplasia held in Vancouver, Canada, in 2012 proposed several provisional/

A. Ozcan (✉)
Gulhane Military Medical Academy, School of Medicine, Department of Pathology, Ankara, Turkey

Yeni Yuzyil University Gaziosmanpasa Hospital, Department of Pathology, Istanbul, Turkey
e-mail: ayhan.ozcan@meditravelist.com

S. Erdogan
Department of Pathology, Cukurova University, School of Medicine, Adana, Turkey

L. D. Truong
Department of Pathology and Genomic Medicine, The Houston Methodist Hospital, Houston, TX, USA

Department of Pathology and Laboratory Medicine, Weill Cornell Medical College of Cornell University, New York, NY, USA

Department of Pathology and Medicine, Baylor College of Medicine, Houston, TX, USA

M. K. Divatia et al. (eds.), *Kidney Cancer*, https://doi.org/10.1007/978-3-030-28333-9_11

Table 11.1 Hereditary RCC syndromes: Molecular mechanisms, related targeted therapies, and extrarenal manifestations

Associated syndrome	Gene(s) (chromosome)	Gene product(s)	Pathway(s)	Renal tumor types	Extrarenal associations	Targeted therapy
VHL	*VHL* (3p25)	pVHL	HIF-α VEGFR	Clear cell RCC	Retinal and CNS hemangioblastomas Pheochromocytoma Pancreatic cysts and neuroendocrine tumors	Bevacizumab Sunitinib Sorafenib Pazopanib Axitinib
HPRCC	*MET* (7q31)	MET	c-MET HGF HGFR RTK PI3K/mTOR	Papillary RCC, type 1	None	Foretinib (for RTK pathway)[b] Everolimus (for mTOR pathway)[b]
BHD	*FLCN* (17p11)	Folliculin	FLCN c-KIT PI3K/mTOR	Hybrid tumor (oncocytoma and chromophobe RCC) Chromophobe RCC	Fibrofolliculoma Trichodiscoma Acrochordon Lung cysts Pneumothorax Colonic polyps and/or cancer	Everolimus
HLRCC	*FH* (1q42)	Fumarate hydratase	HIF-α VEGFR	Papillary RCC, type 2 Clear cell RCC	Cutaneous and uterine leiomyoma and leiomyosarcoma	Bevacizumab
TSC	*TSC1* (9q34) *TSC2* (16p13)	Hamartin Tuberin	PI3K/mTOR	Angiomyolipoma Clear cell RCC	Epilepsy Mental retardation CNS hamartomas (tubers) Adenoma sebaceum Hypomelanotic maculae Shagreen patch Fibrous plaques Facial angiofibroma Subungual fibroma Dental pits Cardiac rhabdomyoma Periventricular hamartomas (tubers) Lymphangioleiomyomatosis	Everolimus Sirolimus Temsirolimus

SDHB-RCC[a]	*SDHB* (1p36)	Succinate dehydrogenase B	HIF-α VEGFR	Clear cell RCC	Paraganglioma, Pheochromocytoma	None
Chromosome 3 translocation-associated RCC	Unknown	Unknown	Unknown	Clear cell RCC	None	None
Familial clear cell RCC	Unknown	Unknown	Unknown	Clear cell RCC	None	None
Hereditary hyperparathyroidism-jaw tumor syndrome	*HRPT2* (1q24–32)	Parafibromin	Beta-catenin RNA polymerase-associated factor-1	Papillary RCC Renal hamartomas Wilms' tumor Cyst	Parathyroid adenoma or carcinoma Fibro-osseous tumors of the jaw bones Benign or malignant uterine tumors	None
Papillary thyroid carcinoma with associated papillary renal neoplasia	*FPTC-PRN* (1q21)	Unknown	Unknown	Papillary RCC multifocal renal papillary adenomas Oncocytoma	Thyroid papillary carcinoma	None

Abbreviations: *BHD* Birt–Hogg–Dubé, *FLCN* folliculin pathway, *HIF-α* hypoxia-inducible factor alpha, *HGF* hepatocyte growth factor, *HGFR* hepatocyte growth factor receptor, *HLRCC* hereditary leiomyomatosis RCC, *HPRCC* hereditary papillary RCC, *HRPT2* hyperparathyroidism type 2, *mTOR* mammalian target of rapamycin, *PI3K* phosphatidylinositol-3-kinases, *RTK* receptor tyrosine kinase, *SDHB* succinate dehydrogenase B, *SDH-RCC* SDHB mutation-associated RCC, *TSC* tuberous sclerosis, *VEGFR* vascular endothelial growth factor receptor, *VHL* von Hippel–Lindau

[a]SDHB RCC is considered an emerging/provisional new tumor entity by the International Society of Urological Pathology (ISUP)

[b]Phase II trial ongoing

emerging entities one of which is succinate dehydrogenase B (SDHB) mutation-associated RCC. This type of RCC is now is a new member of the HRCC syndromes [7]. The rest of the syndromes are very rare, and their molecular pathogenetic mechanisms are currently not known.

The genetic mechanisms for RCC in the most of these syndromes, especially the more frequent ones, have been elucidated, but environmental factors and/or epigenetic mechanisms may also be pathogenetic. These molecular mechanisms may be also applicable in the sporadic context, and this relation has been validated for clear cell RCC. These molecular pathogenetic mechanisms also pave the way for several ongoing clinical trials for sporadic RCCs, in which target molecules are eliminated by their specific antibodies or inhibitors [8].

The purposes of this chapter are to describe (1) the general features of HRCC syndromes; (2) diagnostic approach including morphologic cues recognizable in nephrectomy specimens or tumor biopsy; (3) confirmatory molecular studies and subsequent genetic counseling; (4) pathogenetic relevance to sporadic RCC; and (5) targeted molecular therapy pertinent to sporadic RCC. Herein, we will focus on the six most common HRCC syndromes and summarize the salient features of other rare HRCC syndromes in Table 11.1.

General Diagnostic Approach

Before the discovery of the responsible genes, including *VHL*, *MET*, *FLCN*, *fumarate hydratase*, *TSC1*, *TSC2*, and *SDHB*, HRCC syndromes were identified based on the clinical findings reflecting the phenotypic manifestations of these syndromes. These genes are tumor suppressor genes except *MET*, which is a proto-oncogene. Most affected individuals inherit a germline mutation of gene from an affected parent and a normal "wild-type" gene from their unaffected parent. In hereditary renal carcinogenesis, unlike oncogenes/proto-oncogenes, tumor suppressor genes generally follow Knudson's "*two-hit*" hypothesis, which implies that both alleles of the tumor suppressor gene that codes for a particular protein must be affected before an effect is clinically manifested [9]. On contrary, oncogene/proto-oncogene mutations generally involve a single allele because they are "gain-of-function mutations." These mutations change the gene product, which gains a new and abnormal function. Gain-of-function (activating) mutations change the amino acid sequence of gene protein products, which causes abnormal functions. Many of these mutations affect signaling molecules, leading to activation of constitutive hormonal or other signaling pathways. The inherited germline mutation in HRCC represents the first "hit," which is present in every cell in the body. The second "hit" is a somatic mutation, one that occurs in a specific tissue at some point after birth. It damages the normal or wild-type allele, creating a clonal neoplastic cell of origin, which then transforms to a tumor mass [9].

Although phenotypic manifestations vary within affected members of the same family and among families, these findings are still the best to initiate clinical suspicion for further molecular screening. Renal tumors are often the initial manifestation of HRCC syndromes. These tumors may display distinctive clinical, imaging, or morphologic features, which collectively should raise the possibility of HRCC syndromes for genetic confirmation.

The RCCs in these syndromes, except the SDHB mutation-associated RCC, are more likely to be present at an earlier age (usually before 30 years of age) and tend to be more frequently multifocal and bilateral than the sporadic RCCs [5]. They are also usually associated with extra-renal manifestations. The RCC in each syndrome tends to be of distinctive histologic types. Although the morphology of these types is, in general, similar to that of the same types of RCC that develop sporadically, there are often additional features distinctive for each syndrome (see below), which serve as the first diagnostic clue.

The clinical and/or pathologic suspicion of HRCC syndromes should and can be confirmed by genetic testing. These studies, which are now readily available for routine diagnosis, can be done in blood sample reflecting the pathogenetic germline mutation involving all somatic cell lines of the affected individuals. Although genetic testing is available and is highly reliable, it should be performed by well-established institutes, considering the profound consequences of the findings on the patients and their relatives. Genetic counseling is also important. Potentially affected patients may be intensely interested in genetic testing, but they may not be fully aware of the ethical and legal problems such as informing relatives, impact on spousal relationship, prenatal and infant testing, and discrimination in employment or insurance [10, 11].

Genetic testing is performed on peripheral blood lymphocytes in patients with a strong clinical suspicion, or on other tissues such as skin fibroblasts or exfoliated buccal cells, especially, in the cases without a history of hereditary RCC syndrome in the family members, who have generally somatic mosaicism [1, 12–15]. Somatic mosaicism is a mutation occurring during embryonic development, and some cells are normal whereas others carry the mutation. The mutation may not be detectable in the peripheral blood of these patients because the blood stem cells do not carry the mutation. These patients may be asymptomatic or have less severe disease than offspring and may have negative tests for germline mutation. Phenotypic features and clinical manifestations vary among members within the same family who carry the same germline mutation. This is related to de novo mutation occurring in embryogenesis. De novo mutations may explain genetic diseases in which an affected offspring has a mutation in every cell in the body, but the parents do not, and there is no family history of the disease. In contrary to germline mutations, somatic mosaicism is rare and its identification is likely to be more difficult [1, 12]. To date, among hereditary RCC syndromes, somatic mosaicism is described in VHL-, HLRCC-, and TSC-associated RCCs [1, 12–14].

Some genes are active (on) in some tissues and organs but inactive (off) in others. Which genes are active or inactive discriminate different types of cells. Genes are switched on and off during development in response to environmental changes, such as metabolism and infection. There is no evidence of an organ or target cell specificity of germline mutations; the occasional familial clustering of certain tumor types may reflect the genetic background of the affected family member or the additional influence of environmental and nongenetic host factors [16].

The key points regarding diagnosis and management of each hereditary RCC syndrome and their family member are detailed in the following sections and summarized in Table 11.2.

Table 11.2 Diagnostic key points for hereditary RCC syndromes

Associated syndrome	Diagnostic key points: Morphologic features	Diagnostic key points: Management of affected patients and their family members
VHL	Multifocal and bilateral *clear cell RCCs* Multifocal and bilateral *renal cysts* lined by clear cells forming papillae and epithelial tufting Clear cell *tumorlets*	Surveillance with ultrasound, CT scan, and MRI Surgery recommended for larger than 3 cm For definitive diagnosis, genetic testing[a] essential to demonstrate germline mutation/inactivation of *VHL* gene
HPRCC	Numerous (>100) and bilateral type 1 papillary RCC Numerous microscopic papillary adenomas in the background kidney	Surveillance and surgery recommendations similar to those for VHL disease Genetic testing[a] essential to demonstrate germline mutation of *c-MET* proto-oncogene
BHD	Multifocal renal oncocytic neoplasms (oncocytoma, chromophobe RCC, and HOCT) Renal oncocytosis in the background kidney	Surveillance and surgery recommendations similar to those for VHL disease Genetic testing[a] essential to demonstrate germline mutation of *BHD* gene
HLRCC	Unilateral and solitary renal tumors Papillary (most common), tubulopapillary, tubular, cribriform, and solid patterns Distinctive morphologic appearances in the neoplastic cells with abundant eosinophilic cytoplasm and macronucleoli with perinucleolar halos (*viropathic-like* appearance) Renal cysts lined by eosinophilic epithelial cells in the background kidney	Active surveillance not recommended Surgery promptly recommended whenever tumors detected Genetic testing[a] essential to demonstrate germline mutation of *fumarate hydratase (FH)* gene
TSC	Multifocal and bilateral epithelioid *AMLs* Combination of *AML tumorlets* and *renal cysts* lined by eosinophilic epithelial cells in the background kidney *RCCs* (clear cell, chromophobe, papillary, and unclassified) rare and frequently associated with *intratumoral cysts* and *AML* lesions TSC-associated PRCCs with distinctly abundant clear cytoplasm with delicate thread-like eosinophilic strands and occasionally eosinophilic globules	Surveillance recommended for AMLs and RCCs Surgery recommended for tumors >3 cm (RCC) and 4 cm (AML) Genetic testing[a] essential to demonstrate loss-of-function or inactivating mutations of one of two tumor suppressor genes, *TSC1* and *TSC2* genes

Table 11.2 (continued)

Associated syndrome	Diagnostic key points Morphologic features	Management of affected patients and their family members
SDHB-RCC[b]	Distinctive morphological pattern with nest or tubules consisted of finely granular eosinophilic polygonal cells Distinctive pale eosinophilic intracytoplasmic inclusions, corresponding with giant mitochondria	Surveillance and surgery recommendations similar to HLRCC disease Genetic testing[a] essential to demonstrate germ-line mutation/inactivation *SDHB, SDHC,* and *SDHD* of *succinate dehydrogenase* (*SDH*) complex genes, which are consisted of 5 nuclear genes (*SDHA, SDHB, SDHC, SDHD,* and *SDHAF2)*

Abbreviations: *AML* angiomyolipoma, *BHD* Birt–Hogg–Dubé, *HLRCC* hereditary leiomyomatosis RCC, *HPRCC* hereditary papillary RCC, *HOCT* hybrid oncocytic/chromophobe tumor, *SDH-RCC* SDHB mutation-associated RCC, *TSC* tuberous sclerosis, *VHL* von Hippel–Lindau

[a]Peripheral blood is sufficient for genetic testing in the patients that have clinical diagnosis. However, it has been performed on other tissues, such as skin fibroblasts or exfoliated buccal cells in the patients who have no clinical diagnosis. Genetic tests have also been performed on tissue sections obtained from paraffin blocks of the patients without extra-invasive intervention. For genetic testing, Southern blot analysis or quantitative polymerase chain reaction (PCR) has been usually used. However, new genetic techniques, such as array comparative genomic hybridization (array CGH) and next-generation sequencing, are more powerful tools, especially, in cases of suspected mosaicism with negative genetic tests

[b]SDHB RCC is considered an emerging/provisional new tumor entity by the International Society of Urological Pathology (ISUP)

Von Hippel–Lindau Disease

General Features

Von Hippel–Lindau (VHL) disease, the most common HRCC syndrome, is an autosomal dominant inherited multisystem neoplastic disorder characterized by germline mutation in the *VHL* gene, which leads to benign or malignant tumors, and cysts in many organs including kidney, eye, cerebellum, spine, pancreas, adrenal gland, ear, and epididymis (Table 11.1). Both von Hippel, an ophthalmologist, and Lindau, a pathologist, first described retinal hemangioblastomas in 1904 and 1926, respectively. However, Lindau noted the association of retinal hemangioblastoma and cystic lesions/tumors in other organs. The term "von Hippel–Lindau disease" was first used in 1936 by Davison, but gained popularity starting from the 1970s [17]. In 1964, Melmon and Rosen first proposed criteria for clinical diagnosis of VHL disease, which have been updated and modified [18]. They are listed in Table 11.3. It is emphasized that each of the tumor types seen in VHL disease can

Table 11.3 Clinical criteria of VHL disease

Family history	Manifestations[a]
Positive	Retinal hemangioblastoma (retinal, cerebellar, or spinal) Adrenal or extra-adrenal pheochromocytomas Clear cell RCC Multiple renal and pancreatic cysts
Negative	Two or more hemangioblastomas or single hemangioblastomas in association with one of the visceral tumors (with exception of epididymal and renal cysts) Clear cell RCC Adrenal or extra-adrenal pheochromocytomas Endolymphatic sac tumors (ELST), papillary cystadenomas of the epididymis or broad ligament, or neuroendocrine tumors of the pancreas

[a]The diagnosis of VHL disease requires *two* or more characteristic lesions for *negative* family history; or *one* or more characteristic lesions for *positive* family history

Table 11.4 Genotype–phenotype correlations and clinical classification of VHL disease

		VHL types			
		1	2A	2B	2C
Clinical manifestations (phenotype)	CNS hemangioblastomas	+	+	+	–
	Retinal hemangioblastomas	+	+	+	–
	Clear cell RCC	+	–	+	–
	Adrenal or extra-adrenal pheochromocytomas	–	+	+	+
	Pancreatic neuroendocrine tumors	–	+	+	–
Genotype		Deletion, truncation	Missense	Missense	Missense
Increase of HIF-alpha activity		+++	+	++	Normal

also occur in sporadic cases without family history of VHL disease. Therefore, the diagnosis of VHL disease in a patient without a family history requires the presence of tumors of two different types (Table 11.3).

VHL disease was clinically classified into two types according to the presence of pheochromocytomas: VHL type 1 [75% of VHL families; retinal and central nervous system (CNS) hemangioblastomas, and bilateral clear cell RCC, but *without* pheochromocytomas] and VHL type 2 [tumor types as in VHL1, but with pheochromocytomas] [19]. VHL type 2 is subdivided into subtypes 2A, 2B, and 2C according to other tumor associations (Table 11.4).

About 80% of patients have a positive family, and the rest may represent de novo mutations, *without* other family members being affected [20]. In contrast to other HRCC syndromes, VHL disease demonstrates a high genetic penetrance, with clinical manifestations in over 90% of individuals by 65 years of age [19]. Although these diseases are autosomal *dominant,* tumor development requires inactivation of both copies of the VHL gene. For the development of the tumors, somatic mutation or inactivation of *the remaining wild-type allele* is required in VHL disease, while simultaneous mutation of both *VHL* genes (biallelic inactivation of *VHL* gene) is required for sporadic RCC. VHL patients have a mutated copy of the *VHL* gene, and the second allele is often deleted in the context of VHL-associated RCCs. The inactivation of the wild-type allele in tumors of VHL patients is in keeping with the classic "two-hit" model in tumorigenesis [18, 19, 21].

VHL disease is a life-threatening disorder with the cumulative risk of RCC higher than 70% by the age of 60 years [22]. Although hemangioblastoma is the most common tumor, RCC is the leading cause of death (up to 50% of cases) [18, 21]. Earlier diagnosis RCC in VHL patients afforded by modern imaging, together with rational management, however, has help reduced the morbidity and mortality.

Clinical Features

Renal lesions are the most significant manifestation of VHL disease. Almost all of them are multifocal and bilateral solid/cystic neoplasm composed of clear cells (clear cell RCC) or cysts lined by clear cells (see Pathological Features). Most renal lesions develop between the ages of 25 and 60 years (mean age 40), with RCCs noted in 25–40% of patients and cysts in up to 70% of them. These lesions are even more frequent in older patients, indicating a high genetic penetrance (90% by age 65) and a continuous tumor risk. These tumors, however, rarely develop before 16 years of age [4, 18, 20, 21].

The renal lesions are usually asymptomatic and rarely impair the renal function. VHL patients usually present with extra-renal manifestations, without renal lesions, in early ages (Table 11.1). Thus, the mean age at diagnosis of retinal and cranial hemangioblastomas is 25 years (range 1–68) and 30 years (range 9–70), respectively [21]. Cranial hemangioblastoma develops in 60–80% of patients [21] and may involve cerebellum, brainstem, spinal cord, and nerve roots, but rarely in the brain. It is one main cause of death due to frequent multifocality and high recurrence rate. Retinal hemangioblastoma develops in 50% of patients and causes blindness in 35% of gene carriers [21] and 55% of patients at age of 50 years [18].

These findings serve as the foundation for a rigorous surveillance program aiming at early detection and management of the lesions before they create injury or death.

Pathologic Features

Grossly, kidneys in VHL patients are generally of normal size and weight, especially in younger patients, because most renal cysts and tumor nodules are small. Multiple and bilateral renal cysts are common. It has been estimated that about 600 microscopic tumors and 1100 microscopic clear cell-lined cysts might be seen in each affected kidney in patients under 40 years old [23]. The tumor in about a half of the VHL-associated RCC cases is under 3 cm, which is the general threshold for nephron-sparing surgery [24]. Renal tumors in family members are usually detected early by imaging surveillance. Therefore, larger tumors rarely occur in the kidney. However, larger tumors had increased metastatic risk (0% for ≤3 cm, 6% for 3.2–4 cm, 20% for 4.1–5.5 cm, 33% for 6–10 cm, and 80% for ≥11 cm) [24]. The tumor nodules display the typical features of a low-grade clear cell RCC. They are solid or solid/cystic circumscribed and encapsulated masses, with a homogeneous yellow or orange (due to tumor cell cytoplasmic lipid) cut surface. Hemorrhage, necrosis, and calcification may be seen, imparting a variegated appearance. The transformation of a cortical cyst to a solid lesion is rare, but complex cystic and solid lesions can contain neoplastic tissue [24].

Microscopically, a spectrum of lesions that may represent a continuum of cystic and solid masses is noted, the common feature of which is lesional cells with clear cytoplasm and often low-grade nuclei (Fig. 11.1). These lesions may include (1) simple unilocular cysts lined by one layer of clear cells; (2) cyst with mural nodules, tufting, or small papillations into cyst lumen; (3) uni- or multilocular cysts lined by more than one layer of cells; and (4) solid mass of variable sizes. The smaller ones are often composed of nodular collections or sheets of clear cells with no nuclear atypia, and virtually no stroma. The larger masses tend to display typical features of sporadic clear cell RCC, including alveolar (nested) or acinar growth pattern surrounded arborizing vasculature in thin fibrous septa, with or without associated degenerative changes such as necrosis, hemorrhage, and stromal myxoid changes. In general, there is virtually no or only low-grade nuclear atypia; however, higher nuclear grades can be seen in complex, multilayered cysts, or frank carcinoma. Often, more than one type of lesions is noted in individual kidneys, raising the possibility that these lesions may represent different stages in a continuous growth process. The intervening renal parenchyma is unremarkable. The adenoma/carcinoma demarcation is not well defined for the VHL-associated renal neoplastic lesion. However, it is noted that virtually no tumor that measures less than 3 cm metastasizes [24]. These characteristic renal lesions, especially when encountered in a kidney specimen

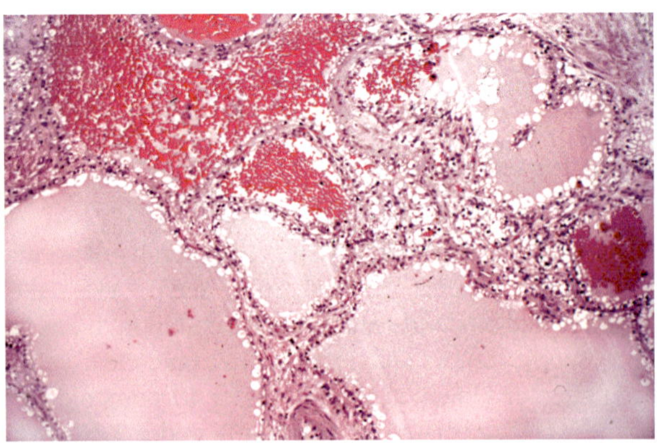

Fig. 11.1 von Hippel–Lindau syndrome: A simple cyst lined by a single layer of clear cells (lower) and a solid neoplastic area representing ISUP nucleolar grade 1 cystic clear cell renal cell carcinoma separated from a simple cyst lined by the same cell type (hematoxylin and eosin, ×200)

from a young patient, should raise the possibility of VHL disease for genetic/molecular confirmation.

The molecular/genetic features, pathogenetic mechanisms, and targeted therapy modalities for the VHL-associated RCC will be discussed together with its sporadic counterpart in Chaps. 18 and 19.

Management, Genetic Counseling, and Treatment

Patients with VHL disease is subjected to a lifelong, continuous risk of development of tumors of multiple organs including kidney. A multidisciplinary comprehensive screening program is essential. This program aims at early detection and management of the lesions before they create injury or death. This program, which should be applicable to all at-risk individuals, includes the following [2]:

1. Annual occular examination starting at 1–4 years (for retinal hemangioma)
2. Biannual CNS imaging starting at 16 years (for CNS hemangiomas)
3. Annual imaging of abdomen starting at 8 years (for kidney and pancreas tumors)
4. Audiology testing every 2–3 years starting at 1 year (for inner ear tumors)
5. Annual plasma metanephrines and normetanephrines starting at 5 years (for pheochromocytoma)

Modifications from this basic program may be needed. Thus, a closer monitoring during the pregnancy is crucial, because it tends to promote the growth of all neoplastic lesions. Family members with VHL disease, who carry a germline *VHL* gene mutation but yet have no tumor, and mild phenotypic changes, can be securely imaged every 2–3 years by MRI, which is often preferred due to lower cumulative radiation load than CT scan. Patients at risk for VHL disease-associated RCC should be assessed more frequently at 6–12 monthly intervals depending on tumor growth rates.

Patients with clinical findings or tissue lesions should undergo confirmatory genetic testing. This should also be applied to all members of the patient's family. Genetic testing, which is widely available, requires only blood, and it has 100% accuracy for well-known mutations. Genetic testing not only confirms the diagnosis but also helps stratify the risk of RCC as well as those of other tumor types [17]. Prenatal genetic testing in conjunction with amniocentesis is also possible.

Management of VHL patients is multidisciplinary. Focus is here directed to the renal lesions. RCC is the most frequent cause of death, and the renal lesions represent the main management concern. Considering the lifelong, continuous risk of development of multifocal bilateral renal tumors, the treatment aims at limited surgery to preserve renal function for avoidance of renal replacement as long as possible, balancing with the need for more definitive surgery before the tumor gives rise to potentially lethal metastasis. Serial imaging of the kidneys is crucial for management. Renal tumors are often small, bilateral, multiple, and asymptomatic for long time. However, these tumors do grow, often slowly at a rate of 0.2–2.2 cm/year (mean 1.6 cm), but can be much faster [25].

The small tumors can be managed conservatively, including MRI-guided percutaneous radiofrequency ablation or cryoablation. Larger tumors call for more definitive surgery. Although the adenoma–carcinoma sequence is not well defined for VHL disease, a demarcation of 3 cm is often proposed. Thus, renal solid tumors larger than 3 cm and confined to the kidney often call for partial (nephron-sparing) nephrectomy, at which time all accessible additional small lesions should also be removed in order to avoid repeated surgery. This approach has been shown to yield results comparable to radical nephrectomy [26]. Recent studies further suggest that partial nephrectomy may be also indicated for bulky (>3 cm) multifocal renal tumors [26, 27]. It is emphasized that most patients will eventually present with a recurrent or de novo tumors even after partial nephrectomy, and some of them may be large at detection, despite serial imaging. Repeated surgery, even conservatively, may finally obliterate functional renal parenchyma, and renal replacement therapy is required [18]. The risk of renal tumor in transplanted kidneys is not well defined [28], but immunosuppression does not affect VHL disease adversely [29].

Current understanding of the molecular mechanism of tumor development including the roles of *VHL* gene and the related signaling pathways has enabled the development of target-specific drugs for the treatment of advanced RCC in VHL and also in sporadic contexts [21]. Bevacizumab, an anti-VEGF monoclonal antibody, was demonstrated to significantly prolong the time interval to progression of metastatic tumor [21]. Inhibitors of VEGFR and PDGFR (sunitinib, sorafenib, pazopanib) were successively shown to confer significant benefit in VHL patients with metastatic clear cell RCC [30]. Sunitinib has been used to reduce the size of multifocal bulky tumor before nephron-sparing surgery [21]. Although significant response to these drugs has been observed in RCC, no improvement has been reported for in retinal and CNS hemangioblastomas [31]. Targeted therapy modalities will be discussed later (see Chap. 19).

Hereditary Papillary Renal Cell Carcinoma

General Features

Hereditary papillary renal cell carcinoma (HPRCC), a rare autosomal dominant hereditary renal cancer syndrome, was first described in 1994 and was later shown to be due to mutations in the *MET* proto-oncogene [32, 33]. HPRCC is highly penetrant (90% possibility of developing RCC at the age of 80 years), but at a lower level than that of VHL disease. The renal tumors in this syndrome tend to develop late in life, progress slowly, rarely metastasize, and do not cause patients' demise.

Clinical Features

HPRCC is characterized by multifocal and bilateral papillary RCC with papillary type-1 histology. Papillary tumors range from microscopic nodules (papillary adenomas) to clinically symptomatic large masses (papillary RCCs). Papillary RCC is typically seen in advanced ages (between 50 and 70 years), but it can develop as early as at 30 years [34]. RCC is generally diagnosed after the age of 50 years [1, 19]. Among affected family members, male/female ratio is 2:1 [1]. It has been estimated that affected family members are at risk of the developing 1100–3400 microscopic tumors in a single kidney throughout their lifetime [34]. CT is a useful screening imaging method, especially for detection of small-sized lesions due to their hypovascularity [35].

Pathologic Features

Grossly, numerous bilateral and multifocal macroscopic well-demarcated tumor nodules are typically noted in the kidneys (Fig. 11.2). Individual nodules are indistinguishable from sporadic papillary RCCs. Their cut surfaces usually have a granular appearance, but hemorrhage and necrosis are also seen, especially in the larger ones.

Microscopically, the renal tumor in HPRCC shares the same histologic features with sporadic type-1 papillary RCCs. Numerous foci of papillary renal neoplasia resembling sporadic renal papillary adenoma with normal intervening renal parenchyma are common (Fig. 11.3a). They are characterized by a large cystic space-lined or filled by complex tumor papillae with fibrovascular stalks, often accompanied by stromal foamy macrophage infiltration. The cystic spaces are usually surrounded by a thick fibrous capsule. Sometimes, tubulopapillary, glomeruloid, trabecular, or solid appearances are seen, as in sporadic papillary RCCs. Psammomatous calcification is also identified in the stroma of the papillary structures. Although type-1 papillary RCC is more common in this setting, type-2 papillary RCC may be seen in same kidney together with type-1 papillary RCC (Fig. 11.3b).

The molecular/genetic features, pathogenetic mechanisms, and targeted therapy modalities of HPRCC will be discussed together with its sporadic counterpart in the later chapters (see Chaps. 18 and 19).

Management, Genetic Counseling, and Treatment

HPRCC patients, like in VHL patients, should be subjected to active screening with serial renal imaging to follow tumor growth. Percutaneous MRI-guided radiofrequency ablation or cryoablation may be suitable for small tumors (<3 cm)

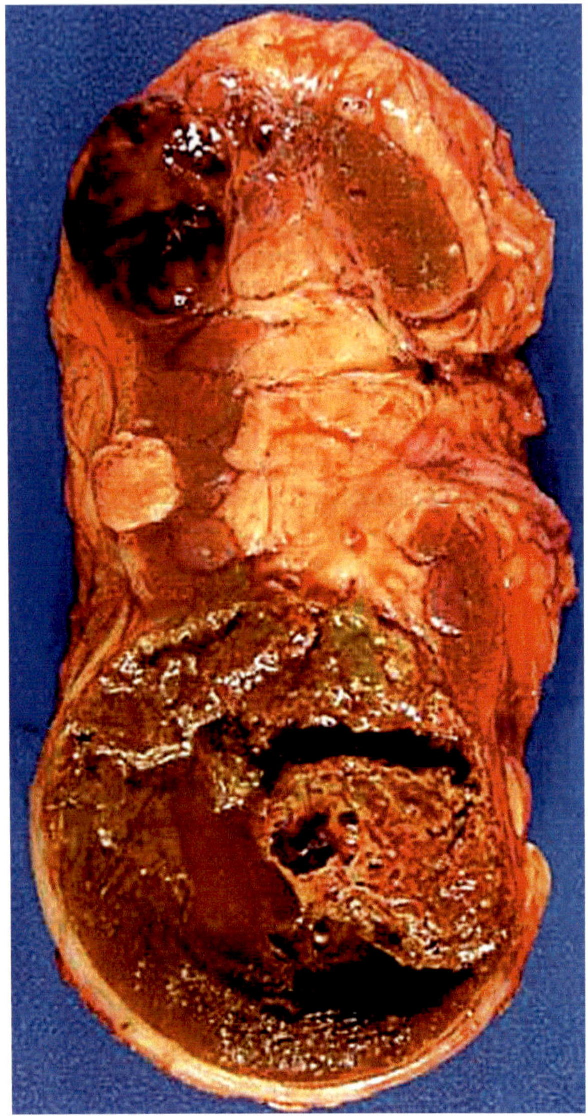

Fig. 11.2 Hereditary papillary RCC: Multiple prominent masses and minute nodules of tumors are noted

[36]. When tumors reach large size (>3 cm) initial, repeat, or salvage nephron-sparing surgery by open, laparoscopic, or robotic approach is indicated to avoid repeated surgery and to mitigate metastatic chance [26, 36, 37].

Over the past 10 years, to avoid surgical intervention, several preclinical and clinical studies on molecular targeted therapy have been conducted for papillary RCC. Nowadays, clinical trial targeting inhibition of both HGF/MET and vascular endothelial growth factor receptor 2 (VEGFR2 [Flk-1/KDR]) in HPRCC patients

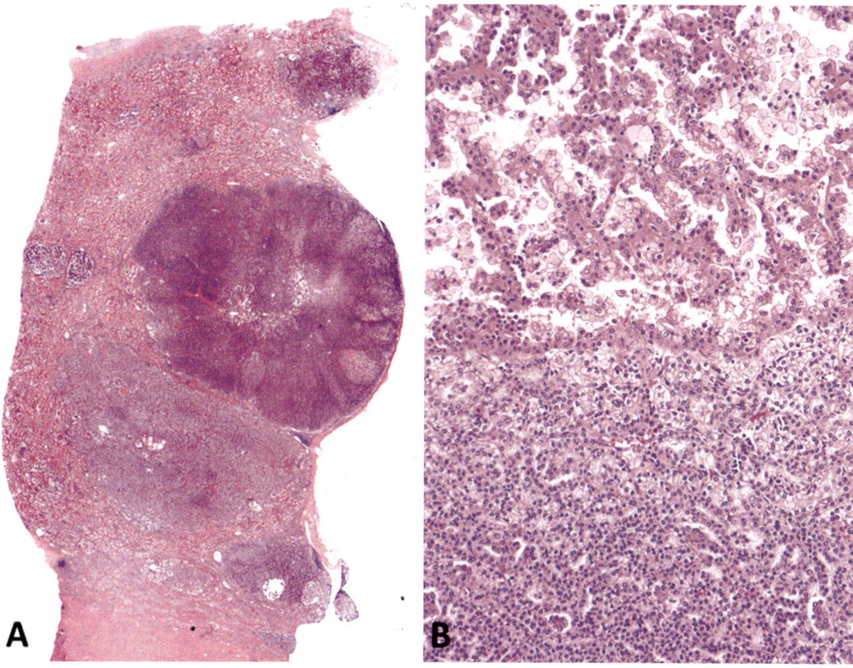

Fig. 11.3 Hereditary papillary RCC: (**a**) The foci of papillary RCC are noted in this tissue section. (**b**) Interface of type 1 (right) and type 2 (left) papillary RCC characterized by tumor cells with abundant eosinophilic cytoplasm (hematoxylin and eosin, ×20 for **a** and ×200 for **b**)

has shown a partial response [34, 37]. Furthermore, foretinib, a novel oral multikinase inhibitor targeting MET, VEGFR2, RON, AXL, and TIE-2 receptors, was shown to confer a high response rate for advanced papillary RCC, with a manageable drug toxicity profile [38].

For early diagnosis and prevention of metastatic disease, all family members of HPRCC patients should be genetically tested for germline MET mutation. Targeted therapy modalities will be discussed later (see Chap. 19).

Birt–Hogg–Dubé Syndrome

General Features

Birt–Hogg–Dubé (BHD) syndrome is a rare hereditary disease (estimated to involve more than 600 families). BHD was first described in 1977 and initially characterized by cutaneous manifestations [39]. In 1993, its association of renal tumors was first described and later confirmed in other reports [40]. Birt–Hogg–Dubé (BHD) gene (also known as *FLCN* gene) locus was mapped to chromosome 17p11.2 in 2001 [41], and 1 year later, the gene product, folliculin, was identified [42]. The clinical spectrum of BHD syndrome has been expanded, and the association of renal tumors and lung cysts was first reported in 2002 [43].

Clinical Features

BHD syndrome is a rare autosomal dominant genodermatosis and characterized by lesions of several organs, including skin tumors (fibrofolliculoma, trichodiscoma, and acrochordon), lung cysts, spontaneous pneumothorax, colonic tumors, medullary thyroid carcinoma, lipoma, and renal tumors (usually bilateral and multifocal). Skin lesions and renal tumors usually appear after the age of 20 and 30 years, respectively [19]. Fibrofolliculoma is the most common (85%) among skin lesions [3]. Renal tumors occur in 25–35% of patients [3, 19]. Lung cysts are a common manifestation (80% of patients) [3, 43]. The diagnosis of BDH syndrome requires one major or two minor criteria (Table 11.5) [44–46].

Pathologic Features

BHD-related renal tumors are histologically distinctive. Most of them are hybrid oncocytic tumor (HOT) (50%) or chromophobe RCC (34%), but other histologic types can be rarely seen, including clear cell RCC (9%), oncocytoma (5%), or papillary RCC (2%) [44]. More than one type can be seen in individual patients [3]. HOT has characteristic features detailed below. The other types of renal tumors are histologically similar to their sporadic counterparts. It is emphasized that HOT can be seen not only in BDH patients but also in a background of renal oncocytosis without any known genetic mutation, or sporadically. HOT, however, displays subtle morphologic difference among these conditions (see below) [3, 7, 45].

Table 11.5 Diagnostic criteria of Birt–Hogg–Dubé syndrome

Major criteria
At least five fibrofolliculomas or trichodiscomas, at least one histologically confirmed, of adult onset
Pathogenic FLCN germ-line mutation
Minor criteria
Multiple lung cysts: Bilateral basally located lung cysts with no other apparent cause, with or without spontaneous primary pneumothorax
Renal cancer: Early onset (<50 yr of age) or multifocal or bilateral renal cancer or renal cancer of mixed chromophobe and oncocytic histology
A first-degree relative with BHD syndrome

Grossly, HOT in BHD patients is multifocal/bilateral (in contrast to a single mass in sporadic or nongenetic oncocytosis background), well demarcated, and comprising nonencapsulated nodules with a homogeneous tan to brown cut surface, which can sometimes display a central scar, or exceptionally, necrosis.

Microscopically, HOT in BHD syndrome is characterized by three morphologic patterns [7]: (1) an admixture of areas with typical features of oncocytoma (Fig. 11.4a) or chromophobe RCC (Fig. 11.4b); (2) scattered tumor cells with typical features of chromophobe RCC in a background of typical oncocytoma; and (3) large eosinophilic cells with prominent cytoplasmic vacuoles. The tumor cell nuclei are frequently more pleomorphic and display a more widespread "raisinoid" feature, compared to HOT in other contexts. Aside from HOT, the kidneys in patients with BHD syndrome often display background changes, including numerous microscopic oncocytic nodules, oncocytic cysts, and aggregates of oncocytic cells with intervening normal renal tissue. These background changes are virtually identical to those of nongenetic renal oncocytosis [1, 4, 6].

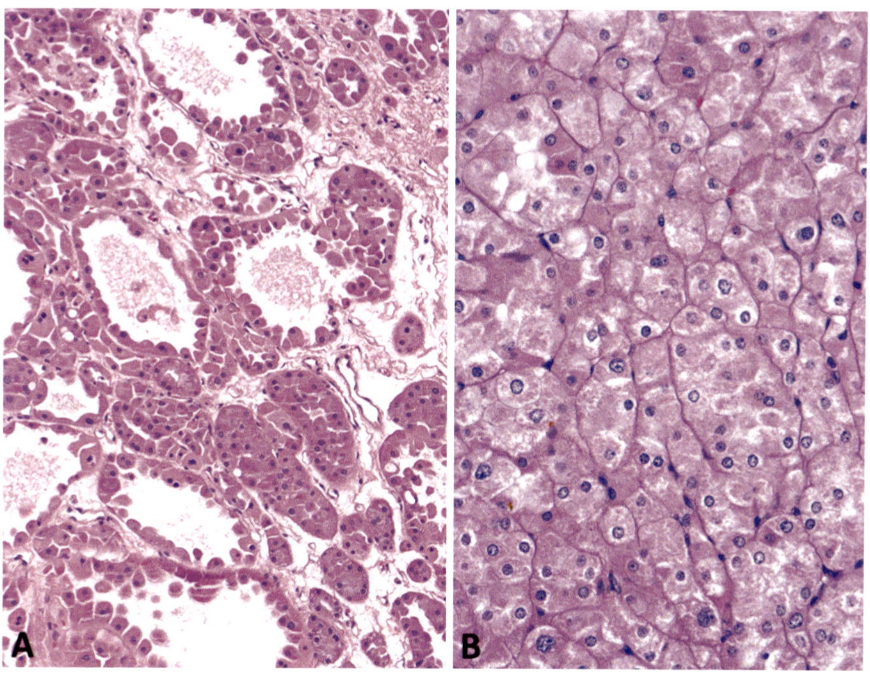

Fig. 11.4 Birt–Hogg–Dubé Syndrome: (**a**) An area from the same tumor displaying typical features of oncocytoma, including abundant eosinophilic cytoplasm, acinar/microcystic growth pattern, myxoid stroma, and round/uniform nuclei. (**b**) Another area from a hybrid tumor showing some features of chromophobe RCC, including reticulated cytoplasm, perinuclear clearing, well-defined cell border, and a tubular-trabecular growth pattern; however, raisinoid nuclei are not seen (hematoxylin and eosin; ×100 for **a** and ×200 for **b**)

The molecular/genetic features, pathogenetic mechanisms, and targeted therapy modalities for BHD-related renal tumor will be discussed together with its sporadic counterparts in the later chapters (see Chaps. 18 and 19).

Management, Genetic Counseling, and Treatment

BHD patients, like in VHL and HPRCC patients, involve active screening with renal imaging until their largest tumor nodule reach 3 cm. At this threshold, nephron-sparing surgery is recommended [26, 36, 37]. For small size tumors (<3 cm), percutaneous radiofrequency ablation or cryoablation can be performed, like in other HRCC syndromes [36, 46].

It should be emphasized that a subset (approximately 10%) of patients with germline mutations of the *FLCN* gene does not have the typical skin lesions [47]. Therefore, multiple, bilateral, and conglomerate renal tumors with a typical morphology should raise the possibility of BHD syndrome.

Molecular understanding of *FLCN* (*BHD*) gene pathway, including the function of FLCN, FNIP1, and FNIP2 protein complex, has enabled the development of target-specific drugs for advanced RCC in BHD patients. Rapamycin, the first inhibitor for mTOR, reduced tumor size and prolonged median survival in animals [35, 48]. Nowadays, new rapamycin analogs with more favorable pharmaceutical profiles, such as everolimus, temsirolimus, deferolimus, and zotarolimus, have been developed and are expected to be more effective with less adverse effects than rapamycin [48]. Targeted therapy modalities will be discussed later (see Chap. 19).

Hereditary Leiomyomatosis and Renal Cell Carcinoma Syndrome

General Features

Hereditary leiomyomatosis and renal cell carcinoma syndrome (HLRCC) is an autosomal dominant hereditary renal cancer syndrome characterized by cutaneous and uterine leiomyomas and RCC. HLRCC was first described in 2001 in two families that have cutaneous and uterine leiomyomas and papillary RCC [49]. HLRCC may be a variant of multiple cutaneous and uterine leiomyomatosis (MCUL) syndrome. First described in 1973 and also known as Reed's syndrome, MCUL includes a rare patient with RCC [50]. Both HLRCC and MCUL syndromes are an autosomal dominant condition with variable organ-dependent penetrance, and both are characterized by *fumarate hydratase (FH)* gene mutation [3]. Although *FH* gene mutation was detected in about 90% of HLRCC family members, this mutation is found only in a rare sporadic RCC [3, 7, 13].

Although cutaneous and uterine leiomyomatosis are highly penetrant with 100% occurrence rate, RCCs have low penetrance with an estimated incidence ranging from 2% to 32% [3, 13, 49]. Most renal tumors associated with *FH* gene mutation are type-2 papillary RCC, followed by a much less frequent collecting duct RCC. These RCCs are usually solitary and unilateral, in contrary to renal tumors associated with VHL, HPRCC, and BHD syndromes [4, 13].

Clinical Features

Multiple cutaneous leiomyomas usually begin to appear in the third decade, and most occur frequently on the trunk and extremities. They are typically grouped, disseminated, or disseminated and segmental, and can be painful [3, 13, 49]. They are histologically similar to its sporadic counterpart. Rare case of cutaneous leiomyosarcoma associated with HLRCC has been reported [13].

Half of the women have undergone hysterectomy for uterine leiomyomas before the age of 30 years [7]. Uterine leiomyomas frequently lead to hypermenorrhea and severe pelvic pain, infertility, and pregnancy complications [4, 50]. Uterine leiomyomas are often cellular and some may have atypical features. Uterine leiomyosarcoma associated with HLRCC is very rare and usually seen in Finnish HLRCC patients with early onset [51].

RCCs associated with HLRCC occur in 2%–20% of affected patients, and they have different biology from other RCCs [4, 13, 50]. Morphologically, they are most frequently papillary type-2 PRCC or, less frequently, collecting duct RCC. Compared with other hereditary RCC syndromes, the renal tumors in HLRCC display aggressive behavior and poor prognosis, including a high stage at presentation [4, 13, 52].

Pathologic Features

Grossly, HLRCC-associated RCCs are often large, unilateral, solitary, and indistinguishable from their sporadic counterparts. They may show extrarenal extension or metastasis at presentation.

Microscopically, HLRCC-associated RCC typically shows features of type-2 PRCC. However, the growth pattern may be highly variable, with solid, alveolar, or tubular architecture. A unique feature regardless of growth pattern is the presence of tall tumor cells with large nuclei and prominent orangeophilic or eosinophilic nucleoli with a peripheral clear halo resembling Cytomegalovirus inclusions and is aptly described as "viropathic-like" (Fig. 11.5). Sometimes, extensive sarcomatoid and rhabdoid features are also seen [53]. Cysts lined by the same type of cells as seen in RCC may be seen in the background kidney (42% of cases) and may serve as tumor precursor [6]. RCCs with features of collecting duct RCC, such as papillary architecture, multinodularity, and desmoplasia, can be less often encountered. However, this tumor type is differentiated from sporadic collecting duct RCC by

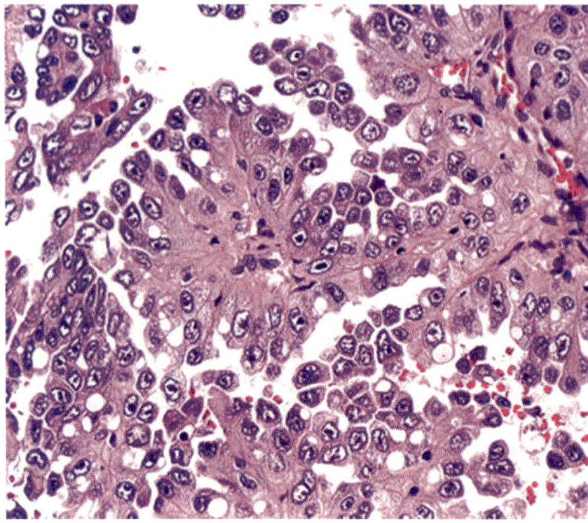

Fig. 11.5 Hereditary leiomyomatosis and renal cell carcinoma syndrome: Type 2 papillary RCC, characterized by tumor cells with abundant eosinophilic cytoplasm forming well-defined papillae. Tumor cells display abundant granular cytoplasm and prominent nucleoli surrounded by a halo, reminiscent of viral change (hematoxylin and eosin, ×200)

the characteristic nucleolar/viropathic-like features and the absence of cytokeratin 7 and *Ulex europaeus* lectin (typically expressed by sporadic collecting duct RCC).

The molecular/genetic features, pathogenetic mechanisms, and targeted therapy modalities of HLRCC-associated RCC will be discussed together with its sporadic counterpart in the later chapters (see Chaps. 18 and 19).

Management, Genetic Counseling, and Treatment

RCCs associated with VHL, HPRCC, or BHD syndromes slowly progress and rarely metastasize when smaller than 3 cm. In contrast, HLRCC-associated RCC is aggressive, with often extrarenal extension or metastasis at presentation even for a primary tumor of small size (less than 1 cm). Most patients have died of metastatic disease within 5 years after diagnosis [5, 19, 37]. As a result, active surveillance is not recommended, and surgery should be immediately performed when RCC is first detected regardless of size.

Several drugs targeting HIF-1α or AMPK (AMP-activated protein kinase) have been studied basing on the molecular premise that activation of HIF-1α or reduction of AMPK in HLRCC patients contributes to invasiveness and growth of FH-deficient cancer cells [54]. Metformin, an oral antidiabetic drug and an activator of AMPK, inhibits tumor invasion in FH-deficient animal model [54]. In addition, there are ongoing clinical trials for the role of bevacizumab, an inhibitor of VEGF, and erlotinib, an inhibitor of EGFR, in patients with metastatic HLRCC-associated RCC [35]. Targeted therapy modalities will be discussed later (see Chap. 19).

Succinate Dehydrogenase-Deficient RCC

General Features

Succinate dehydrogenase-deficient RCC (SDH-RCC) is an autosomal dominant hereditary RCC syndrome with distinctive morphologic features, which are discussed in detail later. Patients with mutated *SDH* gene tend to develop pheochromocytoma/paraganglioma, gastrointestinal stromal tumors, and rarely, RCC (Table 11.1) [37, 55, 56]. SDH-RCC is the second form of hereditary RCC characterized by a Krebs cycle gene mutation, as mentioned earlier. It was first described in 2004, in three patients with *SDHB* gene mutation and associated with paraganglioma [57]. SDH-RCC has been recognized as an emerging/provisional new tumor entity in the most recent classification of renal tumor by the International Society of Urological Pathology [7].

SDH-RCC is associated with germline mutation of subunits B, C, or D of the *SDH* gene, most common among which is that of *SDHB* [5, 6, 56]. These mutations have not yet been identified in sporadic RCCs [19, 57]. To date, 77 cases of *SDH* mutation-associated RCC has been reported: 89.6%, 6.4%, and 4% for *SDHB*, *SDHC* and *SDHD* mutations, respectively [56]. The lifetime risk of renal neoplasia in *SDHB* mutation has been estimated approximately 14%, and this risk is even lower for *SDHC* and *SDHD* mutations [7, 56]. Loss of immunolabeling of cytoplasmic SDHB has been consistently identified in all associated tumors in the setting of *SDHB, SDHC*, and *SDHD* mutations [5, 6, 56]. It is likely to be useful as a screening test before formal genetic testing.

Clinical Features

SDH-RCC is aggressive with a high risk of metastasis and death. The RCC is more common in young adults (median age of 40 years, range 14–76), with an M/F ratio of 1.2/1, and may be bilateral (10–26%) [5, 56]. The renal tumors are often of distinct morphology (see below), but can be of clear cell, chromophobe, or unclassified types, as well as oncocytoma [19, 57, 58]. *SDHC*- and *SDHD*-associated RCCs are very rare and are often of clear cell type with low nuclear grade [5, 6, 58]. Pheochromocytoma/paraganglioma are more common and may be multiple with higher percentage of malignant tumors. Gastrointestinal stromal tumors are often of pediatric type or type 2, which display very characteristic features including earlier onset, multinodular growth, regional lymph node metastasis, and yet rather indolent behavior [59].

Pathologic Features

Grossly, the tumors measure 0.7–20 cm (average size 5.4) [56, 58]. They are usually circumscribed but often unencapsulated with a variegated, tan-brown or red-brown, sometimes hemorrhagic cut surface, which is solid in most cases (Fig. 11.6).

Microscopically, tumors are typically well circumscribed or lobulated with a pushing border, sometimes associated with a pseudocapsule. Prominent stromal myxoid change or hyalinization rarely occurs [58]. Tumor cells arrange into solid nests or tubules, and microcystic and macrocystic spaces with pale eosinophilic fluid are common. Sometimes, neoplastic nests surround cystic spaces forming a pseudoglandular appearance [58]. Tumor cells are cuboidal to oval with round nuclei, centrally placed nucleoli, and inconspicuous nucleoli with granular eosinophilic cytoplasm (Fig. 11.7). Their nuclear grade ranges from grade 2 to grade 4. The cell borders are sometimes indistinct. Tumor cells may have eosinophilic cytoplasm or flocculent but lack the granularity, which associate with true oncocytes, but most have a pale and wispy, generally flocculent appearance. Cuboidal tumor cells have a distinctive features, which consisted of bubbly intracytoplasmic vacuolization with wispy eosinophilic material (inclusion like spaces), which correspond to

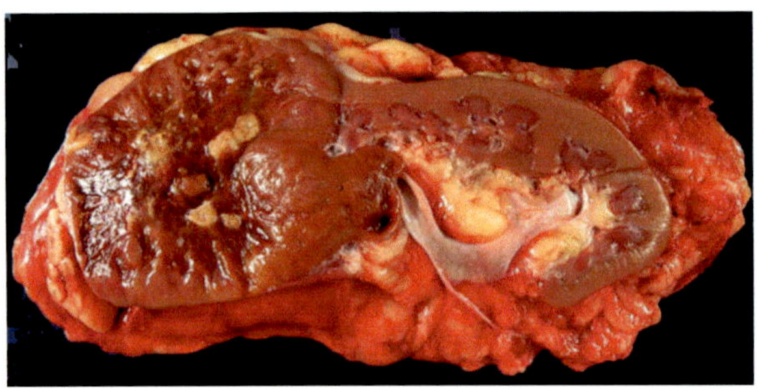

Fig. 11.6 Succinate dehydrogenase B-deficient RCC: The tumor is circumscribed but not encapsulated, with a homogeneous brown cut surface punctuated by focal myxoid/fibrotic areas

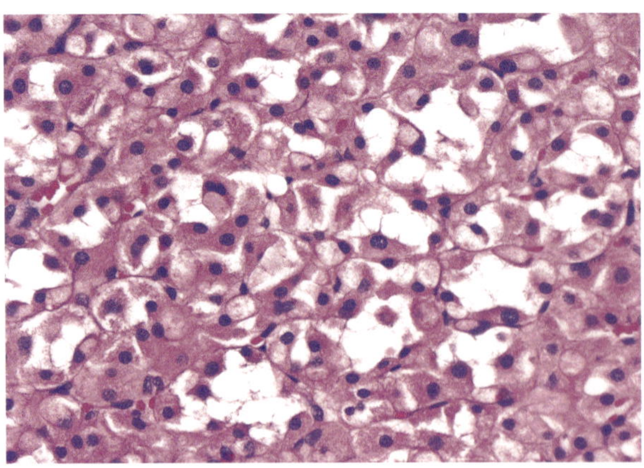

Fig. 11.7 Succinate dehydrogenase B-deficient RCC: Areas of solid growth pattern comprising tumor cells with abundant eosinophilic cytoplasm and low-grade nuclei. Tumor cells with ill-defined cytoplasmic inclusion composed of wispy/flocculated material with clear spaces. (hematoxylin and eosin, ×200)

giant mitochondria (Fig. 11.7). This is a characteristic finding, but it may require diligent search in multiple tissue sections [5, 6, 56, 58]. Clear cytoplasm corresponds to displacement of mitochondria from the cytoplasm and replacement by glycogen or fat [7]. Normal tubules or glomeruli are often entrapped at the periphery of the tumor mass. Sometimes, frank sarcomatoid changes, at least focally, may be identified [56, 58]. Intratumoral mast cells are often seen [56, 58]. Nonneoplastic kidney is normal, except for nonspecific changes such as interstitial inflammation, tubular atrophy, and fibrosis. No dysplastic or precursor lesions are identified in the adjacent renal parenchyma.

Immunohistochemically, CD117, CK7, and SDHB are helpful immunomarkers to differentiate from sporadic chromophobe RCCs and oncocytomas [56]. SDHB-deficient tumors do not express SDHB, whereas endothelial cells and other stromal cells are positive for SDHB. In contrast to the SDH-deficient RCCs, oncocytoma exhibits normal SDHB expression. Although the mechanism of loss of SDH expression in these tumors is unknown, it is useful diagnostic tool before genetic testing [8].

The molecular/genetic features, pathogenetic mechanisms, and targeted therapy modalities of SDH-RCC will be discussed in the later chapters (see Chaps. 18 and 19).

Management, Genetic Counseling, and Treatment

Germline mutations in the subunits (*SDHB, SDHC*, and *SDHD*) of *SDH* genes are not only associated with hereditary paraganglioma syndromes but also with hereditary RCC, especially, under 45 years, even without family history [5].

The management of SDH-RCC is similar to HLRCC and other hereditary renal tumors. SDH-RCCs, like HLRCC-associated RCCs, have propensity to metastasize when primary tumor is very small [5, 56, 58]. Therefore, early detection and prompt surgery are recommended. Surgery should be considered in SDH-deficient patients who have the potential of development of metachronous and bilateral RCCs [5]. SDH-deficient patients may have a lifelong risk to develop renal tumors and may undergo repeated nephron-sparing surgery or partial nephrectomy during their life. Radical surgery instead of nephron-sparing surgery has been recommended, because SDH-RCC more aggressive tumors than other hereditary RCC syndromes [5].

Annual screening for RCC and pheochromocytoma/paraganglioma is recommended.

SDH-deficient tumors are characterized by impaired oxidative phosphorylation and a metabolic shift to aerobic glycolysis, like fumarate hydratase-deficient tumors (HLRCC) [5]. To determine the possible anticancer targets, multiple steps of glycolytic pathway have extensively been evaluated in experimental and clinical studies. To determine the possible anticancer targets, multiple steps of glycolytic pathway have extensively been evaluated in experimental and clinical studies. Nowadays, some agents, including bevacizumab, an inhibitor of VEGF, and erlotinib, an inhibitor of EGFR, have been discovered and entered early clinical trials for SDH-RCC [37, 60]. Targeted therapy modalities will be discussed later (see Chap. 19).

Tuberous Sclerosis Complex

General Features

Tuberous sclerosis complex (TSC) or tuberous sclerosis is a rare autosomal dominant multisystem genetic neurocutaneous disorder characterized by mental retardation, epilepsy, and formation of tumor or tumor-like lesions in multiple organs (Table 11.6). The incidence of TSC is estimated to be about 1/6000–1/10,000 [61]. Although TSC is inherited as an autosomal dominant trait, 60–70% of the cases occur sporadically through a de novo germline mutation [19, 61]. Therefore, an absence of family history does not rule out the diagnosis of TSC [6].

Clinical Features

TSC usually manifests with a combination of distinct clinical signs and symptoms, including epilepsy, intellectual disability, and behavioral problems in association with various tumor and tumor-like lesions in multiple organs (Table 11.6).

Table 11.6 Tumor or tumor-like lesions associated with tuberous sclerosis complex

Affected organs	Tumor or tumor-like lesions
Central nervous system	*Periventricular hamartoma (tubers)* *Subependymoma* *Giant cell astrocytoma*
Skin	*Hypomelanotic macule (ash leaf spots)* *Facial angiofibroma (adenoma sebaceum)* *Shagreen patch* *Forehead fibrous plaque* *Ungual fibroma (Koenen's tumors)*
Lung	*Lymphangioleiomyomatosis* *Clear "sugar" cell tumor*
Heart	*Rhabdomyoma*
Eye	*Retinal hamartomas (phakomas)* *Coloboma* *Angiofibromas of eyelids*
Kidney	*Angiomyolipoma* *Renal cysts* *Oncocytoma* *RCCs (rare)*

Renal manifestations, which are multiple angiomyolipomas (AMLs), cysts, oncocytomas, and RCCs, occur in 50–85% of affected patients [19, 61, 62]. AML is the most common renal manifestation and occurs in approximately 75–80% of affected patients, who are older than 10 years. AML is usually multifocal and bilateral. Renal cysts can be seen in about 45% of affected patients [63]. TSC-associated RCC occurs in 2–4% of affected patients [2, 62, 63], and its mean age at onset is lower (under 30 years) than that in the general population [4, 19]. RCC may occur concurrently with AML, as increasingly reported among women (F/M: 2–5/1) [61, 62], and also rarely in children [64].

Pathologic Features

TSC patients have three types of renal lesions, which are often multiple and bilateral angiomyolipoma, cysts, and much less frequently RCC.

Angiomyolipoma (AML), which is the most common, appears as multiple, variably sized, unencapsulated nodules, with a tan or yellow cut surface, depending on the relative amount of adipose and smooth muscle tissue (Fig. 11.8). Hemorrhage is common, imparting a light or dark brown cut surface. The growth is expansile, and perinephric extension is frequent.

Microscopically, AML is typically triphasic, being composed of adipose tissue, smooth-muscle tissue, and characteristic thick-walled blood vessels that often abut tumor cells without an intervening adventitia (Fig. 11.9). However, other growth patterns can be seen, including lipoma-like, sclerosing, smooth muscle-like/leiomyomatous (monophasic), and epithelioid. Epithelioid AML, composed almost exclusively of epithelioid cells, is more common in TSC than sporadic context (6.2% vs 3.4%) and is often and easily misinterpreted as RCCs [65]. Among differential diagnostic immunomarkers, PAX8 is, perhaps, most useful, since it is expressed by most RCCs, but uniformly absent in AML [6, 66]. AML may also appear as multiple microscopic "tumorlets," a growth pattern strongly suggestive of TSC. Renal cysts are common. They appear as unilocular, variably sized, often multifocal/bilateral cysts lined by large atypical cells with abundant eosinophilic cytoplasm. These cysts may be independent from, but they may be closely associated with AMLs and may represent an integral component of AML.

RCCs are rare (Fig. 11.9) and, thus, not well characterized. Its incidence is, perhaps, not higher than in the general population. RCC often appears as a single mass at a younger age (mean 28 years). The tumor size ranges from 0.1 to 22 cm [62]. A recent multi-institutional study helps expand the morphologic spectrum of TSC-associated RCCs. These tumors display heterogeneous, histologic appearances with clear cell (the most common histologic type), or rarely, papillary, chromophobe, hybrid oncocytic tumor, and unclassified morphology, as well as oncocytoma [62, 64]. HOT may also be identified in TSC syndrome, like in BHD syndrome [62].

The most frequent type is clear cell, similar to the sporadic counterpart; however, a pronounced smooth-muscle component has been reported and thought to be quite

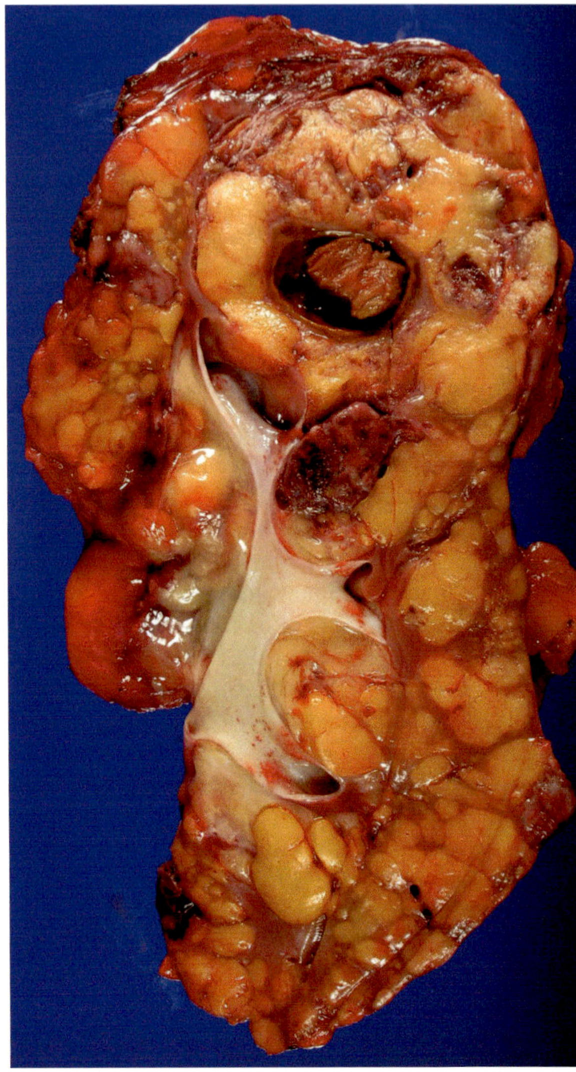

Fig. 11.8 Tuberous sclerosis: Multiple angiomyolipoma (AML) replacing the kidney tissue. There is also a renal cell carcinoma (in upper pole of the kidney) colliding with AML

specific for TSC-related clear cell RCC. Cystic eosinophilic neoplasm characterized by tumor cells with pleomorphic nuclei and large eosinophilic cytoplasm has recently been reported and thought to be TSC specific [62].

TSC-associated papillary RCC, which are similar to Xp11 translocation RCCs, has typically prominent papillary architecture lined by clear cells with eosinophilic globules or delicate thread-like strands and distinct cell membranes. It may also have clear cell papillary RCC-type morphology focally. Psammoma bodies, which are common in Xp11 translocation RCC, are not seen in TSC-associated tumors [62]. TSC-associated papillary RCC displays a characteristic immunoprofile (positive for CAIX, CK7, vimentin and CD10, and uniformly negative for SDHB,

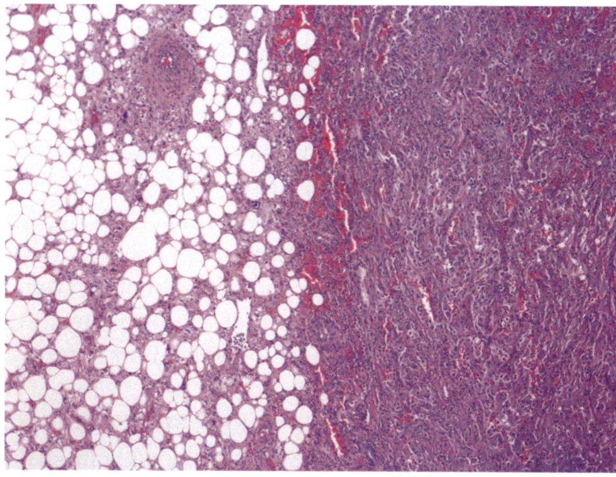

Fig. 11.9 Tuberous sclerosis: RCC (right) colliding with AML (left) composed of adipose tissue, blood vessels, and smooth-muscle cells with a characteristic perivascular condensation. (hematoxylin and eosin, ×100)

TFE3, and AMACR), which helps differentiate it from Xp11 translocation RCC, SDHB-associated RCC, and sporadic papillary RCC [62].

TSC-associated HOT is histologically similar to HOT in other contexts, including BHD syndrome. However, the distinctive cytoplasmic inclusions, which are characteristic for BHD-associated renal tumors, are not seen in TSC-associated RCCs [62].

More than one type of lesions can be seen in individual kidneys. The intervening renal parenchyma is often unremarkable. The following features, often seen in various combinations, especially in a young patient, suggest the diagnosis of TSC:

- Epithelioid, bilateral multiple AMLs
- AML associated with cysts as an integral component or in the background renal parenchyma
- AML tumorlets
- Clear cell RCC with a smooth-muscle component
- Cystic eosinophilic neoplasm (as described earlier)

The molecular/genetic features, pathogenetic mechanisms, and targeted therapy modalities of TSC-associated renal tumors will be discussed together with their sporadic counterparts in the later chapters (see Chaps. 18 and 19).

Management, Genetic Counseling, and Treatment

Renal lesions affect more than 85% of TSC patients and are the main causes of morbidity and mortality [67]. Several clinical, imaging, or histologic findings raise the possibility of TSC, most common among which is perhaps multiple and bilateral AML. These findings should prompt genetic testing for *TSC1* and *TSC2*.

TSC-associated AML is in general more aggressive than sporadic AML [68]. This behavior may be at least, in part, related to an overwhelming epithelioid component. Since AML with a conventional/triphasic morphology is considered benign, this variant of AML should receive active surveillance for asymptomatic small (<4 cm) tumors, whereas angioembolization or nephron-sparing surgery including partial nephrectomy, enucleation, or wedge resection may be needed for symptomatic or larger tumors [69]. Epithelioid AML is usually more aggressive than conventional AML, and therefore, nephron-sparing surgery is first choice. This approach hinges on the AML histologic variants. In this aspect, current renal imaging may help diagnose conventional triphasic AML since adipose tissue can be accurately identified, but this may not help recognize epithelioid AML (which is often devoid of fat) or differentiate it from other types of renal neoplasm. The role of tumor biopsy needs further study in this context. Although RCCs are very rare, nephron-sparing surgery is recommended for tumors <3 cm as in other hereditary RCCs.

Drugs targeting the LKB1/AMPK/TSC2/mTOR pathway are promising [70, 71]. Sirolimus and everolimus, which are rapamycin analogs, can be an effective and safe therapy for TSC-associated renal tumors including AML and advanced RCC [70, 71]. Targeted therapy modalities will be discussed later (see Chap. 19).

Conclusion

Hereditary renal cell carcinoma (HRCC) syndromes involve multiple clinical manifestations, histologic subtypes, genetic alterations, and molecular pathways. Morphologically, the renal tumors associate with these syndromes display distinct features, which, however, may overlap among themselves or with their sporadic counterparts. Although HRCC syndromes are rare and account for only a small portion of RCC, they carry profound biologic and clinical significance. The discovery of the genetic and molecular mechanism of these syndromes represents monumental scientific breakthrough.

These findings provide fundamental pathogenic insights into renal tumor oncogenesis in general and pave the way for modern molecule-targeted therapy. These findings also create a robust framework guiding the care of the affected patients and members of their family.

References

1. Pavlovich CP, Schmidt LS. Searching for the hereditary causes of renal-cell carcinoma. Nat Rev Cancer. 2004;4:381–93.
2. Coleman JA. Familial and hereditary renal cancer syndromes. Urol Clin North Am. 2008;35:563–72.
3. Pfaffenroth EC, Linehan WM. Genetic basis for kidney cancer: opportunity for disease-specific approaches to therapy. Expert Opin Biol Ther. 2008;8:779–90.
4. Axwijk PH, Kluijt I, de Jong D, Gille H, Teertstra J, Horenblas S. Hereditary causes of kidney tumours. Eur J Clin Invest. 2010;40:433–9.

5. Ricketts CJ, Shuch B, Vocke CD, Metwalli AR, Bratslavsky G, Middelton L, Yang Y, Wei MH, Pautler SE, Peterson J, Stolle CA, Zbar B, Merino MJ, Schmidt LS, Pinto PA, Srinivasan R, Pacak K, Linehan WM. Succinate Dehydrogenase Kidney Cancer (SDH-RCC): an aggressive example of the Warburg effect in cancer. J Urol. 2012;188:2063–71.
6. Przybycin CG, Magi-Galluzzi C, McKenney JK. Hereditary syndromes with associated renal neoplasia: a practical guide to histologic recognition in renal tumor resection specimens. Adv Anat Pathol. 2013;20:245–63.
7. Srigley JR, Delahunt B, Eble JN, Egevad L, Epstein JI, Grignon D, Hes O, Moch H, Montironi R, Tickoo SK, Zhou M, Argani P. The ISUP Renal Tumor Panel. The International Society of Urological Pathology (ISUP) Vancouver Classification of renal neoplasia. Am J Surg Pathol. 2013;37:1469–89.
8. Yang OC, Maxwell PH, Pollard PJ. Renal cell carcinoma: translational aspects of metabolism and therapeutic consequences. Kidney Int. 2013;84:667–81.
9. Knudson AG Jr. Mutation and cancer: statistical study of retinoblastoma. Proc Natl Acad Sci U S A. 1971;68:820–3.
10. Brierley KL, Blouch E, Cogswell W, Homer JP, Pencarinha D, Stanislaw CL, Matloff ET. Adverse events in cancer genetic testing: medical, ethical, legal, and financial implications. Cancer J. 2012;18:303–9.
11. Lolkema MP, Gadellaa-van Hooijdonk CG, Bredenoord AL, Kapitein P, Roach N, Cuppen E, Knoers NV, Voest EE. Ethical, legal, and counseling challenges surrounding the return of genetic results in oncology. J Clin Oncol. 2013;31:1842–8.
12. Sgambati MT, Stolle C, Choyke PL, Walther MM, Zbar B, Linehan WM. Glenn GM. Mosaicism in von Hippel-Lindau disease: lessons from kindreds with germline mutations identified in offspring with mosaic parents. Am J Hum Genet. 2000;66:84–91.
13. Toro JR, Nickerson ML, Wei MH, Warren MB, Glenn GM, Turner ML, Stewart L, Duray P, Tourre O, Sharma N, Choyke P, Stratton P, Merino M, Walther MM, Linehan WM, Schmidt LS, Zbar B. Mutations in the fumarate hydratase gene cause hereditary leiomyomatosis and renal cell cancer in families in North America. Am J Hum Genet. 2003;73:95–106.
14. Sancak O, Nellist M, Goedbloed M, Elfferich P, Wouters C, Maat-Kievit A, Zonnenberg B, Verhoef S, Halley D, van den Ouweland A. Mutational analysis of the TSC1 and TSC2 genes in a diagnostic setting: genotype–phenotype correlations and comparison of diagnostic DNA techniques in Tuberous Sclerosis Complex. Eur J Hum Genet. 2005;13:731–41.
15. Shuch B, Vourganti S, Ricketts CJ, Middleton L, Peterson J, Merino MJ, Metwalli AR, Srinivasan R, Linehan WM. Defining early-onset kidney cancer: implications for germline and somatic mutation testing and clinical management. J Clin Oncol. 2014;10:431–7.
16. Kleihues P, Schäuble B, zur Hausen A, Estève J, Ohgaki H. Tumors associated with p53 germline mutations: a synopsis of 91 families. Am J Pathol. 1997;150:1–13.
17. Mario AM, Luis MP, Emilio RG. Renal tumors in patients with von Hippel-Lindau disease: "State of art review". In: Van Poppel H, editor. Renal cell carcinoma. Croatia: InTech; 2011. p. 93–110. Available from: http://www.intechopen.com/books/renal-cell-carcinoma/renaltumors-in-patients-with-von-hippel-lindau-disease-state-of-art-review.
18. Maher ER, Neumann HP, Richard S. Von Hippel–Lindau disease: a clinical and scientific review. Eur J Hum Genet. 2011;19:617–23.
19. Verine J, Pluvinage A, Bousquet G, Lehmann-Che J, de Bazelaire C, Soufir N, Mongiat-Artus P. Hereditary renal cancer syndromes: an update of a systematic review. Eur Urol. 2010;58:701–10.
20. Frantzen C, Links TP, Giles RH. Von Hippel-Lindau disease. In: Pagon RA, Adam MP, Ardinger HH, Bird TD, Dolan CR, Fong CT, Smith RJH, Stephens K, editors. GeneReviews™ [Internet]. Seattle: University of Washington; 2000; updated 2012 Jun 21 . Available from http://www.ncbi.nlm.nih.gov/books/NBK1463/.
21. Richard S, Gardie B, Couvé S, Gad S. Von Hippel-Lindau: how a rare disease illuminates cancer biology. Semin Cancer Biol. 2013;23:26–37.
22. Cho E, Adami HO, Lindblad P. Epidemiology of renal cell cancer. Hematol Oncol Clin North Am. 2011;25:651–65.

23. Walther MM, Lubensky IA, Venzon D, Zbar B, Linehan WM. Prevalence of microscopic lesions in grossly normal renal parenchyma from patients with von Hippel-Lindau disease, sporadic renal cell carcinoma and no renal disease: clinical implications. J Urol. 1995;154:2010–4.
24. Walther MM, Choyke PL, Glenn G, Lyne JC, Rayford W, Venzon D, Linehan WM. Renal cancer in families with hereditary renal cancer: prospective analysis of a tumor size threshold for renal parenchymal sparing surgery. J Urol. 1999;161:1475–9.
25. Choyke PL, Glenn GM, Walther MM, Zbar B, Weiss GH, Alexander RB, Hayes WS, Long JP, Thakore KN, Linehan WM. The natural history of renal lesions in von Hippel-Lindau disease: a serial CT study in 28 patients. AJR Am J Roentgenol. 1992;159:1229–34.
26. Gupta GN, Peterson J, Thakore KN, Pinto PA, Linehan W, Bratslavsky G. Oncological outcomes of partial nephrectomy for multifocal renal cell carcinoma greater than 4 cm. J Urol. 2010;184:59–63.
27. Meister M, Choyke P, Anderson C, Patel U. Radiological evaluation, management, and surveillance of renal masses in von Hippel-Lindau disease. Clin Radiol. 2009;64:589–600.
28. Goldfarb DA, Neumann HP, Penn I, Novick AC. Results of renal transplantation in patients with renal cell carcinoma in Von Hippel-Lindau disease. Transplantation. 1997;64:1726–9.
29. Linehan WM, Srinivasan R, Schmidt LS. The genetic basis of kidney cancer: a metabolic disease. Nat Rev Urol. 2010;7:277–85.
30. Albiges L, Salem M, Rini B, Escudier B. Vascular endothelial growth factor targeted therapies in advanced renal cell carcinoma. Hematol Oncol Clin N Am. *2011*;25:813–33.
31. Jonasch E, McCutcheon IE, Waguespack SG, Wen S, Davis DW, Smith LA, Tannir NM, Gombos DS, Fuller GN, Matin SF. Pilot trial of sunitinib therapy in patients with von Hippel-Lindau disease. Ann Oncol. 2011;22(12):2661–6.
32. Zbar B, Glenn G, Lubensky I, Choyke P, Walther MM, Magnusson G, Bergerheim US, Pettersson S, Amin M, Hurley K. Hereditary papillary renal cell carcinoma: clinical studies in 10 families. J Urol. 1995;153:907–12.
33. Zhuang Z, Park WS, Pack S, Schmidt L, Vortmeyer AO, Pak E, Pham T, Weil RJ, Candidus S, Lubensky IA, Linehan WM, Zbar B, Weirich G. Trisomy 7-harbouring non-random duplication of the mutant MET allele in hereditary papillary renal carcinomas. Nat Genet. 1998;20:66–9.
34. Linehan WM, Pinto PA, Srinivasan R, Merino M, Choyke P, Choyke L, Coleman J, Toro J, Glenn G, Vocke C, Zbar B, Schmidt LS, Bottaro D, Neckers L. Identification of the genes for kidney cancer: opportunity for disease-specific targeted therapeutics. Clin Cancer Res. 2007;13:671s–9s.
35. Choyke PL, Glenn GM, Walther MM, Zbar B, Linehan WM. Hereditary renal cancers. Radiology. 2003;226:33–46.
36. Herring JC, Enquist EG, Chernoff A, Linehan WM, Choyke PL, Walther MM. Parenchymal sparing surgery in patients with hereditary renal cell carcinoma: 10-year experience. J Urol. 2001;165:777–81.
37. Linehan WM, Ricketts CJ. The metabolic basis of kidney cancer. Semin Cancer Biol. 2013;23:46–55.
38. Choueiri TK, Vaishampayan U, Rosenberg JE, Logan TF, Harzstark AL, Bukowski RM, Rini BI, Srinivas S, Stein MN, Adams LM, Ottesen LH, Laubscher KH, Sherman L, McDermott DF, Haas NB, Flaherty KT, Ross R, Eisenberg P, Meltzer PS, Merino MJ, Bottaro DP, Linehan WM, Srinivasan R. Phase II and biomarker study of the dual MET/VEGFR2 inhibitor foretinib in patients with papillary renal cell carcinoma. J Clin Oncol. 2013;31:181–6.
39. Birt AR, Hogg GR, Dube WJ. Hereditary multiple fibrofolliculomas with trichodiscomas and acrochordons. Arch Dermatol. 1977;113:1674–7.
40. Toro JR, Glenn G, Duray P, Darling T, Weirich G, Zbar B, Linehan M, Turner ML. Birt-Hogg-Dube syndrome: a novel marker of kidney neoplasia. Arch Dermatol. 1999;135:1195–202.
41. Schmidt LS, Warren MB, Nickerson ML, Weirich G, Matrosova V, Toro JR, Turner ML, Duray P, Merino M, Hewitt S, Pavlovich CP, Glenn G, Greenberg CR, Linehan WM, Zbar B. Birt-Hogg-Dube syndrome, a genodermatosis associated with spontaneous pneumothorax and kidney neoplasia, maps to chromosome 17p11.2. Am J Hum Genet. 2001;69:876–82.

42. Nickerson ML, Warren MB, Toro JR, Matrosova V, Glenn G, Turner ML, Duray P, Merino M, Choyke P, Pavlovich CP, Sharma N, Walther M, Munroe D, Hill R, Maher E, Greenberg C, Lerman MI, Linehan WM, Zbar B, Schmidt LS. Mutations in a novel gene lead to kidney tumors, lung wall defects, and benign tumors of the hair follicle in patients with the Birt-Hogg-Dube syndrome. Cancer Cell. 2002;2:157–64.
43. Zbar B, Alvord WG, Glenn G, Turner M, Pavlovich CP, Schmidt L, Walther M, Choyke P, Weirich G, Hewitt SM, Duray P, Gabril F, Greenberg C, Merino MJ, Toro J, Linehan WM. Risk of renal and colonic neoplasms and spontaneous pneumothorax in the Birt–Hogg–Dubé syndrome. Cancer Epidemiol Biomarkers Prev. 2002;11:393–400.
44. Pavlovich CP, Grubb RL 3rd, Hurley K, Glenn GM, Toro J, Schmidt LS, Torres-Cabala C, Merino MJ, Zbar B, Choyke P, Walther MM, Linehan WM. Evaluation and management of renal tumors in the Birt-Hogg-Dubé syndrome. J Urol. 2005;173:1482–6.
45. Petersson F, Gatalica Z, Grossmann P, Perez Montiel MD, Alvarado Cabrero I, Bulimbasic S, Swatek A, Straka L, Tichy T, Hora M, Kuroda N, Legendre B, Michal M, Hes O. Sporadic hybrid oncocytic/chromophobe tumor of the kidney: a clinicopathologic, histomorphologic, immunohistochemical, ultrastructural, and molecular cytogenetic study of 14 cases. Virchows Arch. 2010;456:355–65.
46. Menko FH, van Steensel MA, Giraud S, Friis-Hansen L, Richard S, Ungari S, Nordenskjöld M, Hansen TV, Solly J, Maher ER, European BHD Consortium. Birt-Hogg-Dubé syndrome: diagnosis and management. Lancet Oncol. 2009;10:1199–206.
47. Toro JR, Wei MH, Glenn GM, Weinreich M, Toure O, Vocke C, Turner M, Choyke P, Merino MJ, Pinto PA, Steinberg SM, Schmidt LS, Linehan WM. BHD mutations, clinical and molecular genetic investigations of Birt-Hogg-Dubé syndrome: a new series of 50 families and a review of published reports. J Med Genet. 2008;45:321–31.
48. Schmidt LS, Linehan WM. Clinical features, genetics and potential therapeutic approaches for Birt-Hogg-Dubé syndrome. Expert Opin Orphan Drugs. 2015;3(1):15–29.
49. Launonen V, Vierimaa O, Kiuru M, Isola J, Roth S, Pukkala E, Sistonen P, Herva R, Aaltonen LA. Inherited Susceptibility to uterine leiomyomas and renal cell cancer. Proc Natl Acad Sci U S A. 2001;98:3387–92.
50. Alam NA, Barclay E, Rowan AJ, Tyrer JP, Calonje E, Manek S, Kelsell D, Leigh I, Olpin S, Tomlinson IP. Clinical features of multiple cutaneous and uterine leiomyomatosis: an underdiagnosed tumor syndrome. Arch Dermatol. 2005;141:199–206.
51. Lehtonen HJ, Kiuru M, Ylisaukko-Oja SK, Salovaara R, Herva R, Koivisto PA, Vierimaa O, Aittomäki K, Pukkala E, Launonen V, Aaltonen LA. Increased risk of cancer in patients with fumarate hydratase germline mutation. J Med Genet. 2006;43:523–6.
52. Delahunt B, Srigley JR, Montironi R, Egevad L. Advances in renal neoplasia: recommendations from the 2012 International Society of Urological Pathology Consensus Conference. Urology. 2014;83:969–74.
53. Udager AM, Alva A, Chen YB, Siddiqui J, Lagstein A, Tickoo SK, Reuter VE, Chinnaiyian AM, Mehra R. Hereditary leiomyomatosis and renal cell carcinoma (HLRCC): a rapid autopsy report of metastatic renal cell carcinoma. Am J Surg Pathol. 2014;38:567–77.
54. Tong WH, Sourbier C, Kovtunovych G, Jeong SY, Vira M, Ghosh M, Romero VV, Sougrat R, Vaulont S, Viollet B, Kim YS, Lee S, Trepel J, Srinivasan R, Bratslavsky G, Yang Y, Linehan WM, Rouault TA. The glycolytic shift in fumarate-hydratase-deficient kidney cancer lowers AMPK levels, increases metabolic propensities and lowers cellular iron levels. Cancer Cell. 2011;20:315–27.
55. Gill AJ. Succinate dehydrogenase (SDH) and mitochondrial driven neoplasia. Pathology. 2012;44:285–92.
56. Williamson SR, Eble JN, Amin MB, Gupta NS, Smith SC, Sholl LM, Montironi R, Hirsch MS, Hornick JL. Succinate dehydrogenase-deficient renal cell carcinoma: detailed characterization of 11 tumors defining a unique subtype of renal cell carcinoma. Mod Pathol. 2015;28:80–94.
57. Vanharanta S, Buchta M, McWhinney SR, Virta SK, Peçzkowska M, Morrison CD, Lehtonen R, Januszewicz A, Järvinen H, Juhola M, Mecklin JP, Pukkala E, Herva R, Kiuru M, Nupponen NN, Aaltonen LA, Neumann HP, Eng C. Early-onset renal cell carcinoma as a novel extra-

paraganglial component of SDHB-associated heritable paraganglioma. Am J Hum Genet. 2004;74:153–9.
58. Gill AJ, Hes O, Papathomas T, Šedivcová M, Tan PH, Agaimy A, Andresen PA, Kedziora A, Clarkson A, Toon CW, Sioson L, Watson N, Chou A, Paik J, Clifton-Bligh RJ, Robinson BG, Benn DE, Hills K, Maclean F, Niemeijer ND, Vlatkovic L, Hartmann A, Corssmit EP, van Leenders GJ, Przybycin C, JK MK, Magi-Galluzzi C, Yilmaz A, Yu D, Nicoll KD, Yong JL, Sibony M, Yakirevich E, Fleming S, Chow CW, Miettinen M, Michal M, Trpkov K. Succinate dehydrogenase (SDH)-deficient renal carcinoma: a morphologically distinct entity: a clinicopathologic series of 36 tumors from 27 patients. Am J Surg Pathol. 2014;38:1588–602.
59. Miettinen M, Wang ZF, Sarlomo-Rikala M, Osuch C, Rutkowski P, Lasota J. Succinate dehydrogenase-deficient GISTs: a clinicopathologic, immunohistochemical, and molecular genetic study of 66 gastric GISTs with predilection to young age. Am J Surg Pathol. 2011;35:1712–21.
60. Shuch B, Linehan WM, Srinivasan R. Aerobic glycolysis: a novel target in kidney cancer. Expert Rev Anticancer Ther. 2013;13(6):711–9.
61. Leung AK, Robson WL. Tuberous sclerosis complex: a review. J Pediatr Health Care. 2007;21:108–14.
62. Yang P, Cornejo KM, Sadow PM, Cheng L, Wang M, Xiao Y, Jiang Z, Oliva E, Jozwiak S, Nussbaum RL, Feldman AS, Paul E, Thiele EA, Yu JJ, Henske EP, Kwiatkowski DJ, Young RH, Wu CL. Renal cell carcinoma in tuberous sclerosis complex. Am J Surg Pathol. 2014;38:895–909.
63. Rakowski SK, Winterkorn EB, Paul E, Steele DJ, Halpern EF, Thiele EA. Renal manifestations of tuberous sclerosis complex: incidence, prognosis, and predictive factors. Kidney Int. 2006;70:1777–82.
64. Kubo M, Iwashita K, Oyachi N, Oyama T, Yamamoto T. Two different types of infantile renal cell carcinomas associated with tuberous sclerosis. J Pediatr Surg. 2011;46:E37–41.
65. Aydin H, Magi-Galluzzi C, Lane BR, Sercia L, Lopez JI, Rini BI, Zhou M. Renal angiomyolipoma: clinicopathologic study of 194 cases with emphasis on the epithelioid histology and tuberous sclerosis association. Am J Surg Pathol. 2009;33:289–97.
66. Ozcan A, de la Roza G, Ro JY, Shen SS, Truong LD. PAX2 and PAX8 expression in primary and metastatic renal tumors: a comprehensive comparison. Arch Pathol Lab Med. 2012;136:1541–51.
67. Rosser T, Panigrahy A, McClintock W. The diverse clinical manifestations of tuberous sclerosis complex: a review. Semin Pediatr Neurol. 2006;13:27–36.
68. Neumann HP, Schwarzkopf G, Henske EP. Renal angiomyolipomas, cysts, and cancer in tuberous sclerosis complex. Semin Pediatr Neurol. 1998;5:269–75.
69. Koo KC, Kim WT, Ham WS, Lee JS, Ju HJ, Choi YD. Trends of presentation and clinical outcome of treated renal angiomyolipoma. Yonsei Med J. 2010;51:728–34.
70. Henske EP, Rasooly R, Siroky B, Bissler J. Tuberous sclerosis complex, mTOR, and the kidney: report of an NIDDK-sponsored workshop. Am J Physiol Renal Physiol. 2014;306:F279–83.
71. Hasskarl J. Everolimus. Recent Results Cancer Res. 2014;201:373–92.

Chapter 12
Lymphoid Neoplasms of the Kidney

Elizabeth M. Margolskee, Steven P. Salvatore, and Julia T. Geyer

The kidney is one of the most common extranodal sites to be involved by systemic lymphoma. However, because renal biopsies are only performed in a minority of patients, it is likely underdiagnosed. Autopsy series tend to show a higher incidence of renal involvement by lymphoma than clinical or radiological studies. Although data vary by the type of lymphoma. Secondary renal involvement was seen in 48% of patients in a large autopsy series of patients with non-Hodgkin lymphoma (NHL) [1]. Generally, the lymphoma is clinically silent; however, in a minority of patients, the degree of lymphomatous infiltration may compromise renal function, leading to acute renal failure. Renal involvement is most common in B-cell non-Hodgkin lymphoma, with only rare cases of T-cell lymphoma reported in the literature. Primary renal lymphoma appears to be extremely rare, and accounts for approximately 0.7% of all extranodal lymphomas in North America and 0.1% in Japan [2–4]. A large subset (>40%) have bilateral presentation [5].

The existence of primary renal lymphoma is an area of controversy, since the kidney does not contain native lymphoid tissue [6]. Stallone et al. proposed the following three criteria for the diagnosis of primary renal lymphoma:

- There is lymphomatous renal infiltration.
- There is nonobstructive uni- or bilateral renal enlargement.
- There is no extrarenal localization of lymphoma at the time of diagnosis [7].

E. M. Margolskee · J. T. Geyer (✉)
Division of Hematopathology, Department of Pathology and Laboratory Medicine, Weill Cornell Medicine, New York, NY, USA
e-mail: jut9021@med.cornell.edu

S. P. Salvatore
Division of Renal Pathology, Department of Pathology and Laboratory Medicine, Weill Cornell Medicine,
New York, NY, USA

M. K. Divatia et al. (eds.), *Kidney Cancer*, https://doi.org/10.1007/978-3-030-28333-9_12

Although many authors have reported lymphomas, ostensibly limited to the kidney, based on these criteria, it is possible that these are systemic lymphomas which have been inadequately staged. The renal capsule is rich in lymphatics, leading some to suggest that lymphoma penetrates the parenchyma from capsule [8]. Others have suggested that chronic inflammatory processes recruit lymphocytes to the kidney, where they undergo malignant transformation [9]. This chapter will focus on the clinical manifestations and histologic features of lymphoma in the kidney.

The World Health Organization classification of tumors of the hematopoietic and lymphoid system creates a framework for classification of lymphoid neoplasms that relies on integration of clinical features, morphology, immunophenotype, and genetic features to define distinct diseases. A complete evaluation for diagnosis may be extensive; a pathologists' ability to perform a complete diagnostic workup is limited in small needle core biopsies of renal tissue. Lack of adequate material may preclude performance of all the indicated diagnostic and prognostic studies, especially as molecular testing becomes a routine part of the evaluation. Needle biopsies may not be representative of an entire lesion (e.g., demonstrating only the low-grade component at the periphery of an otherwise high-grade neoplasm). Architectural features may be compromised by the small sample size as well. Occasionally, if fresh samples are obtained, material may be set aside for ancillary diagnostic studies, such as direct immunofluorescence, flow cytometry, or cytogenetic analysis. Thus, the diagnostic yield of needle core biopsies of kidney in patients with suspected lymphoma may be suboptimal, although there is little published data addressing this subject [10].

For a renal pathologist who may be routinely dealing with cases of suspected or potential lymphoma in the kidney, a high index of clinicopathologic suspicion is critical in all cases. This may be especially true in patients who are known to have a lymphoma or monoclonal gammopathy with renal disease necessitating biopsy, but new diagnoses of lymphoma on kidney biopsy are certainly possible in patients without a known history. The differential diagnosis for interstitial inflammation in the native kidney includes chronic inflammation, active interstitial nephritis, tubulointerstitial autoimmune diseases, inflammation associated with a glomerular or vascular disease process, or lymphoma among other things. A careful clinical history including serologies, and assessment of the composition of the inflammatory cells by histopathology and possibly immunohistochemistry is critical for arriving at the correct diagnosis. For example, in a clearly reactive inflammatory milieu with numerous interstitial eosinophils, the likelihood of an active interstitial nephritis due to medication hypersensitivity is most likely. If, however, the cells appear either monotonous or high-grade in appearance, consideration of a neoplastic/lymphomatous process should be raised. In most cases, the first step to assess the process may be to gauge the composition of inflammatory cells using CD3 and CD20 stains, or similar T- and B-cell markers. The presence of predominantly T cells or a mixed population would most likely lead to a diagnosis of a reactive process whereas a majority of B cells would require further characterization, as described in further detail below.

Two morphologic patterns have been observed in lymphomas involving the kidney [11]. The most common pattern is a diffuse, interstitial proliferation which spares renal tubules and glomeruli. Distinguishing this pattern from acute interstitial nephritis can be challenging but crucial for determining appropriate treatment. Lymphomatous infiltrates tend to be limited to the interstitium and spare the tubules; in contrast, tubulitis is a common feature of acute interstitial nephritis. Reactive infiltrates are also more commonly T-cell predominant, which classically contain conspicuous clusters of eosinophils in hypersensitivity responses, while most lymphomas are B-cell in origin. For complex cases, polymerase chain reaction (PCR) for immunoglobulin or T-cell receptor gene rearrangement can be helpful in determining B- or T-cell clonality, respectively. Various types of low-grade and high-grade lymphoma can present with this pattern. Immunohistochemical studies (discussed below) may help in assigning a precise diagnosis.

Intraglomerular pattern of lymphoma is a rare and often unexpected finding. Here, there may be considerable morphologic overlap with proliferative glomerulonephritis due to the increased cellularity of the glomeruli [12]. Immunostaining for B-cell markers such as CD20 or PAX-5 will help resolve this differential as all reported cases of intraglomerular lymphoma are large B-cell lymphomas and are best classified as intravascular large B-cell lymphoma (discussed below).

Mechanism/Pathogenesis

Lymphomatous infiltration may cause acute renal failure. It has been suggested that dense tumor infiltrates compress the renal tubules, producing intrarenal obstruction [13]. Tubular atrophy and necrosis can be seen in severe cases, with resolution after the lymphoma is treated [14]. Loss of renal function appears to be linked to the extent of lymphomatous involvement, as renal failure has not been reported in patients with only unilateral disease [11, 15, 16].

Radiology/Gross Features

Lymphoma may not be apparent by radiology. In a study of lymphomas diagnosed by percutaneous kidney biopsies, preprocedure imaging detected abnormalities in only 10 out of 55 (18%) cases [11].

In those cases with detectable abnormalities by imaging, lymphoma can have several patterns of renal involvement. The most common pattern, seen in 50–60% of patients, is multiple parenchymal lesions present bilaterally. Up to 25% of patients may have a solitary mass, which may be confused with renal cell carcinoma. A diffuse enlargement due to extensive parenchymal infiltration may also be seen. Enlargement of the retroperitoneal lymph nodes is present in 25–30% of cases [17, 18]. In contrast CT studies, lymphoma tends to enhance less than normal renal tissue due to the lack of collecting tubules to concentrate contrast media, although administration of contrast may be contraindicated in patients presenting in acute renal failure [17]. On MRI, lymphoma shows intermediate intensity on T1 and T2 weighted images and high signal intensity on diffusion-weighted MR images [19]. Positron emission tomography/computed tomography (PET/CT) imaging is most commonly used in staging lymphoma patients as lymphoma is fluorodeoxyglucose (FDG) avid [20].

Chronic Lymphocytic Leukemia/Small Lymphocytic Lymphoma

Chronic lymphocytic leukemia/small lymphocytic lymphoma (CLL/SLL) is the most common low-grade B-cell lymphoma in developed countries and generally affects elderly individuals. Presentation is generally leukemic although isolated lymphadenopathy may be seen. In autopsy series, renal involvement by CLL/SLL is seen in up to 90% of cases [5, 21–23]. However, renal failure is rare, with only a handful of reported cases [5, 24].

Morphologically, the pattern of renal involvement is generally nodular aggregates, although diffuse and interstitial patterns may also be seen (Fig. 12.1). The

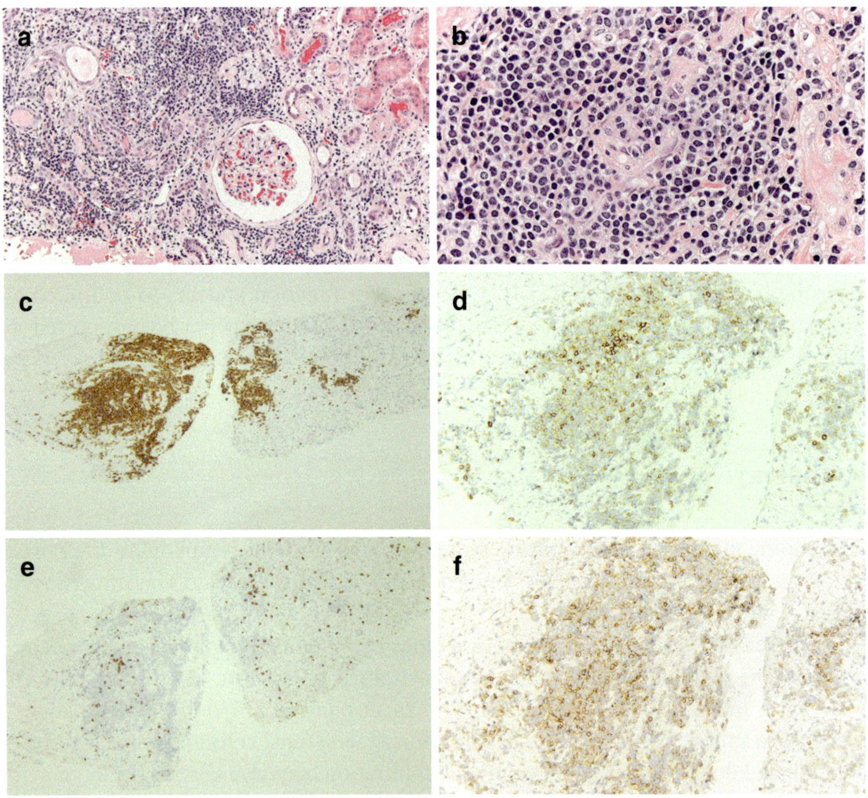

Fig. 12.1 (**a**) Low power image showing infiltrating chronic lymphocytic lymphoma within the interstitium (H&E, 10×). (**b**) High power shows the cells to have a monomorphic appearance with round nuclei and clumped chromatin (H&E, 60×). (**c**–**f**) By immunohistochemistry (IHC) the lymphocytes stain diffusely for CD20 (**c**, 10×), weakly for CD5 (**d**, 20×), with only rare CD3 positive cells (**e**, 10×), and widely for CD23 (**f**, 20×)

neoplastic infiltrate is composed predominantly of small lymphocytes with coarsely clumped chromatin and a small amount of cytoplasm. In a small number of patients, CLL/SLL involves the kidney in conjunction with a granulomatous interstitial nephritis, causing acute renal failure. These patients may respond to steroid treatment without CLL/SLL-directed chemotherapy [25].

By immunohistochemistry, the neoplastic cells express B-cell markers CD20 and PAX5 with dim surface IgM/IgD and aberrant expression of CD5, CD23, and LEF1. The workup for prognostication in CLL (i.e., flow cytometry, *IGH* somatic hypermutation analysis, molecular genetic studies, cytogenetic testing) is most commonly performed on peripheral blood. In general, CLL/SLL is an indolent disease but a small fraction may undergo transformation to diffuse large B-cell lymphoma or classical Hodgkin lymphoma (Richter's transformation), which requires aggressive chemotherapy and confers a poor prognosis [26].

Extranodal Marginal Zone Lymphoma of Mucosa-Associated Lymphoid Tissue (MALT Lymphoma)

Renal MALT lymphoma appears to be rare. In a series from MD Anderson Cancer Center, Garcia et al. identified 10 cases over an 8-year period, 6 of which were limited to kidney and 4 were systemic [27]. Treatment was highly variable, but all patients were alive for 9–53 months after diagnosis. Although MALT lymphoma may be associated with bacterial overgrowth in some anatomic sites (e.g., *H. pylori* in gastric MALT lymphoma), there have been no bacteria linked with renal MALT. However, a few reports have described MALT in association with renal actinomycosis [28, 29].

Morphologically, renal marginal zone lymphoma is characterized by diffuse infiltrate composed of small monocytoid B cells admixed with plasmacytoid lymphocytes and rare, large immunoblasts (Fig. 12.2). Reactive germinal centers may be identified. Although lymphoepithelial lesions are common in MALT lymphoma outside the kidney, they have not been reported in renal MALT lymphoma [27]. There are no immunophenotypic findings specific to marginal zone lymphoma; in general, the neoplastic B cells tend to be negative for CD5, CD10, and Cyclin D1. Aberrant expression of BCL-2 or CD43 can be seen. In situ hybridization for kappa and lambda light chains may be of use in making the diagnosis by identifying the presence of a monotypic plasma cell population.

Translocations involving the *MALT1* gene on chromosome 18 are common in MALT lymphoma in the lung and gastrointestinal (GI) tract. Data on cytogenetic changes in renal MALT is scarce, but one case of presumed renal MALT with t(14,18)(q32;q21) involving the *IGH* and *MALT1* genes has been reported [27].

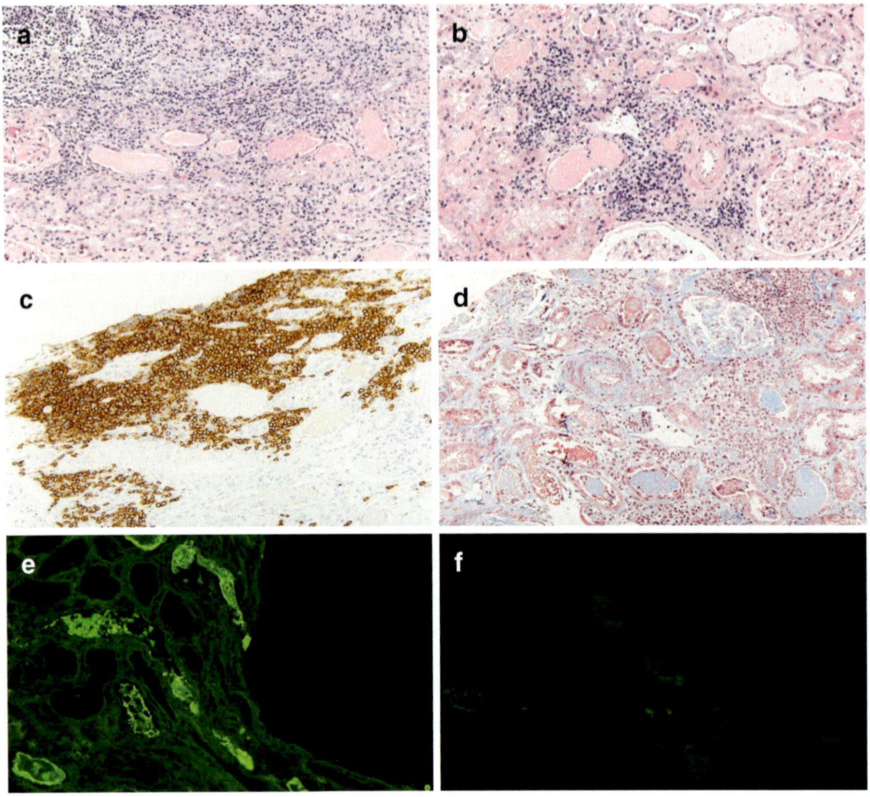

Fig. 12.2 (**a**) A kidney biopsy with low grade infiltrating marginal zone lymphoma within the interstitium (H&E, 10×). In addition to the lymphoma, due to a monoclonal protein elaborated by the cells, the kidney also shows monoclonal cast nephropathy with eosinophilic, brittle intratubular casts (**b**, H&E 20×). The casts were also fuscinophilic and complexed to blue staining uromodulin (**c**) The lymphoma cells are diffusely CD20 positive (20×) (**d**), Trichrome stain, 20×). (**e**) By immunofluorescence (IF), the casts are positive for kappa (**e**, 20×) and negative for lambda (**f**, 20×)

Lymphoplasmacytic Lymphoma

Lymphoplasmacytic lymphoma (LPL) is a low-grade B-cell lymphoma often associated with IgM paraproteinemia. It generally involves the bone marrow and peripheral blood; extranodal disease is rare. In a large cohort study of 1391 patients with LPL, Vos et al. identified LPL-related nephropathy in 44 (3%) patients, with a cumulative incidence of 5.1% over 15 years [30]. The most common pathologies on biopsy were amyloidosis, monoclonal IgM deposition disease/cryoglobulinemia, and LPL infiltration.

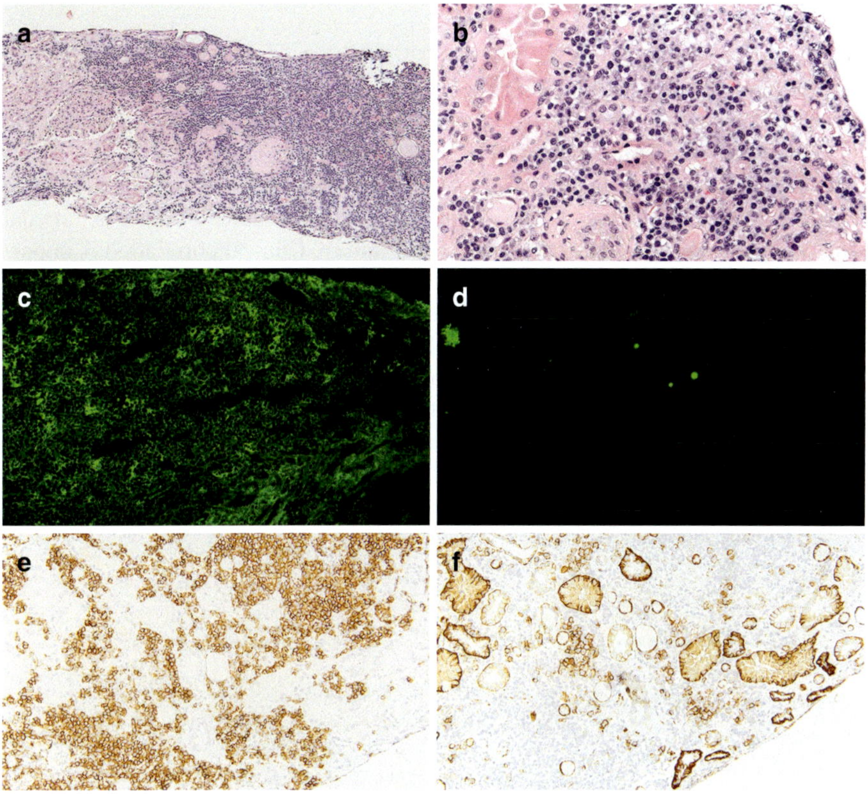

Fig. 12.3 (**a**) At low power, the low grade lymphoplasmacytic lymphoma is seen infiltrating the renal interstitium (H&E, 10×). (**b**) On high power, the cells show a mixture of small lymphocytes and occasional plasma cells (H&E, 40×). With IF, the cells show significant staining for lambda light chain (**c**, 20×) and are negative for kappa light chain (**d**, 20×). CD20 is positive in the B cells (**e**) CD138 is positive in plasma cells and epithelial cells (**f**) (20×)

Morphologically, LPL presents with a diffuse infiltrate of small lymphocytes and plasma cells that spares the renal tubules and glomeruli (Fig. 12.3). Most LPLs express B-cell markers CD20, CD79a, and PAX5 while the plasma cell component expresses CD138 and MUM1 and will show light chain restriction for either kappa or lambda immunoglobulin. As in MALT lymphoma, there are no specific immunophenotypic abnormalities, making morphologic and immunophenotypic discrimination between LPL and MALT lymphoma difficult.

Molecular testing may identify *MYD88* L265P mutation in 90% of cases of LPL. Rarely, *MYD88* mutations other than L265P may be present. In addition, up to 35% of LPLs may have a nonsense or frameshift mutation in *CXCR4* similar to those found in the warts, hypogammaglobulinemia, infections, and myelokathexis (WHIM) syndrome. These mutations are infrequently seen in marginal zone (MALT) lymphoma.

Diffuse Large B-Cell Lymphoma

Diffuse large B-cell lymphoma (DLBCL) is the most common primary renal lymphoma and accounts for slightly more than half of the reported cases [7, 31–35]. On the other hand, in a large series of over 2500 patients with DLBCL, Villa et al. identified renal involvement in 2% of cases by imaging or biopsy [36]. These patients tended to have elevated lactate dehydrogenase and involvement of other extranodal sites. Only a minority, 16%, had severe renal failure. Clinical correlation is important in the diagnosis of DLBCL, as it is the most common lymphoma in patients with HIV, history of transplant, or primary immunodeficiency. There are case reports of patients with primary renal DLBCL and hepatitis C infection [34], patients with a previous diagnosis of multicentric Castleman disease [37] and a patient with history of systemic lupus erythematosus and bilateral renal DLBCL [38].

Morphologically, DLBCL is characterized by diffuse infiltration of the renal parenchyma by sheets of large atypical lymphoid cells which spare the kidney tubules (Fig. 12.4). Frequent mitotic figures, apoptotic debris, and necrosis may be

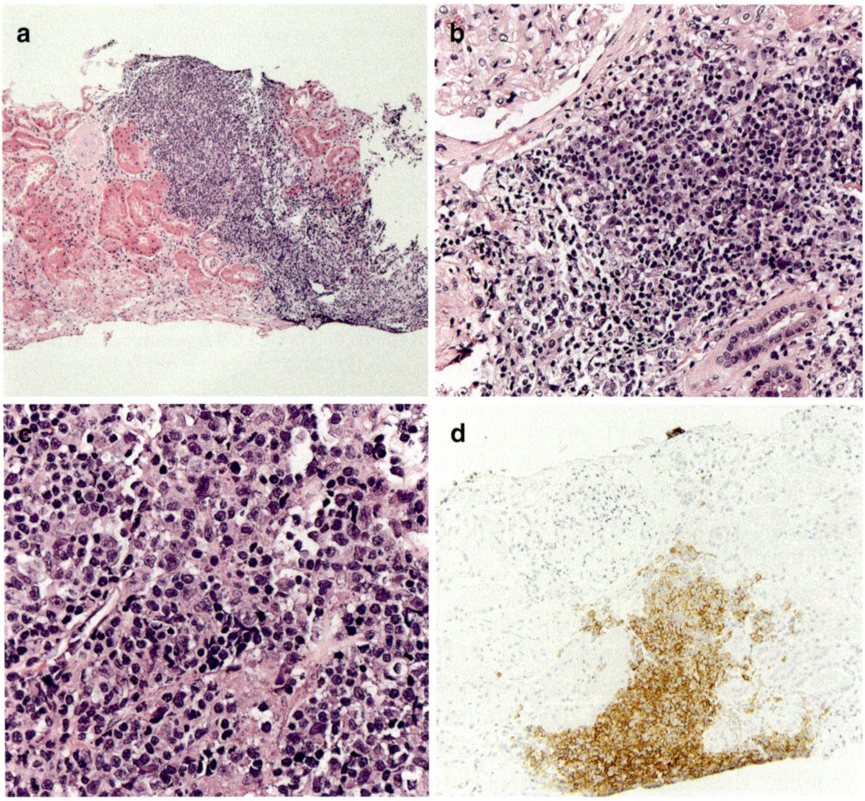

Fig. 12.4 (**a**) Kidney biopsy with infiltrating diffuse large B-cell lymphoma (H&E 10×). (**b**, **c**) On higher power, the cells are large with atypical, pleomorphic nuclei, and occasionally prominent nucleoli (H&E stains, 40× and 60×). (**d**) The lymphocytes were diffusely positive for CD20 (20×)

seen. The large cells express B-cell markers CD20, PAX-5, and CD79a and have a Ki-67 proliferation index over 50%. A subset of DLBCL is Epstein–Barr virus (EBV) driven, not otherwise specified (EBV+ DLBCL, NOS) and are usually associated with some degree of immunosuppression.

Diffuse large B-cell lymphoma is a heterogeneous group and can arise from B-cells at different stages of maturation. Gene expression profiling studies of diffuse large B-cell lymphoma have identified two distinct subgroups with an expression profile characteristic of either normal germinal center cells (GCB-like) or activated blood memory B-cells (ABC-like) and have demonstrated that patients with the ABC subtype have a worse prognosis when treated with chemotherapy. Immunohistochemistry for CD10, BCL-6, and MUM1 can be used to identify GCB and ABC-like subgroups with reasonable accuracy [39]. Expression of MYC and BCL-2 is commonly evaluated by immunohistochemistry and positivity for both may be associated with poor outcomes [40]. Cytogenetic analysis for rearrangements of *MYC, BCL-2,* and *BCL-6* are commonly performed. The presence of *MYC* rearrangement in conjunction with *BCL-2* or *BCL-6* rearrangements is characteristic of "double hit" lymphoma, which is associated with adverse prognosis. These patients are generally treated with more aggressive chemotherapy regimens.

Intravascular Large B-Cell Lymphoma

Intravascular large B-cell lymphoma (IVLBCL) can present in the kidney, with approximately 40 cases reported to date [41]. IVLBCL is a very rare type of non-Hodgkin lymphoma characterized by preferential proliferation of malignant B cells within the lumina of small blood vessels, particularly capillaries (Fig. 12.5). It is usually widely disseminated in extranodal sites, including the bone marrow. Two patterns of clinical presentation have been identified. In the Asian variant, patients present with multiorgan failure, B symptoms, and pancytopenia [42, 43]. The classic or Western variant is characterized by symptoms limited to the involved organ. Both types have a dismal prognosis, usually due to the delay of timely accurate diagnosis. Patients with primary IVLBCL of the kidney presented with fever, renal failure, proteinuria, and/or nephrotic syndrome [41, 43, 44]. The main histologic finding was that of minimal change disease. Lymphoma cells were detected predominantly in glomerular capillaries followed by peritubular and interstitial vessels [41].

Burkitt Lymphoma

Burkitt lymphoma (BL) is a distinct subtype of high-grade B-cell lymphoma which commonly affects children, with peak incidence between ages 4 and 7, although presentation in adults is frequently seen. Burkitt lymphoma is divided into three subtypes: endemic, sporadic, and immunodeficiency-associated. Endemic BL

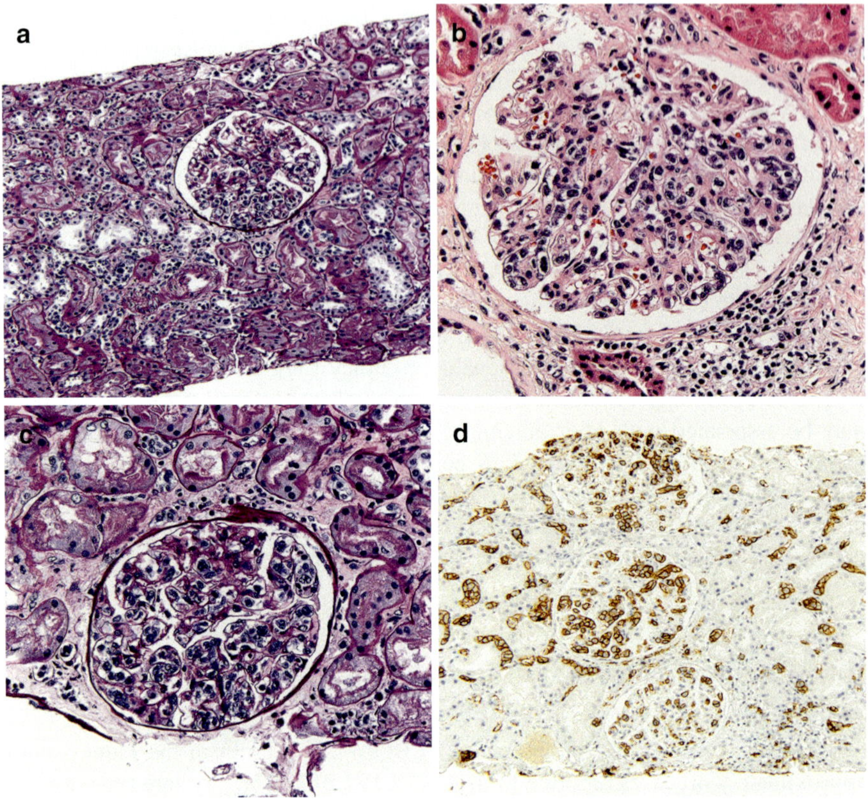

Fig. 12.5 (**a**) A kidney biopsy of intravascular lymphoma is remarkable for large, atypical cells seen almost exclusively within the glomerular capillaries and peritubular capillaries (PAS, 20×). (**b**, **c**) On high power, the cells are marginating along the endothelium and leading to obstruction of the normal capillary loops (H&E and PAS, 40×). (**d**) A CD20 immunohistochemical stain highlights the intravascular lymphoma within the glomeruli and peritubular capillaries (20×)

generally presents in children from equatorial Africa and is associated with EBV infection. Sporadic BL is predominantly diagnosed in children but can also present in older individuals. Immunodeficiency-associated BL is seen in people with HIV with a high CD4 count. Primary Burkitt lymphoma in the kidney is exceptionally rare [45, 46]. Secondary involvement of the kidney is a common finding in patients with BL, with sources suggesting renal involvement in 30–60% of cases based on sonographic or autopsy studies [47–49].

Burkitt lymphoma is classically described as having a "starry sky" appearance, with sheets of monotonous medium-sized neoplastic lymphocytes punctuated by scattered benign histiocytes with clear cytoplasm. The cells have vacuolated cytoplasm, clumped chromatin, and often multiple nucleoli. Mitotic figures and apoptotic debris are frequently seen. The classic immunophenotype is positive for B- cell markers as well as CD10 and BCL-6 with no expression of BCL-2 or TdT. The

Ki-67 proliferation index should be almost 100%. In situ hybridization for EBV-encoded RNA (EBER) should be performed. *MYC* gene rearrangement is a characteristic finding seen in over 90% of cases with fluorescence in situ hybridization (FISH) or conventional karyotype.

Mantle Cell Lymphoma

Mantle cell lymphoma is a mature B-cell lymphoma, which accounts for 3–10% of all non-Hodgkin lymphomas. It frequently presents with disseminated disease and involvement of multiple extranodal sites. Reports of renal involvement by mantle cell lymphoma are rare and correspond to cases with kidney function impairment due to lymphomatous infiltration [50–52]. Presentation includes proliferative glomerulonephritis, focal segmental glomerulosclerosis, acute tubulo-interstitial nephritis, and rarely acute kidney failure [50–52].

Morphologically, the neoplastic cells are small-to-medium-sized lymphocytes with a diffuse infiltration of tubulointerstitial compartment. Tumor cells express B-cell antigens as well as CD5, Cyclin D1, and SOX11. FISH analysis confirms presence of pathognomonic *IGH–CCND1* gene rearrangement.

Follicular Lymphoma

Follicular lymphoma is one of the most common low-grade B-cell lymphomas and generally has a nodal presentation. Renal presentation of follicular lymphoma has been rarely reported in the literature [35, 53]. Data on secondary involvement of the kidney in large studies or autopsy series are lacking.

Morphologically, follicular lymphoma has a nodular appearance and is composed of abnormal lymphoid follicles which are homogeneous in size and shape. They lack polarization, tingible body macrophages, and normal mantle zones. The follicles consist of a mixture of small cells with cleaved nuclei (centrocytes) and larger cells with round nuclei and prominent nucleoli (centroblasts). Grading is determined by the relative proportion of centroblasts in the lymphoid follicles, with more centroblasts seen in higher-grade lesions. However, in small needle core biopsies, assigning a precise grade is challenging and not required. Immunohistochemical staining typically shows expression of germinal B-cell markers CD10, BCL6, and LMO2, with tight CD21+, CD23+ follicular dendritic meshworks. The germinal centers aberrantly express BCL2 due to a rearrangement of *BCL2* with the immunoglobulin heavy chain gene in 80–90% of cases, resulting in a translocation of chromosomes 14 and 18. PCR will identify a monoclonal *IGH* gene rearrangement in 80% of cases.

Posttransplant Lymphoproliferative Disorder

Posttransplant lymphoproliferative disorders (PTLD) are lymphoid and/or plasmacytic proliferations that occur in the setting of solid organ or allogeneic hematopoietic cell transplantation as a result of immunosuppression. While the majority appears to be related to the presence of Epstein–Barr virus (EBV), EBV negative disease does occur. According to the updated 2016 WHO Classification, there are four distinct subtypes. Nondestructive PTLD, including plasmacytic hyperplasia, infectious mononucleosis, and florid follicular hyperplasia, are characterized by architectural preservation with formation of mass lesion and/or EBV reactivity. These lesions typically occur in lymph nodes, tonsils, and adenoids. Polymorphic PTLDs are atypical destructive polyclonal or monoclonal lymphoid infiltrates that do not meet all of the criteria for lymphoma. Monomorphic PTLDs are monoclonal lymphoid proliferations that meet the criteria for lymphomas as recognized in immunocompetent patients. Finally, classical Hodgkin lymphoma PTLD should fulfill the diagnostic criterial for classical Hodgkin lymphoma.

Patients receiving renal allograft have the lowest frequency of PTLD (<1%), compared with all other types of transplant [54]. PTLD may occur at any site of the body, including the renal allograft, raising the differential diagnosis of rejection or infection. Allograft involvement appears more frequently in early-onset (<18 months after transplant), EBV-positive disease. In cases of PTLD confined to the renal allograft, the most frequent clinical manifestations were graft dysfunction and fever [55]. One study of 53 patients with PTLD reported after renal transplant, highlighted 14 patients who developed allograft PTLD [56]. Of these patients, 4 had involvement of renal parenchyma and 10 had involvement confined to the renal hilum. In another study of 9 cases of PTLD presenting as renal allograft dysfunction, 3 patients were diagnosed based on fine-needle aspiration, and 6 with examination of allograft nephrectomy [57]. Polymorphic and monomorphic PTLD morphology has been reported in approximately equal number of cases, while the other two subtypes of PTLD have not been described in the kidney literature [55, 57]. Polymorphic PTLD can be a very challenging diagnosis based on morphology, as it is characterized by a mixed population of small, medium-sized, and large lymphocytes admixed with plasma cells, frequently associated with areas of geographical necrosis (Fig. 12.6). Bizarre Reed–Sternberg-like cells may be seen. Immunophenotypic analysis shows a mixture of B and T lymphocytes. Plasma cells may be polytypic or monotypic. PCR frequently demonstrates clonal IgG gene rearrangement. Presence of numerous EBV-positive cell by in situ hybridization is a very helpful feature that helps to reach the correct diagnosis and rules out allograft rejection. Monomorphic PTLD in the renal allograft usually correspond to cases of DLBCL (Fig. 12.7), although there are rare case reports of other poorly characterized B- and T-/natural killer (NK)-cell neoplasms [55–57].

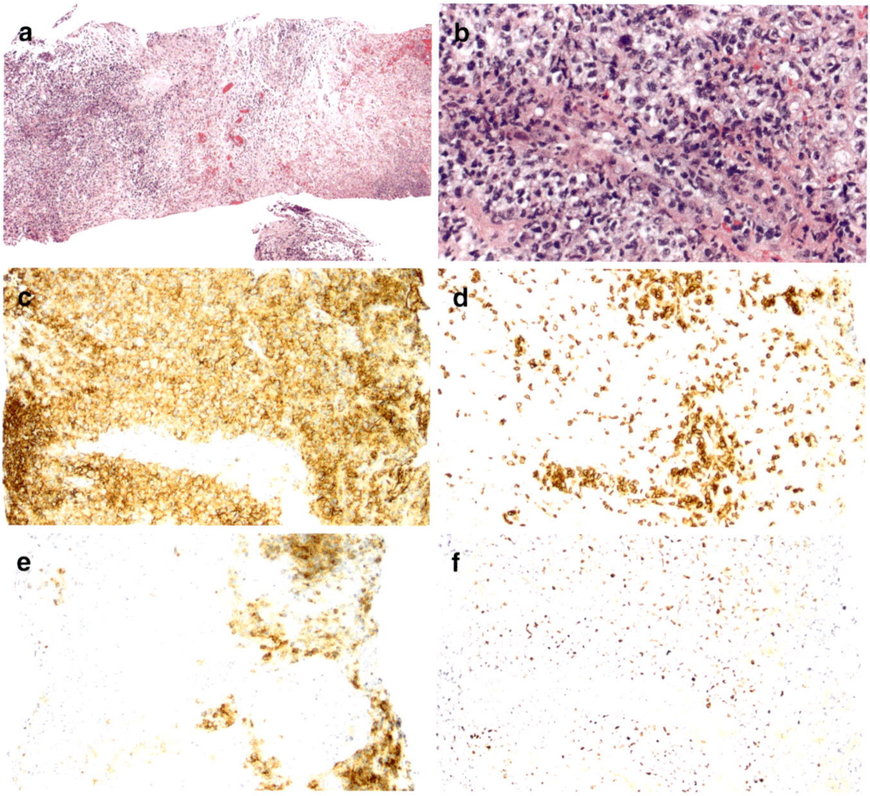

Fig. 12.6 Polymorphic PTLD. (**a**) Low power image of kidney biopsy with a focally dense inflammatory infiltrate and extensive necrosis (H&E, 4×). (**b**) On high power the cells are composed of a heterogeneous/polymorphous mixture of inflammatory cells within the interstitium as well as infiltrating the tubules and vessels (H&E 20×). (**c**) B cells show diffuse staining for CD20 (**c**, 10×), focal T cells express CD3 (**d**, 10×), there are collections of CD30 positive immunoblasts (**e**, 10×), and diffuse positivity with EBER (**f**, 10×)

Lymphoblastic Lymphoma

Cases of B- and T-lymphoblastic leukemia/lymphoma may be primary or secondary, frequently cause bilateral renal enlargement and can occasionally present as acute renal failure (Fig. 12.8) [58–62]. Morphologically, there is a diffuse infiltrate composed of a monotonous population of medium-sized blasts with fine chromatin. Frequently, glomeruli and tubules appear spared [61]. Classically, T lymphoblasts express CD3, CD7, CD34, and TdT, with frequent coexpression of CD4 and CD8. B lymphoblasts typically express B-cell markers like CD20, PAX-5, and CD19 in addition to CD34, TdT, and CD10.

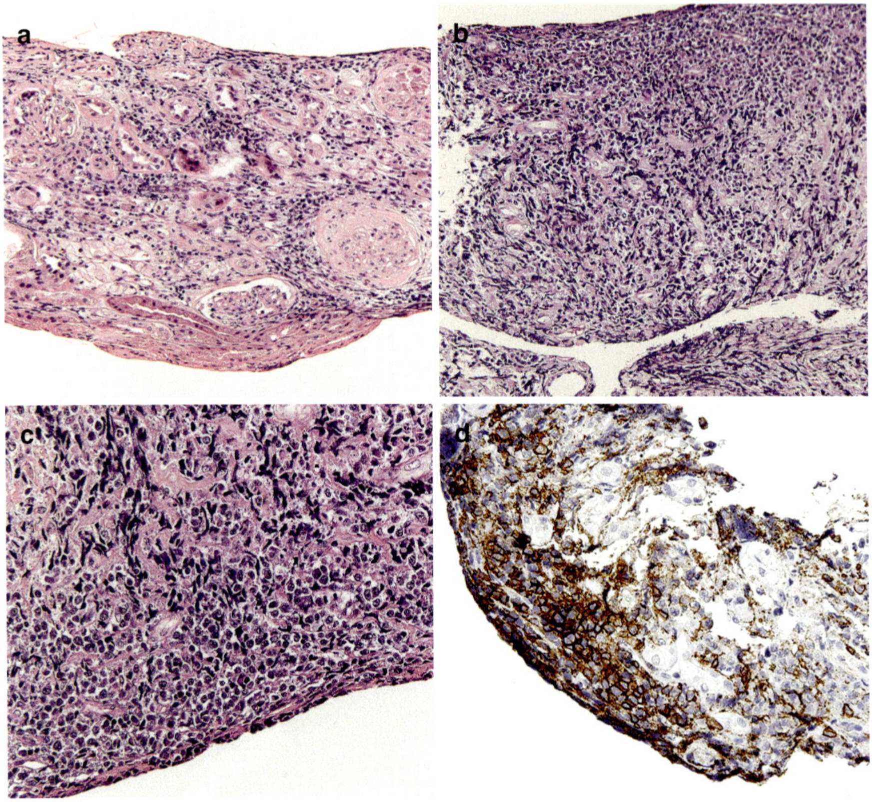

Fig. 12.7 (**a**, **b**) A transplant kidney with infiltrating diffuse large B cell lymphoma/posttransplant lymphoproliferative disease (H&E, 20×). (**c**) On high power, the cells have large, pleomorphic nuclei with a high N:C ratio, and occasional nucleoli present (H&E, 40×). (**d**) By IHC, the inflammatory cells are nearly all positive for CD20 (40×) and are negative for CD3 and EBER (not shown)

T-Cell Lymphoma

Rare cases of T-cell lymphoma in kidney have been documented, including enteropathy associated T-cell lymphoma [63], adult T-cell leukemia/lymphoma [64], NK/T-cell lymphoma [65], angioimmunoblastic T-cell lymphoma [66], and peripheral T-cell lymphoma, NOS [67]. In an autopsy series of five patients with anaplastic large cell lymphoma, only one had renal involvement [68]. Bilateral kidney infiltration is usually seen. Rare cases present with acute renal failure. Morphologically, the neoplastic cells diffusely infiltrate the kidney parenchyma. They express T-cell antigen CD3 and a variety of other T-cell markers, such as CD2, CD4, CD5, CD7, and CD8.

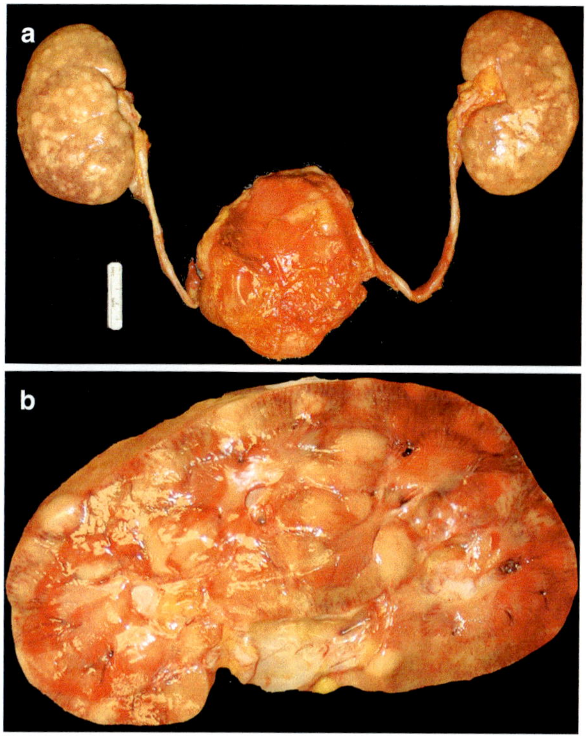

Fig. 12.8 (**a**) Gross images from an autopsy showing both kidneys with nodules of B-Lymphoblastic Lymphoma. On cut section (**b**), the lymphomatous nodules involved both the renal cortex and medulla. The patient died of treatment resistant lymphoma and renal failure

Paraprotein-Related Diseases

These are closely related entities, including primary amyloidosis (PA) and monoclonal immunoglobulin deposition disease (MIDD), also known as light and heavy chain deposition disease (LHCDD). They are characterized by visceral deposition of abnormal immunoglobulin, resulting in organ dysfunction [54]. The underlying disorders are plasma cell or, rarely, lymphoplasmacytic neoplasms. This is frequently an early disease manifestation in patients without overt myeloma or lymphoma. PA is characterized by secretion of abnormal immunoglobulin light chains that deposit in various tissues and form a beta-pleated amyloid structure, which stains red orange with Congo red stain and has apple-green birefringence under polarized light (Fig. 12.9). MIDD/LHCDD is caused by secretion of abnormal light and/or heavy immunoglobulin chains which do not form amyloid beta-pleated sheets or fibrils and do not bind Congo red stain (Fig. 12.10) [54]. Instead of forming fibrils, the abnormal proteins deposit along

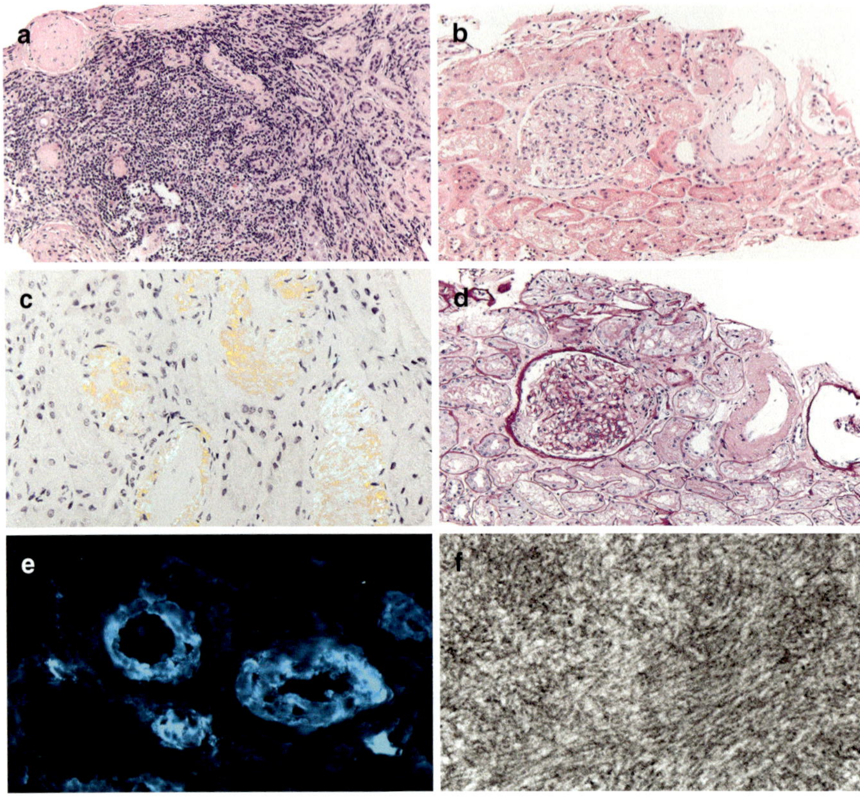

Fig. 12.9 (**a**) Biopsy showing infiltrating low-grade lymphoma within the interstitium (H&E, 10×). (**b**, **d**) Amorphous, PAS-negative material is present within the small arteries (H&E and PAS stains, 20×). (**c**) The amorphous material is Congo red positive with apple green birefringence under polarized microscopy (Congo red stain, 40×). (**e**) On IF, the amyloid was strongly staining for lambda (40×) and was negative for kappa (not shown). (**f**) On electron microscopy (EM), haphazardly arranged fibrils are seen on high power which range in diameter from 8 to 12 nm (120,000×)

the glomerular and tubular basement membrane surfaces leading to renal dysfunction. Renal manifestations are present in >80% of PA patients and up to 96% of MIDD/LHCDD patients and include proteinuria, nephrotic syndrome, and renal failure [69]. The vast majority of the patients have a detectable M protein. Amyloidosis shows a diffuse glomerular deposition of amorphous hyaline material which is periodic acid–Schiff (PAS) and silver negative and Congo red positive, initially in the mesangium and then along the capillary loops. It may also be seen in the surrounding interstitium and small vessels. MIDD/LHCDD may reveal a membrano-proliferative glomerular pattern due to accumulation of punctate usually light chain deposits along the glomerular and tubular basement membranes. In PA, the light chain is lambda in 70% of the cases, while 80% of MIDD/LHCDD express kappa light chain.

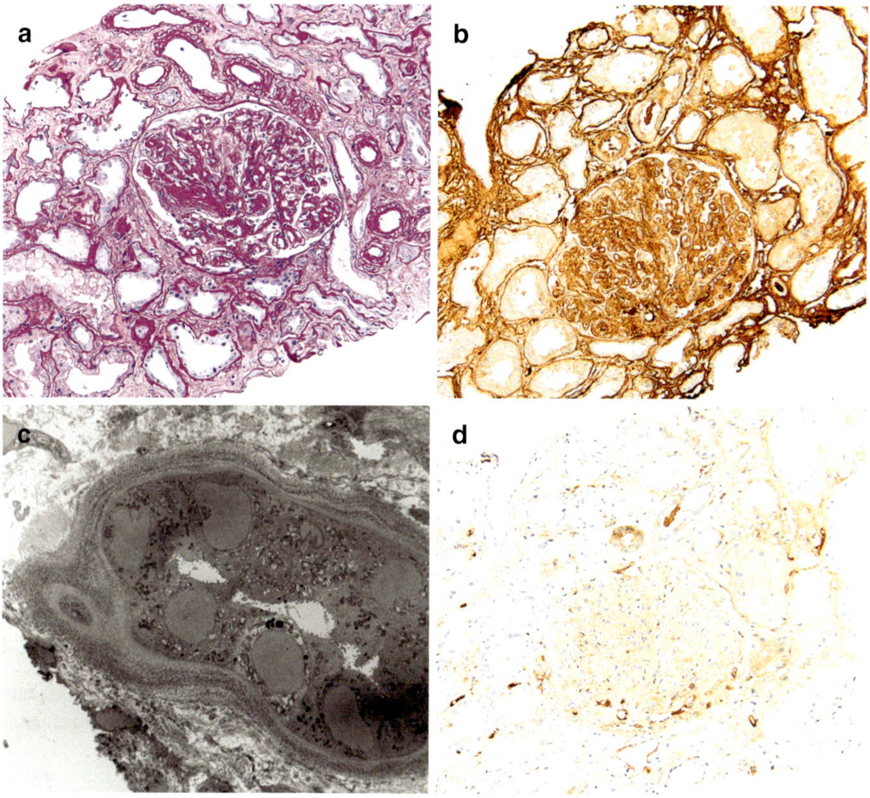

Fig. 12.10 (**a**) A biopsy with monoclonal immunoglobulin deposition disease showing PAS-positive thickening of the glomerular capillary walls, mesangium, and tubular basement membranes (PAS 20×). (**b**, **d**) By immunohistochemistry, the basement membranes show strong staining for kappa light chains (**b**, 20×) which are negative for lambda light chains (**d**, 20×). (**c**) On EM, tubular basement membrane punctate light chain type deposits are seen in layers (3000×)

Histological Findings of Kidney Parenchyma in Patients with Renal Lymphoma

In addition to direct lymphomatous involvement of the kidney, patients with lymphoma may come to clinical attention due to secondary glomerular involvement. Glomerulonephritis (GN) in the course of NHL is one of the causes of acute kidney injury. Many different glomerular diseases have been associated with lymphomas including proliferative glomerular diseases such as membrano-proliferative GN, mesangial proliferative GN, crescentic GN, or proliferative glomerulonephritis with monoclonal deposits. Membranous glomerulonephritis can also be seen, due to monoclonal deposits along the subepithelial basement membrane surfaces. Lymphomas may elaborate cytokines which may damage the podocytes leading to minimal change disease or focal segmental glomerulosclerosis. Overall, there is a wide spectrum of clinical presentations in these patients which may necessitate biopsy, including nephrotic or nephritic syndromes [5]. Start of chemotherapy, resulting in partial remission of lymphoma, correlates with the decrease in the signs of GN and may improve organ function.

References

1. Kandel LB, McCullough DL, Harrison LH, et al. Primary renal lymphoma. Does it exist? Cancer. 1987;60:386–91.
2. Yasunaga Y, Hoshida Y, Hashimoto M, et al. Malignant lymphoma of the kidney. J Surg Oncol. 1997;64:207–11.
3. Freeman C, Berg JW, Cutler SJ. Occurrence and prognosis of extranodal lymphomas. Cancer. 1972;29:252–60.
4. Aozasa K, Tsujimoto M, Sakurai M, et al. Non-Hodgkin's lymphomas in Osaka, Japan. Eur J Cancer Clin Oncol. 1985;21:487–92.
5. Da'as N, Polliack A, Cohen Y, et al. Kidney involvement and renal manifestations in non-Hodgkin's lymphoma and lymphocytic leukemia: a retrospective study in 700 patients. Eur J Haematol. 2001;67:158–64.
6. Farrow GM, Harrison EG Jr, Utz DC. Sarcomas and sarcomatoid and mixed malignant tumors of the kidney in adults. II. Cancer. 1968;22:551–5.
7. Stallone G, Infante B, Manno C, et al. Primary renal lymphoma does exist: case report and review of the literature. J Nephrol. 2000;13:367–72.
8. Betta PG, Bottero G, Cosimi MF, et al. Primary renal lymphoma. Eur Urol. 1986;12:352–4.
9. Duanay P. Linfosarcoma y linfosarcomatosis de los riñones: part II. Rev Med Trop Parasitol Bacteriol Clin Lab. 1940;6:213.
10. Li SJ, Chen HP, Chen YH, et al. Renal involvement in non-Hodgkin lymphoma: proven by renal biopsy. PLoS One. 2014;9:e95190.
11. Tornroth T, Heiro M, Marcussen N, et al. Lymphomas diagnosed by percutaneous kidney biopsy. Am J Kidney Dis. 2003;42:960–71.
12. Wood SM, Boyd SM, Taylor JE, et al. A case of non-Hodgkin lymphoma presenting primarily with renal failure. Nephrol Dial Transplant. 1996;11:535–6.
13. Obrador GT, Price B, O'Meara Y, et al. Acute renal failure due to lymphomatous infiltration of the kidneys. J Am Soc Nephrol. 1997;8:1348–54.
14. Kanfer A, Vandewalle A, Morel-Maroger L, et al. Acute renal insufficiency due to lymphomatous infiltration of the kidneys: report of six cases. Cancer. 1976;38:2588–92.
15. Leung AC, McKean M, Mactier R, et al. Acute oliguric renal failure secondary to lymphomatous infiltration of the kidneys. Postgrad Med J. 1984;60:556–8.
16. Bernard RJ, Thompson C, Verani R, et al. Lymphoma presenting as acute renal failure. Am J Med. 1988;84:366–7.
17. Sheth S, Ali S, Fishman E. Imaging of renal lymphoma: patterns of disease with pathologic correlation. Radiographics. 2006;26:1151–68.
18. Cohan RH, Dunnick NR, Leder RA, et al. Computed tomography of renal lymphoma. J Comput Assist Tomogr. 1990;14:933–8.
19. Pedrosa I, Sun MR, Spencer M, et al. MR imaging of renal masses: correlation with findings at surgery and pathologic analysis. Radiographics. 2008;28:985–1003.
20. Zukotynski K, Lewis A, O'Regan K, et al. PET/CT and renal pathology: a blind spot for radiologists? Part 2–lymphoma, leukemia, and metastatic disease. AJR Am J Roentgenol. 2012;199:W168–74.
21. Barcos M, Lane W, Gomez GA, et al. An autopsy study of 1206 acute and chronic leukemias (1958 to 1982). Cancer. 1987;60:827–37.

22. Schwartz JB, Shamsuddin AM. The effects of leukemic infiltrates in various organs in chronic lymphocytic leukemia. Hum Pathol. 1981;12:432–40.
23. Phillips JK, Bass PS, Majumdar G, et al. Renal failure caused by leukaemic infiltration in chronic lymphocytic leukaemia. J Clin Pathol. 1993;46:1131–3.
24. Uprety D, Peterson A, Shah BK. Renal failure secondary to leukemic infiltration of kidneys in CLL–a case report and review of literature. Ann Hematol. 2013;92:271–3.
25. Nasr SH, Shanafelt TD, Hanson CA, et al. Granulomatous interstitial nephritis secondary to chronic lymphocytic leukemia/small lymphocytic lymphoma. Ann Diagn Pathol. 2015;19:130–6.
26. Parikh SA, Rabe KG, Call TG, et al. Diffuse large B-cell lymphoma (Richter syndrome) in patients with chronic lymphocytic leukaemia (CLL): a cohort study of newly diagnosed patients. Br J Haematol. 2013;162:774–82.
27. Garcia M, Konoplev S, Morosan C, et al. MALT lymphoma involving the kidney: a report of 10 cases and review of the literature. Am J Clin Pathol. 2007;128:464–73.
28. Niwa N, Tanaka N, Horinaga M, et al. Mucosa-associated lymphoid tissue lymphoma arising from the kidney. Can Urol Assoc J. 2014;8:E86–8.
29. Tuzel E, Mungan MU, Yorukoglu K, et al. Primary renal lymphoma of mucosa-associated lymphoid tissue. Urology. 2003;61:463.
30. Vos JM, Gustine J, Rennke HG, et al. Renal disease related to Waldenstrom macroglobulinaemia: incidence, pathology and clinical outcomes. Br J Haematol. 2016;175:623–30.
31. Dimopoulos MA, Moulopoulos LA, Costantinides C, et al. Primary renal lymphoma: a clinical and radiological study. J Urol. 1996;155:1865–7.
32. Ferry JA, Harris NL, Papanicolaou N, et al. Lymphoma of the kidney. A report of 11 cases. Am J Surg Pathol. 1995;19:134–44.
33. Kose F, Sakalli H, Mertsoylu H, et al. Primary renal lymphoma: report of four cases. Onkologie. 2009;32:200–2.
34. Kaya A, Kanbay M, Bayrak O, et al. Primary renal lymphoma associated with hepatitis C virus infection. Leuk Lymphoma. 2006;47:1976–8.
35. Morel P, Dupriez B, Herbrecht R, et al. Aggressive lymphomas with renal involvement: a study of 48 patients treated with the LNH-84 and LNH-87 regimens. Groupe d'Etude des Lymphomes de l'Adulte. Br J Cancer. 1994;70:154–9.
36. Villa D, Connors JM, Sehn LH, et al. Diffuse large B-cell lymphoma with involvement of the kidney: outcome and risk of central nervous system relapse. Haematologica. 2011;96:1002–7.
37. Onishi T, Yonemura S, Sakata Y, et al. Renal lymphoma associated with Castleman's disease. Scand J Urol Nephrol. 2004;38:90–1.
38. Nasr SH, Alobeid B, Jacobs JM, et al. Methotrexate-associated B-cell lymphoma presenting with acute renal failure and bilateral nephromegaly. Kidney Int. 2007;71:272–5.
39. Hans CP, Weisenburger DD, Greiner TC, et al. Confirmation of the molecular classification of diffuse large B-cell lymphoma by immunohistochemistry using a tissue microarray. Blood. 2004;103:275–82.
40. Hu S, Xu-Monette ZY, Tzankov A, et al. MYC/BCL2 protein coexpression contributes to the inferior survival of activated B-cell subtype of diffuse large B-cell lymphoma and demonstrates high-risk gene expression signatures: a report from The International DLBCL Rituximab-CHOP Consortium Program. Blood. 2013;121:4021–31; quiz 4250
41. Desclaux A, Lazaro E, Pinaquy JB, et al. Renal intravascular large B-cell lymphoma: a case report and review of the literature. Intern Med. 2017;56:827–33.
42. Bai X, Li X, Wan L, et al. Intravascular large B-cell lymphoma of the kidney: a case report. Diagn Pathol. 2011;6:86.
43. Kameoka Y, Takahashi N, Komatsuda A, et al. Kidney-limited intravascular large B cell lymphoma: a distinct variant of IVLBCL? Int J Hematol. 2009;89:533–7.
44. Akpinar TS, Ozkok A, Batu D, et al. Isolated renal intravascular lymphoma: a case report and review of the literature. Ren Fail. 2014;36:1125–8.

45. Schniederjan SD, Osunkoya AO. Lymphoid neoplasms of the urinary tract and male genital organs: a clinicopathological study of 40 cases. Mod Pathol. 2009;22:1057–65.
46. Sieniawska M, Bialasik D, Jedrzejowski A, et al. Bilateral primary renal Burkitt lymphoma in a child presenting with acute renal failure. Nephrol Dial Transplant. 1997;12:1490–2.
47. Miller AR, Cipkala DA, Cain MP. Gross hematuria and focal renal masses as initial features of a mature B-cell leukemia in an adolescent male. Urology. 2015;85:470–3.
48. Durodola JI. Pattern of organ involvement in Burkitt's lymphoma in Ibadan: a review. J Natl Med Assoc. 1977;69:319–23.
49. Strauss S, Libson E, Schwartz E, et al. Renal sonography in American Burkitt lymphoma. AJR Am J Roentgenol. 1986;146:549–52.
50. Lubas A, Mroz A, Smoszna J, et al. Membranoproliferative glomerulonephritis, mantle cell lymphoma infiltration, and acute kidney injury. Int Urol Nephrol. 2013;45:1489–94.
51. Peddi S, Ram R, Kataru SR, et al. Acute renal failure in a patient with mantle cell lymphoma. Hemodial Int. 2015;19:E12–5.
52. Lee HJ, Seo JW, Cho HS, et al. Renal involvement of mantle cell lymphona leading to end stage renal disease. Hemodial Int. 2012;16:104–8.
53. Petkovic I, Krstic M, Pejcic I, et al. Renal infiltration of follicular lymphoma. Turk J Haematol. 2014;31:315–6.
54. Swerdlow SHCE, Harris NL, Jaffe ES, Pileri SA, Stein H, Thiele J, editors. WHO classification of tumours of haematopoietic and lymphoid tissues (revised 4th edition). Lyon: IARC; 2017.
55. Cobo F, Garcia C, Talavera P, et al. Diffuse large B-cell lymphoma in a renal allograft associated with Epstein-Barr virus in the recipient: a case report and a review of lymphomas presenting in a transplanted kidney. Clin Transplant. 2008;22:512–9.
56. Caillard S, Lachat V, Moulin B. Posttransplant lymphoproliferative disorders in renal allograft recipients: report of 53 cases of a French multicenter study. PTLD French Working Group. Transpl Int. 2000;13(Suppl 1):S388–93.
57. Randhawa PS, Magnone M, Jordan M, et al. Renal allograft involvement by Epstein-Barr virus associated post-transplant lymphoproliferative disease. Am J Surg Pathol. 1996;20:563–71.
58. Larsen G, Loghman-Adham M. Acute renal failure with hyperuricemia as initial presentation of leukemia in children. J Pediatr Hematol Oncol. 1996;18:191–4.
59. Rajakumar V, Balaraman V, Balasubramaniam R, et al. Lymphoblastic lymphoma presenting as bilateral renal enlargement diagnosed by percutaneous kidney biopsy: report of three cases. Indian J Nephrol. 2016;26:298–301.
60. Shi SF, Zhou FD, Zou WZ, et al. Acute kidney injury and bilateral symmetrical enlargement of the kidneys as first presentation of B-cell lymphoblastic lymphoma. Am J Kidney Dis. 2012;60:1044–8.
61. Kwakernaak AJ, Hazenberg MD, Roelofs JJ, et al. Precursor T-lymphoblastic lymphoma presenting as primary renal lymphoma with acute renal failure. NDT Plus. 2011;4:289–91.
62. Boueva A, Bouvier R. Precursor B-cell lymphoblastic leukemia as a cause of a bilateral nephromegaly. Pediatr Nephrol. 2005;20:679–82.
63. Bakrac M, Bonaci B, Krstic M, et al. A rare case of enteropathy-associated T-cell lymphoma presenting as acute renal failure. World J Gastroenterol. 2006;12:2301–4.
64. Srinivasa NS, McGovern CH, Solez K, et al. Progressive renal failure due to renal invasion and parenchymal destruction by adult T-cell lymphoma. Am J Kidney Dis. 1990;16:70–2.
65. Sem Liew M, Chan AM, Galloway S, et al. Extra-nasal NK/T cell lymphoma masquerading as renal infarction. Leuk Lymphoma. 2010;51:1139–41.
66. Argov O, Charach G, Weintraub M, et al. Angioimmunoblastic T-cell lymphoma presenting as giant kidneys: a case report. J Med Case Reports. 2009;3:9258.
67. Neuhauser TS, Lancaster K, Haws R, et al. Rapidly progressive T cell lymphoma presenting as acute renal failure: case report and review of the literature. Pediatr Pathol Lab Med. 1997;17:449–60.

68. Mosunjac MB, Sundstrom JB, Mosunjac MI. Unusual presentation of anaplastic large cell lymphoma with clinical course mimicking fever of unknown origin and sepsis: autopsy study of five cases. Croat Med J. 2008;49:660–8.
69. Pozzi C, D'Amico M, Fogazzi GB, et al. Light chain deposition disease with renal involvement: clinical characteristics and prognostic factors. Am J Kidney Dis. 2003;42:1154–63.

Chapter 13
Tumors of the Renal Pelvis

Charles C. Guo, Miao Zhang, and Kanishka Sircar

The upper urinary tract (UUT) consists of the renal pelvis and ureter. Tumors of the renal pelvis are relatively uncommon and only account for 5–8% of all renal tumors [1–3]. As the renal pelvic tumors share similar pathologic and clinical features with tumors that arise from the ureter, they are generally grouped together as tumors of the UUT. The vast majority of UUT tumors are composed of urothelial carcinoma (UC) [4–7]. UC occurs about twice more frequently in the renal pelvis than in the ureter [8]. Multifocal tumors are found in 10–20% of new cases of upper urinary tract urothelial carcinoma (UUTUC), and a concomitant bladder UC is present in approximately 20% of cases [9]. However, bilateral synchronous UUTUC represents only 3% of all UC at this site [10]. In spite of some similarities to bladder UC, UUTUC demonstrates distinct clinicopathologic and molecular features [11].

Epidemiology

Tumor of the renal pelvis is a rare disease with an estimated annual incidence of 1–2 cases per 100,000 [12]. The incidence has been increasing in recent years largely due to the improvement of imaging and endoscopic techniques. It is generally a disease of the elderly, with a mean age at diagnosis in the seventh decade [6, 13]. The disease is more common in men than in women with a male-to-female ratio of approximately 2:1 [14]. Although the frequency of UUTUC is increasing, it represents only 5% of all UC of the urinary tract [4–6].

C. C. Guo (✉) · M. Zhang
Department of Pathology, The University of Texas MD Anderson Cancer Center, Houston, TX, USA
e-mail: ccguo@mdanderson.org

K. Sircar
Division of Pathology and Laboratory Medicine, Departments of Pathology and Translational Molecular Pathology, The University of Texas MD Anderson Cancer Center, Houston, TX, USA
e-mail: ksircar@mdanderson.org

M. K. Divatia et al. (eds.), *Kidney Cancer*, https://doi.org/10.1007/978-3-030-28333-9_13

Etiology

Tobacco smoking and aromatic amines exposure are the two most common risk factors for UUTUC in Western countries [15]. Smoking increases the relative risk for developing UUTUC from 2.5 to 7 times, depending on the number of cigarettes smoked every day and the number of years of smoking [16]. Fortunately, the risk for UTUC decreases by 60–70% when smoking cessation has been longer than 10 years [17]. The relative risk for developing upper tract urothelial carcinoma (UTUC) after the exposure to aromatic amines is 8.3, with an average duration of exposure of 7 years and a latency period of approximately 20 years [18]. With the adoption of safety measures, occupational exposure to aromatic amines carcinogen has dramatically decreased in the last several decades.

Balkan endemic nephropathy is another risk factor for UUTUC [19]. The disease affects mainly farmers along the Danube River in the Balkan Peninsula, who are exposed to the degradation products of coal-containing soil [20]. The disease is characterized by chronic tubulointerstitial nephropathy with insidious onset and slow progression to renal failure. The incidence of UUTUC in the Blakan areas may be up to 100 times higher than in the nonepidemic areas. The patients are generally young and present with multiple UC of low grade and stage that may affect bilateral kidneys [21].

Lynch syndrome or hereditary nonpolyposis colorectal cancer syndrome also increases the risk for UUTUC [10]. This autosomal dominant syndrome is caused by germline mutations in the mismatch repair genes, including *hMSH2*, *hMLH1*, *hMSH6*, and *hMLH1*. The most common malignancy in patients with Lynch syndrome is colonic adenocarcinoma, followed by endometrial carcinoma and UUTUC [22]. In people with Lynch syndrome, the risk of UUTUC is increased 14–22 times as compared to the general population [10]. These patients should be referred for genetic counseling and assessment of their family members should also be considered, as they may also be affected by the disease.

Other potential risk factors include renal stones, cyclophosphamide, phenacetin, aristolochic acid (a component in weight-loss pills containing Chinese herbs), and occupational exposures [2, 15, 16].

Clinical Features

Patients usually present with hematuria and dysuria. Hematuria may be gross or microscopic. Flank pain is another common symptom that is present in 10–40% of patients [3]. Computed tomography (CT) urography is the preferred imaging method for the initial evaluation. The presence of a filling defect on imaging is a characteristic finding of the renal pelvic tumor. At an advanced stage, the tumor may metastasize to the lungs, liver, bone, and regional lymph node, leading to constitutional symptoms, such as weight loss, anorexia, fever, night sweats, anemia, malaise, abdominal mass, and bone pain.

Endoscopic biopsy is often performed to evaluate a renal pelvic tumor, particularly when it is equivocal for malignancy on imaging study [23]. In spite of significant improvements in endoscopic techniques of the upper urinary tract, the endoscopic biopsy specimens are usually small and fragmented, typically less than 1 cm in aggregate [24]. Cautery and crushing artifacts are frequently present in the specimens, which may further limit the pathologic interpretation. The sensitivity of a renal pelvic endoscopic biopsy was reported to be 78%, and most errors are due to suboptimal tissue sampling rather than diagnostic errors [23, 24]. Thus, negative biopsies may not completely exclude the possibility of malignancy and a repeat biopsy may be indicated. Grade discordance between endoscopic biopsy specimens and subsequent nephroureterectomy specimens is commonly seen in up to 40% of cases, and the discrepancy is largely due to limited sampling of endoscopic biopsy as well as grade heterogeneity within the tumor [25]. The diagnostic specificity of a renal pelvic biopsy is excellent and near 100%, but rare cases of false positive diagnoses have been reported in literature [23]. To avoid unnecessary nephroureterectomy, the diagnosis of the renal pelvic UC can be made only when the findings are unequivocal for malignancy. Accurate pathologic staging is generally challenging, if not impossible, due to the small and superficial nature of the endoscopic biopsy specimen.

Urinary cytology is another valuable tool in the diagnosis of renal pelvic UC. The sensitivity and specificity of detecting UC in urine cytology depend on specimen type. Voided urine collects exfoliated urothelial cells from the entire urinary tract. Although voided urine has a higher sensitivity for detecting UC, it cannot determine the exact location of the lesion. Selective urine, washing, and brushing samples of the UUT can be obtained by endoscopic ureteral catheterization. The specificity of detecting UC in urine cytology is generally greater than 90% [26]. Although the sensitivity for high-grade UC and urothelial carcinoma in situ (UCIS) can be as high as 80–90%, the sensitivity for detecting low-grade UC is low [27]. The low sensitivity of low-grade UC is due to the fact that low-grade UC by definition has similar cytologic features to normal urothelial cells. Furthermore, low-grade UC cells are not routinely shed into the urine because of their cohesive nature. Therefore, it is exceedingly difficult to make the outright diagnosis of low-grade UC on a urine specimen. Fluorescence in situ hybridization (FISH) and microsatellite analysis may be used to increase the sensitivity of urine cytology, particularly for low-grade UC of the renal pelvis [28–30].

Pathologic Features

More than 90% of the renal pelvic tumors consist of UC, and nonurothelial neoplasms are relatively uncommon at this site [3–7].

Urothelial Tumors

Urothelial tumors of the renal pelvis share similar histopathologic features with their counterparts in the urinary bladder. The renal pelvic urothelial tumors are generally classified using a similar classification system to that for bladder urothelial tumors. The recent World Health Organization (WHO) 2016 Classification System divided urothelial tumors into two broad groups, noninvasive and invasive (Table 13.1) [30]. The noninvasive group is further divided into two subgroups, papillary urothelial neoplasms and flat lesions. Under each subgroup, there are several distinct histologic categories. The invasive group includes conventional UC as well as a number of histologic variants. In invasive UC, pathologic staging is the most important prognostic factor and evaluated according to the criteria by the American Joint Committee of Cancer (AJCC), which are not the same as those for the bladder UC due to different anatomy (Table 13.2) [31].

Table 13.1 2016 World Health Organization histologic classification of urothelial neoplasms

Noninvasive urothelial neoplasms
Papillary tumors
Papillary UC, low-grade
Papillary UC, high-grade
Papillary urothelial neoplasm of low malignant potential
Urothelial papilloma
Flat lesions
UC in situ
Urothelial dysplasia
Invasive urothelial carcinoma
Conventional UC
UC with divergent differentiation
UC with squamous differentiation
UC with glandular differentiation
UC with trophoblastic differentiation
Distinct UC variants
Micropapillary
Nested
Plasmacytoid
Microcystic
Lymphoepithelioma-like
Sarcomatoid
Poorly differentiated
Lipoid-rich
Clear cell

From Humphrey et al. [66], with permission
UC urothelial carcinoma

Table 13.2 Pathologic staging of the renal pelvic tumor

Primary Tumor (T)	
pTx	Primary tumor cannot be assessed
pT0	No evidence of tumor
pTa	Noninvasive papillary urothelial carcinoma
pTis	Urothelial carcinoma in situ
pT1	Tumor invades subepithelial connective tissue
pT2	Tumor invades muscularis propria
pT3	Tumor invades through muscularis propria into peri-pelvic fat or renal parenchyma
pT4	Tumor invades through renal parenchyma into the perinephric fat or adjacent organs
Regional lymph node (N)	
pNx	Regional lymph node metastasis cannot be assessed
pN0	No lymph node metastasis
pN1	Metastasis to a single lymph node, ≤2 cm in greatest dimension
pN2	Metastasis to a single lymph node, >2 cm; or multiple lymph nodes
Distant metastasis (M)	
pMx	Distant metastasis cannot be assessed
pM0	No distant metastasis
pM1	Distant metastasis present

Used with permission of the American College of Surgeons, Chicago, Illinois. The original and primary source for this information is the AJCC Cancer Staging Manual, Eighth Edition (2017) published by Springer International Publishing

Papillary Urothelial Neoplasms

Urothelial papilloma is an extremely rare benign tumor in the renal pelvis with only a few cases reported in literature [32, 33]. It is usually a small, delicate papillary structure that is found incidentally. Sometimes, it may cause hematuria. Microscopically, it consists of thin, delicate fibrovascular cores covered by the urothelium of normal thickness that lacks any noticeable atypical features (Fig. 13.1). Inverted papilloma is a variant of urothelial papilloma [34, 35], which is also detected as an indecent finding in the pelvis by pyelography. It may form a mass, mimicking UC grossly. The tumor often shows an inverted growth pattern and forms complex, anastomosing trabecular structures in the lamina propria. The luminal surface of the lesion is flat. The urothelial cells show minimal atypia but often form small glandular structures with vacuolization in the luminal cells. The prognosis for inverted papilloma is excellent with only occasional recurrence, but they never progress to UC.

Urothelial neoplasm of low malignant potential (PUNLMP) is another uncommon tumor in the pelvis, accounting for less than 5% of all UC at this site [36, 37]. Grossly, it presents as single or multiple discrete exophytic papillary lesions of vari-

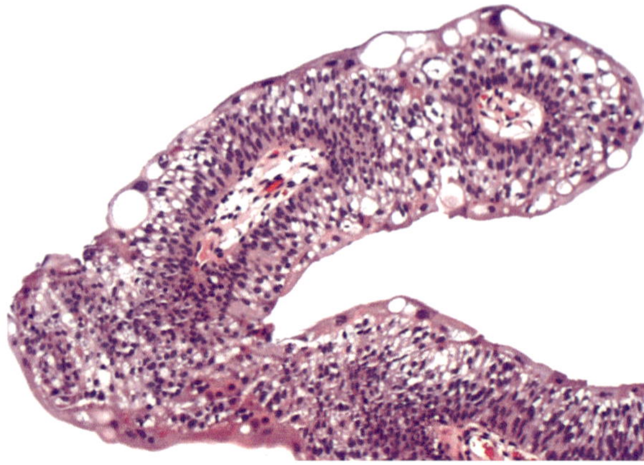

Fig. 13.1 Urothelial papilloma shows slender, delicate papillae lined by normal-appearing urothelium with prominent vacuolization

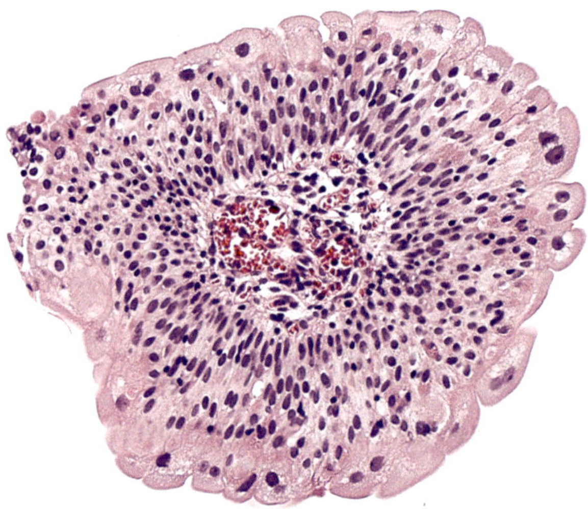

Fig. 13.2 Papillary urothelial neoplasm of low malignant potential (PUNLMP) shows thickened urothelium but minimal cytologic atypia

able size. Microscopically, it shows papillary structures lined by the urothelium that is thicker than normal urothelium, but the urothelial cells do not show apparent cytologic atypia (Fig. 13.2). The papillary fronds are frequently sectioned at random angles, leading to a false impression of increased cellularity. It is important to evaluate the papillary fronds for PUNLMP where they are sectioned lengthwise through the core or perpendicular to the long axis. The prognosis for this lesion is excellent. Interestingly, there is no significant difference in survival between PUNLMP and low-grade papillary UC, when patients are treated with surgery [36]. Therefore, the clinical relevance of separating PUNLMP from low-grade papillary UC in the renal pelvis remains uncertain.

Low-grade papillary urothelial carcinoma is a neoplasm that shows mild architectural and cytologic atypia. Grossly, it shows features similar to PUNLMP, but the tumor may become large and fill up the renal pelvis. Microscopically, it is character-

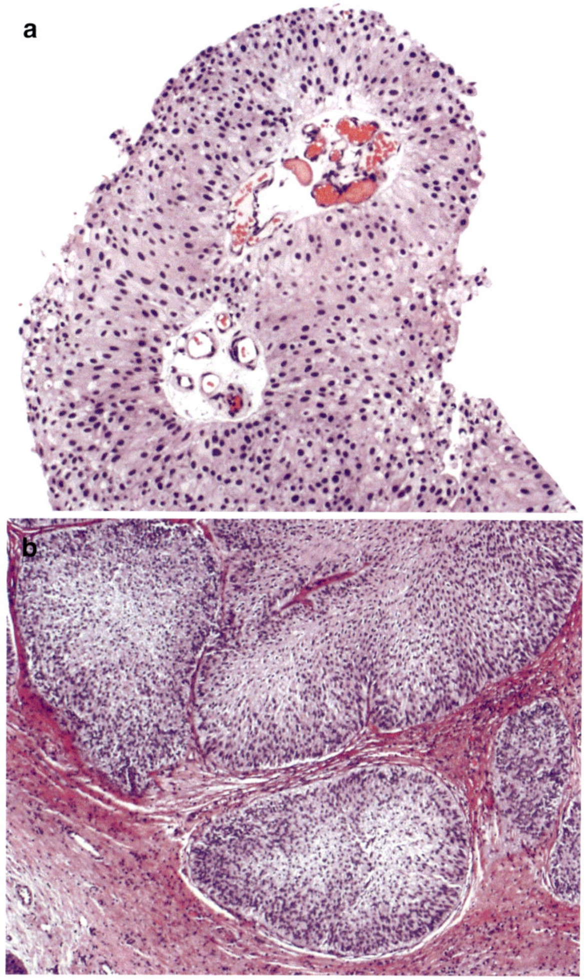

Fig. 13.3 Low-grade papillary urothelial carcinoma. (**a**) The lining urothelium shows easily recognizable cytologic atypia and architectural disorganization. (**b**) Inverted growth pattern is characterized by large tumor nests with smooth, pushing borders in the lamina propria

ized by slender, papillary stalks which show frequent branching but minimal fusion. Unlike PUNLMP, the lining urothelium shows abnormalities in nuclear polarity, size, shape, and chromatin distribution that can be recognized at medium magnification (Fig. 13.3a). Nucleoli may be present, but inconspicuous. Mitoses are infrequent and usually occur near the basal level. In spite of the overall low-grade appearance, some tumors may show focal high-grade areas and these tumor should be classified as high-grade tumors [30].

High-grade papillary urothelial carcinoma demonstrates severe architectural and cytologic atypia. Grossly, it appears from papillary to nodular/solid sessile lesions (Fig. 13.4a). Patients may have single or multiple tumors. Microscopically, the papillae are frequently fused and branching. The urothelial cells exhibit pronounced nuclear pleomorphism with marked variation in size and prominent nucleoli, which are easily recognizable even at low magnification (Fig. 13.4b). Mitoses

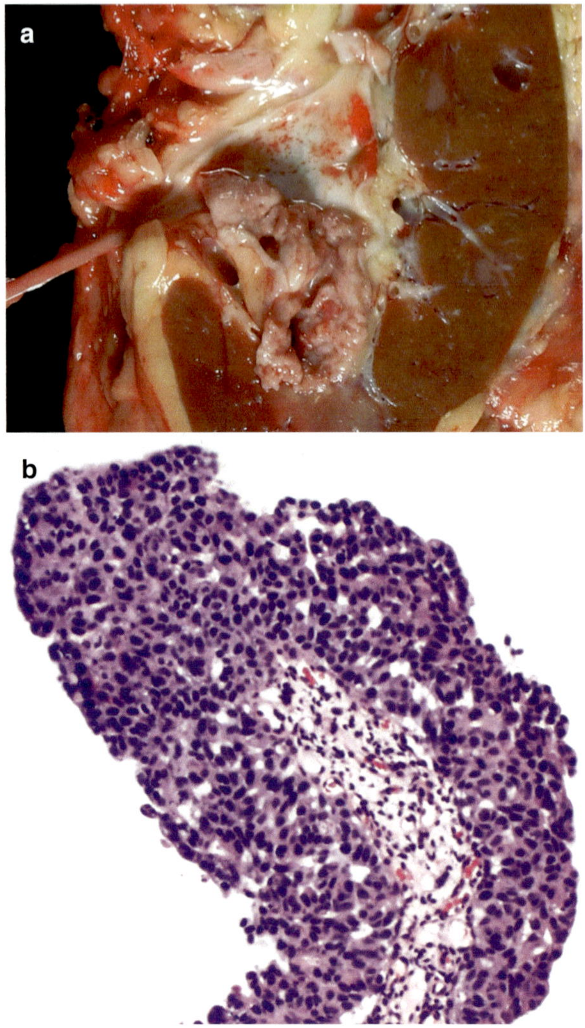

Fig. 13.4 High-grade papillary urothelial carcinoma. (**a**) A tan, papillary tumor occupies the lower portion of the renal pelvis. (**b**) The tumor shows severe cytologic atypia and architectural disorganization

are frequent and may occur at any level, including the surface. The overlying urothelium varies in thickness and often shows cell dyscohesion. High-grade papillary urothelial carcinoma shows significant association with invasive disease and worse prognosis than low-grade papillary urothelial carcinoma. However, histologic grade is not a significant prognostic factor in multivariant analysis, when patients received nephroureterectomy treatment [6, 36].

Papillary UC in the renal pelvis often demonstrates an inverted growth pattern, which is characterized by large, round nests of tumor cells in the stroma with broad base and pushing border (Fig. 13.3b). The nests may become fused but generally maintain the basement membrane. Thus, inverted growth pattern is generally not considered to be a true stromal invasion. The presence of inverted growth pattern in the renal pelvis may be associated with microsatellite instability [38].

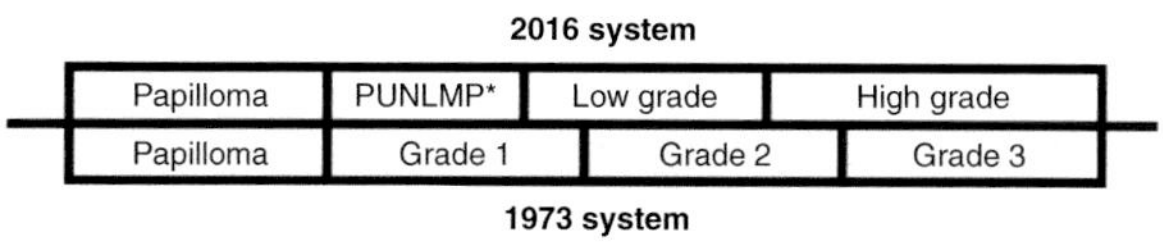

Fig. 13.5 Correlation between 2016 and 1973 World Health Organization grading systems for noninvasive papillary urothelial neoplasms. *PUNLMP papillary urothelial neoplasm of low malignant potential

In addition to the WHO 2016 classification system, another commonly used system is the 1973 WHO system, which divides papillary urothelial neoplasms into benign urothelial papilloma and three numeric grades of carcinoma (Grades 1–3) [39]. Although the 1973 WHO grading system may add some benefit as an independent prognostic factor for pT1 disease, one of the major shortcomings is the lack of precise definition of the various grades and specific histologic criteria for each grade, which has led to a majority of cases falling into an intermediate category (Grade 2). A major misconception in the application of the WHO classification is that there is a one-to-one translation between 1973 and 2016 systems [40]. Only the extreme grades in the 1973 WHO classification have this one-to-one correlation hold true (Fig. 13.5). However, there is no direct correlation of the middle grades between the 1973 and 2016 WHO systems.

Flat Neoplastic Lesions

Urothelial carcinoma in situ (UCIS), also called high-grade intraurothelial neoplasia, is a flat malignant lesion but devoid of papillary structures. Grossly, it often appears as areas of erythema, which may be focal, multifocal, or diffuse. The mucosa may be eroded or raised, with a velvety, granular appearance. Microscopically, it is characterized by malignant urothelial cells with large, pleomorphic, hyperchromatic nuclei, and prominent nucleoli (Fig. 13.6a). There is loss of cell polarity and irregular nuclear crowding. Mitoses may be frequent and sometimes show atypical forms. Sometimes, the presence of scattered malignant cells in the normal urothelium (pagetoid pattern) is sufficient for a diagnosis of UCIS (Fig. 13.6b). Because of the discohesive nature of UCIS, tumor tends to shed neoplastic cells into the urine, resulting in only a few tumor cells attached to the basement membrane (clinging pattern) (Fig. 13.6c). Occasionally, UCIS cells may spread into the lumen of renal tubules with no unequivocal invasion of the renal parenchymal tissue (Fig. 13.6d), and this intratubular spread pattern is not considered as an invasive disease.

Pure form of UCIS is uncommon in the newly diagnosed cases of the renal pelvic UC. UCIS is often present adjacent to high-grade papillary UC and invasive UC. The presence of UCIS has been associated with multifocal disease in the urinary tract and an increased risk for invasive disease [41]. Thus, UCIS should be reported in pathology evaluation, if it is present in the renal pelvis with papil-

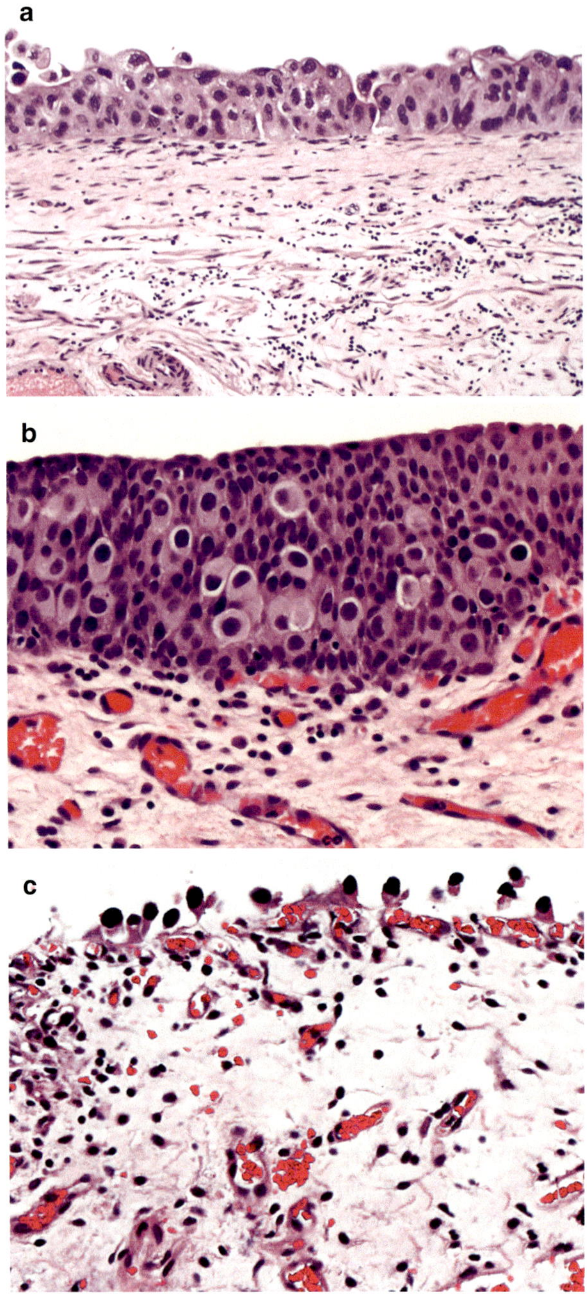

Fig. 13.6 Urothelial carcinoma in situ. (**a**) Malignant cells show enlarged, hyperchromatic nuclei with marked pleomorphism. (**b**) Pagetoid pattern is characterized by malignant cells scattered in the normal urothelium. (**c**) Clinging pattern is characterized by a few malignant cells attached to the basement membrane. (**d**) Intratubular spread is characterized by spread of malignant cells into renal tubules with no invasion into peritubular renal parenchyma

Fig. 13.6 (continued)

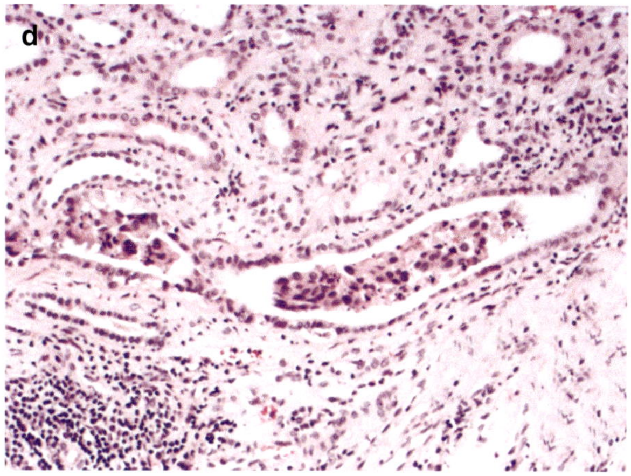

lary UC or invasive UC. However, it is important to distinguish the "shoulder" (lateral extension) of high-grade papillary UC from a focus of true UCIS.

It may be difficult to distinguish UCIS from reactive urothelial atypia. In reactive atypia, the urothelial cells generally show uniform nuclear enlargement, with evenly distributed fine nuclear chromatin, relatively smooth nuclear contours, and pinpoint nucleoli. Inflammatory is often pronounced and involves the urothelium as well as the stroma. A history of bladder infection, indwelling catheter, calculus, or prior therapy is common. However, in some cases, the severity of atypia appears to be out of proportion to the extent of inflammation so that UCIS cannot be confidently excluded (or urothelial atypia of unknown significance). Immunohistochemistry may be useful in the differential diagnosis between UCIS and reactive atypia. The urothelium with reactive atypia typically shows focal immunoreactivity for CK20 and diffuse reactivity for CD44, while UCIS often shows full-thickness immunoreactivity for CK20 and minimal immunoreactivity for CD44. In addition, UCIS often shows more diffuse and stronger nuclear expression of p53 than reactive urothelium. However, the interpretation must always be carried out within the context of the morphologic findings.

Urothelial dysplasia, also called low-grade intraurothelial neoplasia, has appreciable cytological and architectural features that are believed to be preneoplastic but fall short of the diagnostic threshold for UCIS. It is a difficult category to define, due to significant interobserver variability. The presence of nuclear pleomorphism, nuclear size >5–6 lymphocytes, and brisk mitotic activity favor CIS. Urothelial dysplasia generally indicates instability of the urothelium and may be associated with an increased risk for UC, but is difficult to assess its prognostic impact, as urothelial dysplasia is usually found in patients who have a history of urothelial neoplasms [30].

Invasive Urothelial Carcinoma

UC becomes invasive when it grows beyond the basement. Invasive UC accounts for 60% of all UUTUC [42, 43]. Grossly, the tumor may appear papillary, polypoid, fungated, sessile, or solid in the renal pelvis, with or without ulceration. Microscopically, invasive UC is usually featured by irregular small nests or single cells infiltrating beyond the basement membrane (Fig. 13.7). Invasion is often associated with stromal fibrosis and retraction artifacts. Sometimes, invasive UC cells may develop paradoxical differentiation with more abundant eosinophilic cytoplasm in comparison to the noninvasive cells. Pathologic stage is the most important prognostic factor for invasive UC and is based on the depth of tumor invasion and metastasis [6, 36]. Lymphovascular invasion has been associated with diminished clinical outcomes in invasive tumors, but its overall value as an independent factor remains controversial. Accurate pathologic staging can be only performed on a radical nephroureterectomy specimen (Table 13.2).

It is important to differentiate true UC stromal invasion from several mimickers. Noninvasive papillary UC often displays an inverted growth pattern in the renal pelvis, which resembles stromal invasion. Another common mimicker is the intraductal spread of UC cells along the collecting ducts. Although the malignant cells may replace the lining tubular cells in the kidney, they do not infiltrate the peritubular renal stroma. Thus, the intraductal spread of UC cells represents pTis disease. In addition, poor fixation and processing may also result in artificial retraction artifacts, mimicking invasive UC. Sometimes, it may become difficult to distinguish pT1 and pT2 diseases, as the caliber of smooth muscle is often highly variable in the renal pelvis and may be nearly absent in the calyces.

Invasive UC exhibits a high tendency for divergent differentiation. Squamous differentiation is the most common divergent differentiation and may be seen in up to 40% of the renal pelvic UC [44, 45]. Its frequency increases with grade and stage. Another common divergent differentiation is glandular differentiation, which is

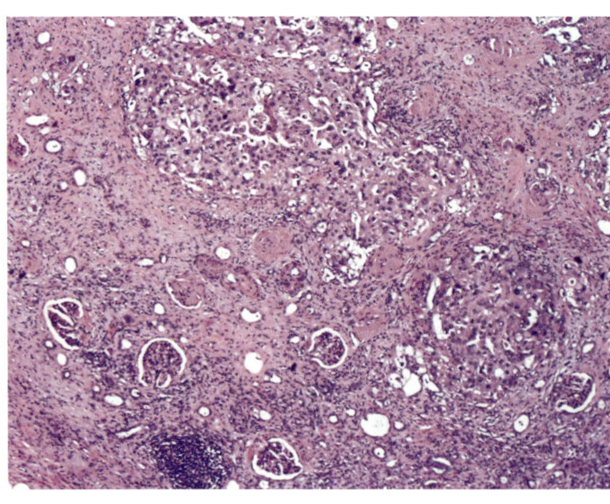

Fig. 13.7 High-grade urothelial carcinoma invades the renal parenchyma

defined as the presence of true glandular spaces within the tumor. Pseudoglandular spaces caused by necrosis or artifact should not be considered glandular differentiation. Cytoplasmic mucin containing cells are present in 14–63% of conventional UC and are not considered to represent glandular differentiation. The diagnosis of squamous cell carcinoma or adenocarcinoma is generally reserved for pure lesions without any associated urothelial component, including UCIS [30]. Tumors with any identifiable urothelial element are classified as UC with squamous or glandular differentiation, and an estimate of the percentage of squamous or glandular component should be provided.

A number of rare, yet distinct, histologic variants have been found in UC of the renal pelvis (Table 13.1) [7, 45]. The micropapillary variant is characterized by small tumor nests or papillae surrounded by retraction spaces (Fig. 13.8a). Micropapillary UC frequently metastasizes to local lymph nodes and distant sites, and the metastases usually contain micropapillary features, even if the variant accounts for only a minute fraction of the primary tumor. The plasmacytoid variant is composed of tumor cells with eccentric nuclei and abundant eosinophilic cytoplasm, resembling plasma cells. The plasmacytoid variant exhibits a strong predisposition for peritoneal spread (Fig. 13.8b). The nested variant is characterized by small nests of tumor cells with bland cytology but demonstrates deep infiltration (Fig. 13.8c). This variant can be difficult to differentiate from florid proliferation of von Brunn nests. Sarcomatoid carcinoma is usually characterized by a marked proliferation of high-grade malignant spindle cells (Fig. 13.8d), sometimes developing heterologous differentiation to chondrosarcoma, osteosarcoma, or rhabdomyosarcoma. UC variants often coexist with conventional UC in the renal pelvis. As some variants show more aggressive clinical behaviors than conventional UC, it is important to recognize these distinct variant morphologies [7, 45, 46].

Several other malignancies may be considered in the differential diagnosis of high-grade UC, particularly when the UC diffusely invades the renal parenchyma. Collecting duct carcinoma (CDC) of the kidney arises from the principal cells of collecting ducts of Bellini and involves the renal medullary, which may mimic high-grade UC. CDC typically shows a predominantly tubular morphology and infiltrates the renal parenchyma with marked desmoplastic stroma reaction. In contrast, invasive UC shows predominantly solid growth pattern, and it is often associated with the presence of UCIS and/or papillary UC. Other high-grade RCC may also show morphologic features overlapping with high-grade UC, but focal areas of typical features of RCC may be found if the tumor is adequately sampled. Immunohistochemistry is helpful in difficult cases. CDC and other RCCs are usually positive for PAX2 and PAX8, while UC is positive for GATA-3, CK903, p63, and uroplakins. Metastatic carcinoma from the lungs, breasts, and other sites may also involve the kidney, mimicking high-grade UC. However, metastatic carcinoma usually shows extensive interstitial growth, bilateral and multifocal diseases, and extensive lymphovascular invasion. Clinical history is helpful. In difficult cases, immunohistochemistry usually leads to the identification of the primary origin of metastasis.

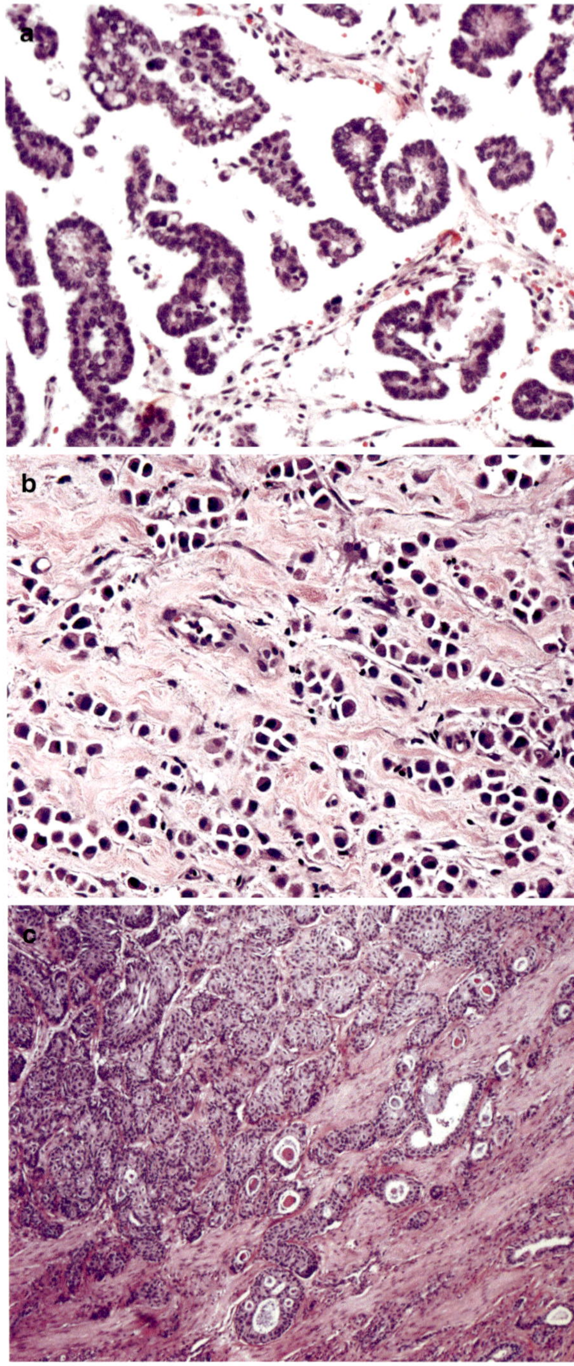

Fig. 13.8 Urothelial carcinoma histologic variants. (**a**) Micropapillary variant shows small nests or papillae in empty spaces. (**b**) Plasmacytoid variant shows discohesive malignant cells with eccentric nuclei and abundant cytoplasm. (**c**) Nested variant shows small nests of tumor cells with bland cytology that infiltrates the stroma. (**d**) Sarcomatoid variant is characterized by high-grade malignant spindle cells

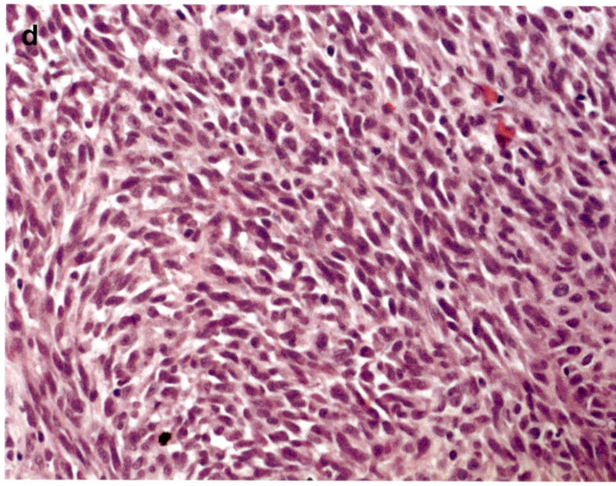

Fig. 13.8 (continued)

Nonurothelial Tumors

Epithelial Malignancies

Squamous cells carcinoma may arise in the renal pelvic tumors [47]. The risk factors for squamous cell carcinoma include chronic infection, nephrolithiasis, and horseshoe kidney. Squamous cell carcinoma is usually characterized by keratin pearls and intercellular bridges. When squamous cell carcinoma becomes poorly differentiated, it may be difficult to distinguish from high-grade UC. Immunohistochemistry may be helpful in the differential diagnosis. CK14 is frequently expressed in squamous cell carcinoma but not in UC, while uroplakins and GATA-3 are frequently expressed in UC but not in squamous cell carcinoma [48]. Squamous cell carcinoma is often present at an advanced stage with extensive infiltration of the renal parenchyma, and as a consequence, it has a poor prognosis. However, when compared stage for stage, the prognosis for pure squamous cell carcinoma is similar to that of UC of the renal pelvis [49].

Adenocarcinomas are even rarer than squamous cell carcinoma [50, 51]. It is also associated with chronic infection and nephrolithiasis. Intestinal metaplasia is a putative precursor as it may be seen in the nonneoplastic mucosa. Like bladder adenocarcinoma, they may show mucinous, intestinal, signet-ring features, but metastatic adenocarcinoma from the colon, lung, pancreas, breast, and gynecologic tract need to be excluded. Multifocal and/or bilateral lesions, extensive lymphovascular invasion, and lack of mucosal involvement should at least raise the possibility of metastasis from another site. Clinicopathologic correlation and history are essential in the differential diagnosis.

Small-cell carcinoma may also affect the renal pelvis [52, 53]. In some cases, renal small-cell carcinoma coexisted with UC of the renal pelvis, suggesting that renal small-cell carcinomas may evolve from a preexisting UC. Renal small-cell carcinoma is a highly aggressive disease that often presents at an advanced stage with widespread metastases. Patients usually have a poor clinical outcome despite multimodal therapy.

Mesenchymal Tumors

Fibroepithelial polyp is the most common mesenchymal tumor of the renal pelvis [54, 55]. It occurs at all ages, especially in the third to fourth decades of life. Signs and symptoms usually associated with ureteral obstruction include flank pain and hematuria, similar to those in the renal pelvic UC. Fibroepithelial polyps have a characteristic appearance as a tan, singular or multiple polyps, or fronds on a common stalk. Microscopically, the polyp consists of a loose fibrovascular stroma with overlying normal urothelium, with a finger-like or polypoid architecture (Fig. 13.9). The stroma is often edematous with inflammatory cells. Care should be taken to differentiate fibroepithelial polyp from urothelial papilloma in the renal pelvis, as the latter is also characterized by a papillary lesion lined by normal urothelium. However, fibroepithelial polyp appears more polypoid rather than the papillary morphology seen in urothelial papilloma. The connective tissue in the stalks of fibroepithelial polyp is often broad and dense, while that in the cores of urothelial papilloma is delicate and loose. Fibroepithelial polyp is a benign tumor and cured by excision.

Other mesenchymal tumors, such as leiomyosarcoma, Ewing's sarcoma, osteosarcoma, rhabdomyosarcoma, and liposarcoma, have also been reported in the renal pelvis, but they are extremely rare [7, 55]. These tumors do not differ histologically from similar lesions at other body sites.

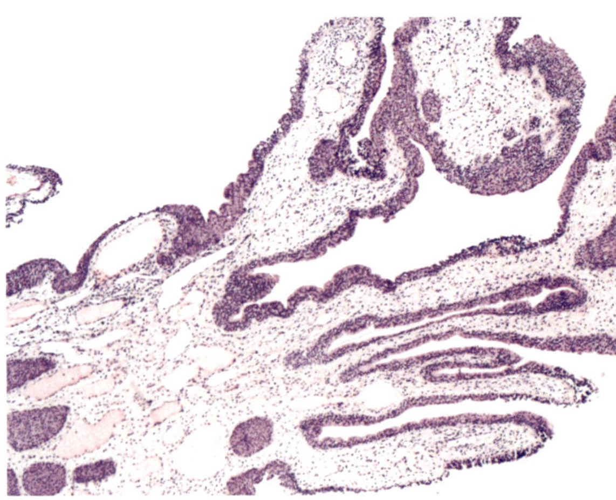

Fig. 13.9 Fibroepithelial polyp shows polypoid and finger-like structures with loose fibrovascular stroma and overlying normal urothelium

Molecular and Genetic Aspects

UC of the renal pelvis often shows deletions on chromosome 9, which are also frequently observed in bladder UC [56]. Some renal pelvic UC demonstrate microsatellite instability and loss of the mismatch repair proteins, particularly in patients with Lynch syndrome [29]. Although UUTUC shows a spectrum of genetic alterations similar to bladder UC, there are significant differences in the prevalence of somatic gene mutations. While *FGFR3*, *HRAS*, and *CDKN2B* genes are altered more commonly in UUTUC, *TP53*, *RB1*, and *ARID1A* genes are less frequently mutated in UUTUC in comparison to bladder UC [57].

A recent comprehensive genomic analysis of the UTUC revealed four different molecular subtypes that exhibit distinct clinical behaviors. Cluster 1 lacked *PIK3CA* mutation, and it was often associated with nonsmokers, high-grade tumors, and frequent recurrences. Cluster 2 was characterized by *FGFR3* mutations and associated with smokers, low-grade tumors, and no recurrence. Cluster 3 displayed FGFR3 and PIK3CA mutations, and it was associated with high-grade tumors at low stage and high recurrence. Cluster 4 exhibited *FGFR3*, *TP53*, and *KMT2D* mutations, and it was associated with high-grade pT2+ disease and shorter survival. However, it remains uncertain if these subtypes have different responses to treatments [58].

Treatment and Prognosis

Radical nephroureterectomy with bladder cuff excision is the gold standard treatment of the renal pelvic UC [2, 59]. Nephron-sparing endoscopic surgery may be considered for patients who would become anephric and require dialysis after nephrouretectomy, including patients with a solitary kidney, renal insufficiency, bilateral UUTUC, and multiple comorbidities [2, 59]. Lymphadenectomy at radical nephroureterectomy may provide survival benefits to locally advanced renal pelvic UC [60]. Efficacy data of BCG treatment for the renal pelvic UC have been mixed, but most of the data show questionable benefit from adjuvant BCG treatment [61]. Adjuvant chemoradiotherapy may be useful for patients with advanced T3/4 or nodal disease [62], but nephroureterectomy often results in postoperative renal insufficiency in most patients, precluding them from adjuvant cisplatin-based chemotherapy.

The prognosis of the renal pelvic UC is closely associated with tumor grade, stage, location, architecture, multifocality, patient age, and treatment modality [6, 13, 63]. Lymphovascular invasion and tumor necrosis (>10% of tumor) may also have a negative impact on patient survival [64]. However, on multivariate analysis, only tumor stage and patient age are independent significant predictors of disease-specific survival [6, 13]. The 5-year disease-specific survival rate varies according to the primary tumor stage: 100% for Ta/cis, 92% for T1, 73% for T2, and 41% for

T3. Patients with primary Stage T4 tumors had a median survival of 6 months [13]. Lymph node status appears to be another strong prognosticator [65]. The 5-year cancer-specific survival rate for patients with nodal involvement was 15% compared to 85% for patients without any nodal involvement.

References

1. Siegel RL, Miller KD, Jemal A. Cancer statistics, 2017. CA Cancer J Clin. 2017;67:7–30.
2. Flanigan RC. Urothelial tumors of the upper urinary tract. In: Wein AJ, Kavoussi LR, Novick AC, et al., editors. Campbell-Walsh urology. 9th ed. Philadelphia: Elsevier; 2007. p. 1638–52.
3. Melamed MR, Reuter VE. Pathology and staging of urothelial tumors of the kidney and ureter. Urol Clin North Am. 1993;20:333–47.
4. Comperat E, Al-ahmadie H. Epithelial tumours of the upper urinary tract. In: Moch H, Humphrey PA, Ulbright TM, et al., editors. World Health Organization Classification of tumours of the urinary system and male genital organs. 4th ed. Lyon: IARC Press; 2016. p. 131.
5. Murphy WM, Grignon DJ, Perlman EJ, editors. AFIP atlas of tumor pathology: tumors of the kidney, bladder, and related urinary structures. 4th ed. Washington D.C.: American Registry of Pathology; 2004. p. 375–82.
6. Olgac S, Mazumdar M, Dalbagni G, et al. Urothelial carcinoma of the renal pelvis: a clinicopathologic study of 130 cases. Am J Surg Pathol. 2004;28:1545–52.
7. Gupta R, Paner GP, Amin MB. Neoplasms of the upper urinary tract: a review with focus on urothelial carcinoma of the pelvicalyceal system and aspects related to its diagnosis and reporting. Adv Anat Pathol. 2008;15:127–39.
8. Favaretto RL, Shariat SF, Chade DC, et al. The effect of tumor location on prognosis in patients treated with radical nephroureterectomy at Memorial Sloan-Kettering Cancer Center. Eur Urol. 2010;58:574–80.
9. Cosentino M, Palou J, Gaya JM, et al. Upper urinary tract urothelial cell carcinoma: location as a predictive factor for concomitant bladder carcinoma. World J Urol. 2013;31:141–5.
10. Rouprêt M, Yates DR, Comperat E, et al. Upper urinary tract urothelial cell carcinomas and other urological malignancies involved in the hereditary nonpolyposis colorectal cancer (lynch syndrome) tumor spectrum. Eur Urol. 2008;54:1226–36.
11. Green DA, Rink M, Xylinas E, et al. Urothelial carcinoma of the bladder and the upper tract: disparate twins. J Urol. 2013;189:1214–21.
12. Raman JD, Messer J, Sielatycki JA, et al. Incidence and survival of patients with carcinoma of the ureter and renal pelvis in the USA, 1973–2005. BJU Int. 2011;107:1059–64.
13. Hall MC, Womack S, Sagalowsky AI, et al. Prognostic factors, recurrence, and survival in transitional cell carcinoma of the upper urinary tract: a 30-year experience in 252 patients. Urology. 1998;52:594–601.
14. Shariat SF, Favaretto RL, Gupta A, et al. Gender differences in radical nephroureterectomy for upper tract urothelial carcinoma. World J Urol. 2011;29:481–6.
15. Soria F, Shariat SF, Lerner SP, et al. Epidemiology, diagnosis, preoperative evaluation and prognostic assessment of upper-tract urothelial carcinoma (UTUC). World J Urol. 2017;35:379–87.
16. Colin P, Koenig P, Ouzzane A, et al. Environmental factors involved in carcinogenesis of urothelial cell carcinomas of the upper urinary tract. BJU Int. 2009;104:1436–40.
17. McLaughlin JK, Silverman DT, Hsing AW, et al. Cigarette smoking and cancers of the renal pelvis and ureter. Cancer Res. 1992;52:254–7.
18. Shinka T, Miyai M, Sawada Y, et al. Factors affecting the occurrence of urothelial tumors in dye workers exposed to aromatic amines. Int J Urol. 1995;2:243–8.

19. Stefanovic V, Radovanovic Z. Balkan endemic nephropathy and associated urothelial cancer. Nat Clin Pract Urol. 2008;5:105–12.
20. Stefanovic V, Toncheva D, Polenakovic M. Balkan nephropathy. Clin Nephrol. 2015;83(7 Suppl 1):64–9.
21. Jankovic Velickovic L, Hattori T, et al. Upper urothelial carcinoma in Balkan endemic nephropathy and non-endemic regions: a comparative study of pathological features. Pathol Res Pract. 2009;205:89–96.
22. Koornstra JJ, Mourits MJ, Sijmons RH, et al. Management of extracolonic tumours in patients with Lynch syndrome. Lancet Oncol. 2009;10:400–8.
23. Vashistha V, Shabsigh A, Zynger DL. Utility and diagnostic accuracy of ureteroscopic biopsy in upper tract urothelial carcinoma. Arch Pathol Lab Med. 2013;137:400–7.
24. Tavora F, Fajardo DA, Lee TK, et al. Small endoscopic biopsies of the ureter and renal pelvis: pathologic pitfalls. Am J Surg Pathol. 2009;33:1540–6.
25. Smith AK, Stephenson AJ, Lane BR, et al. Inadequacy of biopsy for diagnosis of upper tract urothelial carcinoma: implications for conservative management. Urology. 2011;78:82–6.
26. Badalament RA, Kimmel M, Gay H, et al. The sensitivity of flow cytometry compared with conventional cytology in the detection of superficial bladder carcinoma. Cancer. 1987;59:2078–85.
27. Gregoire M, Fradet Y, Meyer F, et al. Diagnostic accuracy of urinary cytology, and deoxyribonucleic acid flow cytometry and cytology on bladder washings during followup for bladder tumors. J Urol. 1997;157:1660–4.
28. Mian C, Mazzoleni G, Vikoler S, et al. Fluorescence in situ hybridisation in the diagnosis of upper urinary tract tumours. Eur Urol. 2010;58:288–92.
29. Liang JF, Zheng HX, Li N, et al. Fluorescent microsatellite analysis of urine sediment in patients with urothelial carcinoma. Urol Int. 2010;85:296–303.
30. Moch H, Humphrey PA, Ulbright TM, et al., editors. World Health Organization Classification of tumours of the urinary system and male genital organs. 4th ed. Lyon: IARC Press; 2016. p. 77–133.
31. McKiernan JM, Hansel DE, Bochner BH, et al. Renal pelvis and ureter. In: Amin MB, Edge SB, Greene FL, et al., editors. AJCC cancer staging manual. 8th ed. Berlin: Springer; 2017. p. 749–55.
32. Kanamori S, Okumura S, Nishimura T, et al. Papilloma of renal pelvis in childhood. Urology. 1990;35:523–5.
33. Dounis A, Mitropoulos D. Recurrence of papilloma of renal pelvis on ureteral stump thirty years after nephrectomy. Urology. 1988;32:50–1.
34. Luo JD, Wang P, Chen J, et al. Upper urinary tract inverted papillomas: report of 10 cases. Oncol Lett. 2012;4:71–4.
35. Spevack L, Herschorn S, Srigley J. Inverted papilloma of the upper urinary tract. J Urol. 1995;153:1202–4.
36. Holmäng S, Johansson SL. Urothelial carcinoma of the upper urinary tract: comparison between the WHO/ISUP 1998 consensus classification and WHO 1999 classification system. Urology. 2005;66:274–8.
37. Maxwell JP, Wang C, Wiebe N, et al. Long-term outcome of primary Papillary Urothelial Neoplasm of Low Malignant Potential (PUNLMP) including PUNLMP with inverted growth. Diagn Pathol. 2015;10:3. https://doi.org/10.1186/s13000-015-0234-z.
38. Hartmann A, Dietmaier W, Hofstädter F, et al. Urothelial carcinoma of the upper urinary tract: inverted growth pattern is predictive of microsatellite instability. Hum Pathol. 2003;34: 222–7.
39. Mostofi FK, Sobin LH, Torloni H. Histological typing of urinary bladder tumours. Geneva: World Health Organization; 1973.
40. May M, Brookman-Amissah S, Roigas J, et al. Prognostic accuracy of individual uropathologists in noninvasive urinary bladder carcinoma: a multicentre study comparing the 1973 and 2004 World Health Organisation classifications. Eur Urol. 2010;57:850–8.

41. Redrow GP, Guo CC, Brausi MA, et al. Upper urinary tract carcinoma in situ: current knowledge, Future Direction. J Urol. 2017;197:287–95.
42. Lughezzani G, Jeldres C, Isbarn H, et al. Temporal stage and grade migration in surgically treated patients with upper tract urothelial carcinoma. BJU Int. 2010;105:799–804.
43. Rouprêt M, Babjuk M, Compérat E, et al. European Association of Urology Guidelines on upper urinary tract urothelial cell carcinoma: 2015 update. Eur Urol. 2015;68:868–79.
44. Martin JE, Jenkins BJ, Zuk RJ, et al. Clinical importance of squamous metaplasia in invasive transitional cell carcinoma of the bladder. J Clin Pathol. 1989;42:250–3.
45. Perez-Montiel D, Wakely PE, Hes O, et al. High-grade urothelial carcinoma of the renal pelvis: clinicopathologic study of 108 cases with emphasis on unusual morphologic variants. Mod Pathol. 2006;19:494–503.
46. Rink M, Robinson BD, Green DA, et al. Impact of histological variants on clinical outcomes of patients with upper urinary tract urothelial carcinoma. J Urol. 2012;188:398–404.
47. Blacher EJ, Johnson DE, Abdul-Karim FW, et al. Squamous cell carcinoma of renal pelvis. Urology. 1985;25:124–6.
48. Gulmann C, Paner GP, Parakh RS, et al. Immunohistochemical profile to distinguish urothelial from squamous differentiation in carcinomas of urothelial tract. Hum Pathol. 2013;44: 164–72.
49. Holmäng S, Lele SM, Johansson SL. Squamous cell carcinoma of the renal pelvis and ureter: incidence, symptoms, treatment and outcome. J Urol. 2007;178:51–6.
50. Lai C, Teng XD. Primary enteric-type mucinous adenocarcinoma of the renal pelvis masquerading as cystic renal cell carcinoma: a case report and review of the literature. Pathol Res Pract. 2016;212:842–8.
51. Ye YL, Bian J, Huang YP, et al. Primary mucinous adenocarcinoma of the renal pelvis with elevated CEA and CA19-9. Urol Int. 2011;87:484–8.
52. Si Q, Dancer J, Stanton ML, et al. Small cell carcinoma of the kidney: a clinicopathologic study of 14 cases. Hum Pathol. 2011;42:1792–8.
53. Miller RJ, Holmäng S, Johansson SL, et al. Small cell carcinoma of the renal pelvis and ureter: clinicopathologic and immunohistochemical features. Arch Pathol Lab Med. 2011;135: 1565–9.
54. Nowak MA, Marzich CS, Scheetz KL, et al. Benign fibroepithelial polyps of the renal pelvis. Arch Pathol Lab Med. 1999;123:850–2.
55. Tamboli P, Ro JY, Amin MB, et al. Benign tumors and tumor-like lesions of the adult kidney. Part II: benign mesenchymal and mixed neoplasms, and tumor-like lesions. Adv Anat Pathol. 2000;7:47–66.
56. Rigola MA, Fuster C, Casadevall C, et al. Comparative genomic hybridization analysis of transitional cell carcinomas of the renal pelvis. Cancer Genet Cytogenet. 2001;127: 59–63.
57. Sfakianos JP, Cha EK, Iyer G, et al. Genomic characterization of upper tract urothelial carcinoma. Eur Urol. 2015;68(6):970–7.
58. Moss TJ, Qi Y, Xi L, et al. Comprehensive genomic characterization of upper tract urothelial carcinoma. Eur Urol. 2017;72:641–9.
59. Raman JD, Scherr DS. Management of patients with upper urinary tract transitional cell carcinoma. Nat Clin Pract Urol. 2007;4:432–43.
60. Roscigno M, Shariat SF, Margulis V, et al. Impact of lymph node dissection on cancer specific survival in patients with upper tract urothelial carcinoma treated with radical nephroureterectomy. J Urol. 2009;181:2482–9.
61. Schnapp DS, Weiss GH, Smith AD. Fever following intracavitary bacillus Calmette-Guerin therapy for upper tract transitional cell carcinoma. J Urol. 1996;156:386–8.
62. Seisen T, Krasnow RE, Bellmunt J, et al. Effectiveness of adjuvant chemotherapy after radical mephroureterectomy for locally advanced and/or positive regional lymph node upper tract urothelial carcinoma. J Clin Oncol. 2017;35:852–60.

63. Mbeutcha A, Rouprêt M, Kamat AM, et al. Prognostic factors and predictive tools for upper tract urothelial carcinoma: a systematic review. World J Urol. 2017;35:337–53.
64. Zigeuner R, Shariat SF, Margulis V, et al. Tumour necrosis is an indicator of aggressive biology in patients with urothelial carcinoma of the upper urinary tract. Eur Urol. 2010;57:575–81.
65. Kondo T, Nakazawa H, Ito F, et al. Primary site and incidence of lymph node metastases in urothelial carcinoma of upper urinary tract. Urology. 2007;69:265–9.
66. Humphrey PA, Moch H, Cubila AL, et al. The 2016 WHO Classification of tumours of the urinary system and male genital organs—part B: prostate and bladder tumours. Eur Urol. 2016;70:106–19.

Chapter 14
Nonneoplastic Changes in Nephrectomy Specimens for Tumors

Ngoentra Tantranont, Boonyarit Cheunsuchon, Lillian W. Gaber, and Luan D. Truong

Nonneoplastic renal changes are frequent in nephrectomy specimens for tumor. These changes display a wide morphologic and diagnostic range. They often carry profound clinical implications, but are often underappreciated or even ignored. This chapter reviews the clinicopathogenetic attributes of these lesions and details their morphologic spectrum.

Clinical Considerations

Chronic kidney disease (CKD) is frequent (about 26%) in patients with renal cell carcinoma (RCC) even before surgery [1]. Since the serum creatinine is not elevated until about 75% of the functional renal mass is lost, the high incidence of preoperative CKD indicates a much higher incidence of nonneoplastic renal changes in these patients. Indeed, these changes are noted in up to 90% of nephrectomy specimens, either partial or radical, for tumors [2–4]. Although these lesions represent a broad

N. Tantranont · B. Cheunsuchon
Department of Pathology, Faculty of Medicine, Siriraj Hospital, Mahidol University, Bangkok, Thailand

L. W. Gaber
Departments of Pathology and Genomic Medicine, The Houston Methodist Hospital, Weill-Cornell Medical College, Houston, TX, USA

L. D. Truong (✉)
Department of Pathology and Genomic Medicine, The Houston Methodist Hospital, Houston, TX, USA

Department of Pathology and Laboratory Medicine, Weill Cornell Medical College of Cornell University, New York, NY, USA

Department of Pathology and Medicine, Baylor College of Medicine, Houston, TX, USA
e-mail: ltruong@houstonmethodist.org

M. K. Divatia et al. (eds.), *Kidney Cancer*, https://doi.org/10.1007/978-3-030-28333-9_14

Table 14.1 Nonneoplastic changes in nephrectomy specimens for neoplasm

Localized changes adjacent to the tumor	
Chronic tubulointerstial injury	
Fibro-muscular proliferation	
"Medical renal diseases" [1]	
Normal	10%
Arterionephrosclerosis	
Vascular changes with normal/near normal parenchyma	29%
Vascular changes with parenchymal scarring	22%
Diabetic nephropathy	23%
Others	8%
Atheroembolism	
Acute tubulointerstitial nephritis	
BCG-related granulomatous interstitial nephritis	
IgA nephropathy	
Collapsing glomerulopathy	
End-stage renal disease	
Thin glomerular basement membrane disease	
Amyloidosis	
Chronic thrombotic microangiopathy	
Sickle cell nephropathy	
Focal segmental glomerulosclerosis	
Glomerulonephritis	
Changes due to urinary obstruction	
Changes related to end-stage renal disease	
End-stage renal disease	
Acquired cystic kidney disease	
Changes related to specific genetic/hereditary renal tumors	
Nephroblastoma associated with WAGR or Denys–Drash syndrome (neoadjuvent chemotherapy-induced changes; nephrogenic rests; diffuse mesangial hyperplasia; focal segmental glomerulosclerosis)	
Von Hippel–Lindau syndrome (mutiple simple/complex cysts lined by clear cells)	
Hereditary papillary renal cell carcinoma syndrome (multiple microscopic papillary adenomas)	
Birt–Hogg–Dubé syndrome (microscopic oncocytic cell nodules, aggregates, or cysts)	
Hereditary leiomyomatosis and renal cell carcinoma syndrome (microscopic oncocytic cysts)	
Tuberous sclerosis complex (eosinophilic tubular microcysts, multiple microscopic angiomyolipomas, polycystic changes)	

Data compiled from Ref. [2–4]

morphologic spectrum, as listed in Table 14.1 and detailed later, it is stressed that the vast majority of them (up to 80%) are arterionephrosclerosis and/or diabetic nephropathy [2–4]. The high incidence of these two diagnoses accounts for most of the clinical significance of the nonneoplastic changes in nephrectomy specimens for tumor, described in details below.

Recognizing these lesions can be very significant [1–8]. In a small but significant percentage of cases (about 8%), specific diseases, often of significant therapeutic/

prognostic implications, are first diagnosed in the nephrectomy specimens, and are later confirmed clinically [2–4]. More importantly, it is now known that these lesions may determine the renal outcome and patient survival, better than the tumor itself, at least for the RCCs of lower stage/grade [3]. Bijol et al. found that at 6 months postoperatively, the renal function was stable if the nonneoplastic renal parenchyma was normal/near normal. In contrast, renal function deteriorated to high-grade CKD if the nonneoplastic renal parenchyma showed arterionephrosclerosis or diabetic nephropathy and the severity of the renal function loss correlated with that of these renal changes [2]. Salvatore et al. confirmed these observations [4]. In both studies, the histologic types of the renal tumors did not carry any impact [2, 4].

The better renal outcome of partial nephrectomy versus total nephrectomy (CKD in 3.7–20% versus 20–65% for partial and total nephrectomy, respectively), regardless of preoperative clinical background including renal function, was first emphasized by Huang et al. in 2006, and was repeatedly confirmed [5–9]. These observations also strongly imply the high incidence of the nonneoplastic renal lesions in nephrectomy specimens and their clinical significance. If the background kidney tissue is normal, unilateral nephrectomy is not associated with any subsequent clinically significant morphologic or functional changes of the remaining kidney tissue [10]. This, however, may not be the case for those with CKD. Patients with RCC often also develop CKD, since many risk factors for RCC, for example, hypertension, smoking, diabetes, obesity, and aging are also risk factors for CKD [2, 3, 11]. Nephrectomy for tumor leading to additional nephronic loss is therefore expected to further erode the renal reserve of these patients whose renal function was already impaired by CKD [7, 8, 11, 12]. These observations at least partially explain why the less nonneoplastic renal tissue removed, that is, partial nephrectomy, the better the renal outcome. Against this background, it is also obvious that an early diagnosis and prompt treatment of the associated nonneoplastic diseases may prevent progressive renal failure.

In spite of their high incidence and profound clinical significance, nonneoplastic lesions in nephrectomy specimens are often missed. The diagnoses were not initially made in 62–88% of cases [3, 4]. A survey reported that 25% of pathologists did not evaluate these lesions [13]. To improve this limitation, the College of American Pathologist checklist for RCC now includes a section on nonneoplastic lesions [14]. This evaluation is also formally recommended in the 2017 American Urologic Association Guideline for localized renal cancer [15]. To facilitate the diagnosis, it is recommended that tissue samples are taken from the parenchyma away from the tumor mass, since the areas adjacent to the tumor almost always show nonspecific chronic changes. Routine histochemical staining including periodic acid-Schiff and Masson's trichome stains should be performed [2, 3]. Awareness of these associated conditions and perhaps renal pathology consultation should lead to a correct diagnosis in most cases. Immunofluorescent (IF) and/or electron microscopic (EM) studies are rarely needed, but can be effectively performed on routinely processed tissue samples, obviating the need for tissue being snap-frozen for IF or fixed in specialized EM fixatives [16].

Pathologic Findings

A large spectrum of changes has been described in summary in Table 14.1 and described in detail below.

Localized Changes Adjacent to the Tumor

These changes include tubular atrophy, interstitial fibrosis, and interstitial mild chronic inflammation, with or without glomerulosclerosis. They are noted in the renal parenchyma adjacent to the tumor, but not elsewhere (Fig. 14.1a). They are observed in most renal tumors and are of no clinical significance [2, 3, 10]. Although the most possible cause is local ischemic/obstructive mass effects, this type of changes is not seen in some tumor types (histologically normal tumor/renal

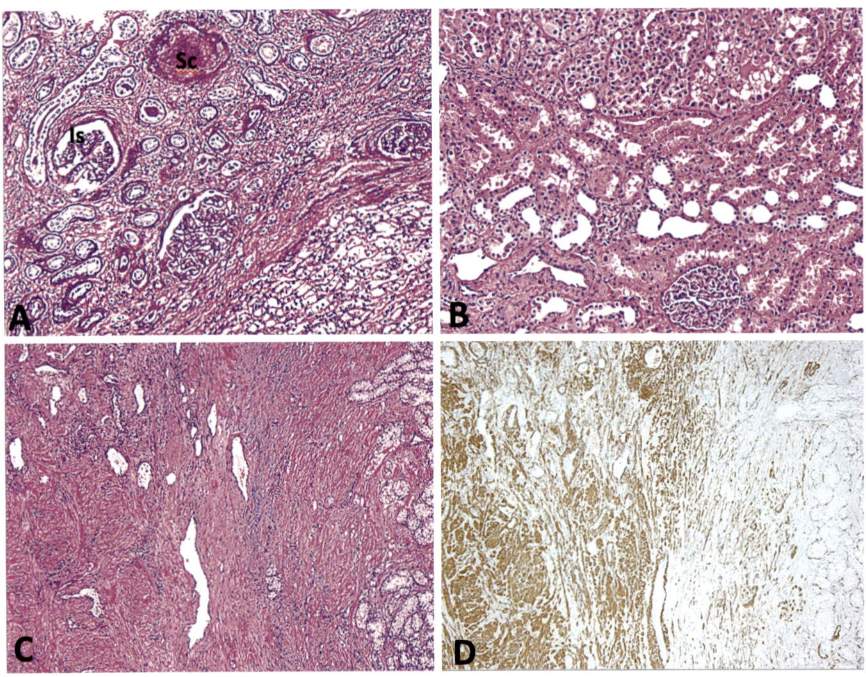

Fig. 14.1 *Tumor–parenchyma interface*. (**a**) The renal tissue adjacent to a clear cell renal cell carcinoma (lower right) shows severe changes including glomeruli with sclerosis (Sc) or ischemia (Is), tubular atrophy, and interstitial fibrosis. The renal tissue away from this area is, however, normal (periodic acid-Schiff, ×200). (**b**) The kidney tissue adjacent to an oncocytoma (upper) is well preserved (hematoxylin & eosin, ×200). (**c**, **d**) The tissue adjacent to a clear cell papillary renal cell carcinoma (right) is composed of large smooth muscle bundles and dilated vessels (**c**), which is confirmed by an immunostain for smooth muscle actin (**d**) (hematoxylin & eosin, ×200 for panel **c**; immunostain, ×200 for panel **d**)

parenchyma interface) (Fig. 14.1b), such as oncocytoma, chromophobe RCC, or angiomyolipoma, suggesting that additional mechanisms, for example, tumor immunity, may play a role [2, 10].

In rare cases, a peculiar peritumoral changes composed of smooth muscle bundles and blood vessels of capillary type termed "angioleiomyoma-like proliferation" is noted (Fig. 14.1c). This change has been most often described in clear cell papillary RCC (previously termed angiomyoadenomatous tumor), a type of RCC that may feature smooth muscle as a component of the tumor. This has no clinical significance and is perhaps related to the localized cytokine effects of the tumor cells [17].

"Medical Renal Diseases"

The nonneoplastic renal tissue may be normal, but frequently displays pathologic changes (15–90%) (Table 14.1) [2, 3, 4]. The different incidences most probable reflect variable diagnostic criteria. If only well-developed, "specific" diseases such as advanced arterionephrosclerosis (AN) or diabetic nephropathy (DN) are included, the lower frequency emerged [3, 4] However, inclusion of the cases with minor arterionephrosclerosis or vascular sclerosis without renal scarring resulted in the higher frequency [2]. Regardless of this diagnostic threshold, the uniform finding is that AN and/or DN accounted for the majority of the reported diseases (>85%), with the rest of cases distributing a long list of diagnoses [2–4]. In fact, the predominance of AN and DN accounts for most of the clinical relevance of the nonneoplastic changes in nephrectomy specimens for tumors [2–4].

Normal

About 10% of specimens display no or minimal changes [2]. These cases tend to be associated with specific tumor types. Thus, about 83% of these cases are associated with oncocytoma or chromophobe RCC, regardless of tumor sizes [2]. The reason for this association is not clear. Interestingly, a lack of peri-tumoral changes is also noted for the same tumor types (see above).

Arterionephrosclerosis (AN)

AN is perhaps the most frequent lesion, together without (29%) or with (22%) renal tissue scarring [2]. AN is characterized by vascular changes including hyalinosis, involving predominantly arterioles (Fig. 14.2a–c) and intimal fibrous thickening

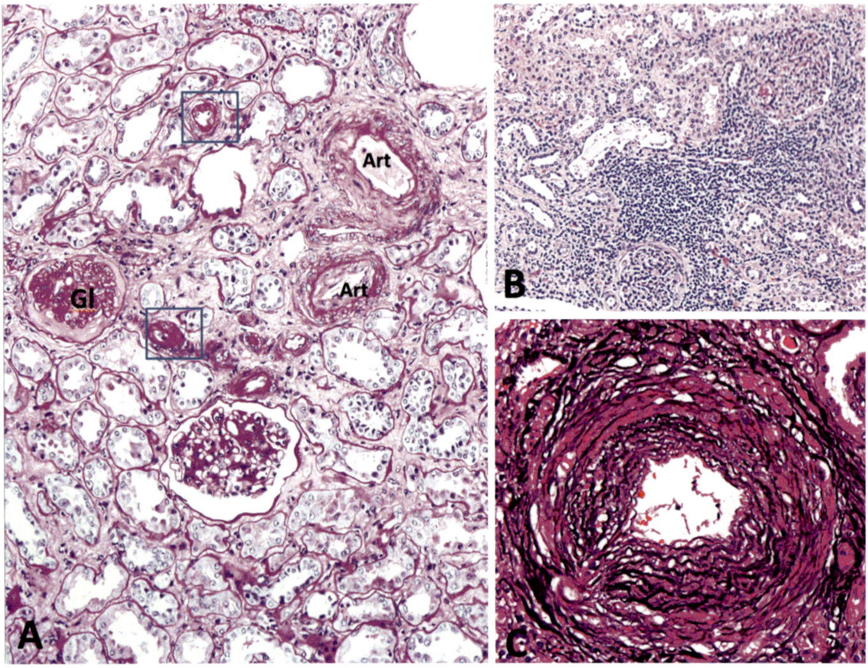

Fig. 14.2 *Arterionephrosclerosis*: (**a**) The changes include glomerular sclerosis with subcapsular fibrosis (Gl); patchy tubular atrophy and interstitial fibrosis, with mild/minimal interstitial mononuclear inflammatory cell infiltrate; intimal fibrous thickening of small arteries (Art); and arteriolar hyalinosis (box) (periodic acid-Schiff, ×100). (**b**) The interstitial inflammatory cell infiltrate may be focally heavy, but still is composed of mononuclear inflammatory cells (hematoxylin & eosin, ×200). (**c**) Arterial intimal thickening characteristically displaying multilayering of the internal elastic lamina (VVG stain, ×400)

with multilayering of internal elastic lamina, and also involving arteries regardless of size. The renal parenchyma may be normal or displays chronic ischemic injury of variable severity. This is characterized by focal global glomerulosclerosis, patchy tubular trophy, interstitial fibrosis, and mild mononuclear inflammatory cell infiltrates. The inflammatory cell infiltrate may be rarely heavy, at least locally, the etiology of which is not clear, but importantly, does not include renal infection (Fig. 14.2b). These changes are most pronounced in the subcapsular areas or in the vicinity of the arterial blood vessels with fibrointimal thickening (Fig. 14.2a). In addition to rendering this specific diagnosis, the severity of the changes, such as percentage of sclerotic glomeruli, level of intimal fibrosis/hyalinosis, and extent of tubular atrophy/interstitial fibrosis, should be evaluated, since it prognostically correlates with the postoperative renal functional changes [4].

AS is pathogenetically linked to chronic ischemia, which is in turn related to the characteristic vascular changes. These vascular lesions may be a manifestation of aging, reflecting the older age of those with renal neoplasms [2–4, 8], or due to hypertension often seen in this group of patients [2–4]. The association of AS and RCC may be more than just coincidental, since CKD, which can be caused by many condition including AS, is a risk factor for RCC [11, 18].

Diabetic Nephropathy (DN)

DN is as frequent as AS [2]. It can develop as an independent lesion or together with AS [2]. This is perhaps the most frequent clinically significant but asymptomatic renal lesion first diagnosed in nephrectomy specimens for tumor [2–4].

The diabetic changes may be mild with mild global or segmental mesangial sclerosis and hypercellularity (Fig. 14.3a), marked with severe mesangial changes including Kimmelsteil's mesangial nodules and thickened glomerular capillaries without endocapillary cell proliferation (Fig. 14.3b). Vascular changes, as noted in AS, and chronic tubulointerstitial changes are also frequent (Fig. 14.3a), which may be due to diabetes itself or the frequently associated hypertension, or both. As in AS, and for the same reason, not only the diagnosis is made, but also the severity of DN should be evaluated [2].

The high incidence of DN in nephrectomy specimens for tumor may be due the fact that DN and RCC share several common risk factors including old age, hypertension, obesity, and smoking [2]. Beyond coincidence, pathogenetic relation is possible. DN is significantly more frequent in tumor nephrectomy specimens than in the general population, even in those with risk factors (24% versus 18%) [2]. Furthermore, DN is more frequently associated with clear cell RCC (30%) than with other histologic types (11%) [2].

Other Kidney Diseases

Kidney diseases other than AS and DN can be encountered (Table 14.1). They are relatively unusual, accounting for about 8% of cases [2–4]. They, however, run the entire gamut of medical renal diseases encountered in the general population and do not show any significant morphologic deviation from their respective sporadic counterparts [2–4].

A specific diagnosis may be quite obvious as in the cases of atheroembolism (Fig. 14.4a) or granulomatous tubulointerstitial nephritis, but is often problematic for the general pathologists who may be relatively unfamiliar with diagnosing medical renal diseases. These cases may benefit from renal pathology consultation, together with special studies including immunofluorescence and electron microscopy. As in the case for "medical" kidney biopsies, aside from light microscopic morphologic clues, which can be quite subtle, clinical information suggesting an underlying medical disease, such as hematuria, heavy proteinuria, pertinent serologic findings, or a family history of medical disease, is very helpful for initiating a comprehensive diagnostic study.

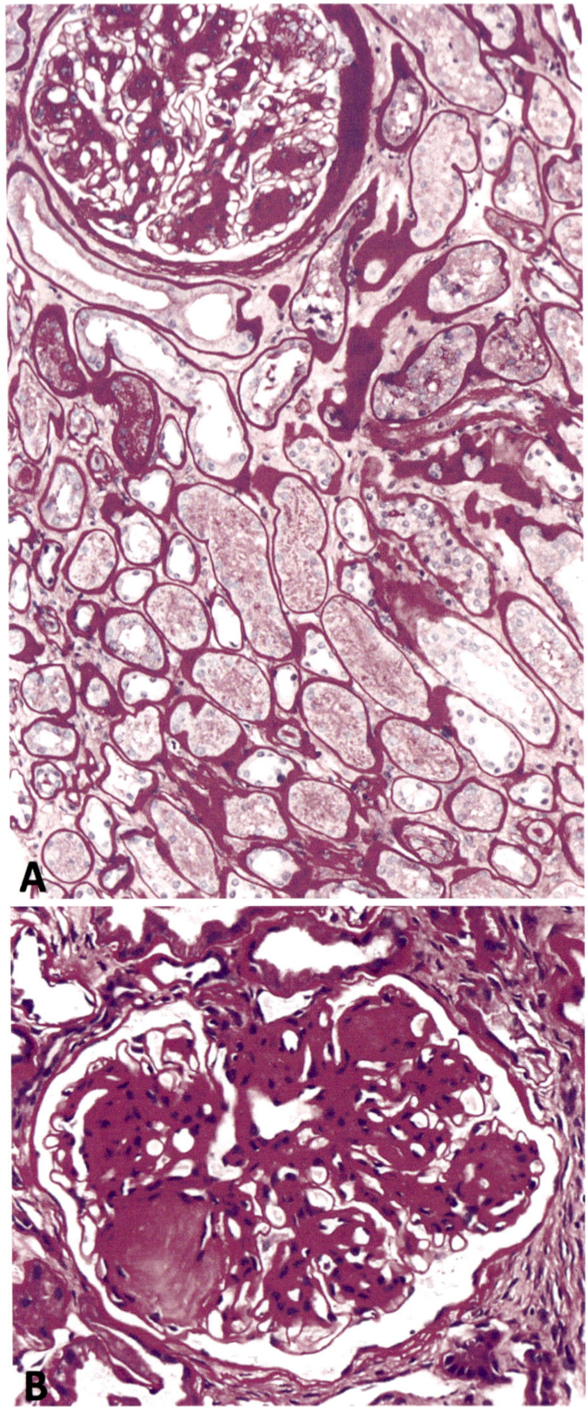

Fig. 14.3 *Diabetic nephropathy*. (**a**) A glomerulus shows moderate mesangial sclerosis and hypercellularity involving all mesangial areas. The tubular basement membrane is thickened, even in tubules without atrophy (periodic acid-Schiff, ×200). (**b**) The mesangial expansion forms poorly cellular nodules (periodic acid-Schiff, ×400)

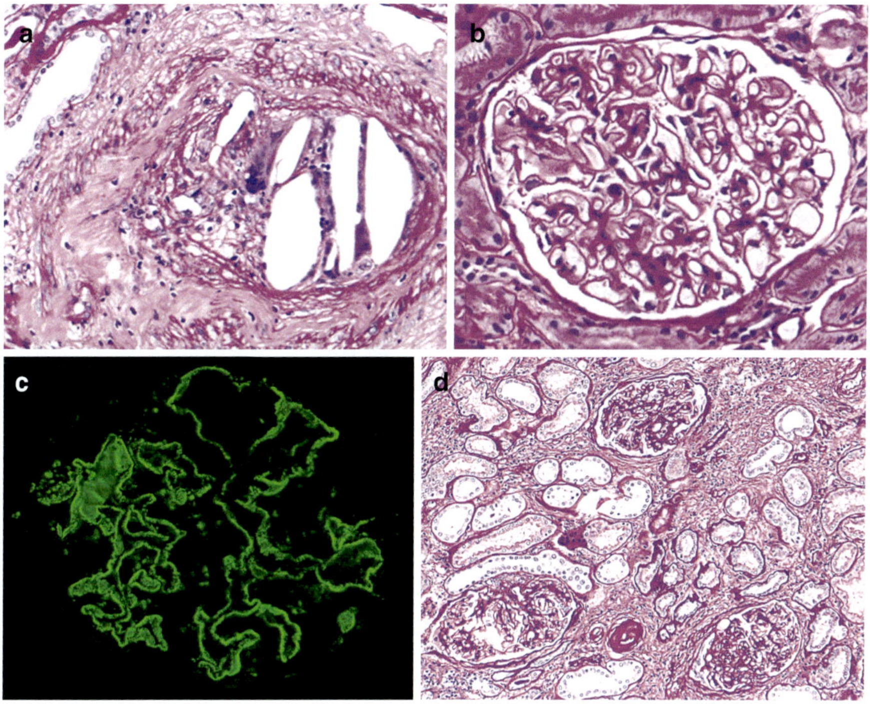

Fig. 14.4 *"Medical" renal diseases*. (**a**) *Atheroembolism* characterized by cholesterol crystals in arterial lumen, associated with inflammatory cell infiltration and intimal fibrous thickening (periodic acid-Schiff, ×400). The patient was a 65-year-old man with a preoperative history of hypertension, peripheral vascular disease, and chronic kidney injury (serum creatinine 2.3 mg/dL). End-stage renal disease developed 5 months after a partial nephrectomy for clear cell renal cell carcinoma (RCC). (**b**, **c**) Membranous glomerulonephritis characterized by thickening of glomerular capillary wall (**b**). The diagnosis was confirmed by granular deposition of immunoglobulin G along the glomerular capillaries revealed by immunofluorescent staining on paraffin tissue (**c**). (Periodic acid-Schiff, ×400 for panel **b**, immunofluorescence ×400 for panel **c**). The patient was a 63-year-old woman with normal renal function and heavy proteinuria (3.3 g/day) preoperatively. The proteinuria was improved after partial nephrectomy for a clear cell RCC. (**d**) Secondary focal segmental glomerulosclerosis, characterized by segmental sclerosis of a glomerulus (lower right), there is also focal chronic tubulointerstitial injury (periodic acid-Schiff, ×200). The patient was a 53-year-old man who had a history of partial nephrectomy for clear cell renal cell carcinoma, followed 2 years later by partial nephrectomy for clear RCC in the contralateral kidney, at which time there was both chronic kidney injury and heavy proteinuria

The pathogenesis of these diseases is as varied as their morphology (Figs. 14.4 and 14.5). Some of them are perhaps mere coincidental, such as IgA nephropathy or thin basement membrane disease. Some others share pathogenesis with the associated renal tumor; thus, sickle cell disease is known as the underlying pathogenetic factor for both sickle-cell nephropathy and renal medullary carcinoma [19]. Still some others share quite convincing pathogenetic link with the associated renal tumors; yet, the molecular connection remains enigmatic, as is the answer to the

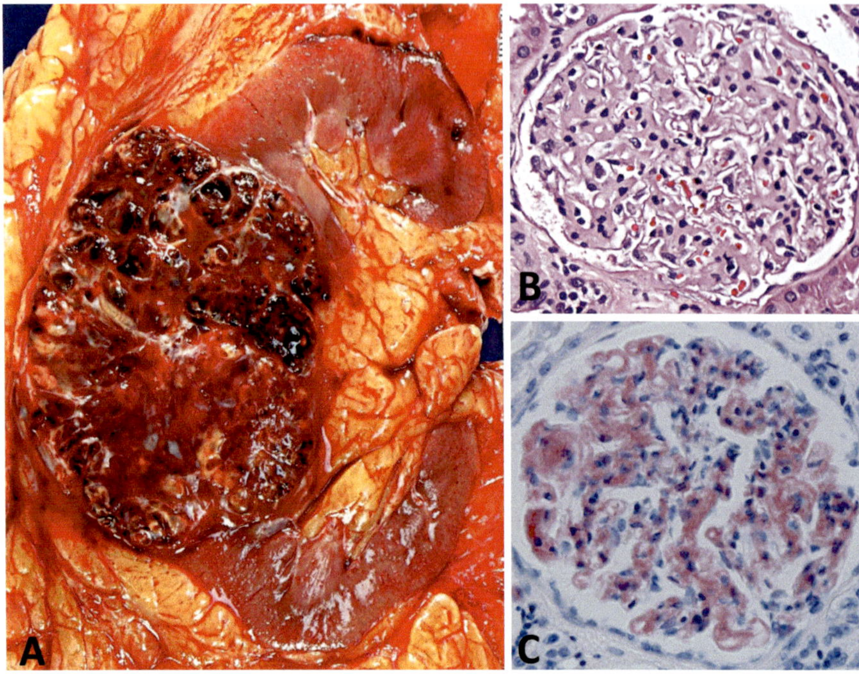

Fig. 14.5 *"Medical" renal diseases. Leukocyte cell-derived chemotaxin 2 amyloidosis*. (**a**) Clear cell renal cell carcinoma surrounded by unremarkable renal tissue. (**b**, **c**) Glomerular amyloid deposition is noted (**b**), and confirmed by a Congo red stain (**c**) (hematoxylin & eosin, ×400 for panel **b**; Congo red, ×400 for panel **c**). The chemical type of amyloidosis was revealed by mass spectrometry study of laser-assisted resected tissue from the paraffin block. This is a 54 Hispanic man with normal renal function and minimal proteinuria preoperatively

obvious question why only a rare patient develops such paraneoplastic renal disease. For example, glomerulonephritis has long been described in association with various cancers, prominent among which is indeed RCC (Fig. 14.4b,c), but the pathogenetic links as well as the rarity of such association remain unexplained [20]. Renal amyloidosis has been reported in association with RCC (Fig. 14.5), and this association recently came to the forefront: Leukocyte cell-derived chemotaxin-2 (LECT2) amyloidosis first recognized in 2008, represents the third most frequent type of systemic amyloidosis in USA, and 6% of these cases are associated with RCC, mostly of clear cell type. What causes this association is yet to be uncovered [21].

The clinical significance of these diseases is perhaps also variable. Most of the time, they are not suspected or diagnosed before surgery for tumors. Their diagnosis thus affords the first opportunity for treatment, since many of them are indeed of clinical and prognostic importance. Even for the diseases known to be traditionally indolent such as thin basement membrane disease or some forms of IgA nephropathy, the loss of functional nephron mass due to nephrectomy may introduce a more aggressive course worthy of active management.

Renal Changes Due to Urine Obstruction

Large renal cell neoplasms, especially those which are centered in renal medulla or urothelial carcinoma, may be associated with changes in nonneoplastic renal parenchyma secondary to urine obstruction. These changes may be diffuse, but are often segmental, reflecting the tumor-induced urine obstruction effect limited to the affected segment of the kidney. Thus, areas of pronounced changes can be seen in adjacent to unremarkable renal tissue (Fig. 14.6).

The renal parenchymal changes include marked chronic tubulointerstitial nephritis, with disproportionately milder glomerular or vascular changes. The tubulointerstitial changes include tubular atrophy, thickened tubular basement membrane, tubular hyaline casts, interstitial fibrosis, and interstitial mononuclear inflammatory cell infiltrates (Fig. 14.6a). Uromodulin (previous called Tamm–Horsfall protein) with a characteristic morphology (glassy pale in H&E, and strongly PAS-positive) (Fig. 14.6c) is often seen either in tubular lumen or interstitium (Fig. 14.6a). The glomeruli, which appear crowded as the result of the tubulointerstitial tissue loss, are either normal, or show compensatory hypertrophy, chronic ischemic and/or "obstructive" changes (small size, mild collapse and wrinkling of glomerular capillaries, and enlarged urinary spaces) (Fig. 14.6a). The blood vessels are either normal in early course, or display marked fibrointimal thickening, reflecting either intrarenal, or systemic hypertension, rather than obstructive effects, and perhaps, accounting for some of the glomerular changes [22, 23]. These changes are rather uniform within the affected renal segment, in contrast to a patchy involvement typical for arterionephrosclerosis. Against this common background, some rare changes may be seen, including superimposing acute bacterial infection (neutrophil infiltration, abscess formation), urine polyp (Fig. 14.6c) [24, 25] (uromodulin forming a microscopic mass in the lumen of intrarenal lymphatic or venous channels), granulomatous pyelitis [26] (granulomatous inflammation limited to the pyelocaliceal wall, without involvement of the renal parenchyma), and papillary necrosis.

Renal Changes Related to End-Stage Renal Disease (ESRD)

Kidneys of patient with ESRD maintained on long-term dialysis display characteristic changes. These changes can also give rise to acquired cystic kidney disease (ACKD), characterized by cystic dilatation of renal tubules. The incidence of ACKD increases in parallel with the duration of dialysis (87% after 9 years). ESRD is a risk factor for RCC and ACKD enhances this risk. Renal neoplasms, including RCC, thus develop in patients with ESRD at a frequency of eight- to tenfold compared to for the general population [27–29]. These renal neoplasms are associated with ESRD changes alone (22%) or with ESRD and ACKD (78%) [30].

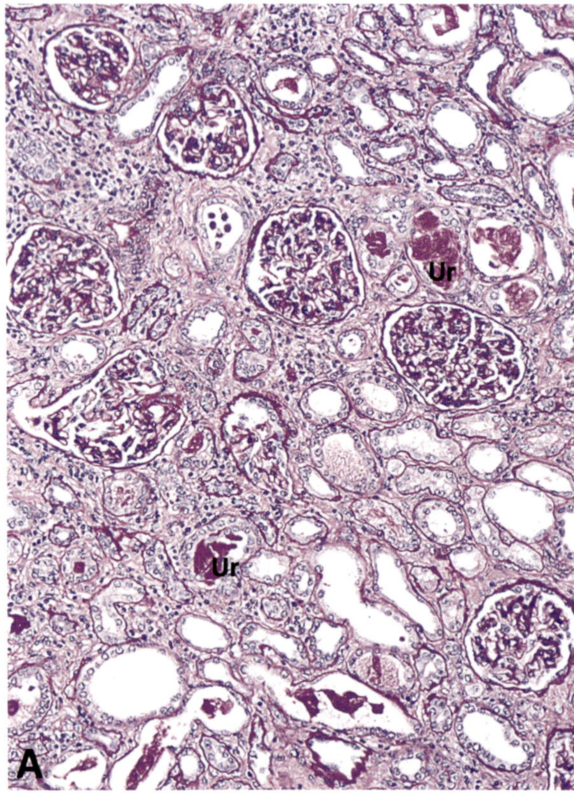

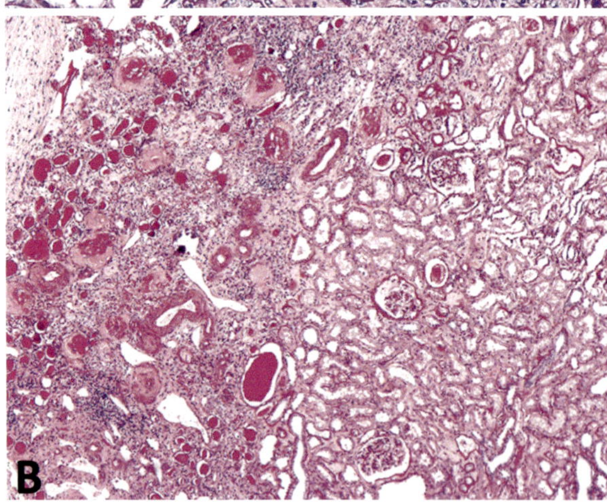

Fig. 14.6 *Urine obstruction*. (**a**) The glomeruli, which appear crowded as the result of the tubulointerstitial tissue loss, are normal or show mild chronic ischemic changes. The tubulointerstitial changes include tubular atrophy, interstitial fibrosis, and mild interstitial mononuclear inflammatory cell infiltrates. Uromodulin is seen in lumens of several tubular profiles (Ur) (periodic acid-Schiff, ×200). (**b**) Kidney with severe obstructive changes adjacent to well-preserved renal tissue, indicating localized tumor-mediated urine obstruction (periodic acid-Schiff, ×100). (**c**) Urine polyp characterized by uromodulin forming nodular collections in dilated arcuate veins (upper), but sparing arteries (lower). Uromodulin appears homogeneous pale gray (Hematoxylin & eosin, ×200). (**d**) Uromodulin is strongly PAS-positive (×200)

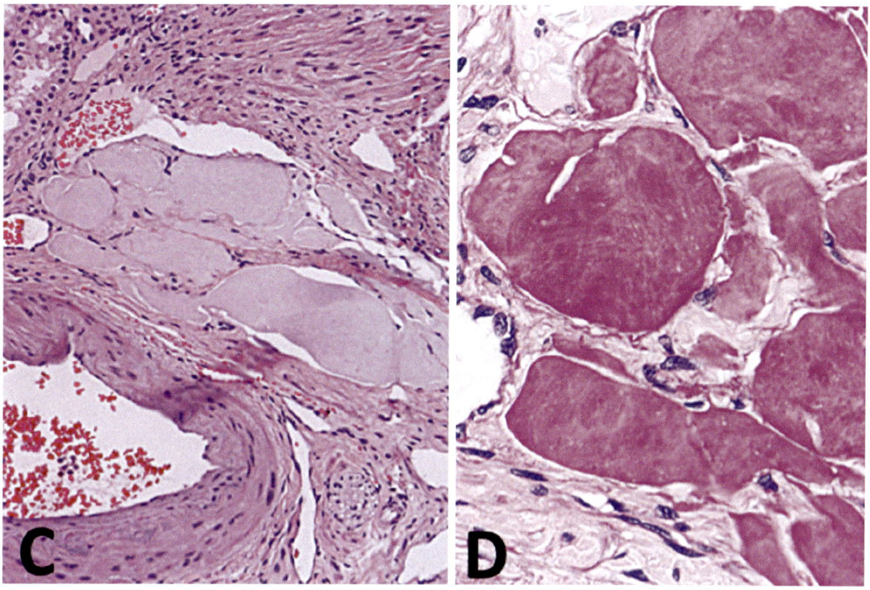

Fig. 14.6 (continued)

Nephrectomy is recommended for tumor measuring more than 3 cm, or those of smaller sizes but associated with persistent hematuria or rapid growth, since, on nephrectomy, many of the latter tumors turn out to be unequivocal RCCs [27–29]. This type of specimen is expected to be more numerous since the number of patients with ESRD on dialysis is increasing, they survive longer, and the incidence of ACKD increases with the duration of dialysis to reach virtually 100% after 10 years, leading to a concomitant increase in the incidence of the associated renal neoplasms [27–29]. It should be noted that nephrectomy is also indicated for ACKD kidneys without RCC, but with complications such as bleeding or infection [31].

Although somewhat irrelevant to the focus of this chapter, the histologic types of the RCCs in ESRD patients are of interest. Two distinct histologic types of RCC, clear cell papillary RCC and acquires cystic-disease-associated RCC, predominate those developed in kidneys with ESRD and ACKD, whereas the histologic spectrum of those in kidneys with only ESRD is similar to that in the general population [30].

The nonneoplastic changes in the nephrectomy specimens may include ESRD changes only or ESRD and ACKD.

End-Stage Renal Disease

Kidneys with ESRD are often are small. They remain small, even in the presence of tumor, perhaps reflecting early detection through serial imaging and timely removal when the tumor is still small. They retain a reniform appearance with finely granular surface. The combined cortical and medullary thickness is marked decreased, with enlargement of the renal sinus, but the pyelocaliceal system is normal.

Most glomeruli are globally sclerotic with or without hyalinosis, and do not reveal the primary disease (Fig. 14.7a). However, in many cases, the nature of the primary glomerular disease can still be recognized in glomeruli with less advanced changes [32, 33]. More frequent examples include chronic ischemic/hypertensive changes, diabetic glomerulosclerosis, or glomerulonephritis. Other rare but distinctive changes, albeit of no diagnostic significance, may present, for example, periglomerular or tubular proliferation of cells with scant cytoplasm, and small hyperchromatic nuclei, imparting an "embryonic" appearance (Fig. 14.7b).

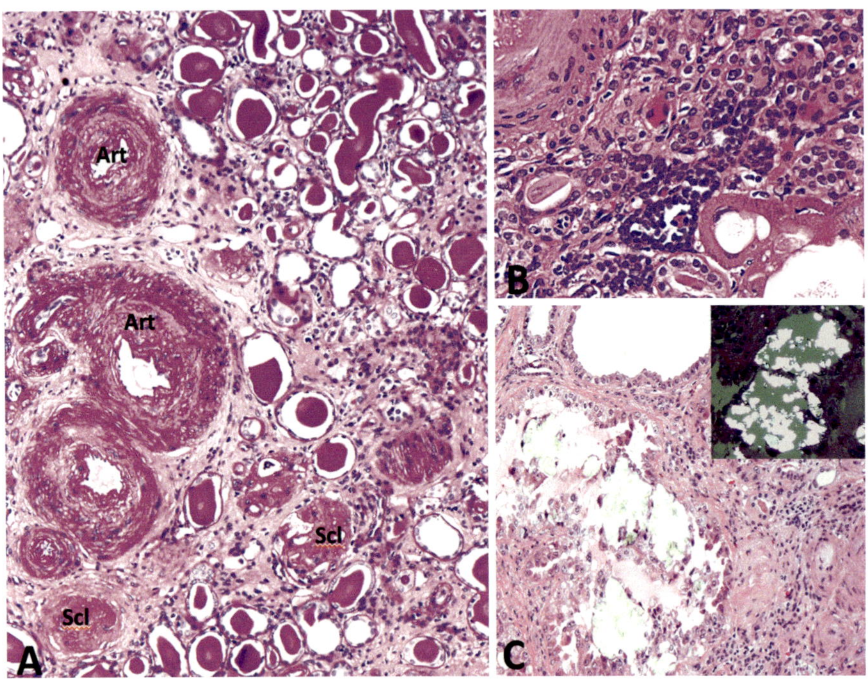

Fig. 14.7 *End-stage renal disease*. (**a**) The arterial blood vessels (Art) show marked concentric fibrous intimal thickening and mild medial hyperplasia. Tubular atrophy, tubular hyaline casts, interstitial fibrosis, and mild interstitial mononuclear inflammatory cell infiltrates are noted. The glomeruli show advanced sclerosis with loss of Bowman capsule (Scl) (periodic acid-Schiff, ×200). (**b**) Focal proliferation of cells with scant cytoplasm and nuclear hyperchromasia ("embryonic" appearance) (hematoxylin & eosin, ×400). (**c**) Colorless but refractile calcium oxalate crystals in dilated tubular lumens, highlighted under polarized light (insert) (Hematoxylin & eosin, ×400)

The tubulointerstitial compartment shows diffuse chronic changes [32, 33]. There is tubular atrophy, dilatation, thickened tubular basement membrane, and hyaline casts (Fig. 14.7a), but acute changes such as necrosis, cellular disruption, or apoptosis, are not obvious. In most case, a few tubular cross-sections without changes or even with compensatory hypertrophy are noted. There is diffuse interstitial fibrosis and inflammation involving both cortex and medulla. The interstitial inflammatory cell infiltrates, which include predominantly lymphocytes and monocytes, with fewer plasma cells, is often mild, but can be marked, but this does not imply infection. However, marked neutrophilic infiltration suggests superinfection. One of the most characteristic tubulointerstitial changes seen in most cases is calcium oxalate crystal deposition, which can be extensive [32, 33]. These crystals can be seen in tubular lumens, tubular cells, or interstitium (Fig. 14.7c). Oxalate, which is normally excreted by the kidney, could not be effectively removed by dialysis in the context of ESRD, leading to high serum level and tissue deposition.

The arterial blood vessels show characteristic changes, such as by marked concentric fibrous or fibromyxoid intimal thickening, intact internal elastic lamina, and mild medial hyperplasia, involving blood vessels of all sizes (Fig. 14.7a). These changes are most probably related to prolonged dialysis, and are thus seen in virtually every case, regardless of the nature of the primary renal diseases or the blood pressure levels.

Acquired Cystic Kidney Disease

Grossly, cystic changes indicate the development of ACKD from the background of ESRD. The kidneys with ACKD are usually *small* (weight range 5–458 g, mean 99 g), with about 87% of them weighing less than normal (about 150 g) (Fig. 14.8). The low weight in spite of the presence of cysts and often tumor reflects the fact that cysts develop not from a normal kidney but from a severely atrophic kidney associated with ESRD. Exceptionally, a kidney with ACKD may reach a large size, looks similar to a fully developed autosomal polycystic kidney, and weighs as much as 1250 g, a value highly unusual for ACKD but average for kidneys with autosomal polycystic kidney disease. *Heavier weights, however, usually imply bleeding complication or neoplastic transformation* [28, 29, 31] (see below).

The kidney with ACK is composed of cysts with a size range from microscopic to about 2 cm, but about 60% of them are smaller than 0.2 cm [34, 35]. Larger cysts, a frequent feature of autosomal polycystic kidney disease, can occur but are distinctly rare. The cut surface may display a few scattered larger cysts involving only cortex (Fig. 14.8a), diffuse small cysts imparting a spongy appearance to the kidney, or variably sized cysts dispersed throughout parenchyma (Fig. 14.8b). The highly variable extent of cystic changes among kidneys with ACKD is expected considering the fact that the severity of cystic change is continuously progressive and is determined by several factors including the duration of dialysis. This variation, however, raises questions concerning the degree of cystic change that establishes

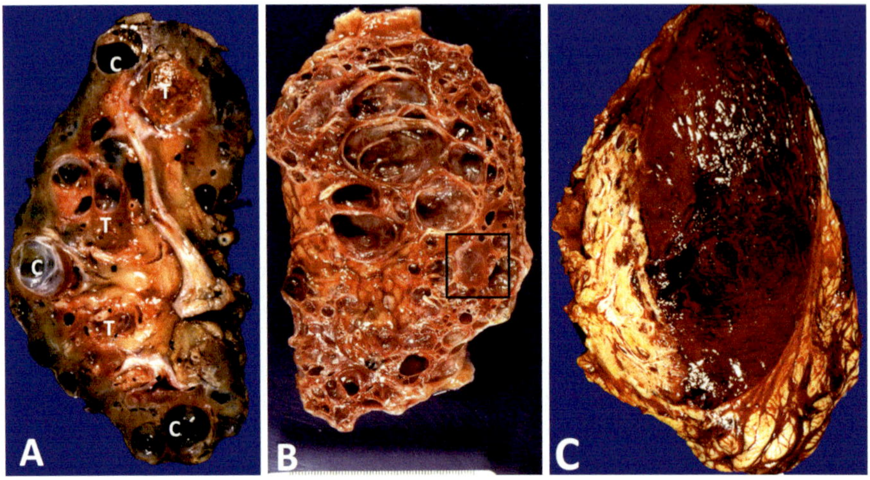

Fig. 14.8 *Nephrectomy specimens for tumors associated with end-stage renal disease and acquired cystic kidney disease*. (**a**) Multiple tumor masses are seen (T), admixed with a few cysts (C), against the background of diffusely atrophic kidney tissue. (**b**) One tumor mass (box) is noted against the background of diffuse cystic change. The kidney, however, remain small (8 cm). (**c**) Massive hematoma compressing kidney with end-stage renal disease (left). A 5 cm renal cell carcinoma was found, but is masked in this profile by hematoma

the diagnostic threshold for ACK. Although the continuous progression of cystic changes in ACK renders any reported threshold somewhat arbitrary, which, indeed, ranges from a few cysts to cystic changes involving 40% of the renal tissue [34–36], the suggestion of Grantham et al. that a minimum of five grossly observable cysts seems to be a reasonable requirement [37]. Such a criterion would exclude cases of multiple, incidental simple cysts, the only other cystic condition that, in theory, can arise from the background of ESRD. The cysts are unilocular and contain clear, straw-colored, or less frequently gelatinous fluid. Bleeding is a frequent finding. Bleeding, seen in about 17% of cases, may appear in the form of intact cysts with bloody or dark putty-like content representing degenerated blood, but can be so massive that the entire nephrectomy specimen looks like a hematoma (Fig. 14.8c). However, bleeding often indicates an underlying tumor [31, 38].

Microscopically, almost all cysts derive from tubules and they are noted against the constant background of ESRD described above (Fig. 14.9a). They are lined by a single layer of epithelium, which is variously composed of flat, nondescript cells, cells with abundant cytoplasm containing hyaline droplets similar to those seen in hypertrophic proximal tubules, or small cuboidal cells resembling distal tubular or collecting duct cells (Fig. 14.9a). *Virtually every kidney with ACKD displays some cysts with atypical features of the cyst lining cells*, which include cellular atypia (enlarged, hyperchomatic nuclei with irregular contour and loss of polarity), multilayering, intracystic papillary formations, or microscopic mural nodules (Fig. 14.9a–c). These atypical cysts may be preneoplastic and are more frequent in cases with renal tumors. Cysts usually show secondary changes including intracystic bleeding,

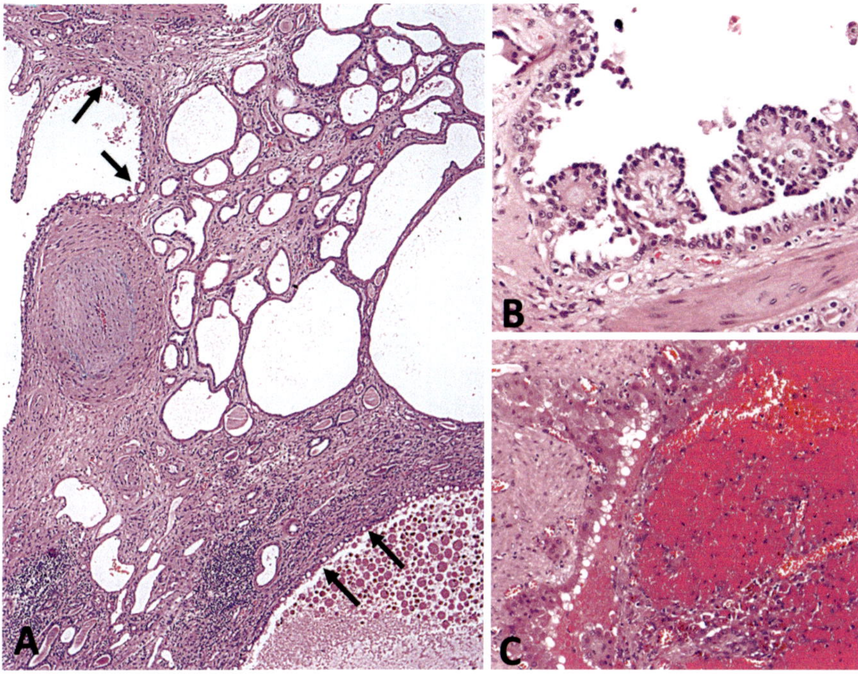

Fig. 14.9 *Acquired cystic kidney*. (**a**) Many tubules are cystically dilated and lined by flattened epithelial cells. Some cysts are lined by enlarged atypical cells (arrows). The cystic changes develop against a background of end-stage renal disease (hematoxylin & eosin, ×100). (**b**) A cyst lined by multilayered atypical epithelial cells forming short papillary structures (hematoxylin & eosin, ×200). (**c**) A cyst lined by atypical eosinophilic cells, together with lumenal hematoma (Hematoxylin & eosin, ×200)

and deposition of necrotic cell debris, hemosiderin, macrophages, or calcium oxalate deposition (Fig. 14.9c). In some cases, as mentioned above, these degenerative changes, especially the bleeding, are extensive and create mass lesion including hematoma. Careful examination is needed since these "masses" may be nonneoplastic, but in about 30% of cases there is neoplasm associated with but masked by the hematomas [31, 38, 39].

Changes Related to Specific Genetic/Hereditary Renal Tumors

Nephrectomy may be performed for renal tumors associated with specific hereditary syndromes [40–47]. The nonneoplastic portion of these nephrectomy specimens may show changes of pathogenetic/clinical interest, but they have not been well characterized chiefly due to the fact that these specimens are rare (Fig. 14.10). The types of lesions described above perhaps can be encountered, but those related to aging perhaps are unusual, reflecting the observations that hereditary renal tumors

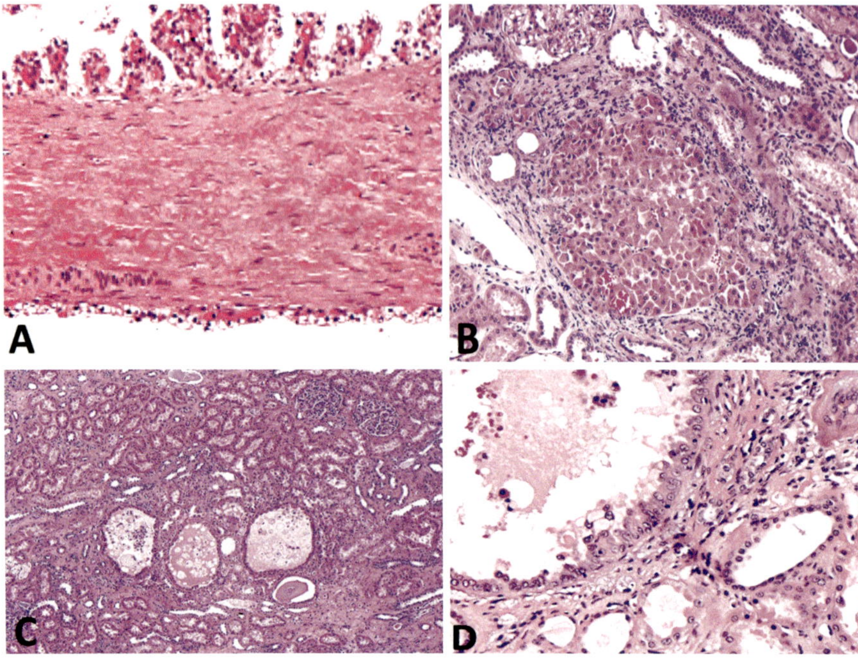

Fig. 14.10 *Nonneoplastic changes in genetic/hereditary renal tumor syndromes.* (**a**) Cysts lined by clear cells forming single linear array (lower), or focally multilayered and papillary (upper) (hematoxylin & eosin, ×200). (**b**) An oncocytic cell nodule in a kidney with Birt–Hogg–Dube syndrome (hematoxylin & eosin, ×200). (**c**) Microscopic cysts lined by oncocytic cells against a background of unremarkable renal parenchyma (hematoxylin & eosin, ×100). (**d**) A cyst lined by atypical oncocytic cells in a kidney with tuberous sclerosis (hematoxylin & eosin, ×200)

tend to develop and are excised at a relatively younger age of patients. On the other hand, several distinctive lesions, some of which is perhaps preneoplastic, have been described. They are listed in Table 14.1 [40–47], and described in more detail in Chap. 11. It is also emphasized that, with few exceptions, these lesions are microscopic and develop against a background of otherwise normal renal parenchyma, thus are often not associated with the usual clinical manifestations of medical renal diseases [40–47].

References

1. Huang WC, Levey AS, Serio AM, et al. Chronic kidney disease after nephrectomy in patients with renal cortical tumors: a retrospective cohort study. Lancet Oncol. 2006;7:735–40.
2. Bijol V, Mendez GP, Hurwitz S, et al. Evaluation of the nonneoplastic pathology in tumor nephrectomy specimens: predicting the risk of progressive renal failure. Am J Surg Pathol. 2006;30:575–84.
3. Henriksen KJ, Meehan SM, Chang A. Non-neoplastic renal diseases are often unrecognized in adult tumor nephrectomy specimens: a review of 246 cases. Am J Surg Pathol. 2007;31:1703–8.

4. Salvatore SP, Cha EK, Rosoff JS, Seshan SV. Nonneoplastic renal cortical scarring at tumor nephrectomy predicts decline in kidney function. Arch Pathol Lab Med. 2013;137:531–40.
5. Ito K, Nakashima J, Hanawa Y, et al. The prediction of renal function 6 years after unilateral nephrectomy using preoperative risk factors. J Urol. 2004;171:120–5.
6. McKiernan J, Simmons R, Katz J, et al. Natural history of chronic renal insufficiency after partial and radical nephrectomy. Urology. 2002;59:816–20.
7. Ohishi A, Suzuki H, Nakamoto H, et al. Status patients who underwent uninephrectomy in adulthood more than 20 years ago. Am J Kidney Dis. 1995;26:889–97.
8. Shirasaki Y, Tsushima T, Nasu Y, et al. Long-term consequence of renal function following nephrectomy for renal cell cancer. Int J Urol. 2004;11:704–8.
9. Leppert JT, Lamberts RW, Thomas IC, Chung BI, Sonn GA, Skinner EC, Wagner TH, Chertow GM, Brooks JD. Incident CKD after radical or partial nephrectomy. J Am Soc Nephrol. 2018;29:207–16.
10. Bonsib SM, Pey Y. The non-neoplastic kidney in tumor nephrectomy specimens. What can it show and what is important. Adv Anat Pathol. 2010;17:235–50.
11. Budin RE, McDonnell PJ. Renal cell neoplasms: their relationship to arteriolonephrosclerosis. Arch Pathol Lab Med. 1984;108:138–41.
12. Epstein M. Aging and the kidney. J Am Soc Nephrol. 1996;7:1106–22.
13. Algaba F, Delahunt B, Berney DM, et al. Handling and reporting of nephrectomy specimens for adult renal tumours: a survey by the European Network of Uropathology. J Clin Pathol. 2012;65:106–13.
14. Srigley JR, Amin MB, Delahunt B, et al. Protocol for the examination of specimens from patients with invasive carcinoma of renal tubular origin. Arch Pathol Lab Med. 2010;134:e25–30.
15. Campbell S, Uzzo RG, Allaf ME, Bass EB, Cadeddu JA, Chang A, Clark PE, Davis BJ, Derweesh IH, Giambarresi L, Gervais DA, Hu SL, Lane BR, Leibovich BC, Pierorazio PM. Renal mass and localized renal cancer: AUA guideline. J Urol. 2017;198:520–9.
16. Nasr SH, Galgano SJ, Markowitz GS, et al. Immunofluorescence on pronase-digested paraffin sections: a valuable salvage technique for renal biopsies. Kidney Int. 2006;70:2148–51.
17. Kuhn E, Anda JD, Manoni S, Netto G, Rosai J. Renal cell carcinoma associated with prominent angioleiomyoma-like proliferation. Report of 5 cases and review of the literature. Am J Surg Pathol. 2006;30:1372–81.
18. Kompotiatis P, Thongprayoon C, Manohar S, Cheungpasitporn W, Gonzalez Suarez ML, Craici IM, Mao MA, Herrmann SM. Association between urologic malignancies and end-stage renal disease: a meta-analysis. Nephrology. 2019;24(1):65–73.
19. Amin MB, Merino MJ. Renal medullary carcinoma. In: Moch H, Humphrey PA, Ulbright TM, Reuter VE, editors. WHO classification of tumours of the urinary system and male genital organs. 4th ed. Lyon: International Agency for Research on Cancer (IARC); 2016. p. 31.
20. Bacchetta J, Juillard L, Cochat P, Droz J-P. Paraneoplastic glomerular diseases and malignancies. Crit Rev Oncol Hematol. 2009;70:39–58.
21. Nasr SH, Dogan A, Larsen CP. Leukocyte cell-derived chemotaxin 2-associated amyloidosis: a recently recognized disease with distinct clinicopathologic characteristics. Clin J Am Soc Nephrol. 2015;10:2084–93.
22. Weis M, Liapiz H, Tomaszewski JE, et al. Pyelonephritis and other infection, reflux nephropathy, hydronephrosis, and nephrolithiasis. In: Jennette JC, Olson JL, Schwartz MM, Silva FG, editors. Heptinstall's pathology of the kidney. 6th ed. Philadelphia: Lippincott, Williams & Wilkins; 2007. p. 992–1065.
23. Pais VM, Strandhoy JW, Assimos DG. Pathophysiology of urinary tract obstruction. In: Walsh PC, Retik AB, Vaughan ED, Wein AJ, Kavoussi LR, Partin AW, Peters CA, editors. Campbell's urology. 4th ed. Philadelphia: Elsevier; 2007. p. 1195–226.
24. Solez K, Heptinstall RH. Intrarenal urinary extravasation with formation of venous polyps containing Tamm-Horsfall protein. J Urol. 1978;119:180–3.
25. Bhagavan BS, Wenk RE, Dutta D. Pathways of urinary backflow in obstructive uropathy. Demonstration by pigmented gelatin injection and Tamm-Horsfall uromucoprotein markers. Hum Pathol. 1979;10:669–83.

26. Gonlusen G, Truong A, Shen SS, et al. Granulomatous pyelitis associated with urinary obstruction: a comprehensive clinicopathologic study. Mod Pathol. 2006;19:1130–8.
27. Truong LD, Choi Y-J, Shen SS, et al. Renal cystic neoplasms and renal neoplasms associated with cystic renal diseases: pathogenetic and molecular links. Adv Anat Pathol. 2003;10:135–59.
28. Matson M, Cohen E. Acquired cystic kidney disease: occurrence, prevalence, and renal cancers. Medicine. 1990;69:217–42.
29. Truong L, Krishnan B, Cao J, et al. Renal neoplasm in acquired cystic kidney disease. Am J Kidney Dis. 1995;26:1–12.
30. Tickoo SK, dePeralta-Venturina MN, Harik LR, et al. Spectrum of epithelial neoplasms in end-stage renal disease: an experience from 66 tumor-bearing kidneys with emphasis on histologic patterns distinct from those in sporadic adult renal neoplasia. Am J Surg Pathol. 2006;30:141–53.
31. Ishikawa I. Hemorrhage versus cancer in acquired cystic disease. Semin Dial. 2000;13:56–64.
32. Sule N, Yakupoglu U, Shen SS, et al. Calcium oxalate deposition in renal cell carcinoma associated with acquired cystic kidney disease: a comprehensive study. Am J Surg Pathol. 2005;29:443–51.
33. Hughson MD. End-stage renal disease. In: Jennette JC, Olsen JL, Schwartz MM, Silva FG, editors. Heptinstall's pathology of the kidney. 6th ed. Philadelphia: Lippincott Williams & Wilkins; 2007. p. 1308–37.
34. Neureiter D, Frank H, Kunzendorf U, et al. Dialysis-associated acquired cystic kidney disease imitating autosomal dominant polycystic kidney disease in a patient receiving long-term peritoneal dialysis. Nephrol Dial Transplant. 2002;17:500–3.
35. Ishikawa I. Uremic acquired renal cystic disease. Nephron. 1991;58:257–67.
36. Levine E. Acquired cystic kidney disease. Radiol Clin North Am. 1996;34:947–52.
37. Granthem J. Acquired cystic kidney disease. Kidney Int. 1991;40:143–52.
38. Moore AE, Kujubu DA. Spontaneous retroperitoneal hemorrhage due to acquired cystic kidney disease. Hemodial Int. 2007;11:S38–40.
39. Schwarz A, Vatandaslar S, Merkel S, et al. Renal cell carcinoma in transplant recipients with acquired cystic kidney disease. Clin J Am Soc Nephrol. 2007;2:750–6.
40. Walther MM, Lubensky IA, Venzon D, Zbar B, Linehan WM. Prevalence of microscopic lesions in grossly normal renal parenchyma from patients with von Hippel-Lindau disease, sporadic renal cell carcinoma and no renal disease: clinical implications. J Urol. 1995;154:2010–4.
41. Verine J, Pluvinage A, Bousquet G, Lehmann-Che J, de Bazelaire C, Soufir N, Mongiat-Artus P. Hereditary renal cancer syndromes: an update of a systematic review. Eur Urol. 2010;58:701–10.
42. Petersson F, Gatalica Z, Grossmann P, Perez Montiel MD, Alvarado Cabrero I, Bulimbasic S, Swatek A, Straka L, Tichy T, Hora M, Kuroda N, Legendre B, Michal M, Hes O. Sporadic hybrid oncocytic/chromophobe tumor of the kidney: a clinicopathologic, histomorphologic, immunohistochemical, ultrastructural, and molecular cytogenetic study of 14 cases. Virchows Arch. 2010;456:355–65.
43. Pavlovich CP, Grubb RL 3rd, Hurley K, Glenn GM, Toro J, Schmidt LS, Torres-Cabala C, Merino MJ, Zbar B, Choyke P, Walther MM, Linehan WM. Evaluation and management of renal tumors in the Birt-Hogg-Dubé syndrome. J Urol. 2005;173:1482–6.
44. Udager AM, Alva A, Chen YB, Siddiqui J, Lagstein A, Tickoo SK, Reuter VE, Chinnaiyian AM, Mehra R. Hereditary leiomyomatosis and renal cell carcinoma (HLRCC): a rapid autopsy report of metastatic renal cell carcinoma. Am J Surg Pathol. 2014;38:567–77.
45. Neumann HP, Schwarzkopf G, Henske EP. Renal angiomyolipomas, cysts, and cancer in tuberous sclerosis complex. Semin Pediatr Neurol. 1998;5:269–75.
46. Yang P, Cornejo KM, Sadow PM, Cheng L, Wang M, Xiao Y, Jiang Z, Oliva E, Jozwiak S, Nussbaum RL, Feldman AS, Paul E, Thiele EA, Yu JJ, Henske EP, Kwiatkowski DJ, Young RH, Wu CL. Renal cell carcinoma in tuberous sclerosis complex. Am J Surg Pathol. 2014;38:895–909.
47. Aydin H, Magi-Galluzzi C, Lane BR, Sercia L, Lopez JI, Rini BI, Zhou M. Renal angiomyolipoma: clinicopathologic study of 194 cases with emphasis on the epithelioid histology and tuberous sclerosis association. Am J Surg Pathol. 2009;33:289–97.

Chapter 15
Application of Immunohistochemistry in Diagnosis of Renal Cell Neoplasms

Fang-Ming Deng and Qihui Jim Zhai

Diagnosis and classification of renal tumors are usually straightforward based on gross and routine hematoxylin and eosin (H&E) microscopic examination of the biopsy and resection specimens. Immunohistochemistry (IHC), however, has been increasingly used in the workup of challenging cases [1–8]. IHC markers are used to verify histological subtypes, distinguish primary renal cell carcinomas (RCC) from other nonrenal cell tumor types that can occur in the kidney, or from the rare metastasis to the kidney. Metastatic RCCs to distant sites often require confirmation of its renal origin by IHC. Finally, needle biopsies with limited material often require IHC stains to establish diagnosis and classification [9, 10].

In this chapter, we will discuss immunophenotypes of major renal tumors and IHC markers that are commonly used in clinical laboratories. In addition, algorithms incorporating morphology and IHC profiles in the differential diagnosis of major RCC histological subtypes will also be discussed.

Immunohistochemical (IHC) Markers Commonly Used in the Diagnosis of Renal Tumors

Markers That Support the Renal Origin

These markers are expressed in the different parts of the nephron structures and majority of renal cell neoplasms, but infrequently in non-renal cell neoplasms. Because of their

F.-M. Deng (✉)
Department of Pathology, New York University Langone Medical Health, New York, NY, USA
e-mail: Fang-Ming.Deng@nyumc.org

Q. J. Zhai
Department of Laboratory Medicine and Pathology, Mayo Clinic, Jacksonville, FL, USA

M. K. Divatia et al. (eds.), *Kidney Cancer*, https://doi.org/10.1007/978-3-030-28333-9_15

relative specificity in renal tumors, they are often used to distinguish renal and nonrenal cell neoplasms and to confirm the renal origin of metastatic RCC at distant sites. These markers include cytokeratins (CKs), vimentin, CD10, RCC marker (RCCMa), human kidney injury molecule-1 (hKIM-1), PAX2, and PAX8. It should be noted that several commonly used IHC markers are almost always negative in RCC. These include TTF-1, CDX2, P63, GATA3, NKX3.1, and PSA. Labeling any of these markers is a strong argument against the diagnosis of RCC. The International Society of Urological Pathology (ISUP) recommended that PAX8 is the most useful IHC marker for establishing the diagnosis of metastatic RCC. One can use IHC for other markers such as ER, CDX2, NKX3.1, PSA, TTF-1, GATA3, and P63 to help exclude other nonrenal origin carcinomas, including those that also label for PAX8. The other IHC markers in common practice are more valuable in RCC classification (see below), can be also supportive of metastatic RCC but usually not indicated or useful [6].

PAX2 and PAX8 are both nuclear transcriptional factors mediating embryonic development of the kidney, Mullerian and other organ systems [11, 12]. Their expression in human tissues is similar except PAX8 is also expressed in thyroid follicular cells while PAX2 is not. They are expressed diffusely in normal kidney with higher level in the distal tubules than the proximal tubules (Fig. 15.1a) and patchy and weakly in the urothelium of the collecting system (Fig. 15.1b). They

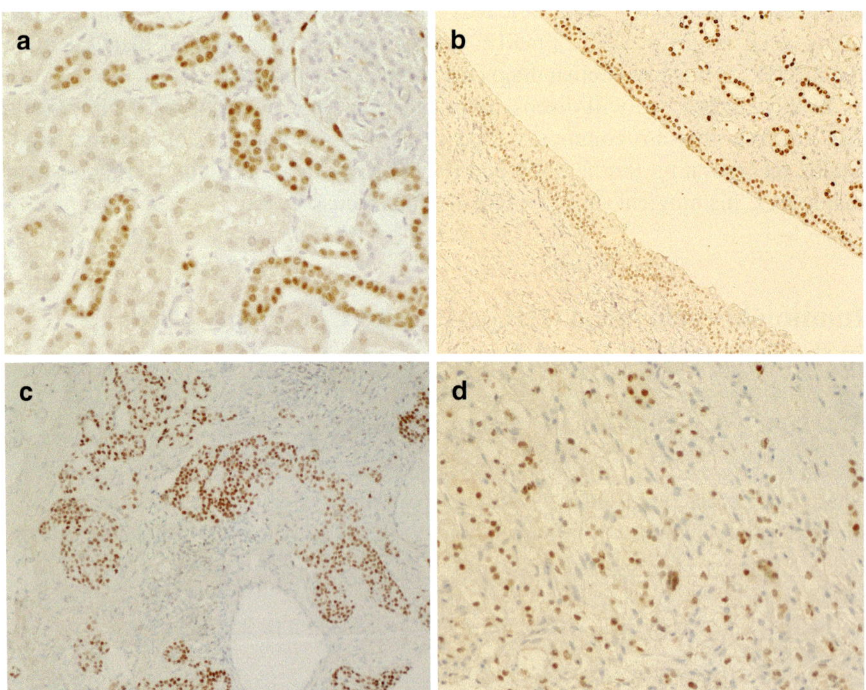

Fig. 15.1 Expression of PAX8 in normal and neoplastic renal tissues. PAX8 is expressed throughout renal tubules, but more intensely in distal tubules and collecting ducts (**a**), and weakly in urothelial lining the renal papillae and minor calyx/renal pelvis (**b**). PAX8 expresses in the majority of renal cell neoplasms, including medullary RCC and metastatic RCCs (**c**, **d**), and therefore PAX8 is considered the most useful marker to confirm a diagnosis of renal cell origin

have a similar expression profile and are found in approximately 90% of all the histological subtypes of renal cell neoplasms, including the high-grade sarcomatoid and metastatic RCCs (Fig. 15.1c, d). PAX2 and PAX8 are therefore considered the most useful markers to confirm a diagnosis of renal cell neoplasms both in the kidney and at distant sites due to their high sensitivity, high percentage of positive tumor cells in positive cases and discrete nuclear staining pattern. These two markers do have some differences. For example, some renal tumors that may be negative or infrequently positive for PAX2, including oncocytoma and chromophobe RCC (chRCC), are often positive for PAX8. Another diagnostic pitfall is occasional expression of PAX2 and PAX8 in other nonrenal neoplasms, including 10–15% of pelvic urothelial carcinoma, parathyroid tumor, and tumors derived from the Mullerian and Wolffian duct systems. PAX8 is also expressed in pancreatic well-differentiated neuroendocrine tumors, thyroid follicular cells, and thyroid neoplasms. However, PAX2 is usually negative in thyroid neoplasms, making itself a better marker to use in the distinction between RCC and thyroid carcinoma. Positive staining is also reported in neuroendocrine tumors and B-cell lymphoma due to antibody cross-reactivity with other members of the PAX gene family.

RCC Marker (RCC Ma)

RCC Ma is a monoclonal antibody raised against a glycoprotein on the brush border of proximal renal tubules. It is considered a "renal" marker as its expression is found in approximately 80% of renal cell neoplasms, present in almost all low-grade clear cell (cc) and papillary (p) RCC [13]. Its expression in other renal tumors is widely variable and the staining is often focal. It is absent in oncocytoma and collecting duct carcinoma (CDC). Its main disadvantage is the poor specificity with expression reported in many other nonrenal tumors, including neoplasms of parathyroid, salivary gland, breast, lung, colon, adrenal gland, testicular germ cell tumors, and mesothelioma. Its use to support the renal origin of a poorly differentiated tumor is now largely supplanted by other more sensitive and specific renal markers (i.e., PAX8 and PAX2).

CD10

CD10 is a cell-surface glycoprotein expressed on the proximal renal tubular epithelial cells and podocytes and many renal tumors with the expression pattern similar to that of RCC Ma. It was therefore considered a useful marker to support the renal origin of a poorly differentiated neoplasm. Almost all ccRCCs and pRCCs are positive for this marker while other types of renal cell neoplasms are negative. Unfortunately, CD10 is even less specific than RCC Ma. Its expression is reported in wide array of nonrenal tumors, including carcinomas of lung, colon, ovary, and urinary bladder, and mesenchymal tumors such as atypical fibroxanthoma, fibrous histiocytoma, endometrial stromal sarcoma, and lymphomas. CD10 has fallen out of favor with the advent of PAX8/PAX2.

Human Kidney Injury Molecule-1 (hKIM-1)

hKIM-1 is a type I transmembrane glycoprotein expressed in injured proximal renal tubules. Its expression is also detected in the majority of ccRCCs and pRCCs [14]. None or rare cases of chRCC and oncocytoma express this marker. It is therefore a relatively sensitive (80%) and specific (90%) marker for ccRCC and pRCC, and metastatic RCCs. However, its expression is also detected in the majority (93.8%) of ovarian clear cell carcinoma, one-third of endometrial clear cell carcinoma, and infrequently in colonic adenocarcinoma, limiting its use to narrow clinical circumstances.

Vimentin

Vimentin is found in majority of proximal origin RCCs, such as ccRCC and pRCC, but it is negative on oncocytoma and chRCC. It by itself is not a specific renal marker as it is a broad mesenchymal marker and its expression is found in wide range of neoplasms. Co-expression of vimentin and CK, however, is limited to RCC and a few other carcinomas including endometrioid carcinoma, thyroid carcinoma, and mesothelioma. Therefore, co-expression of vimentin and CK suggests RCC as one of the possible diagnoses.

Cytokeratins (CKs)

As an epithelial marker, pan-CK expressed in most RCCs while down expressed in high grade, sarcomatoid RCC, succinate dehydrogenase deficient (SDH) RCC and MiTF translocation RCCs. Differential CKs are mainly used to discriminate different types of renal neoplasms. The most widely expressed CK was CK7 that was present in 87% pRCCs, 73% of chRCCs, 83% of CDCs and almost 100% clear cell papillary (ccp) RCCs (Fig. 15.2a–c) and mucinous tubular and spindle cell carcinomas (MTSCCs). Lower expression of CK7 was found in ccRCC (20%) and tubulocystic RCC (33%). CK7 was negative or very focally/scattered positive in oncocytoma (Fig. 15.2d). CK5/6 were expressed in 75% of urothelial carcinoma, 17% CDC/medullary RCC, while negative in most other renal tumor types.

Markers That Are Differentially Expressed in Different RCC Subtypes

Different histological subtypes of RCC are postulated to be derived from, or differentiate toward, different parts of nephron units which have distinct immunoprofiles. Therefore, renal tumors may be classified based on their immunoprofiles that

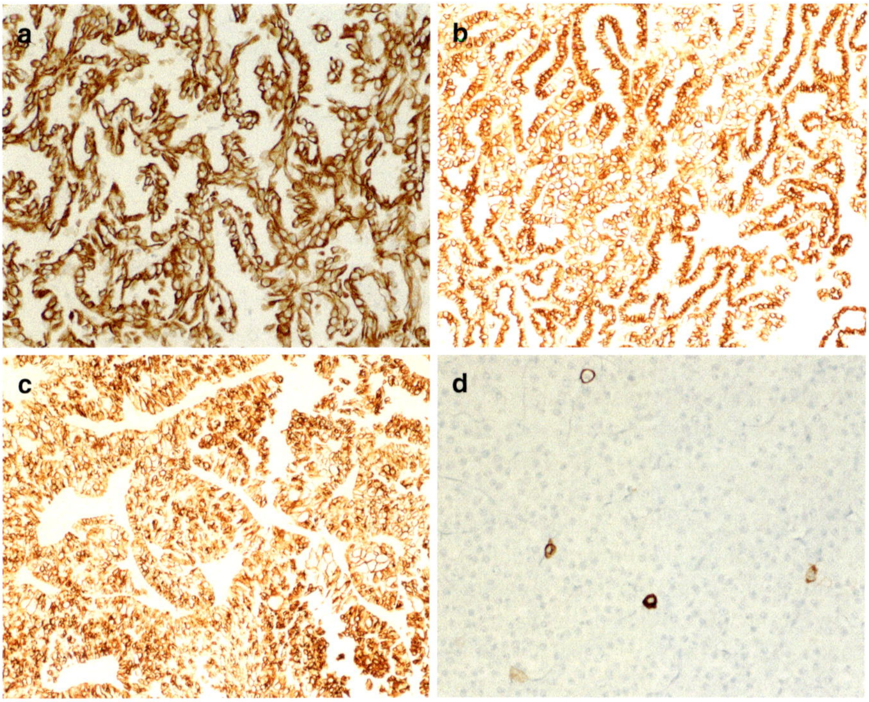

Fig. 15.2 Expression of CK7 in renal cell neoplasms. CK7 expression is diffusely and strongly positive in pRCCs, ccpRCCs, and chromophobe RCCs (**a–c**), while only in rare, scattered tumor cells positive in oncocytoma (**d**)

recapitulate those of the normal nephrons. For example, CD10 and RCC Ma are found on the proximal renal tubules and in ccRCC and pRCC that are derived from the proximal renal tubules. Kidney-specific cadherin (Ksp-cadherin), parvalbumin, claudins, and S100A are found on the distal nephrons and corresponding chRCC and oncocytomas. High molecular weight (HMW) CKs are detected on collecting ducts of Bellini and the namesake CDCs. However, caution is required, because morphology–-immunophenotype concordance is not necessarily perfect. Such discordance occurs as the result of heterogeneity in tumor biology and technicality of IHC. Furthermore, most published studies utilized morphologically straightforward cases but not genetically confirmed difficult cases with ambiguous morphology. One has also to bear in mind that the published immunoprofiles are generally derived from studies of renal tumors of typical morphology. A poorly differentiated often retains at least partially the characteristic immunoprofile of the renal tumors of the same histological class. However, significant deviation from the "typical" immunoprofile of a particular renal tumor type can occur and may impact the utility of these IHC markers in the classification of renal tumors. It should be emphasized that IHC plays a supportive, rather than primary and definitive, role in the histological classification of RCC, and is best applied in the context of differential diagnosis.

Therefore, while a concordant immunoprofile supports classifying the tumor under study into the subtype with that immunoprofile, a lack of concordance does not invalidate that classification.

Carbonic Anhydrase IX (CA9)

CA9 is a transmembrane protein of the carbonic anhydrase family that regulates intracellular pH as well as the transfer of CO_2 across the renal tubules. It is regulated by hypoxia inducible factor (HIF) and considered a marker for tissue hypoxia. CA9 is not expressed in healthy renal tissue as opposed to other carbonic anhydrase family members. It is instead expressed in most cc RCC through HIF-1α accumulation driven by hypoxia or inactivation of the VHL gene [11, 15]. The staining pattern in ccRCC is circumferential membranous, "box shape" and is usually diffusely positive in most or all tumor cells (Fig. 15.3a). Focal staining is seen in up to one-fourth of cases, typically in high-grade cancer. Its expression is also detected in ccpRCC with a unique "cup-like" pattern with staining decorating the basolateral, but not the apical portion of cells lining glandular and cystic spaces (Fig. 15.2b). Its expression may also be detected in other high-grade tumors in the kidney including CDC and pelvic urothelial carcinoma, and can be seen adjacent to tumor necrosis due to ischemia and hypoxia. CA9 is usually not expressed in chRCCs and oncocytomas.

CA9 expression is also seen in many non-renal tumors, including tumors of endometrium, stomach, cervix, breast, lung, liver, neuroendocrine tumors, mesotheliomas, and brain tumors. Therefore, CA9 has limited value in distinguishing renal versus nonrenal carcinomas. It is mainly used to confirm a diagnosis of ccRCC or ccpRCC.

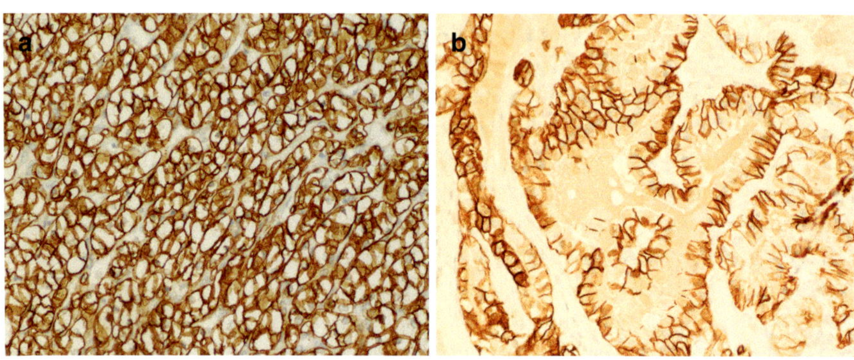

Fig. 15.3 Expression of carbonic anhydrase IX (CA9) in renal cell neoplasms. CA9 expression is diffuse and circumferential membranous (box-shaped) in ccRCC (**a**). In ccpRCC, CA9 stains the basolateral, but not the apical portion of tumor cells (so-called "cup-shaped" pattern or shark teeth pattern) (**b**)

α-Methylacyl Coenzyme A Racemase (AMACR)

AMACR is a mitochondrial enzyme involved in the oxidation of branched chain fatty acids and bile acid [16]. In the kidney, it is expressed in the proximal renal tubules. Majority of pRCC, both type 1 and 2, are positive for AMACR as granular cytoplasmic staining [17] (Fig. 15.4). Its expression is also found in MTSCCA, tubulocystic RCC, MiTF translocation RCC, but not in ccRCC, ccpRCC, oncocytomas, and chRCC. Therefore, a positive AMACR staining provides support for a morphological diagnosis of papillary RCC.

AMACR is found in a wide array of non-renal tumors, most commonly in prostate adenocarcinoma, rendering itself of little use in distinguishing renal from non-renal tumors.

Parvalbumin

Parvalbumin is a calcium-binding protein involved in the intracellular calcium homeostasis. In the kidney, its expression is limited to the distal nephrons from which chRCC and oncocytomas are postulated to be derived. In support of such a histogenic derivation, parvalbumin expression is detected in these two subtypes of renal cell neoplasms, but is absent in other subtypes [18]. Therefore, parvalbumin immunostains may be used to differentiate oncocytoma and chRCC from other renal tumors with similar "oncocytic" cytoplasm.

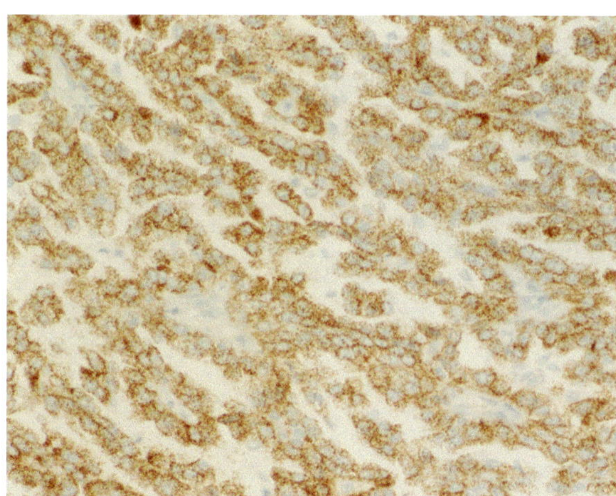

Fig. 15.4 Expression of α-methyl acyl coA racemase (AMACR) in pRCC. Note its granular cytoplasmic staining pattern

E-Cadherin and Kidney-Specific Cadherin (Ksp-Cadherin)

E-cadherin is a calcium-dependent cell–cell adhesion glycoprotein. It is normally expressed in many cell types including renal tubular epithelial cells. Ksp-cadherin is an isoform of E-cadherin whose expression is exclusively found on the basolateral cell membranes of the distal convoluted tubules and collecting ducts [19]. Both E-cadherin and ksp-cadherin are expressed in almost all chRCC and oncocytomas, but variably in other subtypes, including CDC, MiTF translocation RCC, MTSCCA, and urothelial carcinoma. They are usually negative in ccRCC and pRCC. Therefore, E-cadherin and ksp-cadherin may be used to distinguish chRCC and oncocytoma from other renal tumors with "oncocytic cytoplasm."

E-cadherin expression is commonly seen in other nonrenal tumors, often with positive staining in high percentage of tumor cells, including lung, breast, and bladder carcinomas, rendering it unsuitable for differentiating renal from nonrenal tumors.

CD117

CD117, or c-Kit, is a receptor tyrosine kinase that, upon binding to its ligands, phosphorylates and activates signal transduction molecules that propagate signals in cells and plays a critical role in cell survival, proliferation, and differentiation. Most chRCC and oncocytomas are positive for CD117 [20] (Fig. 15.5). However, no mutations were identified in exons 9 and 11 of c-Kit gene the presence of which corresponds to the therapeutic response to Gleevec in gastrointestinal stromal tumors. ccRCC and pRCC are in general negative for CD117. Its expression has also been described in sarcomatoid RCC [21] and a small portion of pelvic urothelial carcinomas.

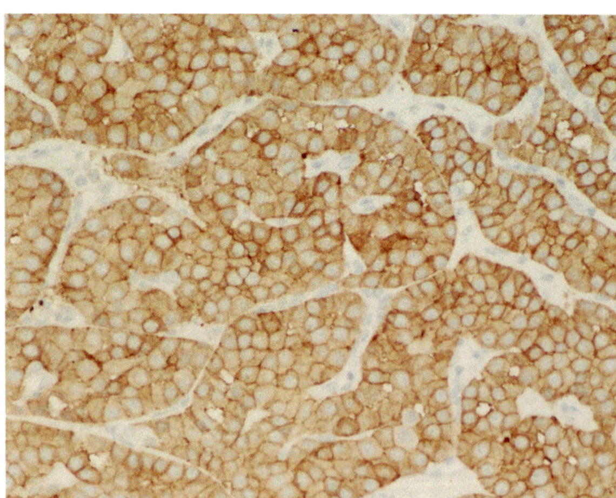

Fig. 15.5 Diffuse expression of CD117 in chRCC and oncocytoma. This represents an example of oncocytoma

S100A1

A member of S100 gene family, S100A1 is a calcium-binding protein and its expression is found in nephrons in the adult kidney. It is expressed in most oncocytomas, but in significantly lower percentage of chRCC cases. Such a differential expression pattern may aid the distinction of these two tumors. Its expression, however, is also found in majority of ccRCC and pRCC.

TFE3, TFEB, and Cathepsin K

TFE3 protein is encoded by TFE3 gene on chromosome Xp11.2, and TFEB protein is encoded by TFEB gene on chromosome 6p21. Both genes are members of "microphthalmia transcription factor/transcription factor E (MiTF/TFE)" gene family. RCCs harboring chromosomal translocations involving respective genes overexpresses TFE3 and TFEB proteins which can be detected by IHC [22–24]. Although molecular genetic analysis for the chromosomal translocation involving TFE3 and TFEB genes provides the most definitive evidence, IHC stains for TFE3 and TFEB proteins are simple, sensitive, specific, and highly correlate with the TFE3 and TFEB gene status in these tumors. TFE3 is undetectable in normal kidney tissues. TFE3 fusion protein, in contrast, is overexpressed in Xp11 translocation RCC and is detected in over 95% of Xp11.2 translocation RCC confirmed molecularly (Fig. 15.6). However, TFE3 immunostaining can rarely be seen in tumors other than Xp11.2 translocation RCC, as its expression is detected in many perivascular epithelioid cell tumors (PECOMA) of soft tissue and gynecological tract, a subset of which indeed harbors TFE3 gene alteration. Rarely, TFE3 immunostain is also

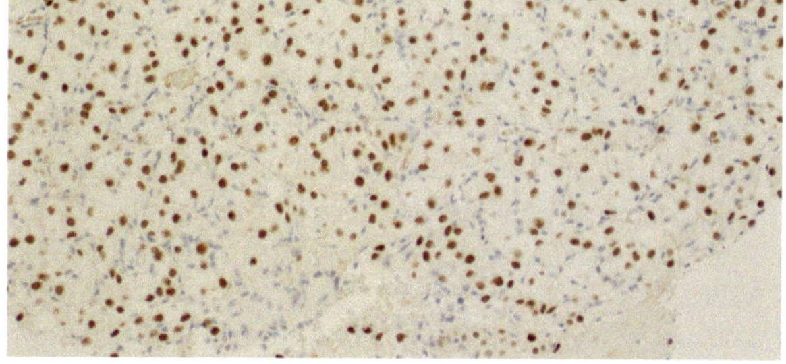

Fig. 15.6 Expression of TFE3 in a Xp11.2 translocation renal cell carcinoma. Note the nuclear stain of TFE3 in tumor cells and internal negative control of stromal cells

detected in other tumors, including adrenal cortical carcinoma, granular cell tumor, bile duct carcinoma, and high-grade myxofibrosarcoma. The IHC stain for TFEB protein is both sensitive and specific for RCC associated with TFEB translocation, and is not detectable in other neoplasms. Weak nuclear staining for TFEB is rarely detected in scattered normal lymphocytes. The most significant issue with the IHC detection of TFE3 and TFEB proteins is that the staining is susceptible to tissue fixation. Inconsistent staining results are often encountered, especially when the staining is performed on an automatic stainer. Some staining protocols call for manual staining.

Cathepsin K is transcriptionally regulated by members of the MiTF/TFE gene family. Its overexpression is seen in all TFEB RCC and 60% of TFE3 RCC, but none of the other RCC subtypes [25, 26]. Its expression in nonrenal carcinomas is rare (2.7%), although very common in mesenchymal tumors (>50%). These findings suggest that cathepsin K may be used as a surrogate marker for TFE3 and TFEB overexpression and is a highly specific marker for translocation RCC.

Markers for Urothelial Lineage Differentiation

Markers for urothelial lineage differentiation, including p63, thrombomodulin, uroplakin and GATA3, are expressed in high percentage of urothelial carcinoma but not in RCC, and therefore, can be used in the diagnosis of a poorly differentiated carcinoma where the differential diagnosis is between a urothelial carcinoma and RCC [27]. One caveat is that some of these “urothelial” markers including uroplakin, GATA3, and p63 have found to be expressed in a small fraction of RCC, particularly CDC, but usually weak and focal.

Differential Cytokeratins (CKs)

Different types of CK are expressed in different renal tumors and can be taken advantage of for the purpose of differential diagnosis (also see above). For example, CK18, a low molecular weight cytokeratin expressed in simple epithelia, is detected while CK20 is virtually absent in all major renal tumors except the newly described eosinophilic solid cystic RCC [28, 29] CK7, a low molecular weight cytokeratin, is expressed in pRCC (predominantly type 1), ccpRCC, chRCC, CDC, and urothelial carcinoma. It is usually negative in oncocytoma and ccRCC. High molecular weight cytokeratins (HMWCKs), detected by antibody clone 34βE12 and CK5/6, in contrast, are expressed in the majority of CDC and almost all urothelial carcinoma and significant proportion of ccpRCC, but uncommonly in other RCC subtypes.

Clinically several CK monoclonal antibody clones are used, including AE1/3, CAM5.2, 34βE12, and CK5/6. AE1/3 is considered a pan-CK as it detects both LMW (CK7, 8, and 19) and HMW (CK10, 14–16) CKs, but it lacks reactivity to CK18, a CK almost ubiquitously present in simple epithelia, including renal tumors.

Notably, AE1/3 is positive in only one-third ccRCC and one-fourth of translocation RCC. If one wishes to confirm the carcinomatous nature of a poorly differentiated tumor in the kidney, a panel of markers, including AE1/3, CAM5.2, and CK18, is recommended to be used.

Immunophenotype of Common Renal Tumors

Clear Cell Renal Cell Carcinomas (ccRCCs)

ccRCCs are commonly reactive for kidney-specific transcriptional factors including PAX2 and PAX8 (Fig. 15.1). Most also react with brush border antigens such as RCC Ma and CD10, low molecular weight cytokeratins (LMWCKs), epithelial membrane antigen (EMA), and vimentin. HMWCKs are rarely expressed. CA9, a downstream target gene of hypoxia inducible pathway, is expressed in the majority of cases (Fig. 15.3). CK7, CK20, CD117, epithelial cadherin, parvalbumin, and CD117 are usually negative. Some ccRCCs demonstrate a focal "pseudopapillary" growth pattern secondary to tumor cell dropout sparing the cells at the periphery of blood vessels. Unlike pRCC, histiocytes, and intracellular hemosiderin are usually absent from the papillae. Classic ccRCC foci are usually evident elsewhere, but if necessary, CK7, and CA9 may be useful as CK7 often is expressed in pRCC, but not by ccRCC and CA9 has a reverse expression pattern.

Multilocular Cystic Renal Cell Neoplasm of Low Malignant Potential

It has almost identical immunoprofiles with classic low-grade ccRCC. The clusters of epithelial cells within the septa react with antibodies to CKs, EMA, CK7, and CA9, but not histiocytic markers.

Clear Cell (Tubulo) Papillary Renal Cell Carcinomas (ccpRCCs)

ccpRCCs have a characteristic immunophenotype. Tumor cells are diffusely positive for CK7 (Fig. 15.2b), and positive for CA9 with a "cup-shaped" staining pattern (Fig. 15.3b), but negative for CD10, AMACR, and TFE-3. Due to the presence of papillary structures lined with clear cells, ccRCCs, and pRCCs often enter into the differential diagnosis for ccpRCC. However, ccRCC does not contain extensive papillary structures, and are positive for CD10 but negative for CK7. pRCC, on the other hand, does not harbor a prominent clear cell component, and is positive for

CD10 and AMACR. RCC associated with Xp11.2/TFE3 translocation typically affects children and young adults. Papillae lined with tumor cells with abundant clear and granular cytoplasm are characteristic. However, tumor cells have high-grade nuclei and are positive for TFE-3 and negative for CKs.

Papillary Renal Cell Carcinomas (pRCCs)

pRCCs are usually strongly reactive with antibodies to panCKs and LMWCKs, but only rarely with antibodies to HMWCKs. CK7 expression is more frequent in type 1 (87%) than in type 2 (20%) (Fig. 15.2a). Reactivity for vimentin and EMA is variable and inconsistent. CD10, AMACR, RCC Ma, PAX2, and PAX8 are expressed in pRCC. Several other renal tumors should be differentiated from pRCC. Lesions 1.5 cm or less than 1.5 cm with low grade (Fuhrman grade 1 or 2) and lacking of distinct capsule have been designated papillary adenomas while those larger than 1.5 cm are classified as pRCCs. ccpRCCS are small tumors arising frequently in end-stage kidney disease with cystic and fibrotic background. ccpRCC characteristically has low-grade tumor cells and clear cytoplasm. Nuclei are characteristically linearly polarized away from the basement membrane toward the luminal surface (reverse polarization of nuclei). Tumor cells are diffusely positive for CK7, positive for CA9 with "cup-like" staining pattern, and negative for CD10. pRCC can be confused with ccRCC exhibiting a pseudopapillary growth pattern. Such pseudopapillae are typically devoid of the fibrovascular cores of pRCCs. ccRCC is also much less likely to show calcification, cytoplasmic hemosiderin and islands of foamy macrophages expanding papillae. Tumor cells of ccRCC express CA9, but lack CK7 and AMACR expression which is frequently seen in the pRCCs. CDC with papillary features can be distinguished from pRCC by its medullary location in the kidney, desmoplastic stromal reaction, its high-grade features, and intracytoplasmic, and luminal mucin. In contrast to CDC, pRCC rarely demonstrates a desmoplastic stroma. Immunohistochemically, unlike most pRCCs, CDC reacts with CEA, and HMWCKs. Metanephric adenoma is well circumscribed, but does not have a tumor capsule. Tumor cells have scant cytoplasm and uniform and round nuclei, and are negative for cytokeratin but positive for WT-1. WT-1 is frequently detectable in the nuclei of metanephric adenomas. The cells of metanephric adenoma are positive for PAX2, PAX8, and CD57, frequently negative for EMA, CK7, cytokeratin CK AE1/AE3, CD56, and AMACR. CD57 and WT1 are positive, and BRAF V600E is positive in 90% metanephic adenoma [30, 31].

Therefore, before to render the diagnosis of metanephric adenoma, pan-CK, and CK7 should be performed and if CK is positive, this tumor is most likely not metanephric adenoma.

Chromophobe Renal Cell Carcinoma (chRCC)

Antibody to cytokeratin 7 is useful in diagnosing chRCC. It typically reacts strongly with the great majority of cells and the reaction is accentuated at the cell membrane (Fig. 15.2c). E-cadherin, kidney-specific cadherin, parvalbumin, and CD117 are also diffusely positive in chRCCs (Fig. 15.5). Vimentin, CA9, and AMACR are negative. Classic chRCC including distinct plant-like cell membrane, raisinoid nuclei, and perinuclear clearing often can be diagnosed with confidence on hematoxylin and eosin sections. ccRCC occasionally enters into the differential diagnosis and the correct diagnosis is usually achieved by adequate sampling, diffusely positive CK7 and E-cadherin staining, and negative CA9 staining. Eosinophilic chRCC closely resembles renal oncocytoma. In oncocytomas, Hale's colloidal iron stain is negative and only scattered cells or small clumps of cells react with antibody to cytokeratin 7.

MiT Family Translocation RCC

This tumor underexpresses epithelial markers such as CKs and EMA. CD10, RCC Ma, PAX2, and PAX8 are consistently expressed. Melanocytic markers such as HMB-45 and Melan A are positive in some tumors. Nuclear immunoreactivity for TFE3 gene product is confirmatory (Fig. 15.6). Cathepsin K, whose expression is modulated by MiTF and other members of MIT family including TFE3, is detected in 60% of Xp11.2/TFE3 translocation RCCs.

Collecting Duct Carcinoma (CDC) of Bellini

There is no specific immunoprofile for CDCs. Most cases stain with LMWCK and broad-spectrum CKs, CEA, peanut lectin agglutinin (PNA) and *Ulex europaeus* agglutinin (UEA). The majority expresses HMWCK 34βE12, CK7, PAX2, and PAX8. CD10 and P63 are usually negative. The differential diagnosis includes pRCC (discussed earlier), hereditary leiomyomatosis RCC syndrome, urothelial carcinoma with glandular differentiation, medullary carcinoma, and metastatic carcinoma. Urothelial carcinoma presents the most difficult challenge since it shares many features with CDC such as the propensity to form tubular glands, desmoplastic stroma, tumor cells in adjacent collecting tubules, and intracytoplasmic mucin. The finding of in situ urothelial carcinoma within adjacent calyces or the renal pelvis is supportive of the diagnosis of urothelial carcinoma. Therefore, generous sampling of renal pelvis and proximal ureter with careful microscopic examination is mandatory. Additionally, the immunohistochemical profile of urothelial carcinoma is PAX8-/P63+/GATA3+. Hereditary leiomyomatosis RCC syndrome typically affects young patients who may also be afflicted with multiple cutaneous leiomyomas and early-onset uterine fibroids. Tumor cells characteristically have very prominent nucleoli that resemble melanoma nuclei or cytomegalovirus inclusions.

Renal Medullary Carcinoma

The main differential diagnosis of renal medullary carcinoma includes CDC and high-grade invasive urothelial carcinoma. The tumor cells are positive for keratin AE1/AE3, PAX2, and PAX8, and variably for EMA and CEA. They are negative for HMWCK and immunohistochemical loss of expression of the nuclear transcriptional regulator SMARCB1 (INI1) is seen in all renal medullary carcinoma but not in other types of RCCs except a small portion of CDCs [32] (Fig. 15.7). OCT3/4 also stains medullary carcinoma, usually not for CDC or urothelial carcinomas [33].

Tubulocystic RCC

The immunoprofile is closely related to pRCC with diffuse positivity with AMACR, CD10, PAX2, and PAX8 staining. CK 7 staining is positive in all cases, but is often heterogeneous and weak.

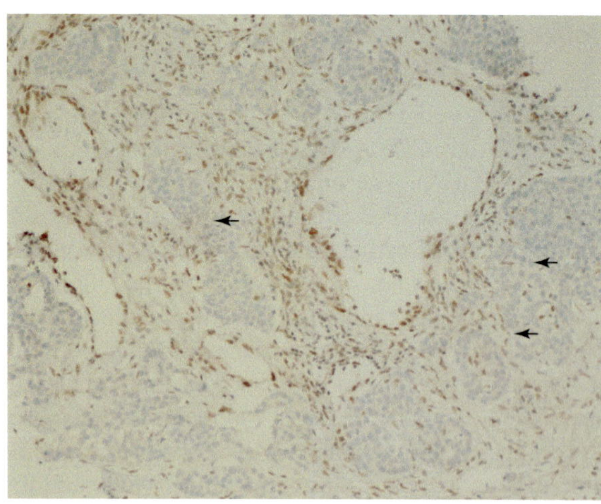

Fig. 15.7 Immunohistochemical loss of expression of transcriptional regulator SMARCB1 (INI1) in a renal medullary carcinoma. Note the loss of nuclear stain of INI1 in tumor cells (indicate with arrows) and preserved INI1 in adjacent nonneoplastic inflammatory and stromal cells

Acquired Cystic Disease-Associated RCC

A consistent immunoprofile is not yet known, but the morphology is so distinct and in general, no immunostains are required. This tumor is known to express AE1/3, CD10, RCC Ma, and AMACR. CK7 is negative, or at most, focally positive.

Hereditary Leiomyomatosis RCC (HLRCC RCC)

The epithelial component of the tumor showed positive immunoreactivity for CK7, CAM 5.2, and CD-10, and negative for smooth muscle actin (SMA). The stromal component is positive for α-SMA and negative for HMB45, CD117, CKs, ER, and PR. Loss of fumarate hydratase (FH) is specific for HLRCC RCC. Loss of FH expression can be confirmed by immunohistochemistry if specific antibody is available. Recently, immunoexpression of S-(2-succinyl cysteine (2SC) has been shown to be of diagnostic utility for HLRCC RCC. 2SC results from the reaction of accumulate fumarate with the cysteine sulfhydryl group of proteins and shows strong nuclear and cytoplasmic expression in these tumors. Most of other types of RCCs are negative for 2SC, although some cytoplasmic staining can be seen in type 2 pRCCs. Together with the loss of FH and high expression of 2SC a very useful ancillary tool in the differentiation of HLRCC RCCs from other high-grade RCCs [34] (Fig. 15.8).

Succinate Dehydrogenase-Deficient Renal Cell Carcinoma (SDH-Deficient RCC)

The tumor cells show variable CK expression and are positive for PAX8 and kidney-specific cadherin. Loss of IHC staining for SDHB is considered a requirement for the diagnosis of SDH-deficient RCC. One should be cautious in interpreting SDHB

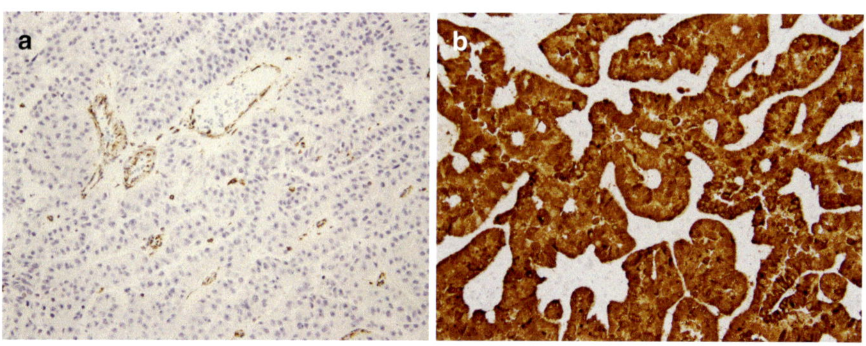

Fig. 15.8 (**a**, **b**) Loss of fumarate hydratase and accumulation of 2SC in a FH-deficient (HLRCC) RCC. Note the loss of FH in tumor cells and preserved FH in adjacent nonneoplastic (**a**), accumulation/over expression of 2-SC in the tumor cells

immunohistochemistry in renal tumors and markedly decreased or weak SDHB staining should not be interpreted as SDHB-deficient RCC [35, 36].

Oncocytoma

Oncocytomas are immunoreactive with antibodies to EMA, most CKs, CD117, E-cadherin, and kidney-specific cadherin. Their CK7 reactivity is focal, decorating scattered single cells and small clusters of cells (Fig. 15.2d). Vimentin is invariably negative.

Metanephric Adenomas

WT-1 is frequently detectable in the nuclei of metanephric adenomas. The cells of metanephric adenoma are positive for PAX2, PAX8, and CD57, frequently negative for EMA, CK7, CK AE1/AE3, CD56, and AMACR. CD57 and WT1 are positive, and BRAF V600E is positive in 90% metanephic adenoma. It is recommended that all adult cases histologically resembling metanephric adenoma have WT1, CD57, CK7, and AMACR immunohistochemical staining performed. If the staining pattern is characteristic for metanephric adenoma (CK7-, AMACR-, WT1+, and CD57+, including membranous staining), then no other diagnostic tests are indicated. However, if there is a different immunostaining pattern, then we recommend FISH analysis [31].

Utility of Immunohistochemistry in Morphological Classification of Renal Tumors

With the exception of TFE3, TFEB, FH, 2-SC, and SDHB, none of the above-mentioned markers are specific for a specific type of renal tumors. Immunostains should then be used to corroborate, rather than to establish, the morphological classification. One should always carefully examine the H&E morphology of the tumor first to generate a differential diagnosis and then apply appropriate markers. A panel of markers is preferred to include markers that support the favored diagnosis and markers that rule out other diagnoses included in the differential diagnosis.

Renal Tumors with Predominantly Clear Cell Nests and Sheets

Besides, ccRCC, many other renal tumors have clear, or pale-staining, cytoplasm at least focally but often as the predominant morphological feature. Their characteristic morphological features should lead to the correct diagnosis, or at least narrow down the differential diagnosis in most cases. An initial panel of markers, including CK7, CA9, and ksp-cadherin (or CD117), is recommended for working up of difficult cases. Additional markers can be performed judiciously based on the differential diagnosis. For example, urothelial markers, including p63, GATA-3, and HMWCK can be stained if urothelial carcinoma is suspected. Adrenal cortical markers including inhibin, calretinin, and MelanA can be performed to rule out intrarenal adrenal cortical tissue. TFE3, TFEB, Cathepsin K, and melanoma-associated markers can be used for the diagnosis of MiTF translocation RCC. HMB45, MART-1 as well as cathepsin K are quite valuable in the diagnosis of epithelioid angiomyolipoma (AML) when initial CK is negative. One important clinical question frequently raised by clinicians is whether a poorly differentiated RCC is a ccRCC or a non-ccRCC for treatment purpose. The tumor should be extensively sampled to look for areas with classical ccRCC morphology. The latter may be minute, but if present and possessing a characteristic immunoprofile (CK7-, CA9+, ksp-cadherin-, p63-), supports the diagnosis of ccRCC.

Renal Tumors with "Oncocytic" Cytoplasm (Pink Cell Tumor)

Oncocytic cytoplasm can be seen in many renal tumors and may pose significant diagnostic challenges. In ccRCC, high-grade tumor cells tend to lose cytoplasmic clarity and acquire oncocytic cytoplasm. The initial panel to work up on a challenging tumor with oncocytic cytoplasm includes CK7, CA9, AMACR, and ksp-cadherin (or CD117). Additional markers can be added if other tumors are suspected, including melanocytic markers for oncocytic AML, and TFE3, TFEB, and cathepsin K for translocation RCC. One frequently faced diagnostic issue is the distinction between an oncocytoma and chRCC, eosinophilic variant. Oncocytomas are characteristically negative or positive in single or small clusters of cells for CK7, diffusely positive CD117, ksp-cadherin, and E-cadherin. ChRCC, on the other hand, is diffusely positive for CK7, CD117, ksp-cadherin, and E-cadherin. Deviation from these characteristic immunoprofiles may justify labeling the tumor as "oncocytic tumor" without further subclassification. For example, an oncocytoma with diffuse CK7 staining is not characteristic and may be labeled as "oncocytic tumor, not otherwise specified," especially when other atypical features, such as diffuse nuclear atypia, are present. Recently, some new entities of RCCs with oncocytic/eosinophilic cytoplasm have been described and these include SDH-deficient RCC, FH-deficient RCC (HLRCC RCC), and eosinophilic cystic solid RCC (ESC). Li et al. reviewed 33 unclassified RCCs with predominantly eosinophilic cytoplasm in patients aged 35 years or younger and performed IHC for SDHB, FH, and CK20 (a marker of ESC RCC) on all cases. 30% cases were reclassified as ESC RCCs; 24% as SDH-deficient RCCs. 12% as FH-deficient RCCs; and 33% remained unclassified. The authors suggested that pathologists should have a low threshold for performing FH, SDHB, and CK20 IHC when confronted with unclassified eosinophilic RCC or "oncocytoma" in young patients [37].

Renal Tumors with Predominantly Papillary Components

Renal tumors with predominantly papillary components are pRCC, ccpRCC, and MiTF translocation RCCs, although focally papillary pattern is seen in many other renal tumors, especially in high-grade tumors [38]. The initial panel of markers should include CK7, AMACR, and CA9. A high-grade renal tumor with predominantly papillary architecture should elicit a differential diagnosis of type 2 pRCC, CDC, HLRCC RCC, and metastatic adenocarcinoma to the kidney. Except for lineage-specific markers (CDX2, TTF-1, etc.), other markers are considerably variable in their expression pattern in these tumors; therefore, offer little help in the classification of these tumors. Classification of these tumors therefore depends largely on morphology and clinical manifestation.

Renal Tumors with Papillae Covered with Clear Cells as Predominant Features

The differential diagnosis includes ccpRCC, pRCC, and translocation RCC. Characteristic morphological features and immunoprofiles can readily distinguish these three lesions. ccpRCC is a recently described new subtype which behaves in a benign or indolent fashion [39]. Therefore, it is important to distinguish it from ccRCC and pRCC. It has characteristic morphology and immunoprofile (CK7+, CD10-, CA9+ with "cup-shaped" staining pattern," and AMACR-) [39].

Renal Tumors with Tubulopapillary Architecture in Children and Young Adults

If a renal tumor has tubulopapillary architecture in children and young adults, the differential diagnosis should include pRCC, metanephric adenoma, and epithelial predominant Wilms tumor. With appropriate clinical history and morphology, translocation RCC and metastatic adenocarcinoma may also be considered.

Renal Tumors with High-Grade Infiltrative Growth Pattern

Renal tumors with multinodular growth, desmoplastic stroma, and invasive borders (tumor cells infiltrating between renal tubules and glomeruli at the advancing front) are difficult to classify based on morphology alone. One has to first rule out a metastasis to the kidney. PAX8 and PAX2 are probably the most useful markers owing to their relatively high sensitivity and specificity. If a tumor is deemed likely to originate in the kidney, urothelial carcinoma should always be considered and ruled out as the management for urothelial carcinoma and RCC is drastically different. The presence of urothelial carcinoma in pelvic mucosa and typical staining pattern (CK7+, CK20+, PAX8-, HMWCK+, and p63+) supports a diagnosis of an urothelial carcinoma. Clinical history of hemoglobin disease and loss of INI1 make the diagnosis of medullary RCC. To make a diagnosis of CDC we need to rule out other possibilities, particularly urothelial carcinoma, HLRCC RCC (FH-deficient RCC) and metastatic tumors [32].

Use of Immunohistochemical Markers in the Interpretation of Needle Biopsies of Renal Masses

Needle biopsy of renal masses has recently become more popular in the management of patients with renal masses owing to several reasons. The biopsy aims to clarify at least three questions. (A) Is the renal mass a neoplasm? (B). Is it a primary RCC, or metastatic cancer/lymphoma? (C). What is the histological classification of a primary RCC?

The most significant limitation of renal mass needle biopsy is the small quantity of tissue procured which may limit the morphological evaluation of the renal mass lesion. Consequently, IHC is often employed to supplement the morphological evaluation. A recent study found that standard morphological evaluation and judicious use of five markers (CK7, CD10, CA9, AMACR, and CD117) yielded accurate diagnoses in >90% of cases in an ex vivo needle biopsy study after nephrectomy [9]. When using IHC to work-up a renal mass biopsy, one should use the same, if not more, due diligence as in the workup of nephrectomy specimens. Careful morphological examination should be performed first to generate a list of differential diagnoses. Appropriate markers are then applied and the results are used to corroborate, rather than to establish, the morphological diagnosis.

Prognostic and Predictive Markers

The roles of several genetic pathways, including mammalian target of rapamycin (mTOR) and hypoxia inducible factor (HIF), in renal carcinogenesis and progression have been increasingly elucidated. Key components of these pathways have been investigated for their prognostic and predictive value for targeted therapies. For example, von Hippel–Lindau gene (VHL), a tumor suppressor gene on chromosome 3p25–26, plays a crucial role in HIF pathway. In normal cells, VHL targets HIF for proteasome-mediated degradation and therefore keeps HIF at low level. When VHL gene is inactivated, by gene mutation or promoter hypermethylation,

HIF accumulates and activates the downstream target genes, including vascular endothelial growth factor (VEGF) and CA9. Many of these molecules contribute to carcinogenesis in ccRCC. Functional loss of VHL is implicated in hereditary and sporadic ccRCC. However, studies have shown conflicting data on the prognostic value of VHL gene alteration. Loss of function mutation in VHL gene correlated with response to anti-VEGF therapy in some studies.

Several studies have found that the level of CA9 expression seems to have prognostic significance, with low expression (≤85% of tumor cells) correlated with worse overall survival in metastatic RCC, and high CA9 expression (>85%) was predictive of response to IL-2 [40, 41]. In addition, high CA9 expression (>85%) is associated with greater tumor shrinkage in response to sorafenib, a VEGF inhibitor, treatment [42]. However, more recent data from the TARGET study did not find CA9 expression status to be either predictive of clinical benefit for treatment with sorafenib or of prognostic value in patients with metastatic ccRCC following cytokine therapy [43].

Other molecules that have been investigated for their prognostic and predictive roles in RCC include key components of mTOR pathway, B7 family members that are coregulatory molecules inhibiting T-cell-mediated immunity, IMP3 which is a member of the insulin-like growth factor II mRNA-binding protein [44], p53, histone-modifying and chromatin-remodeling genes [45]. However, vast majority of published studies are of single-center research and comprise small number of cases. No marker has so far emerged as being reproducible and consistent across published studies. Therefore, no markers are ready to be recommended in routine clinical use for prognosis and prediction of therapy response. Large, multicenter prospective studies are needed to validate some promising markers. CA9 may be performed at clinician's request and expression can be quantified as ≤85% or >85%.

Summary

Diagnosis and classification of renal cell neoplasms, based primarily on the routine H&E morphological features, are usually straightforward. IHC markers, however, play an important role in several clinical settings, including distinguishing renal from nonrenal tumors, subtyping of renal cell neoplasms and working up renal mass needle biopsy with limited tissue quantity. These markers include those whose expression supports a renal origin (PAX2/PAX8, RCC Ma, CD10, HKIM-1, and vimentin) and those with differential expression in different renal tumor subtypes (CA9, AMACR, parvalbumin, E-cadherin, ksp-cadherin, claudin 7/8, CD117, S100A1, TFE3, TFEB, cathepsin K, markers of urothelial differentiation, and various CKs). Each marker has its utility in a specific diagnostic setting. A panel of markers should be used to corroborate, but not to supplant, the morphological diagnosis and classification. So far, no markers have proven clinical utility in the prediction of clinical outcomes and response to novel targeted therapy.

References

1. Zhou M, Roma A, Magi-Galluzzi C. The usefulness of immunohistochemical markers in the differential diagnosis of renal neoplasms. Clin Lab Med. 2005;25(2):247–57.
2. Skinnider BF, Amin MA. An immunohistochemical approach to the differential diagnosis of renal tumors. Semin Diagn Pathol. 2005;22(1):51–68.
3. Hammerich KH, Ayala GE, Wheeler TM. Application of immunohistochemistry to the genitourinary system (prostate, urinary bladder, testis, and kidney). Arch Pathol Lab Med. 2008;132(3):432–40.
4. Truong LD, Shen SS. Immunohistochemical diagnosis of renal neoplasms. Arch Pathol Lab Med. 2011;135(1):92–109.
5. Shen SS, Truong LD, Scarpelli M, Lopez-Beltran A. Role of immunohistochemistry in diagnosing renal neoplasms: when is it really useful? Arch Pathol Lab Med. 2012;136(4):410–7.
6. Reuter VE, Argani P, Zhou M, Delahunt B, et al. Best practices recommendations in the application of immunohistochemistry in the kidney tumors: report from the International Society of Urologic Pathology consensus conference. Am J Surg Pathol. 2014;38(8):e35–49.
7. Zhou M, Deng FM. The utility of immunohistochemistry in the differential diagnosis of renal cell carcinoma. In: Magi-Galluzzi C, Przybycin G, editors. Genitourinary pathology: practical advances. New York: Springer Science; 2015. p. 383–99.
8. Deng FM, Zhou M. Molecular genetics and immunohistochemistry of renal tumours: translation into clinical practice. Diagn Histopathol. 2016;22(2):73–9.
9. Al-Ahmadie HA, Alden D, Fines SW, Gopalan A, Touijer KA, Russo P, et al. Role of immunohistochemistry in the evaluation of needle core biopsies in adult renal cortical tumors: an ex vivo study. Am J Surg Pathol. 2011;35(7):949–61.
10. Alderman MA, Daignault S, Wolf JS Jr, Palapattu GS, Weizer AZ, et al. Categorizing renal oncocytic neoplasms on core needle biopsy: a morphologic and immunophenotypic study of 144 cases with clinical follow-up. Hum Pathol. 2016;55:1–10.
11. Gupta R, Balzer B, Picken M, Osunkoya AO, Shet T, Alsabeh R, et al. Diagnostic implications of transcription factor Pax 2 protein and transmembrane enzyme complex carbonic anhydrase IX immunoreactivity in adult renal epithelial neoplasms. Am J Surg Pathol. 2009;33(2):241–7.
12. Ozcan A, de la Roza G, Ro JY, Shen SS, Truong LD. PAX2 and PAX8 expression in primary and metastatic renal tumors: a comprehensive comparison. Arch Pathol Lab Med. 2016;136(12):1541–51.
13. McGregor DK, Khurana KK, Cao C, Ayala G, Krishnan B, et al. Diagnosing primary and metastatic renal cell carcinoma: the use of the monoclonal antibody 'Renal Cell Carcinoma Marker'. Am J Surg Pathol. 2001;25(12):1485–92.
14. Lin F, Zhang PL, Yang XJ, Shi J, Blasick T, Han WK, et al. Human kidney injury molecule-1 (hKIM-1): a useful immunohistochemical marker for diagnosing renal cell carcinoma and ovarian clear cell carcinoma. Am J Surg Pathol. 2007;31(3):371–81.
15. Ivanov S, Liao SY, Ivanova A, Danilkovitch-Miagkova A, Tarasova N, Weirich G, et al. Expression of hypoxia-inducible cell-surface transmembrane carbonic anhydrases in human cancer. Am J Pathol. 2001;158(3):905–19.
16. Zhou M, Chinnaiyan AM, Kleer CG, Lucas PC, Rubin MA. Alpha-Methylacyl-CoA racemase: a novel tumor marker over-expressed in several human cancers and their precursor lesions. Am J Surg Pathol. 2002;26(7):926–31.
17. Molinie V, Balaton A, Rotman S, Mansouri D, De Pinieux I, Homsi T, et al. Alpha-methyl CoA racemase expression in renal cell carcinomas. Hum Pathol. 2006;37(6):698–703.
18. Young AN, de Oliveira Salles PG, Lim SD, Cohen C, Petros JA, Marshall FF, et al. Beta defensin-1, parvalbumin, and vimentin: a panel of diagnostic immunohistochemical markers for renal tumors derived from gene expression profiling studies using cDNA microarrays. Am J Surg Pathol. 2003;27(2):199–205.

19. Shen SS, Krishna B, Chirala R, Amato RJ, Truong LD. Kidney-specific cadherin, a specific marker for the distal portion of the nephron and related renal neoplasms. Mod Pathol. 2005;18(7):933–40.
20. Huo L, Sugimura J, Tretiakova MS, Patton KT, Gupta R, Popov B, et al. C-kit expression in renal oncocytomas and chromophobe renal cell carcinomas. Hum Pathol. 2005;36(3):262–8.
21. Castillo M, Petit A, Mellado B, Palacín A, Alcover JB, Mallofré C. C-kit expression in sarcomatoid renal cell carcinoma: potential therapy with imatinib. J Urol. 2004;171(6 Pt 1):2176–80.
22. Argani P, Lal P, Hutchinson B, Lui MY, Reuter VE, Ladanyi M. Aberrant nuclear immunoreactivity for TFE3 in neoplasms with TFE3 gene fusions: a sensitive and specific immunohistochemical assay. Am J Surg Pathol. 2003;27(6):750–61.
23. Argani P, Lae M, Hutchinson B, Reuter VE, Collins MH, Perentesis J, et al. Renal carcinomas with the t(6;11)(p21;q12): clinicopathologic features and demonstration of the specific alpha-TFEB gene fusion by immunohistochemistry, RT-PCR, and DNA PCR. Am J Surg Pathol. 2005;29(2):230–40.
24. Camparo P, Vasiliu V, Molinie V, Couturier J, Dykema KJ, Petillo D, et al. Renal translocation carcinomas: clinicopathologic, immunohistochemical, and gene expression profiling analysis of 31 cases with a review of the literature. Am J Surg Pathol. 2008;32(5):656–70.
25. Martignoni G, Pea M, Gobbo S, Brunelli M, Bonetti F, Segala D, et al. Cathepsin-K immunoreactivity distinguishes MiTF/TFE family renal translocation carcinomas from other renal carcinomas. Mod Pathol. 2009;22(8):1016–22.
26. Martignoni G, Bonetti F, Chilosi M, Brunelli M, Segala D, Amin MB, et al. Cathepsin K expression in the spectrum of perivascular epithelioid cell (PEC) lesions of the kidney. Mod Pathol. 2012;25(1):100–11.
27. Albadine R, Schultz L, Illei P, Ertoy D, Hicks J, Sharma R, et al. PAX8 (+)/p63 (−) immunostaining pattern in renal collecting duct carcinoma (CDC): a useful immunoprofile in the differential diagnosis of CDC versus urothelial carcinoma of upper urinary tract. Am J Surg Pathol. 2010;34(7):965–9.
28. Trpkov K, Abou-Ouf H, Hes O, Lopez JI, Nesi G, Comperat E, et al. Eosinophilic Solid and Cystic Renal Cell Carcinoma (ESC RCC): further morphologic and molecular characterization of ESC RCC as a distinct entity. Am J Surg Pathol. 2017;41(10):1299–308.
29. Palsgrove DN, Li Y, Pratilas C, Lin MT, Pallavajjalla A, Gocke C, et al. Eosinophilic Solid and Cystic (ESC) renal cell carcinomas harbor TSC mutations: molecular analysis supports an expanding clinicopathologic spectrum. Am J Surg Pathol. 2018; https://doi.org/10.1097/PAS.0000000000001111.
30. Choueiri TK, Cheville J, Palescandolo E, Fay AP, Kantoff PW, Atkins MB, et al. BRAF mutations in metanephric adenoma of the kidney. Eur Urol. 2012;62(5):91722.
31. Kinney SN, Eble JN, Hes O, Williamson SR, Grignon DJ, Wang M, et al. Metanephric adenoma: the utility of immunohistochemical and cytogenetic analyses in differential diagnosis, including solid variant papillary renal cell carcinoma and epithelial-predominant nephroblastoma. Mod Pathol. 2015;28(9):1236–48.
32. Ohe C, Smith SC, Sirohi D, Divatia M, de Peralta-Venturina M, Paner GP, et al. Reappraisal of morphologic differences between renal medullary carcinoma, collecting duct carcinoma, and fumarate hydratase-deficient renal cell carcinoma. Am J Surg Pathol. 2018;42(3):279–92.
33. Rao P, Tannir NM, Tamboli P. Expression of OCT3/4 in renal medullary carcinoma represents a potential diagnostic pitfall. Am J Surg Pathol. 2012;36(4):583–8.
34. Chen YB, Brannon AR, Toubaji A, Dudas ME, Won HH, Al-Ahmadie HA, et al. Hereditary leiomyomatosis and renal cell carcinoma syndrome-associated renal cancer: recognition of the syndrome by pathologic features and the utility of detecting aberrant succination by immunohistochemistry. Am J Surg Pathol. 2014;38(5):627–37.
35. Gill AJ, Pachter NS, Clarkson A, Tucker KM, Winship IM, Benn DE, et al. Renal tumors and hereditary pheochromocytoma-paraganglioma syndrome type 4. N Engl J Med. 2011;364:885–6.

36. Gill AJ, Hes O, Papathomas T, Šedivcová M, Tan PH, Agaimy A, et al. Succinate dehydrogenase (SDH)-deficient renal carcinoma: a morphologically distinct entity: a clinicopathologic series of 36 tumors from 27 patients. Am J Surg Pathol. 2014;38(12):1588–602.
37. Li Y, Reuter VE, Matoso A, Netto GJ, Epstein JI, Argani P. Re-evaluation of 33 'unclassified' eosinophilic renal cell carcinomas in young patients. Histopathology. 2018;72(4):588–600.
38. Deng FM, Kong M, Zhou M. Papillary or pseudopapillary tumors of the kidney. Semin Diagn Pathol. 2015;32:124–39.
39. Aydin H, Chen L, Cheng L, Vaziri S, He H, Ganapathi R, et al. Clear cell tubulopapillary renal cell carcinoma: a study of 36 distinctive low-grade epithelial tumors of the kidney. Am J Surg Pathol. 2010;34(11):1608–21.
40. Atkins M, Regan M, McDermott D, Mier J, Stanbridge E, Youmans A, et al. Carbonic anhydrase IX expression predicts outcome of interleukin 2 therapy for renal cancer. Clin Cancer Res. 2005;11(10):3714–21.
41. Stillebroer AB, Mulders PF, Boerman OC, Oyen WJ, Oosterwijk E. Carbonic anhydrase IX in renal cell carcinoma: implications for prognosis, diagnosis, and therapy. Eur Urol. 2010;58(1):75–83.
42. Choueiri TK, Regan MM, Rosenberg JE, et al. Carbonic anhydrase IX and pathological features as predictors of outcome in patients with metastatic clear-cell renal cell carcinoma receiving vascular endothelial growth factor-targeted therapy. BJU Int. 2010;106:772–8.
43. TK C, Cheng S, Qu AQ, Pastorek J, Atkins MB, Signoretti S. Carbonic anhydrase IX as a potential biomarker of efficacy in metastatic clear-cell renal cell carcinoma patients receiving sorafenib or placebo: analysis from the treatment approaches in renal cancer global evaluation trial (TARGET). Urol Oncol. 2013;8:1788–93.
44. Jiang Z, Chu PG, Kang Y, Lee SS. Analysis of RNA-binding protein IMP3 to predict metastasis and prognosis of renal-cell carcinoma: a retrospective study. Lancet Oncol. 2006;7(7):556–64.
45. Hakimi AA, Chen YB, Wren J, Gonen M, Abdel-Wahab O, Heguy A, et al. Clinical and pathologic impact of select chromatin-modulating tumor suppressors in clear cell renal cell carcinoma. Eur Urol. 2013;63(5):848–54.

Chapter 16
Cytology of Kidney Tumors

Suzanne M. Crumley

Fine needle aspiration (FNA) with cytologic evaluation of renal masses has traditionally been underutilized. This is largely due to the high accuracy of radiologic evaluation of kidney tumors and the predominance of surgical resection by radical nephrectomy in nearly all kidney tumors. However, cytology evaluation, often in concert with concurrent core needle biopsy (CNB), has an increasingly important role in directing management, particularly for small or incidentally detected renal tumors in which radical nephrectomy may not be indicated [1]. A preoperative biopsy is recommended by the American Society of Clinical Oncology (ASCO) 2017 guidelines for small renal tumors (defined as less than or equal to 4 cm) when the results may alter management [2]. The indications include kidney tumors with indeterminate characteristics by imaging, patients who are poor surgical candidates, tumors that could benefit from ablative therapies or a nephron-sparing surgery (partial nephrectomy), consideration of active surveillance, exclusion of nonrenal tumors involving the kidney, exclusion of inflammatory etiologies, and in renal cysts with indeterminate characteristics [1, 2]. The renal tumor biopsy may include a touch preparation for adequacy and triage purposes and/or a dedicated fine-needle aspiration specimen.

Knowledge of the cytological features of kidney tumors is also important in cases of tissue procurement from a metastatic site in patients with widespread metastatic disease. There are targeted therapies for vascular endothelial growth factor receptor and tyrosine kinase inhibitors that have efficacy in certain histologic subtypes (clear cell renal cell carcinoma: ccRCC) but not in other histologic subtypes [3]. Therefore, the importance of identification and histologic subtype classification on a FNA/CNB from a metastatic lesion is increasing.

S. M. Crumley (✉)
Department of Pathology and Genomic Medicine, Houston Methodist Hospital, Weill Medical College of Cornell University, Houston, TX, USA
e-mail: smcrumley@houstonmethodist.org

M. K. Divatia et al. (eds.), *Kidney Cancer*, https://doi.org/10.1007/978-3-030-28333-9_16

A recent systematic review and meta-analysis of diagnostic accuracy of percutaneous renal tumor biopsy that included 5228 patients [4] found that the median diagnostic rate of renal tumor biopsy was excellent (92%) [4]. The sensitivity and specificity was higher for CNB (99.1% and 99.7%) and lower for FNA (93.2% and 89.8%) [4]. The best sensitivity and specificity is achieved when both FNA and CNB are utilized. In one recent study of 247 cases of FNA and/or CNB, the diagnostic rate of FNA and CNB in combination was superior to either FNA alone (92% versus 72%; $P < 0.05$) or CNB alone (92% versus 87%) [5]. The increased sampling area achieved by FNA as well as the ability of FNA to direct the CNB toward the areas of viable identifiable tumor complements the ability of CNB to evaluate preserved architecture and improved histologic subtyping with immunoperoxidase stains on CNB [5, 6].

However, it is also important to understand the limitations of FNA/CNB in the evaluation of kidney tumors. Although concordance of up to 90.3% has been reported in small studies using FNA alone [7], the diagnostic accuracy by FNA alone was reported as 77% in another large study [8]. False positive diagnoses, although rare, have been reported in the presence of inflammatory and benign lesions [7, 8], and assigning a definitive histologic subtype can be challenging with FNA alone [7, 8]. Challenges in histologic classification can arise on FNA, particularly with papillary renal cell carcinoma (pRCC), tumors with oncocytic features, renal cell carcinoma (RCC) with sarcomatoid component, urothelial carcinoma, and angiomyolipoma [8]. False negative FNA has also been reported as ranging from 0% to as high as 36% in the literature and can occur in small lesions or those with abundant necrosis [4, 9]. A CNB is not immune from challenges of sampling, with nondiagnostic rates in CNB ranging from 0 to 22.6% [4]. The importance of immediate onsite adequacy evaluation is essential to help minimize the false negative rate for both FNA and CNB. If the FNA is performed without CNB, obtaining adequate material for a cell block preparation is advised to facilitate the use of immunohistochemical stains, if necessary.

FNA and CNB are typically performed by the radiologist with image guidance by computed tomography (CT) and/or ultrasound, with FNA generally performed first (using 21 gauge or smaller needle) and preparation of Diff-Quik Romanowsky–Giemsa stain and/or Papanicolaou-stained slides. Core needle biopsy typically uses 18–20 gauge needles for sampling. Complications from renal tumor biopsies are low, with the median overall complication rate as low as 8.1% [4], and comprised predominantly of perirenal hematoma, hematuria, lumbar pain, pneumothorax, and one case of septic shock after aspiration of a pyelonephritic kidney has been reported [4]. The risk of tumor seeding is very rare [4].

There are no standard adequacy criteria for sampling of renal masses. In general, a specimen is considered adequate for a solid lesion if the smears are cellular and diagnostic for a lesion, while unsatisfactory if scant, necrotic, or technically poor preparations [10]. A recent large study of 290 cases of renal FNA/CNB suggested that unsatisfactory be used only if there was inadequate cellularity for evaluation, while nondiagnostic if all cells were consistent with normal renal elements and not representative of a lesion. This is important in cases of benign kidney lesions or benign cysts, which may be non-diagnostic at the time of adequacy assessment and negative at the time of final sign-out, rather than unsatisfactory [6]. Cystic lesions can be considered satisfactory if fluid is present, regardless of cellularity, and unsatisfactory if soft tissue and/or normal kidney or blood only [10].

Normal Elements

Familiarity with the appearance of normal kidney on FNA is essential, as it is one of the recognized pitfalls in identification of kidney masses [8, 10]. Each of the normal kidney elements can mimic renal neoplasms. Aspiration of glomerular elements is identified by the overall architecture and capillary loops that may contain red blood cells. They can be densely cellular with bland cells present, and the distorted glomeruli can mimic papillae of an RCC (Fig. 16.1a, b). Renal tubular cells have bland round nuclei with smooth nuclear borders and surrounding granular cytoplasm (Fig. 16.1c, d). They can be present as single cells or in small clusters [10]. The renal tubular cells can mimic oncocytoma, chromophobe RCC (chRCC),

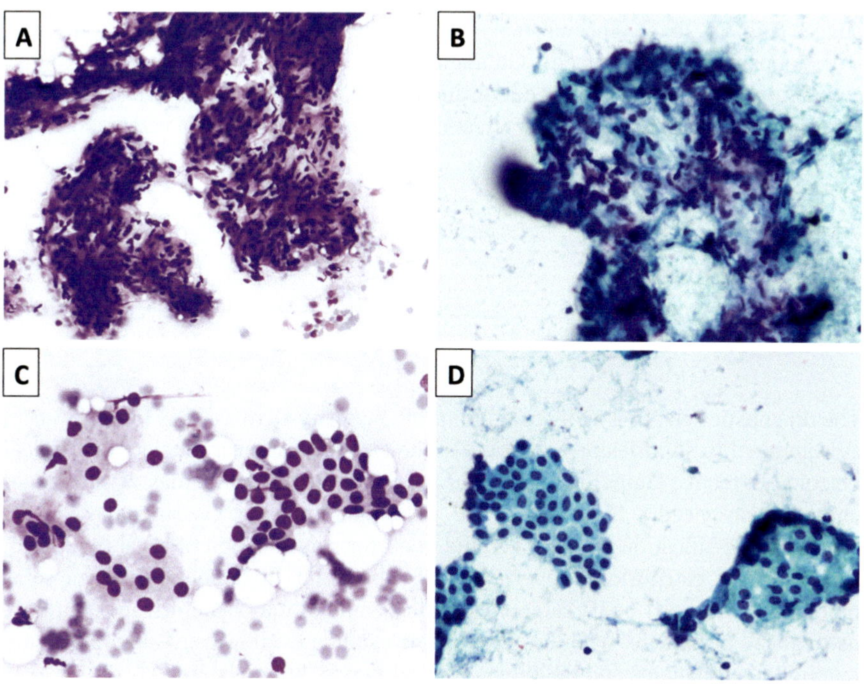

Fig. 16.1 Normal kidney elements. The aspirates of normal kidney can be cellular on cytologic preparations. The glomerulus is seen (**a**, DQ, 10× and **b**, Papanicolaou, 20×) and can mimic papillary tumors. In addition, the renal tubules (**c**, DQ, 20× and **d**, Papanicolaou, 10×) can mimic oncocytic neoplasms

or even a low-grade ccRCC in a cystic lesion. In addition, inadvertent sampling of hepatocytes or adrenal cortical cells can occur and mimic a renal neoplasm.

Inflammatory/Nonneoplastic Conditions

Renal abscess/pyelonephritis typically presents with a clinical history or urinary tract infection and has abundant neutrophils on fine needle aspiration, with similar features to abscess in other sites (Fig. 16.2a). Two chronic pyelonephritic conditions, xanthogranulomatous pyelonephritis or malakoplakia, can cause a radiologic appearance of a mass and mimic an RCC on fine needle aspiration [7, 11], predominantly due to the presence of necrosis, histiocytes, and admixed proximal collecting tubules. Xanthogranulomatous pyelonephritis is an uncommon destructive chronic granulomatous process that is more common in females and typically caused by *Escherichia coli* and *Proteus mirabilis* [12]. Fine needle aspiration will show a mixed inflammatory infiltrate with histiocytes, lymphocytes, plasma cells, neutrophils, and multinucleated giant cells. Necrosis can be present. In cases of malakoplakia, the pathognomonic intracytoplasmic Michaelis–Gutmann bodies can be seen on Diff-Quick (DQ) and Papanicolaou-stained preparations within macrophages (Fig. 16.2b, c). Special stains for periodic acid-Schiff (PAS) and von Kossa will be positive. The Michaelis–Gutmann bodies are the result of phagolysosomes containing undigested bacteria due to ineffective macrophage bactericidal activity [11]. Immunosuppressed patients are at risk and malakoplakia has been reported in the setting of renal transplant [11].

Benign Tumors

Renal Cysts

The diagnostic sensitivity for renal tumor biopsy in cystic masses is lower (83.6%) as compared to solid lesions (98%) [4]. The current American Society of Clinical Oncology Practice Guidelines suggest that predominantly cystic masses should not undergo core needle biopsy [2]. The radiologic imaging classification system (Bosniak Classification System) is quite good for classification of renal cysts [13], and in general, categories I (benign) and IV (malignant) do not need cytologic sampling. Cysts in the II or III categories (indeterminate) may benefit from sampling, particularly in patients who are nonsurgical candidates; however, sampling is not required in all patients and radiologic follow-up may be considered [13].

The majority of renal cysts sampled in one large series were benign simple cysts (41 of 113 renal FNAs, 36%) [14]. These characteristically show cystic macrophages and scant small bland epithelial cells without atypia (Fig. 16.3). Of note, sampling of the renal tubules can be seen and can give a cellular appearance to the smears. Macrophages can also cluster together and mimic an epithelial cell compo-

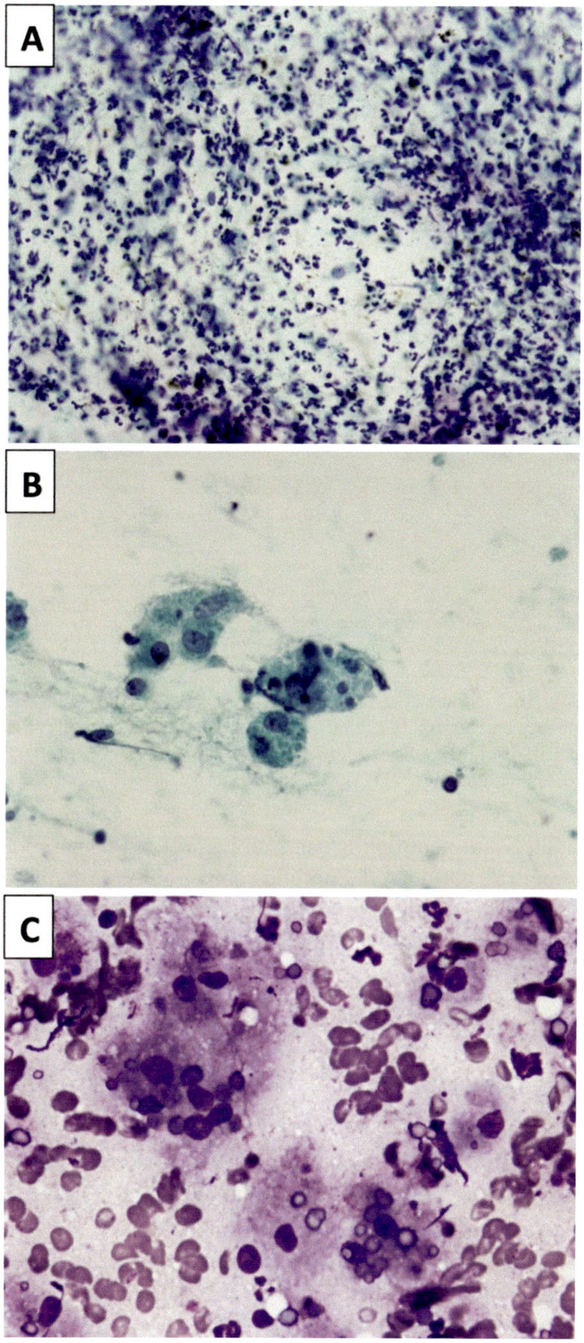

Fig. 16.2 Inflammatory/non-neoplastic conditions. Renal abscess shows abundant neutrophils present and reactive atypia can be seen (Papanicolaou, **a**, 20×). The refractile intracytoplasmic Michaelis–Gutman bodies are seen on Papanicolaou (**b**, 40×) and DQ (**c**, 40×) and Papanicolaou (**b**, 40×) preparations. (Photos courtesy of Zulfia McCroskey, MD)

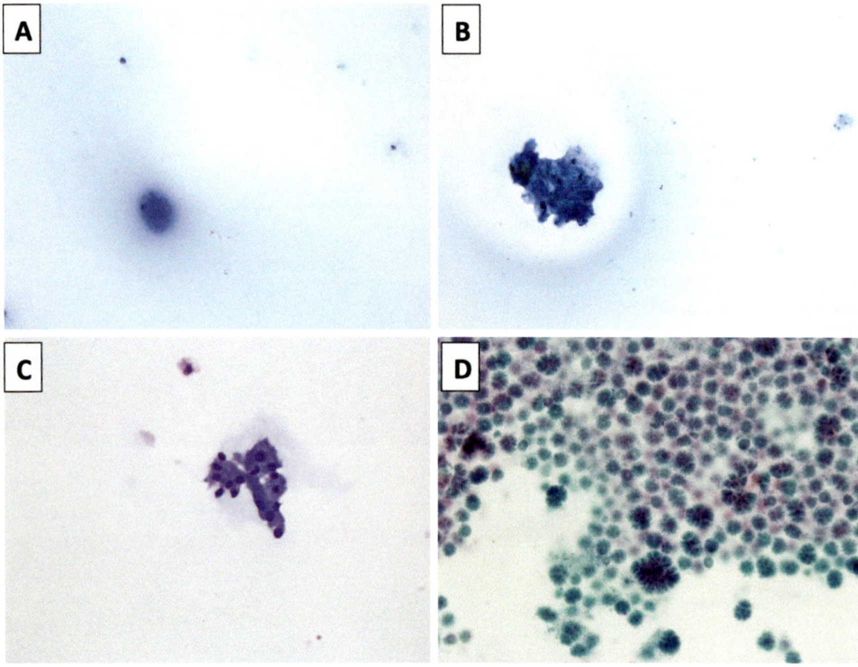

Fig. 16.3 Renal cyst. A benign renal cyst shows proteinaceous material and scattered macrophages and amorphous debris and benign renal tubular cells (**a**, Diff-Quik 40×, **b**, Diff-Quik 20×, **c** Diff-Quik 40×). Liesegang rings can sometimes be seen (**d**, Papanicolaou, 20×, Courtesy of Zulfia McCroskey, MD)

nent. Scant neutrophils can also be present; if markedly increased, a renal abscess should be considered. Sampling can be an issue in multilocular cysts and correlation with corresponding imaging findings is essential. Liesegang rings (concentrically lamellar strongly cyanophilic structures) can be seen as a component of a renal cyst [14] (Fig. 16.3).

Angiomyolipoma

Angiomyolipoma is considered a benign mesenchymal tumor that is part of the family of perivascular epithelioid cell tumors (PEComas). These typically arise in adults and can be associated with tuberous sclerosis [15, 16]. The tumors have a varying component of adipose tissue, smooth muscle/spindled cells, and abnormal thick-walled vessels. The current World Health Organization (WHO) classification 2016 considers epithelioid angiomyolipoma as a separate entity due to its potential for aggressive biologic behavior and requires a diagnosis of at least 80% of epithelioid cells within the tumor to qualify for this diagnosis [15].

The cytologic diagnosis of angiomyolipoma can be quite challenging [17]. Tumors with classical adipose tissue component or those in association with tuberous sclerosis are typically not biopsied. Therefore, the tumors that are received on FNA are infrequent and often have indeterminate radiological findings. The largest reported series of angiomyolipoma on FNA reviewed the findings in 25 cases and found that the smears are typically of moderate to high cellularity (88% of cases), and predominantly comprised of spindled cells (76% of cases) [17] (Fig. 16.4). Epithelioid cells were also noted, as well as adipose tissue and vascular components (Fig. 16.4). Correlation with clinical and imaging findings, as well as obtaining sufficient material for a cell block preparation to perform immunoperoxidase staining is advised. This is of particular importance in cases with predominant epithelioid morphology, which can be highly atypical and lead to misdiagnosis as a ccRCC, sarcomatoid RCC, or other malignancies [8, 17]. The tumor cells show epithelial markers' negativity (cytokeratin, EMA, CAM5.2) and positivity for HMB45, melan A, cathepsin K, CD10, ER, PR, and smooth muscle markers, with cathepsin K typically showing diffuse positive staining [15, 18].

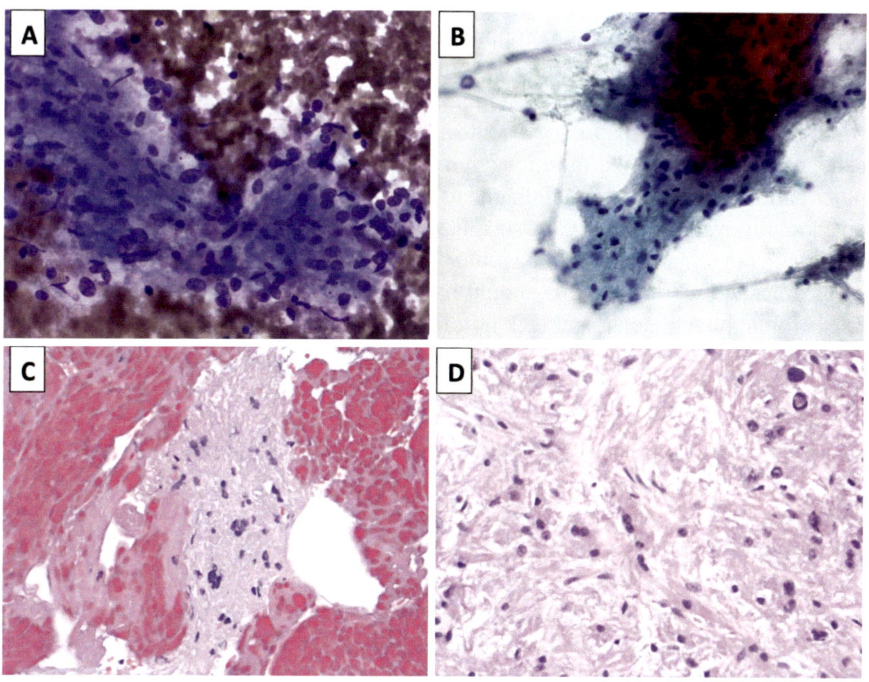

Fig. 16.4 Angiomyolipoma. The cytologic smears show clusters of spindled to epithelioid cells with an occasional nucleolus and nuclear atypia (**a** Diff-Quik 40×, **b** Pap 40×). The cell block shows a cluster of spindled to epithelioid cells (**c** H&E 40×). The corresponding core biopsy had similar spindled to epithelioid cells with intranuclear inclusion (**d** H&E 40×). The tumor cells were positive for HMB45 and smooth muscle actin (not pictured)

Metanephric Adenoma

Metanephric adenoma is a benign tumor that is typically well circumscribed and can present in a wide age range, with the median age of presentation about 50 years and a female predominance [15]. On fine needle aspiration, the cells are round to oval and bland with scant cytoplasm, fine chromatin, nuclear grooves, and absent nucleoli [19]. Mitotic activity is not seen. Nuclear pleomorphism or necrosis not typically seen, and if present, should raise concern for a low-grade pRCC. Psammoma bodies can be present in both metanephric adenoma and pRCC. Immunoperoxidase stains show that the tumor cells are positive for CD57, WT-1, AE1/AE3, and PAX-8, while negative for CK7 (focal positivity can be seen) and epithelial membrane antigen (EMA) [19]. This staining pattern aids in the differential diagnosis, which includes a pRCC or an epithelial predominant Wilms' tumor.

Oncocytoma

A renal oncocytoma is a benign tumor of the kidney that accounts for approximately 6% of all renal neoplasms [20]. The tumor cells are characterized by eosinophilic cytoplasm and round bland monotonous nuclei with fine chromatin [20, 21] (Fig. 16.5). Necrosis, papillary architecture, significant nuclear irregularity, clear cells, or readily identified mitotic activity is not seen and should raise concern for other entities in the differential diagnosis [21], which includes chromophobe RCC, eosinophilic variant of pRCC, succinate dehydrogenase (SDH)-deficient RCC, hybrid oncocytoma-chromophobe tumor, and epithelioid angiomyolipoma [18]. On surgical resection, oncocytoma should have the classic nested pattern with edematous stroma, bland nuclei, and lack mitotic activity.

Immunoperoxidase stains, in particular CK7 and CD117 (c-kit), can aid in the differential diagnosis [18, 21]. CK7 staining should be rare to focal in oncocytoma and positivity is often near the fibrotic area of the tumor with generally <5% of staining [18]. In contrast, CK7 will be typically diffuse in chRCC and completely absent in SDH-deficient RCC. CD117 is positive in oncocytoma, while this will be negative in SDH-deficient RCC. Of note, eosinophilic variant of papillary RCC can also have lack or decreased staining for CK7, but will have more atypia than seen in oncocytoma [18]. As sampling by FNA/CNB is limited, caution is advised with diagnosis of oncocytoma by cytology alone and consensus evaluation and cell block preparations should be obtained before rendering a definitive diagnosis. Another important exclusion is to confirm that normal renal tubules or liver parenchyma have not been sampled, which can also mimic oncocytoma. Bile and lipofuscin pigment will be seen in hepatocytes, if present [22].

The diagnosis of oncocytoma can also be quite challenging on cytology, core needle biopsy, and even surgical resection specimens. However, it is important to understand the cytologic features to aid in the management of these patients,

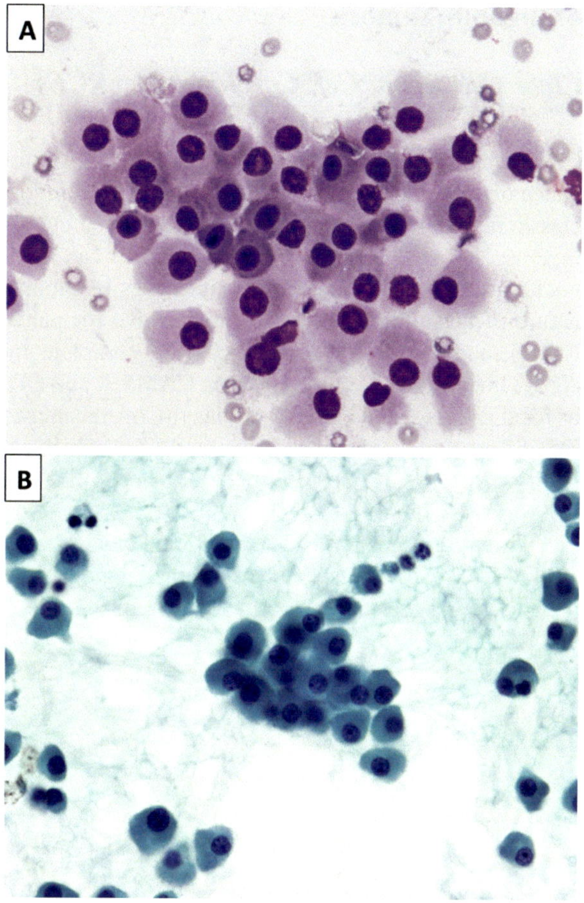

Fig. 16.5 Oncocytoma. The tumor cells have eosinophilic cytoplasm and round bland monotonous nuclei. Nuclear atypia, nuclear irregularity, necrosis, and mitotic activity are not seen (**a**, Diff-Quik and **b**, Pap stains, both 40×)

particularly in those who can avoid surgery if other entities in the differential diagnosis are ruled out. A series of FNA of 11 oncocytomas with comparison to eosinophilic variant of pRCC and chRCC was performed [22] and found that the FNA of oncocytoma has cells with densely granular cytoplasm, round bland nuclei, and arranged singly or in small loose clusters with a uniform appearance. However, this study also found that on cytologic evaluation alone, the diagnosis of "oncocytic neoplasm" may be best rendered if findings are not conclusive, with a suggestion of the differential diagnosis [22]. On core needle biopsies, others have suggested that if the classic features of oncocytoma are seen, the diagnosis of "oncocytic tumor, favor oncocytoma" can be rendered [21]. If a case has nuclear features that are beyond what is typical for oncocytoma but insufficient for a diagnosis of RCC, the diagnosis of "oncocytic tumor, cannot exclude RCC" can be utilized, although ideally this diagnosis should be infrequently utilized [21].

Malignant Tumors

Clear Cell Renal Cell Carcinoma (ccRCC)

Clear cell renal cell carcinoma (ccRCC) is an entity with good diagnostic concordance on fine needle aspiration sampling with resection specimens [7, 8, 10]. The classic features on cytology include vacuolated cytoplasm and a delicate arborizing vascular pattern (Fig. 16.6). Tumor cells can lose their cytoplasm with naked nuclei present [10]. Smears can sometimes be bloody due to the highly vascular nature of these tumors. ccRCC are positive for paired-box genes 8 & 2 (PAX8, PAX2), carbonic anhydrase IX (CAIX; complete membranous staining), AE1/AE3, vimentin, RCC marker, EMA, CAM5.2, and CD10. CK7 should be negative or focal positive, and alpha-methylacyl-CoA racemase (AMACR) is negative [15]. The differential diagnosis includes ccpRCCs, which will have low-grade clear cells but have diffuse CK7 positivity, CAIX in a cup-like distribution, and are also negative for AMACR [23].

Fuhrman grading (WHO/International Society of Urologic Pathology (ISUP) grading) on cytology specimens is challenging. A large meta-analysis of 5228 patients found that the concordance of tumor grade on renal tumor biopsies and

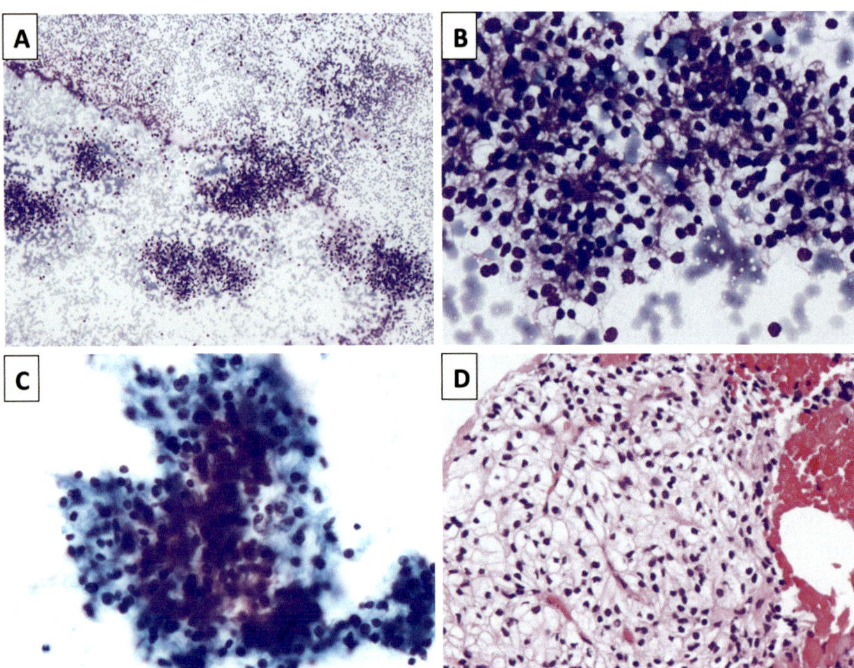

Fig. 16.6 Clear cell renal cell carcinoma. The smears can be bloody with clusters of tumor cells with clear cytoplasm (**a**, Diff-Quik, 4×). On higher power, the tumor cells have clear and vacuolated cytoplasm with delicate vasculature present (**b**, Diff-Quik, 20×). On Pap-stained slides, visible nucleoli can be seen (**c**, Pap 40×). A cell block preparation can show similar morphology and is useful for confirming the diagnosis and attempt at Fuhrman nuclear grading (**d**, Hematoxylin and eosin (H&E), 20×)

surgical specimens (including FNA and CNB) is only fair (median $k = 0.34$), with a median concordance rate of 62.5% [4]. This assessment is limited by tumor heterogeneity and limited sampling. Improvement of concordance with a two-tier system is possible (Fuhrman I/II versus III/IV); however, the limitations in this area are recognized [4]. In general, an attempt to give a Fuhrman grade can be assigned; however, as these tumors will undergo surgical resection, there should be awareness that the Fuhrman grade may change after examination of the surgical specimen.

Papillary Renal Cell Carcinoma

Papillary RCC (pRCC) is the second most common renal carcinoma subtype, comprising up to 18.5% of renal tumors [15]. The smears in pRCC are cellular, and the cytologic features include papillary architecture with fibrovascular cores, foamy macrophages, and intracytoplasmic hemosiderin [24]. Psammoma bodies and nuclear grooves have also been described, but may be infrequent. The morphology will differ in the pRCC type 1 versus type 2 subtypes, with type 1 pRCC showing smaller basophilic low-grade nuclei arranged in a single layer with scant cytoplasm (Fig. 16.7). Type 2 pRCC shows abundant eosinophilic cytoplasm,

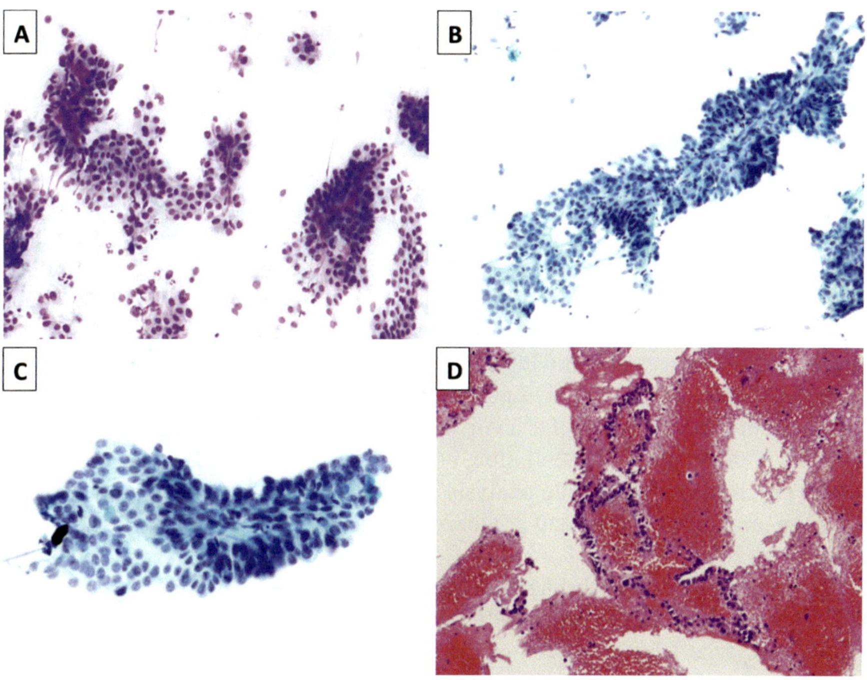

Fig. 16.7 Papillary renal cell carcinoma, type 1. Papillary renal cell carcinoma, type 1, typically has cellular smears with readily evident fibrovascular cores noted (**a**, Diff-Quik, 10×). The Pap slide shows nuclear irregularity, occasional nucleoli, and mitotic activity present (**b** and **c**, Pap, 10× and 20×). A cell block preparation also shows papillary cells present (**d**, H&E, 10×)

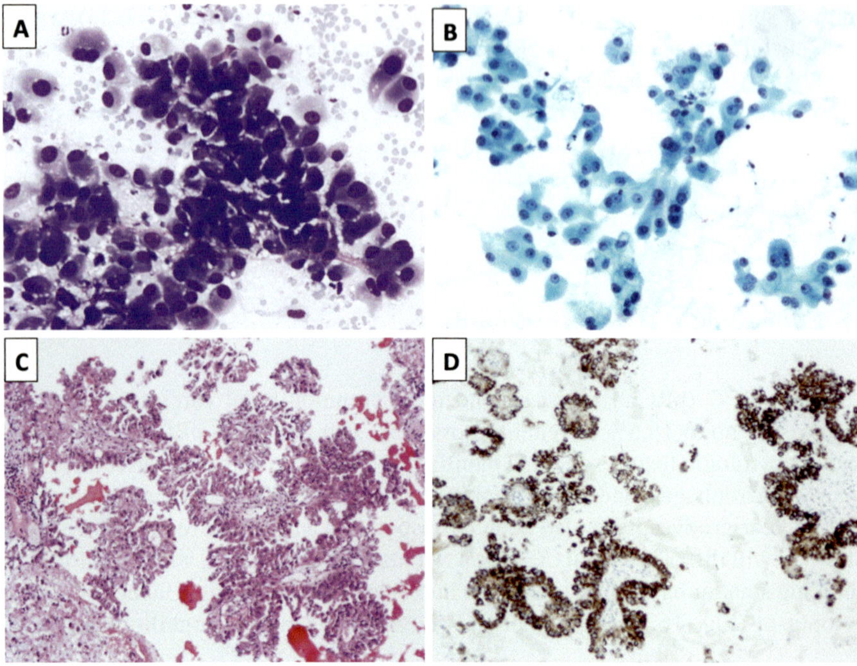

Fig. 16.8 Papillary renal cell carcinoma, type 2. Papillary renal cell carcinoma type 2 has a papillary architecture, however, the cells show more abundant eosinophilic cytoplasm and higher-grade nuclear features (**a**, Diff-Quik, 10× and **b**, Pap, 10×). The nuclear atypia and pseudostratification can be seen on cell block preparations (**c**, H&E, 10×). The tumor showed diffuse staining for AMACR (**d**, 4×), while negative for cathepsin K, TFE3, CAIX, and CK7 (not pictured)

nuclear stratification, and high-grade nuclei with pleomorphic nuclei and visible nucleoli (Fig. 16.8). pRCCs are typically positive for AMACR/racemase and CK7 (diffuse), while negative for CAIX, cathepsin K, and CD117. The immunoperoxidase staining profile can differ slightly between type 1 and type 2 pRCC. In type 2 pRCC, the staining for CK7 can be variable or even negative [25]. Fuhrman grading has been associated with a worse prognosis in pRCC [26]. In one study of 395 patients with pRCC; symptoms at presentation, renal vein tumor thrombus, perinephric/renal sinus fat involvement, advanced stage, coagulative tumor necrosis, sarcomatoid differentiation, and pRCC subtype were associated with a worse prognosis on univariate analysis. Multivariate analysis showed that clinical symptoms, stage group, and grade were maintained as associated with a worse prognosis [26].

Fluorescence in situ hybridization (FISH) for the trisomy 7 and 17, which has been shown to be characteristic of pRCC, can be performed on renal FNA specimens [27]. pRCC type 1 has also been reported to be associated with *MET* gene alterations and treatment with Crizotinib has been shown to be effective in those patients with advanced/metastatic tumors [28].

Chromophobe Renal Cell Carcinoma

Chromophobe renal cell carcinoma (chRCC) is an uncommon variant of RCC, comprising 5–7% of all RCC cases [15]. The cytologic features on fine needle aspiration are characterized by the wrinkled and irregular nuclei with occasional binucleation. There can be nuclear enlargement, hyperchromasia, and pleomorphism that contribute to a koilocytic appearance of the cells [29] (Fig. 16.9). The perinuclear haloes are characteristic on the surgical pathology/histologic sections, but may be subtle to nonexistent in cytology preparations [29]. The cytoplasm is abundant and granular in appearance and can show small cytoplasmic vacuoles that can be accentuated in the perinuclear zone [29]. Distinguishing chRCC from an oncocytoma can be challenging on cytology and core needle biopsies, and has been discussed above under oncocytoma. chRCC can have areas that mimic oncocytoma-type morphology and combined tumors, known as hybrid tumor "oncocytoma–chRCC," can occur, particularly in Birt–Hogg–Dube syndrome and renal oncocytosis [15].

chRCC is positive for CK7 (usually diffuse) and CD117 is also positive, while vimentin is negative. The behavior of these tumors is generally overall favorable (78–100% 5-year survival) [15], however; certain features can portend a worse outcome, including tumor size (>7 cm), small vessel invasion, sarcomatoid differentiation, and microscopic tumor necrosis [30].

Clear Cell Papillary Renal Cell Carcinoma

Clear cell papillary renal cell carcinoma (ccpRCC) is a subtype of RCC that is described as the fourth most common kidney tumor (4% of renal cell carcinomas) [31]. ccpRCC has a very good prognosis, typically presenting with low stage disease and indolent behavior [31].

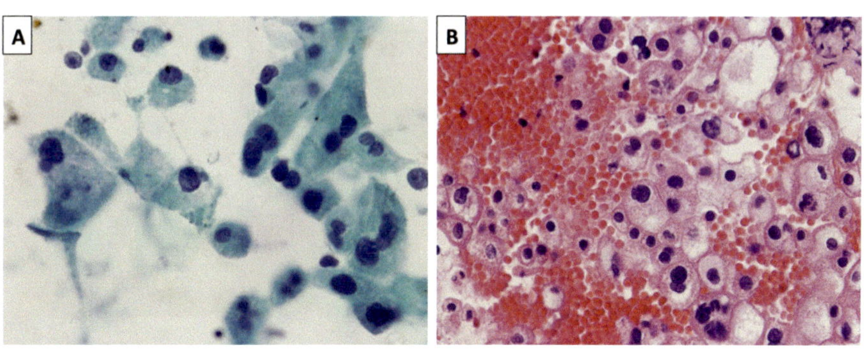

Fig. 16.9 (**a**, **b**) Chromophobe renal cell carcinoma. Chromophobe renal cell carcinoma has cells with abundant eosinophilic cytoplasm, nuclear irregularity, and occasional nucleoli (**a**, Pap 40×). Perinuclear haloes are not necessarily seen on cytology preparations, but can be seen on cell block, which also highlights the nuclear irregularity (**b**, Cell block, 40×)

The tumors are characteristically comprised of clear cells with bland nuclear features, clear cytoplasm, and tumor cell nuclei placed in a linear arrangement away from the basement membrane [31]. The cytologic features most commonly show a nested, papillary, or tubular/acinar growth pattern, columnar to polygonal cell shape, moderate amount of clear to wispy cytoplasm, low-grade nuclei (Fuhrman grades 1–2), and nuclear location at one aspect of the cell [23] (Fig. 16.10). The linear arrangement of the tumor cell nuclei is one of the most helpful and distinctive features. Macrophages have been noted (up to 57% of cases in one study), but are seen scattered in the background and not associated with papillary cores as in pRCC [23].

The differential diagnosis by morphology includes a low-grade ccRCC or pRCC, type 1. The immunoperoxidase staining pattern assists in the differential diagnosis. ccpRCC is typically diffusely positive for CK7, while negative for RCC-marker, and has negative to focal staining for AMACR. In contrast, pRCC will be positive for AMACR and CK7, while negative for RCC-marker. ccRCC will be positive for RCC-marker, while negative for CK7 and AMACR [23, 31]. CAIX is positive in ccpRCC, with characteristically a cup-shaped membranous staining pattern. ccRCC will also be positive for CAIX with complete membranous staining, while pRCC is negative [23].

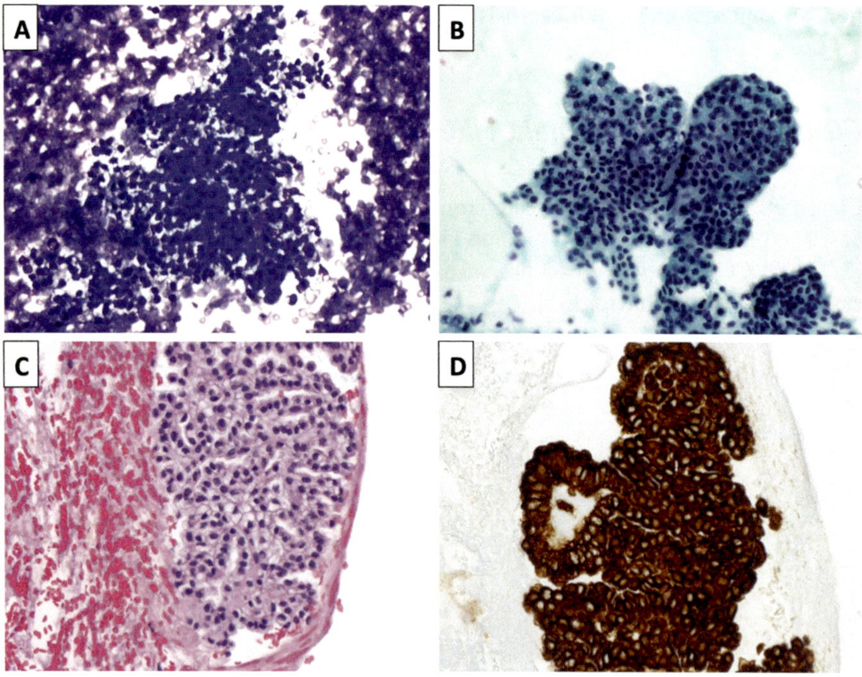

Fig. 16.10 Clear cell papillary renal cell carcinoma. The tumor cells show clusters of cells with clear cytoplasm (**a**, Diff-Quik, 40×). The linear arrangement of the tumor cells and bland nuclear features can be seen on the Pap-stained slides as well as the cell block preparations (**b** and **c**, Pap 40× and H&E 40×). An immunoperoxidase stain for CK7, performed on the cell block preparation, is diffusely positive (**d**, 40×)

MiT Family Translocation Renal Cell Carcinoma

The microphthalmia transcription factor (MiT) family translocation RCC is a category included in the 2016 WHO classification that includes RCCs with gene fusions involving the *TFE3* and *TFEB* gene members of the MiT family of transcription factors [15]. These tumors include most commonly those with Xp11 translocation RCC as well as those with the t(6;11) RCC [32, 33].

These tumors can be challenging to identify due to the broad range of morphology present and are increasingly recognized. The Xp11 translocation RCC classically show high-grade tumor cells with coexistent areas of cells with abundant clear to eosinophilic cytoplasm as well as papillary and nested morphology [32, 33]; cases with oncocytic morphology and papillary morphology have been described. The t(6;11) translocation RCC classically has a predominance of cells with clear to eosinophilic cytoplasm with areas showing small eosinophilic cells with hyperchromatic nuclei and areas of hyalinized structures with basement membrane material with surrounding rosette-like structures, mimicking Call–Exner Bodies. There have been reported examples of both Xp11 translocation RCC and t(6;11) RCC that are indistinguishable from classic ccRCC [32].

The immunoperoxidase staining pattern aids in the differential diagnosis. Xp11 RCC and t(6;11) RCC are negative for pancytokeratin, CAIX, and CK7, and CD117, while both tumors show positivity for cathepsin K. The t(6;11) translocation RCC will also show positivity for melan A and HMB45. Immunoperoxidase staining for transcription factor F3 (TFE3) or transcription factor EB (TFEB), along with FISH testing, will confirm the diagnosis [32, 33]. We recommend pancytokeratin in any RCCs in persons under 30 years of age. If the stain is negative or only weakly/focally positive, the possibility of translocation tumor should be considered and TFE3 or TFEB immunostain or FISH performed to rule out this entity.

The cytologic features of Xp11 translocation RCC have been described in single case reports. Two recent cytologic case reports have described that the tumors have papillary clusters with clear cytoplasm, hyperchromatic nuclei with prominent nucleoli, and rare psammoma bodies [34]. In addition, acellular hyaline nodules can be seen on cytologic smears and within the cell block [34, 35]. Underexpression of cytokeratin and EMA is an important clue if the diagnosis is suspected.

Mucinous Tubular and Spindle Cell Carcinoma

Mucinous tubular and spindle cell carcinoma is a rare renal tumor that occurs more commonly in females. This is another kidney tumor more commonly seen in females than in males. The other tumors with female predominance all begin with the letter "m" and include metanephric adenoma, mixed epithelial and stromal tumor of kidney, and MiT family translocation RCC. The tumor cells of mucinous tubular and spindle cell carcinoma are comprised of bland tubular structures and bland spindled cells that are present in a mucinous stroma [15]. The cytologic features have been described only in rare case reports [36]. FNA shows cellular smears with uniform round to ovoid nuclei in the epithelial (tubular) component, and bland spindled cells in the spindle cell component. Mucoid magenta-colored material can be seen on the Diff-Quik stains [36]. The immunoperoxidase staining pattern is similar to pRCC, with positivity for CK7, AMACR, and PAX2 [15, 37], and may represent a subtype of pRCC [37].

Collecting Duct Carcinoma and Medullary Carcinoma

Collecting duct carcinoma of the kidney is a rare entity (1–2% of renal tumors) [15]. The findings on fine needle aspiration have only been described in small case series and case reports. These tumors are cytologically high-grade tumors with high nuclear to cytoplasmic ratios and show cohesive groups with tubular, solid, or papillary-like growth patterns [38] (Fig. 16.11). Arborizing transgressing epithelium, hobnail nuclear appearance, basal membrane-like substance, and fibrous tissue fragments have also been described [38].

Histologically, these tumors are required to show involvement of the medulla of the kidney, predominant tubular or tubulopapillary morphology, desmoplastic stroma, infiltrating growth, high-grade cytology, and absence of other RCC subtypes or urothelial carcinoma [15]. Most importantly, this diagnosis should be made after exclusion of metastatic tumors, particularly from the lung, colorectum, or breast. It is also important to note if there is a history of sickle cell trait or disease, as renal medullary carcinoma is likely with this morphology. Renal medullary carcinoma has loss of SMARCB1/INI-1 and acquires OCT3/4 expression [15, 39]. PAX-8 can be helpful in excluding urothelial carcinoma (positive in collecting duct/medullary carcinoma, while negative in urothelial carcinomas).

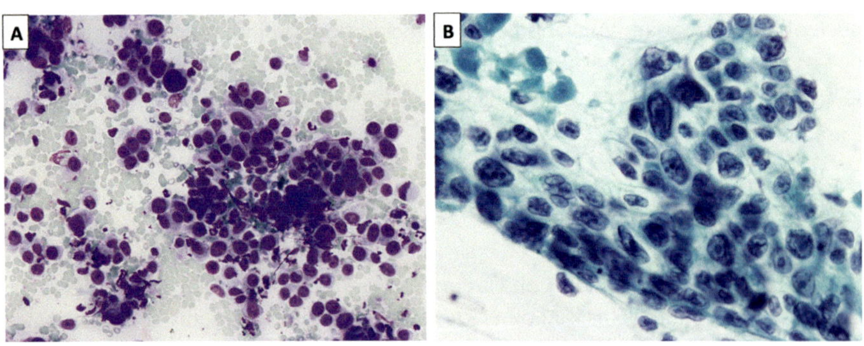

Fig. 16.11 (**a, b**) Medullary carcinoma. The tumor cells show high-grade nuclear cytomorphology with increased nuclear size, pleomorphism, nuclear irregularity, hyperchromasia, and nucleoli (Diff-Quik 40× and Pap 40×). (Photos courtesy of Zulfia McCroskey, MD)

Metastasis/Lymphoma

Involvement of the kidney by metastasis or lymphoma is an important contribution by FNA or core needle biopsy to avoid a potentially unnecessary nephrectomy. In a recent study of 151 patients with metastatic disease to the kidney, the most common sites were lung (43.7%), colorectal (10.6%), head and neck (6%), breast (5.3%), soft tissue (5.3%), and thyroid (5.3%). Interestingly, in this study, the renal metastases were typically solitary (77.5%) [40]; therefore, a helpful clue of bilateral or multifocal masses may not be present. The morphology of the metastatic tumor varies by the primary site; however, immunoperoxidase staining and clinical and imaging history may be necessary to arrive at the correct diagnosis.

Renal lymphoma is uncommon, and can present as either secondary involvement of the kidney by a systemic lymphoma, or as a primary lesion in the kidney, including posttransplant primary renal lymphoma in the transplant population [41]. FNA and/or core needle biopsy can help in confirming the diagnosis. The majority of renal lymphomas are B-cell type [41]. Triage at the time of immediate adequacy is essential in order to obtain material for concurrent flow cytometry. In the case of posttransplant primary renal lymphoma, confirmation by Epstein–Barr virus in situ hybridization (EBV ISH) is important. The cytomorphology seen on the aspirates will vary according to the type of lymphoma. Lymphoglandular bodies can be seen but are not specific. Potential cytologic pitfalls include mistaking spindled cells or the large irregular cells of a large cell lymphoma as carcinoma [41].

Urothelial Carcinoma

Urothelial carcinoma is rarely encountered on FNA, and more likely diagnosed on renal pelvis washings. If present in a FNA, the cytology will show cellular smears with frequent necrosis, papillary clusters, and spindled cells. Nuclear atypia is evident, and occasionally the "cercariform" cellular morphology can be seen (Fig. 16.12). The differential diagnosis will include other high-grade renal tumors (collecting duct carcinoma) or metastasis [10]. Immunoperoxidase staining and clinical and imaging correlation is necessary to reach the correct diagnosis. Urothelial carcinoma is positive for CK7 (up to 100% of cases), CK20 (67% of cases), although there are cases that can be negative for CK7 and CK20 (14% of cases) [15]. GATA-3, uroplakin, high molecular weight keratin, and S-100P are also positive, while PAX-8 and RCC-markers will be negative [15].

Washings or brushings of the renal pelvis or ureter are more commonly encountered as part of the diagnosis for an urothelial carcinoma, or to evaluate for recurrent disease. In general, cytology is not generally reliable for the diagnosis of low-grade lesions (unless well-defined fibrovascular cores with capil-

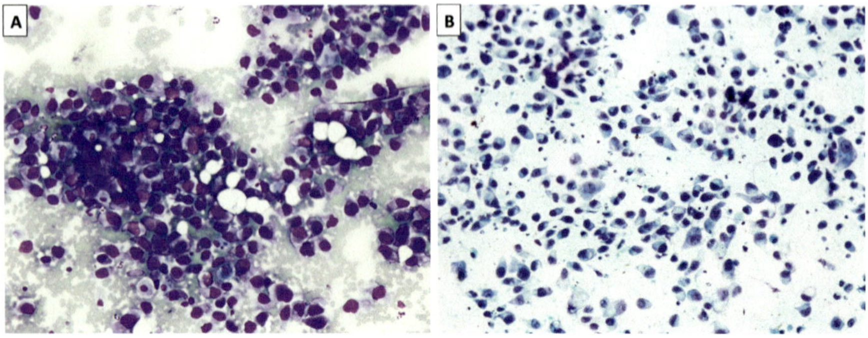

Fig. 16.12 (**a**, **b**) Urothelial carcinoma. The tumor cells show high-grade nuclear cytomorphology, with increased nuclear size and pleomorphism. They can also show a cercariform cytomorphology with nuclear tails (Diff-Quik and Pap stains, both 10×)

laries are present) and should be made with caution [42]. Cytologic evaluation can identify high-grade urothelial lesions with good sensitivity, but cannot distinguish between invasive high-grade urothelial carcinoma versus urothelial carcinoma in situ. According to the Paris System, the criteria for the diagnosis as positive for high-grade urothelial carcinoma/carcinoma in situ include at least 5–10 abnormal cells, although they specifically recommend at least 10 abnormal cells fulfilling the criteria when evaluating the upper urothelial tract. The Paris System also requires a nuclear to cytoplasmic ratio of 0.7 or greater, moderate-to-severe hyperchromasia, markedly irregular nuclear membranes, and coarse/clumped chromatin. Other features can be seen, including squamous or glandular differentiation, cellular pleomorphism with marked variation in size and shape, scant cytoplasm, prominent nucleoli, mitoses, necrosis, or inflammation [42]. Clinical correlation and correlation with concurrent surgical biopsy specimens, if available, are recommended.

Conclusion

Cytology can play an important role in the diagnosis and triage of renal tumors, and immediate assessment is an important component for successful classification and management. Familiarity with the variety of kidney tumors is necessary to provide an accurate differential diagnosis. However, knowledge of the pitfalls and limitations is important, and correlation with clinical, imaging, and concurrent surgical specimens (if available) is essential. Urinary cytology plays an important role in diagnosis of high-grade urothelial tumors, and guidance by the recently released *Paris System for Reporting Urinary Cytology* [41] provides an important framework for evaluation.

References

1. Ha SC, Zlomke HA, Cost N, Wilson S. The past, present, and future in management of small renal masses. J Oncol. 2015;2015:364807.
2. Finelli A, Ismaila N, Russo P. Management of small renal masses: American Society of Clinical Oncology Clinical Practice Guideline Summary. J Oncol Pract. 2017;13(4):276–8.
3. Tannir NM, Jonasch E, Albiges L, Altinmakas E, Ng CS, Matin SF, et al. Everolimus versus sunitinib prospective evaluation in metastatic non-clear cell renal cell carcinoma (ESPN): a randomized multicenter phase 2 trial. Eur Urol. 2016;69(5):866–74.
4. Marconi L, Dabestani S, Lam TB, Hofmann F, Stewart F, Norrie J, et al. Systematic review and meta-analysis of diagnostic accuracy of percutaneous renal tumour biopsy. Eur Urol. 2016;69(4):660–73.
5. Yang CS, Choi E, Idrees MT, Chen S, Wu HH. Percutaneous biopsy of the renal mass: FNA or core needle biopsy? Cancer Cytopathol. 2017;125(6):407–15.
6. Parks GE, Perkins LA, Zagoria RJ, Garvin AJ, Sirintrapun SJ, Geisinger KR. Benefits of a combined approach to sampling of renal neoplasms as demonstrated in a series of 351 cases. Am J Surg Pathol. 2011;35(6):827–35.
7. Masoom S, Venkataraman G, Jensen J, Flanigan RC, Wojcik EM. Renal FNA-based typing of renal masses remains a useful adjunctive modality: evaluation of 31 renal masses with correlative histology. Cytopathology: Off J Br Soc Clin Cytol. 2009;20(1):50–5.
8. Adeniran AJ, Al-Ahmadie H, Iyengar P, Reuter VE, Lin O. Fine needle aspiration of renal cortical lesions in adults. Diagn Cytopathol. 2010;38(10):710–5.
9. Volpe A, Kachura JR, Geddie WR, Evans AJ, Gharajeh A, Saravanan A, et al. Techniques, safety and accuracy of sampling of renal tumors by fine needle aspiration and core biopsy. J Urol. 2007;178(2):379–86.
10. Truong LD, Todd TD, Dhurandhar B, Ramzy I. Fine-needle aspiration of renal masses in adults: analysis of results and diagnostic problems in 108 cases. Diagn Cytopathol. 1999;20(6):339–49.
11. Merritt AJ, Thiryayi SA, Rana DN. Malakoplakia diagnosed by fine needle aspiration (FNA) and liquid-based cytology (LBC) presenting as a pararenal mass in a transplant kidney. Cytopathology: Off J Br Soc Clin Cytol. 2014;25(4):276–7.
12. Li L, Parwani AV. Xanthogranulomatous pyelonephritis. Arch Pathol Lab Med. 2011;135(5):671–4.
13. Bosniak MA. The Bosniak renal cyst classification: 25 years later. Radiology. 2012;262(3):781–5.
14. Todd TD, Dhurandhar B, Mody D, Ramzy I, Truong LD. Fine-needle aspiration of cystic lesions of the kidney. Morphologic spectrum and diagnostic problems in 41 cases. Am J Clin Pathol. 1999;111(3):317–28.
15. PAH HM, Ulbright TM, Reuter VE, editors. WHO classification of tumours of the urinary system and male genital organs. 4th ed. Lyon: International Agency for Research on Cancer; 2016.
16. Aydin H, Magi-Galluzzi C, Lane BR, Sercia L, Lopez JI, Rini BI, et al. Renal angiomyolipoma: clinicopathologic study of 194 cases with emphasis on the epithelioid histology and tuberous sclerosis association. Am J Surg Pathol. 2009;33(2):289–97.
17. Zhou H, Guo M, Gong Y. Challenge of FNA diagnosis of angiomyolipoma: a study of 33 cases. Cancer Cytopathol. 2017;125(4):257–66.
18. Wobker SE, Williamson SR. Modern pathologic diagnosis of renal Oncocytoma. J Kidney Cancer VHL. 2017;4(4):1–12.
19. Blanco LZ Jr, Schein CO, Patel T, Heagley DE, Cimbaluk DJ, Reddy V, et al. Fine-needle aspiration of metanephric adenoma of the kidney with clinical, radiographic and histopathologic correlation: a review. Diagn Cytopathol. 2013;41(8):742–51.

20. Perez-Ordonez B, Hamed G, Campbell S, Erlandson RA, Russo P, Gaudin PB, et al. Renal oncocytoma: a clinicopathologic study of 70 cases. Am J Surg Pathol. 1997;21(8):871–83.
21. Wu A. Oncocytic renal neoplasms on resections and core biopsies: our approach to this challenging differential diagnosis. Arch Pathol Lab Med. 2017;141(10):1336–41.
22. Liu J, Fanning CV. Can renal oncocytomas be distinguished from renal cell carcinoma on fine-needle aspiration specimens? A study of conventional smears in conjunction with ancillary studies. Cancer. 2001;93(6):390–7.
23. Lin X. Cytomorphology of clear cell papillary renal cell carcinoma. Cancer Cytopathol. 2017;125(1):48–54.
24. Granter SR, Perez-Atayde AR, Renshaw AA. Cytologic analysis of papillary renal cell carcinoma. Cancer. 1998;84(5):303–8.
25. Reuter VE, Argani P, Zhou M, Delahunt B. Best practices recommendations in the application of immunohistochemistry in the kidney tumors: report from the International Society of Urologic Pathology consensus conference. Am J Surg Pathol. 2014;38(8):e35–49.
26. Sukov WR, Lohse CM, Leibovich BC, Thompson RH, Cheville JC. Clinical and pathological features associated with prognosis in patients with papillary renal cell carcinoma. J Urol. 2012;187(1):54–9.
27. Roh MH, Dal Cin P, Silverman SG, Cibas ES. The application of cytogenetics and fluorescence in situ hybridization to fine-needle aspiration in the diagnosis and subclassification of renal neoplasms. Cancer Cytopathol. 2010;118(3):137–45.
28. Schoffski P, Wozniak A, Escudier B, Rutkowski P, Anthoney A, Bauer S, et al. Crizotinib achieves long-lasting disease control in advanced papillary renal-cell carcinoma type 1 patients with MET mutations or amplification. EORTC 90101 CREATE trial. Eur J Cancer (Oxford, England : 1990). 2017;87:147–63.
29. Granter SR, Renshaw AA. Fine-needle aspiration of chromophobe renal cell carcinoma. Analysis of six cases. Cancer. 1997;81(2):122–8.
30. Przybycin CG, Cronin AM, Darvishian F, Gopalan A, Al-Ahmadie HA, Fine SW, et al. Chromophobe renal cell carcinoma: a clinicopathologic study of 203 tumors in 200 patients with primary resection at a single institution. Am J Surg Pathol. 2011;35(7):962–70.
31. Zhou H, Zheng S, Truong LD, Ro JY, Ayala AG, Shen SS. Clear cell papillary renal cell carcinoma is the fourth most common histologic type of renal cell carcinoma in 290 consecutive nephrectomies for renal cell carcinoma. Hum Pathol. 2014;45(1):59–64.
32. Argani P. MiT family translocation renal cell carcinoma. Semin Diagn Pathol. 2015;32(2):103–13.
33. Magers MJ, Udager AM, Mehra R. MiT family translocation-associated renal cell carcinoma: a contemporary update with emphasis on morphologic, immunophenotypic, and molecular mimics. Arch Pathol Lab Med. 2015;139(10):1224–33.
34. El Naili R, Nicolas M, Gorena A, Policarpio-Nicolas ML. Fine-needle aspiration findings of Xp11 translocation renal cell carcinoma metastatic to a hilar lymph node. Diagn Cytopathol. 2017;45(5):456–62.
35. Manucha V, Sessums MT, Lewin J, Akhtar I. Cyto-histological correlation of Xp11.2 translocation/TFE3 gene fusion associated renal cell carcinoma: report of a case with review of literature. Diagn Cytopathol. 2018;46(3):267–70.
36. Huimiao J, Chepovetsky J, Zhou M, Sun W, Simsir A, Cohen D, et al. Mucinous tubular and spindle cell carcinoma of the kidney: diagnosis by fine needle aspiration and review of the literature. CytoJournal. 2015;12:28.
37. Shen SS, Ro JY, Tamboli P, Truong LD, Zhai Q, Jung SJ, et al. Mucinous tubular and spindle cell carcinoma of kidney is probably a variant of papillary renal cell carcinoma with spindle cell features. Ann Diagn Pathol. 2007;11(1):13–21.
38. Sironi M, Delpiano C, Claren R, Spinelli M. New cytological findings on fine-needle aspiration of renal collecting duct carcinoma. Diagn Cytopathol. 2003;29(4):239–40.

39. Amin MB, Smith SC, Agaimy A, Argani P, Comperat EM, Delahunt B, et al. Collecting duct carcinoma versus renal medullary carcinoma: an appeal for nosologic and biological clarity. Am J Surg Pathol. 2014;38(7):871–4.
40. Zhou C, Urbauer DL, Fellman BM, Tamboli P, Zhang M, Matin SF, et al. Metastases to the kidney: a comprehensive analysis of 151 patients from a tertiary referral centre. BJU Int. 2016;117(5):775–82.
41. Truong LD, Caraway N, Ngo T, Laucirica R, Katz R, Ramzy I. Renal lymphoma. The diagnostic and therapeutic roles of fine-needle aspiration. Am J Clin Pathol. 2001;115(1):18–31.
42. Rosenthal EMW DL, Kurtycz DFI, editors. The Paris system for reporting urinary cytology. Switzerland: Springer; 2016.

Part III
Diagnostic Imaging

Chapter 17
Diagnostic Imaging in Renal Tumors

Mi-hyun Kim and Kyoung-Sik Cho

Kidney cancer is the sixth and tenth most common malignancy in males and females expected to occur in the United States in 2018, with estimated 73,820 new cases of kidney cancer (44,120 in men and 29,700 in women) in 2019. The total number of estimated deaths from kidney cancer is 14,770 people (9,820 men and 4,950 women) in the United States, in 2019 [1]. Kidney cancer is more common in men, with an approximate ratio of 2:1 (male: female), and rare in children. Multidetector computed tomography (MDCT) is the most commonly used method for evaluation and staging of kidney cancer. In addition to computed tomography (CT), magnetic resonance imaging (MRI) or ultrasound (US) are also used. US is a classic screening method of renal tumors, and MRI is used for more detailed analysis.

Computed Tomography

MDCT examination is routinely used for the evaluation of renal tumors in the clinical practice. It is possible to estimate the degree of enhancement and the presence of macroscopic fat, calcification, and hemorrhagic or proteinaceous material within the tumor by using unenhanced scans [2]. In addition to unenhanced scans, dynamic time-delay contrast-enhanced CT images can be obtained at different combinations of corticomedullary, nephrographic, and excretory phases. Helical CT, which enables rapid coverage of the abdominopelvic cavity and intravenous administration of iodinated contrast agent, has improved the diagnostic performance of CT in the evaluation of renal masses [3]. The multiplanar reconstruction capabilities, such

M.-h. Kim · K.-S. Cho (✉)
Department of Radiology, Research Institute of Radiology, Asan Medical Center, University of Ulsan College of Medicine, Seoul, South Korea
e-mail: kscho@amc.seoul.kr

M. K. Divatia et al. (eds.), *Kidney Cancer*, https://doi.org/10.1007/978-3-030-28333-9_17

as coronal and sagittal directions of MDCT, enable accurate analysis of renal tumor location and size.

Renal Cell Carcinoma Subtypes

Renal cell carcinoma (RCC) is the most common malignant renal tumor, accounting for more than 90% of all renal cancers, and 2–3% of all adult cancers [4]. RCC is now regarded as a clinicopathologically heterogeneous lesion, which is categorized as a clear cell, papillary, chromophobe, multilocular cystic renal neoplasm of low malignancy potential, collecting duct carcinoma (CDC), renal medullary carcinoma, and other miscellaneous cancers on the revised 2016 World Health Organization (WHO) classification [5] (Table 17.1). The histopathological entities differ in their prognosis, biologic behavior, and response to available therapies. According to the histologic subtypes of RCCs, imaging findings are also different (Fig. 17.1). Clear cell RCC is the most common adult RCC, and typically enhances strongly and heterogeneously in MDCT scans. Several investigators have shown that clear cell RCC is enhanced to a greater extent, and is more heterogeneous than other histologic subtypes in MDCT scans. While the larger parts of clear cell RCCs show these characteristics, other areas enhance poorly and homogeneously, overlapping with imaging features of the non-clear cell RCCs, such as papillary or chromophobe types [6]. Papillary RCC is usually hypovascular and demonstrates homogeneous enhancement, which is less than in the clear cell subtype, during the corticomedullary phase on dynamic CT scans [7]. Chromophobe RCCs also are less hypervascular than clear cell RCCs and have a propensity for higher peripheral enhancement. However, these characteristics are not sufficient to differentiate

Table 17.1 WHO classification of renal cell tumors

Clear cell RCC
Multilocular cystic renal cell neoplasm of low malignant potential
Papillary RCC
Hereditary leiomyomatosis and RCC-associated RCC
Chromophobe RCC
Collecting duct carcinoma
Renal medullary carcinoma
MiT family translocation RCC
Succinate dehydrogenase-deficient RCC
Mucinous tubular and spindle cell carcinoma
Tubulocystic RCC
Acquired cystic disease-associated RCC
Clear cell papillary RCC
RCC, unclassified
Papillary adenoma
Oncocytoma

From Moch et al. [5], with permission

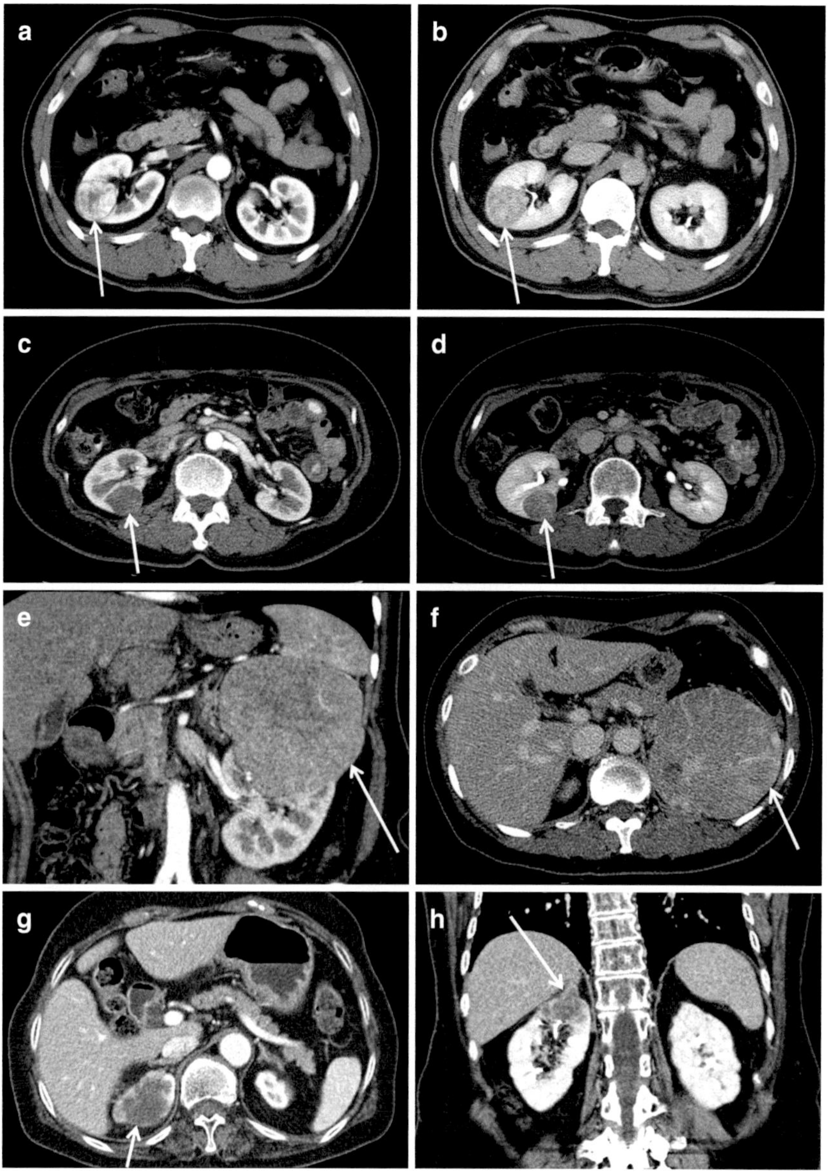

Fig. 17.1 CT appearances of various RCCs. (**a**, **b**) Clear cell RCC in 50-year-old man. CT scans of TNM stage T1a tumor in corticomedullary (**a**) and excretory (**b**) phases show typical hypervascularity of tumor (arrow, **a**) and subsequent washout (arrow, **b**). (**c**, **d**) Papillary RCC in 52-year-old woman. CT scans of TNM stage T1a tumor in corticomedullary (**c**) and excretory (**d**) phases show typical hypovascularity of tumor (arrows, **c, d**). (**e**, **f**) Chromophobe RCC in 42-year-old woman. CT scans of TNM stage T2b tumor in coronal corticomedullary (**e**) and axial excretory (**f**) phases scans show hypovascularity of tumor (arrows, **e**, **f**). (**g**, **h**) Collecting duct carcinoma in 72-year-old woman. CT scans of TNM stage T4 tumor in the axial corticomedullary (**g**) and coronal excretory (**h**) phases scans show infiltrative growth pattern and heterogeneous enhancement with areas of necrosis (arrow, **g**). Direct extension of the tumor to the ipsilateral adrenal gland is noted (arrow, **h**)

between chromophobe and other types of RCCs. Despite their large size, chromophobe RCCs are classically known to show relatively homogeneous enhancement at CT [8]. However, in a recent study, chromophobe RCCs have been found to have a wider spectrum of CT features than previously reported, although they have a greater propensity for homogeneity and the presence of a central scar or necrosis [9]. CDC of the kidney is a highly aggressive subtype, and shows an infiltrative growth pattern and heterogeneous enhancement with intratumoral necrosis, hemorrhage, and calcification on imaging [8].

RCC Staging

Accurate radiological staging of RCC is crucial to allow appropriate management decisions. The *American Joint Committee on Cancer Staging Manual*, 8th edition, TNM staging is commonly used to stage renal cell cancer [10]. The primary tumor T stages are listed in Table 17.2. CT is the modality of choice in RCC staging. In patients with RCC confined to the kidney, differentiation between T1 and T2 depends on tumor size. The recent modification of the T stage, separating tumors 7 cm or less in diameter (stages T1a and T1b) from those greater than 7 cm (stages T2a and T2b) reflects the importance of tumor size on survival and prognosis [10]. Therefore, accurate measurement of tumor size on CT is crucial. Radiologic findings suggesting perinephric fat tissue invasion (T3a stage) consist of large tumor

Table 17.2 Definition of primary tumor (T)

T categories for kidney cancer	
Tx	Primary tumor cannot be assessed
T0	No evidence of primary tumor
T1	*Tumor 7 cm or less in greatest dimension, limited to kidney*
T1a	Tumor 4 cm or less in greatest dimension, limited to kidney
T1b	Tumor more than 4 cm but not 7 cm in greatest dimension, limited to kidney
T2	*Tumor more than 7 cm in greatest dimension, limited to kidney*
T2a	Tumor more than 7 cm but less than or equal to 10 cm in greatest dimension, limited to kidney
T2b	Tumor more than 10 cm in greatest dimension, limited to kidney
T3	*Tumor extends into major veins or perinephric tissues but not into the ipsilateral adrenal gland and not beyond Gerota's fascia*
T3a	Tumor extends into the renal vein or its segmental veins branches, or invades pelvicalyceal system, or invades perirenal and/or renal sinus fat but not beyond Gerota's fascia
T3b	Tumor grossly extends into the vena cava below the diaphragm
T3c	Tumor grossly extends into the vena cava above the diaphragm or invades the wall of the vena cava
T4	*Tumor invades beyond Gerota's fascia (including contiguous extension into the ipsilateral adrenal gland)*

size, fat infiltration with a nodular appearance, irregular tumor margin, collateral vessels, and fascial thickening [11]. RCC has a tendency to extend into the venous system, and accurate preoperative evaluation of the renal vein and inferior vena cava (IVC) extension is essential. Findings of the renal vein (stage T3a) or vena cava extension of tumor (stages T3b or T3c) are low attenuation filling defect within the renal vein or vena cava (Fig. 17.2). Other helpful ancillary signs include abrupt change in the diameter of the renal vein and presence of a clot within the collateral veins. The presence or absence of thrombus enhancement assists in distinguishing malignant tumor thrombus from bland thrombus. Heterogeneous enhancement of the thrombus on contrast-enhanced CT scan indicates neovascularity, thus suggesting tumoral thrombus. Direct continuity of the thrombus with the primary renal tumor also suggests tumoral thrombus. If the tumor extends within the IVC, accurate delineation of the superior margin of the thrombus is pivotal for differentiation between stages T3b and T3c. In stage T4, loss of tissue planes and irregular margins between the tumor and surrounding structures can be seen on the contrast-enhanced CT scan (Fig. 17. 3).

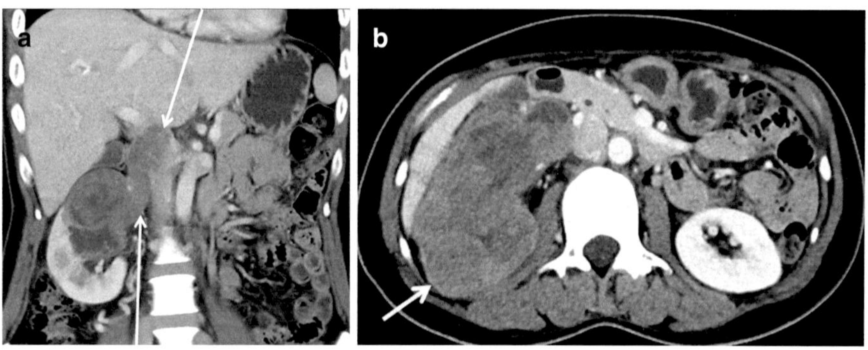

Fig. 17.2 Venous involvement of renal vein and IVC. (**a**) Enhanced coronal CT scan of 46-year-old man shows enhancing tumor thrombus (arrows, **a**) in the expanded right renal vein and IVC (TNM stage T3b). (**b**) Mixed clear cell and papillary renal cell RCC (12 cm) in the right kidney on axial nephrogenic (**b**) phase (arrow, **b**)

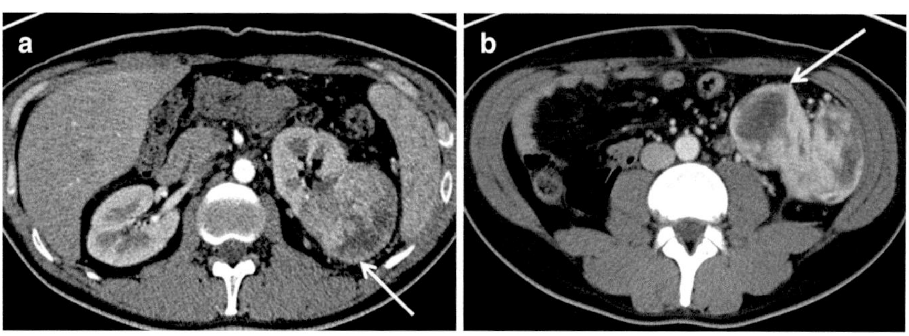

Fig. 17. 3 Tumor invasion beyond Gerota's fascia (TNM stage T4). (**a**) Axial corticomedullary CT scan in 33-year-old man shows heterogeneous enhancing mass in the left kidney (arrow, **a**). (**b**) Enhanced axial CT scan of the left lower perinephric space shows anterior bulging of tumor with high suspicion of Gerota's fascial invasion by the tumor (arrow, **b**)

Lymph node metastasis of RCC is relatively infrequent. For CT diagnosis of lymph node metastases, the nodal size should be greater than 1 cm in the short-axis diameter. However, in RCC, reactive nodal hyperplasia is often seen, likely due to reactive immune response associated with extensive tumoral necrosis or venous thrombosis. The enhancement pattern of the lymph node may also help differentiate reactive from malignant adenopathy. The metastatic nodes can show avid enhancement, especially if the primary tumor is very vascular. RCCs usually metastasize to the lungs, mediastinum, bones, and liver. Less common sites are the contralateral kidney, adrenal gland, brain, pancreas, mesentery, and abdominal wall [12].

Small Renal Tumors

With the rapidly growing use of imaging studies, particularly during follow-up testing for another tumor, the incidental detection of small renal tumors (less than 4 cm in size) also continues to increase. Pathologically, small renal tumors can be characterized as RCCs and benign tumors, such as oncocytomas and angiomyolipomas (AMLs). According to a previous report [13], the likelihood of a benign lesion increases with decreasing size of the tumor. There is a direct relationship between malignancy and the size of the mass: The smaller the renal mass, the greater the percentage of benign causes. When stratified according to size, the proportion of benign masses is 25% among masses smaller than 3 cm, 30% among masses less than 2 cm, and 44% among masses smaller than 1 cm [14]. However, current imaging techniques have low accuracy in differentiating between RCCs and a number of benign tumors. Imaging findings alone are not sufficient to predict the biologic behavior of renal tumors.

In one study, 43% of the patients underwent unnecessary radical nephrectomy because their benign tumors were incorrectly diagnosed as malignant on preoperative imaging [15]. In the series of Frank et al. [16], 65% of benign lesions were treated with radical nephrectomy. Various clinical and imaging findings, such as the patient's sex, tumor growth rate, special imaging studies including MRI, and the presence of central scar in the oncocytoma were helpful but insufficient to differentiate between malignant and benign tumors [13]. Therefore, in the clinical practice, percutaneous biopsy of small renal mass is steadily increasing to avoid unnecessary surgery. According to the tumor location or tumor size, biopsy is performed with the guidance of ultrasound (US) or CT (Fig. 17.4 and 17.5). The most important task in small renal tumor biopsy is the extraction of sufficient and adequate specimen, which ensures accurate histologic diagnosis. Radiologists should always strive to acquire sufficient sample with optimizing patient position and angle of inserted needle and choosing the adequate modality for the biopsy (including US or CT). Accurate tumor targeting is mandatory for optimal diagnosis, which depends on the tumor size, location, the patient's weight, and the patient's ability to hold breath. To some extent, endophytic renal masses are special in clinical management and choice

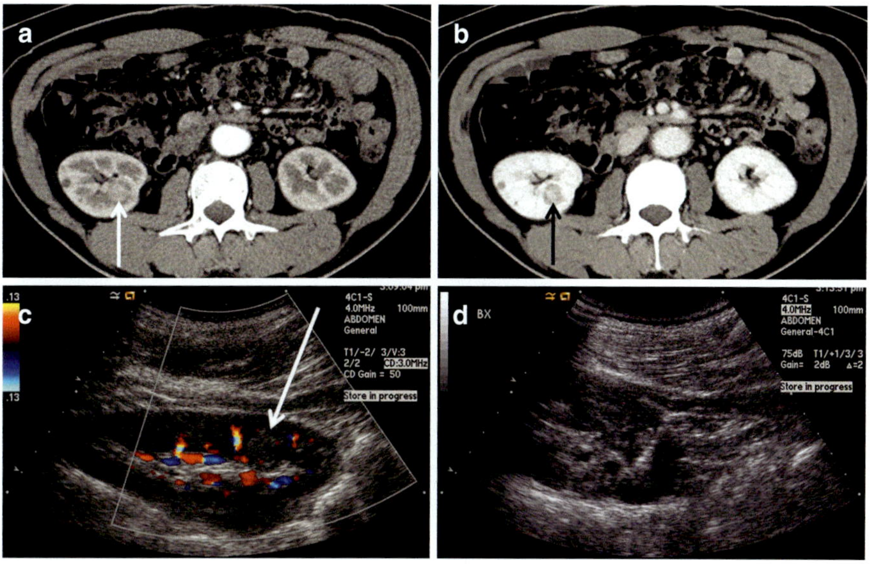

Fig. 17.4 US-guided biopsy of small renal mass in 50-year-old man. (**a, b**) Corticomedullary (**a**) and nephrogenic (**b**) phases of CT scan show an enhancing mass (1.4 cm) in the right kidney lower pole (arrows **a**, **b**). (**c**) Doppler US image shows a subtle hyperechoic mass (1.4 cm) in the right kidney (arrow). (**d**) US-guided percutaneous biopsy was performed, and pathology showed clear cell RCC

of biopsy technique. It is generally agreed on that partial nephrectomy is more challenging for endophytic than exophytic lesions [17]. Challenging tumors are endophytic, hilar, or posterior upper pole masses, and laparoscopic partial nephrectomy of these tumors resulted in higher rates of collecting system repair [18]. From a radiological point of view, it is nearly impossible to detect an isoechoic, endophytic small renal mass on US due to similar echogenicity with the normal renal parenchyma. Therefore, in these cases, CT-guided biopsy instead of US-guided biopsy should be considered. Although hypo- or hyperechoic renal masses can be detected on US, it is difficult to perform biopsy percutaneously under the US-guidance for medial or upper located tumors because the liver, basal lung, or lower ribs can shield the renal tumor along the ultrasound beam pathway. In these cases, CT-guided biopsy with the patient in prone position is useful. The possible advantages of CT guidance compared with US guidance for renal mass biopsy are 1) better visualization of detailed anatomic structures, which avoids inadvertent puncture of vascular elements and other solid organs, and 2) accurate detection and targeting of small renal masses with or without contrast enhancement. However, CT-guided biopsy has two main drawbacks: Patients receive a radiation dose and an injection of contrast medium. The goal of CT at the time of biopsy is only to distinguish between a small renal mass and the renal parenchyma—not to characterize the small renal mass; hence, the radiation dose and amount of contrast medium should be low and adverse impact to the patient is negligible. In a previous report [19], biopsy was

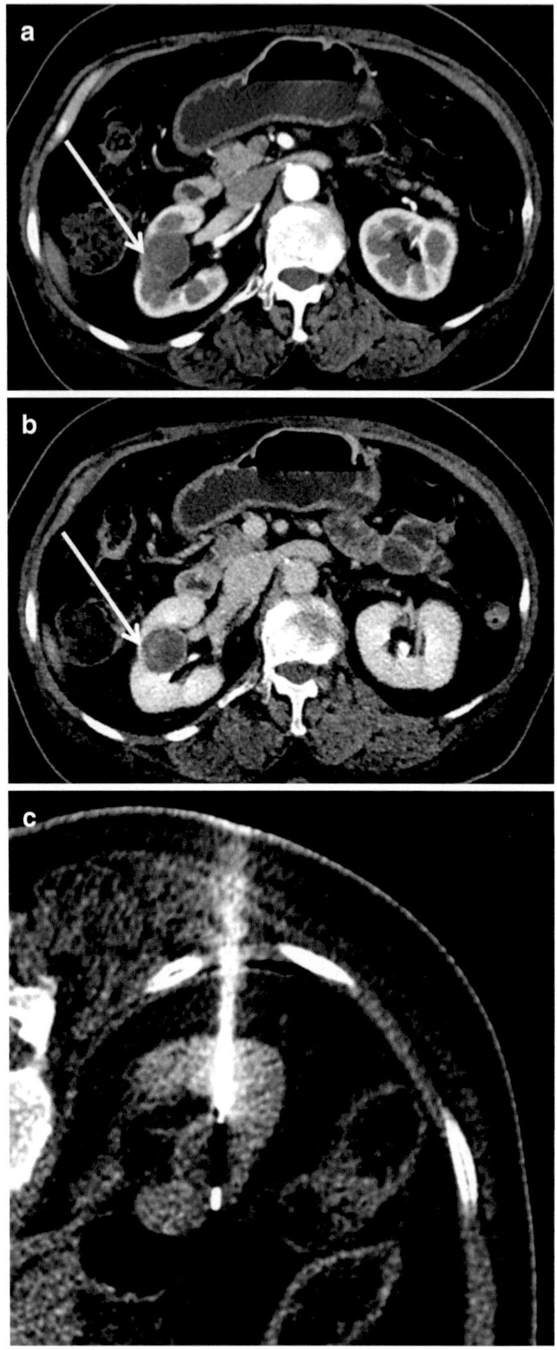

Fig. 17.5 CT-guided biopsy of small renal mass in 69-year-old woman. (**a**, **b**) Corticomedullary (**a**) and excretory (**b**) phases show a hypovascular mass (2.4 cm) in the right kidney mid pole, protruding to the renal sinus fat and abutting the renal venous branch and calyx (arrows, **a**, **b**). (**c**) CT-guided biopsy was performed with 18-gauge needle in prone position

performed with guidance using a reduced-dose CT protocol, and gives diagnostic results similar to a standard-dose CT protocol without any increase in complication rate or procedure duration. Skilled radiologists using both US- and CT-guided biopsy techniques can perform biopsies of almost all small renal masses. However, solid masses smaller than 1 cm are challenging. It is often difficult to characterize a solid and enhancing mass smaller than 1 cm, despite an advanced technique using MDCT and MR. Accurate targeting of biopsy for the small renal masses less than 1 cm in size is nearly impossible. Therefore, if there is a solid mass less than 1 cm in size, imaging follow-up is recommended until the mass reaches ≥1 cm in size. The most probable diagnosis of small renal tumor between 1 cm and 3 cm is RCC, and surgical removal is recommended. However, if the mass showed hyperattenuation and homogeneous enhancement, further evaluation with MR or percutaneous biopsy can be considered to rule out AML with minimal fat [20].

Magnetic Resonance Imaging (MRI)

The kidney MRI protocols generally consist of T2-weighted imaging, diffusion-weighted imaging (DWI), and T1-weighted dual echo in-phase and opposed-phase imaging. If the patients already have performed contrast-enhanced CT scan, contrast-enhanced MRI is optional because contrast-enhanced CT scan is enough for the evaluation of the renal tumor. T2-weighted images are most helpful in distinguishing simple renal cysts from other lesions. A homogeneous hyperintense lesion with a thin wall on T2-weighted images can be accurately characterized as a simple cyst. The presence of enhancement within a renal lesion after the administration of gadolinium-based contrast agent is the most reliable finding for distinguishing solid masses from pure cysts. In-phase and opposed-phase T1-weighted imaging is useful in the detection of intratumoral microscopic fat. Subtraction imaging is a technique whereby an unenhanced T1-weighted sequence is digitally subtracted from the identical sequence performed after gadolinium administration. By performing this technique, any native T1 signal is removed and the remaining signal on the subtracted images is only due to enhancement [21]. Subtraction images can facilitate the detection of small enhancing components within a cystic renal lesion, particularly when intralesional hemorrhagic or proteinaceous contents generate high signal intensity on unenhanced T1-weighted images, thereby making the detection of enhancement within the lesion challenging (Fig. 17.6) [22].

RCC Subtype Analysis

Differentiation among the RCC subtypes is important, because prognosis and management are different depending on the RCC subtype. For example, papillary RCC tends to have a more favorable prognosis than clear cell RCC. Therefore, preoperative diagnosis and differentiation of RCC subtype can help clinicians select the

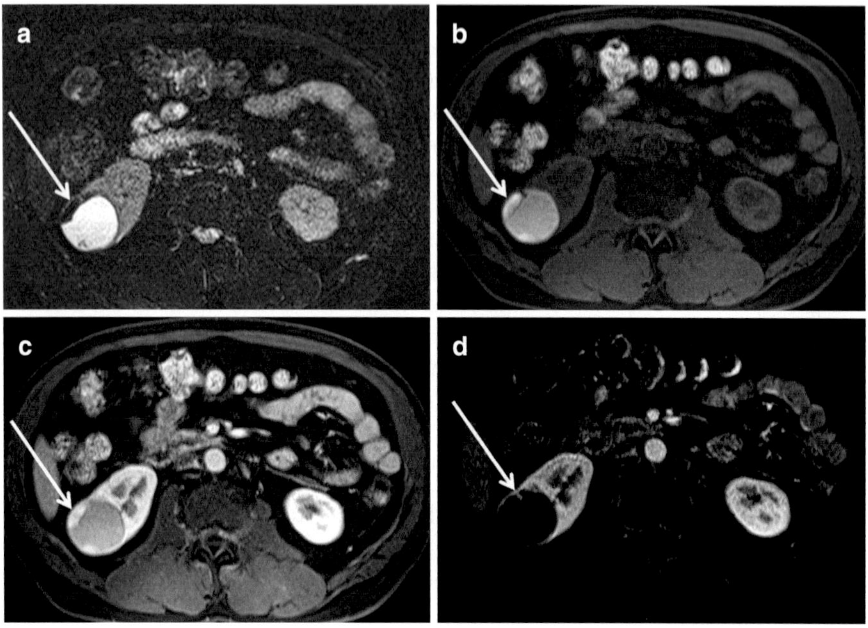

Fig. 17.6 Predominantly hemorrhagic cystic mass in 59-year-old man. (**a**) Axial fat-suppressed T2-weighted MR image shows mass in the right kidney upper pole with predominantly high signal intensity, suggestive of fluid content. Eccentric T2 dark signal intensity mural nodule is also noted (arrow, **a**). (**b**, **c**) Axial unenhanced T1 volumetric interpolated breath-hold examination (VIBE) fat saturated image (**b**) and corticomedullary phase of an axial T1 VIBE fat saturated image (**c**) show T1 high signal intensity mass (arrows, **b**, **c**). Evaluation of the enhancing portion within the mass is limited due to T1 high signal intensity on unenhanced T1 VIBE image. (**d**) Axial subtraction of images (contrast-enhanced corticomedullary phase image (**c**) – unenhanced image (**b**)) shows septal enhancement at the periphery of the mass (arrow, **d**). On the basis of this finding, this hemorrhagic cyst is characterized as Bosniak category III

appropriate treatment modality, such as percutaneous ablation, cryosurgery, cyberknife, active surveillance, and surgical resection. According to previous studies, most papillary RCCs and clear cell RCCs are hypointense and hyperintense on T2-weighted images, respectively. T2 hypointensity of papillary RCCs correlated with predominant papillary architecture on pathology [23]. Clear cell RCCs usually demonstrate increased signal intensity on T2-weighted images and signal intensity similar to that of the renal parenchyma on T1-weighted images. Focal loss of signal intensity within the solid portion of clear cell RCCs on T1 opposed-phase imaging compared to T1 in-phase imaging is attributed to intracytoplasmic fat, and has been observed in up to 60% of tumors [24]. Central necrosis is common, and presents as a moderate to high signal intensity on T2-weighted imaging, although occasionally it can appear hypointense. Intratumoral hemorrhage can occur, and has a variable MR appearance depending on the stage of degradation and oxygenation of blood products. Clear cell RCCs tend to be hypervascular, with heterogeneous enhancement during the arterial phase. Renal vein tumor thrombi can be seen, especially in large tumors. On MR imaging, papillary RCCs show homogeneous low signal intensity on T2-weighted images, with homogeneous low-grade enhancement (Fig. 17.7). Chromophobe RCCs account for about 4–11% of RCCs. Central necrosis is usually absent, even in very large chromophobe RCCs [22]. On dynamic contrast-enhanced MRI, the relative signal intensity of clear cell RCCs was significantly greater than that of non-clear cell RCCs in the corticomedullary, nephrographic, and excretory phases. Similar to CT images, clear cell and papillary RCCs exhibited the most and least avid enhancement on the three contrast-enhanced phases, respectively. Chromophobe RCCs exhibited intermediate enhancement in avidity across the three contrast-enhanced phases [25]. In addition,

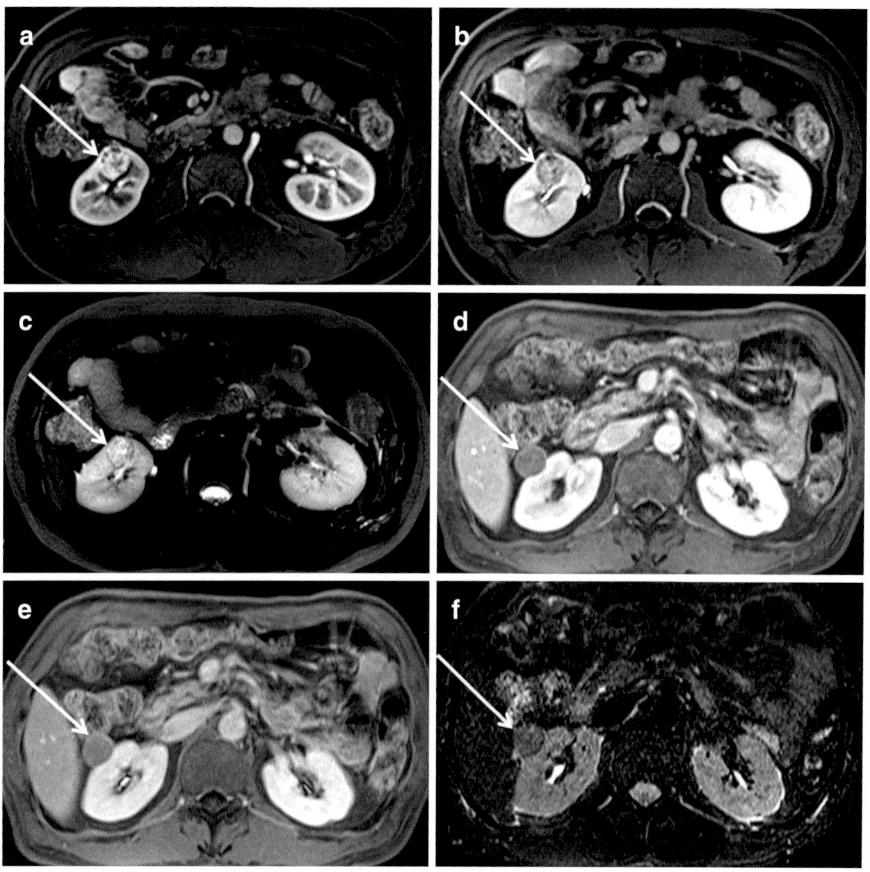

Fig. 17.7 MR appearances of various RCCs. (**a**–**c**) Clear cell RCC in 37-year-old man. MR images of TNM stage T1a tumor in corticomedullary (**a**) and excretory phases (**b**) show typical hypervascularity of tumor (arrow, **a**) and subsequent washout (arrow, **b**). On fat-suppressed T2-weighted image (**c**), the tumor shows heterogeneous hyperintensity (arrow, **c**). (**d**–**f**) Papillary RCC in 57-year-old woman. MR images of TNM stage T1a tumor in corticomedullary (**d**) and excretory (**e**) phases show typical hypovascularity of tumor (arrows, **d**, **e**). On fat-suppressed T2-weighted image (**f**), the tumor shows homogeneous hypointensity

hypervascular and hypovascular renal tumors demonstrate different patterns of enhancement. On both corticomedullary and nephrographic phase images, hypervascular tumors such as clear cell RCCs showed greater changes in signal intensity than hypovascular tumors such as papillary RCCs. Chromophobe RCCs showed intermediate changes in signal intensity [26]. In addition to the T2 signal intensity and enhancement pattern, DWI is also helpful to differentiate RCC subtypes and evaluate tumor grade/aggressiveness. DWI reflects the degree of water motion within the tumor, which is affected by cellularity or tissue organization. On the basis of the DWI principles, the degree of water motion is associated with the WHO/International Society of Urological Pathology (ISUP) nuclear grading system (Fuhrman grade) of RCCs. In a recent study, DWI showed moderate diagnostic performance in differentiating high- from low-grade clear cell RCCs [27]. The apparent diffusion coefficient (ADC) provides a measure of water diffusion within the tumor and it is commonly calculated using MRI with DWI. Clear cell RCCs had significantly higher ADC values, higher peak enhancement, and higher washout rates than non-clear cell RCCs [28]. Among clear cell RCCs, ADC values of high-grade clear cell RCCs were statistically significantly lower than those of low-grade clear cell RCCs [29]. Multiparametric MRI is helpful in differentiating RCC subtypes and grades on the basis of T2 signal intensity, ADC map values, and enhancement patterns.

Differentiation of RCC from AML with Minimal Fat

Diagnosis is challenging when an AML does not show macroscopic fat on unenhanced CT scan due to minimal fat content within the tumor. Several CT and MR imaging studies have reported helpful findings in differentiating AML with minimal fat from RCC [30–35]. Favorable imaging findings for AMLs with minimal fat include high-attenuation mass at unenhanced CT compared with the adjacent renal parenchyma, homogeneous enhancement, low T2 signal intensity on MR imaging, and loss of signal intensity within the tumor on T1 opposed-phase imaging, as compared to T1 in-phase imaging, which is attributed to minimal fat. However, clear cell RCCs often contain intracytoplasmic fat, and loss of signal intensity within tumors on T1 opposed-phase images has also been observed. Fat-suppressed T2-weighted images can be helpful in differentiating clear cell RCCs from AMLs with minimal fat, which show focal loss of signal intensity within the tumor on T1 opposed-phase images [36]. On T2-weighted images, AMLs with minimal fat show homogeneous hypointensity, whereas clear cell RCCs show heterogeneous hyperintensity. However, T2 low signal intensity of the AMLs with minimal fat is similar to papillary or chromophobe RCCs. Multiparametric MRI, including DWI and T1-weighted dual echo in-phase and opposed-phase imaging, is useful in differentiating small renal tumors with predominantly low SI on T2-weighted images [37]. Comprehensive analysis of multiple MR imaging parameters is useful in differentiating small renal tumors (Fig. 17.8).

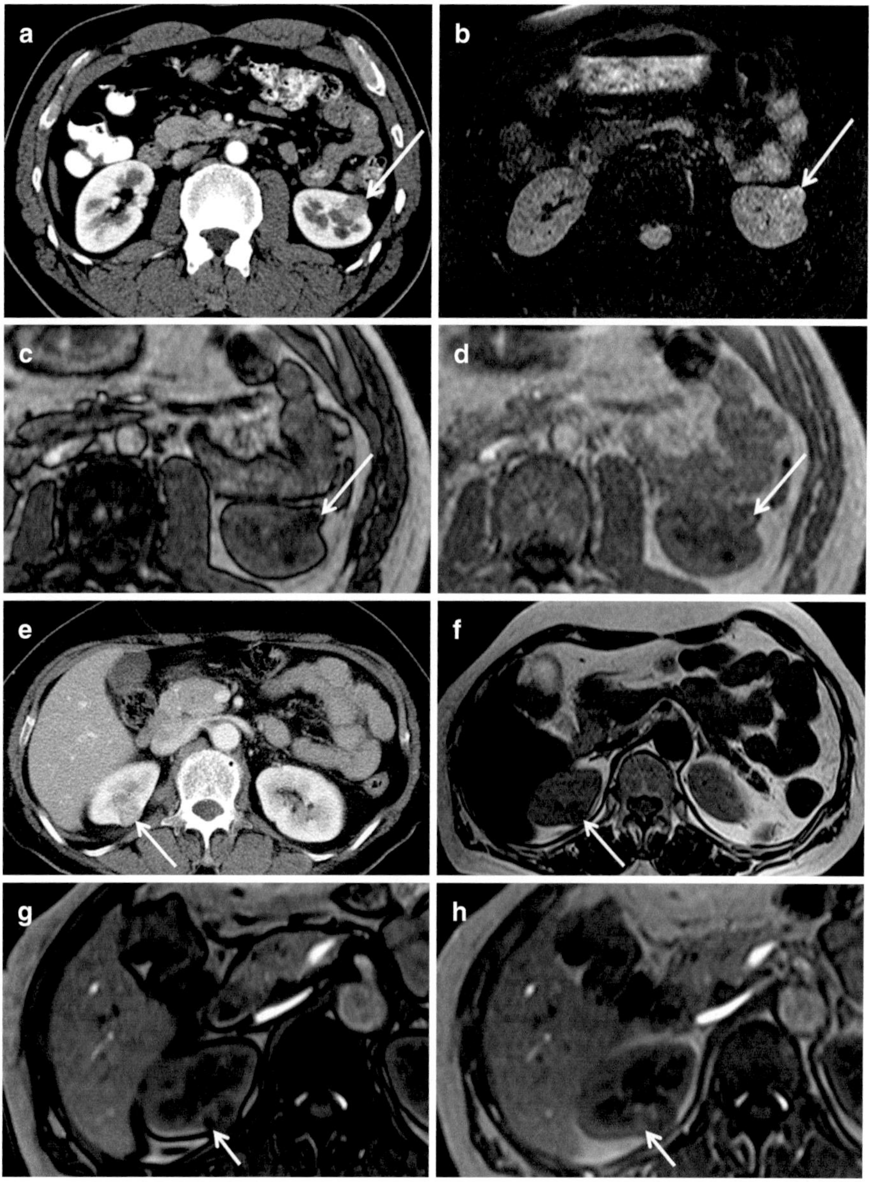

Fig. 17.8 Multiparametric MRI for the evaluation of small renal masses. (**a–d**) Clear cell RCC in 41-year-old man. Relatively homogeneous enhancing mass (1.7 cm) in the left kidney on enhanced CT scan (**a**). On fat-suppressed T2-weighted image (**b**), the tumor shows heterogeneous hyperintensity. MR image of T1 opposed-phase (**c**) shows focal signal drop within the tumor (arrow, **c**), compared with T1 in-phase (**d**) image (arrow, **d**). (**e–h**) Angiomyolipoma with minimal fat in 57-year-old woman. Relatively homogeneous enhancing mass (1.6 cm) in the right kidney on enhanced CT scan (arrow, **e**). On T2-weighted image (**f**), the tumor shows homogeneous hypointensity (arrow, **f**). MR image of T1 opposed-phase (**g**) shows focal signal drop within the tumor (arrow, **g**), compared with T1 in-phase (**h**) image (arrow, **h**)

Tumor Thrombus

MRI has been reported to have similar staging accuracy to CT. MRI is generally used when CT cannot be performed due to severe allergy to the iodinated contrast agent or pregnancy. MRI is not commonly used in diagnosis and staging of RCC. However, it is regarded as the most accurate method to evaluate the extent of venous tumor thrombus (Fig. 17.9). RCC has a propensity to spread through the venous system. In patients with RCC, the most frequent sites of venous involvement are the renal veins and IVC. In patients with venous extension, surgical resection is the primary method of treatment, with reported improved survival rates as compared to patients who did not undergo surgical resection. Accurate detection and evaluation of venous tumor thrombus is crucial in determining an operative approach. The multiplanar capability of MRI is particularly useful to delineate the upper and lower margins of a tumor in IVC [38].

Ultrasound (US)

On US, most RCCs are hypoechoic or isoechoic to renal parenchyma, with hyperechoic tumors being less common. However, several previous reports on US evaluation of renal tumors demonstrated that RCCs can have many different appearances, spanning from hypoechoic, isoechoic, to markedly hyperechoic, and occasionally simulating AMLs (Fig. 17.10 and 17.11) [39]. US is a commonly used screening method of renal tumors; however, the sonographic appearances span a wide spectrum and are nonspecific. If a solid mass is diagnosed on kidney US, RCC or AML should be initially considered, given the high frequency of occurrence of these tumors. Usually, RCCs are less echogenic than AMLs. A number of RCCs, however, are more echogenic than the normal renal parenchyma, and these tumors can be misdiagnosed as AMLs. The anechoic halo of RCCs, observed on US, indicates a different tissue composition, and is usually associated with a pseudocapsule composed of compressed surrounding tissue. The anechoic halo on kidney US is a useful characteristic to differentiate hyperechoic RCCs from AMLs, because it is exclusively encountered in RCCs. At histologic examination, thick pseudocapsules, formed by compression of the normal renal parenchyma, were observed around the tumors in small RCCs with hypoechoic rims. The presence of a capsule can assist in evaluating the aggressiveness of the tumor [40]. The degrees of echogenicity of RCCs and AMLs overlap considerably, indicating that the two entities are indistinguishable by their type of echogenicity. The incidence of hyperechoic RCCs, particularly of smaller ones, appears to be on the rise. CT or MRI can achieve higher specificity in diagnosing hyperechoic renal tumors. Presence of an anechoic rim and/or intratumoral cyst strongly suggests RCC, and these characteristics are useful in differentiating RCC from AML [41]. Contrast-enhanced US (CEUS) agents are small gas bubbles encapsulated in a stabilizing shell, with a typical diameter on the

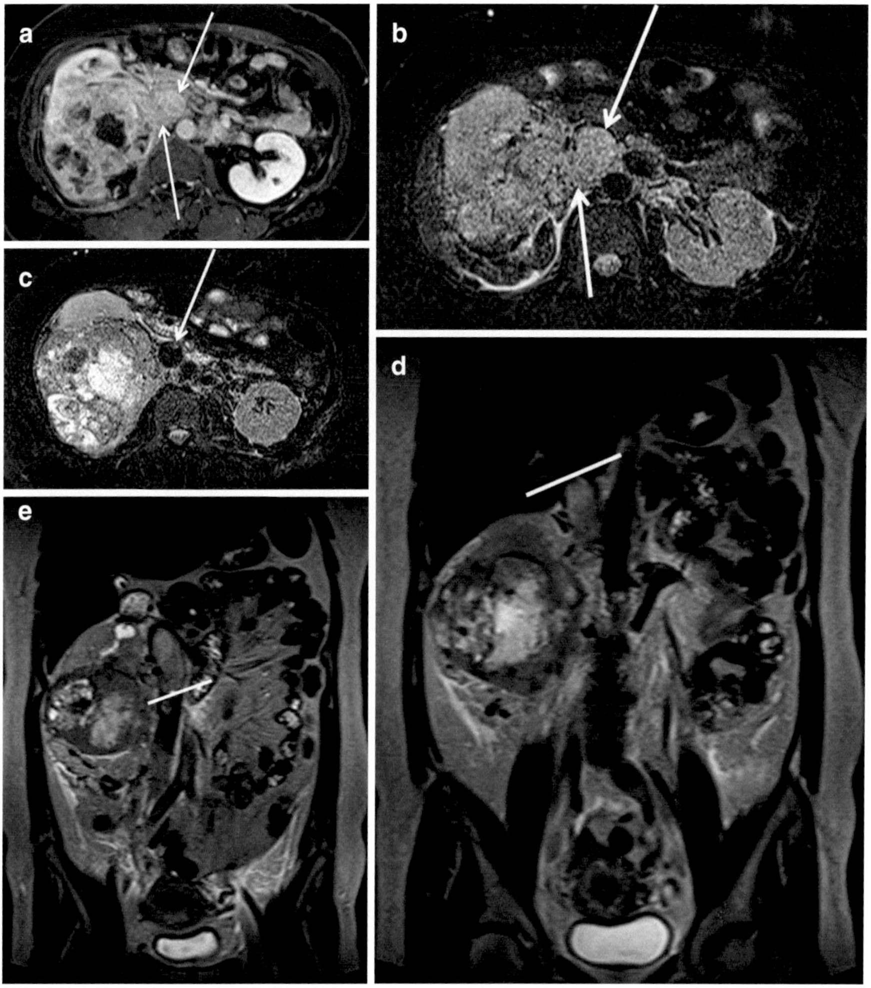

Fig. 17.9 Venous involvement of renal vein and IVC of RCC (TNM stage T3b). (**a**) Enhanced axial T1 VIBE fat-saturated image in 52-year-old woman shows a heterogeneous enhancing mass (10.5 cm) in the right kidney. Enhancing tumor thrombus in the expanded right renal vein and IVC are also noted (arrows, **a**). (**b**, **c**) On fat-suppressed T2 weighted images, tumor thrombus in the dilated right renal vein and IVC show heterogeneous hyperintensity (arrows, **b**), compared with the normal IVC of T2 dark signal intensity (arrow, **c**). (**d**, **e**) Thrombus in the expanded IVC on coronal T2-weighted images with clearly identified upper (white line, **d**) and lower (white line, **e**) margins of thrombus

order of microns. Considering their intravascular nature and their inability to pass the interstitial tissue, these agents appear to be a good measure of vascularity and intravascular volume [42]. A study on the accuracy of CEUS in the evaluation of renal masses has been reported [43]. In this study, hypovascularity of small solid renal masses relative to the cortex in the arterial phase was a helpful characteristic

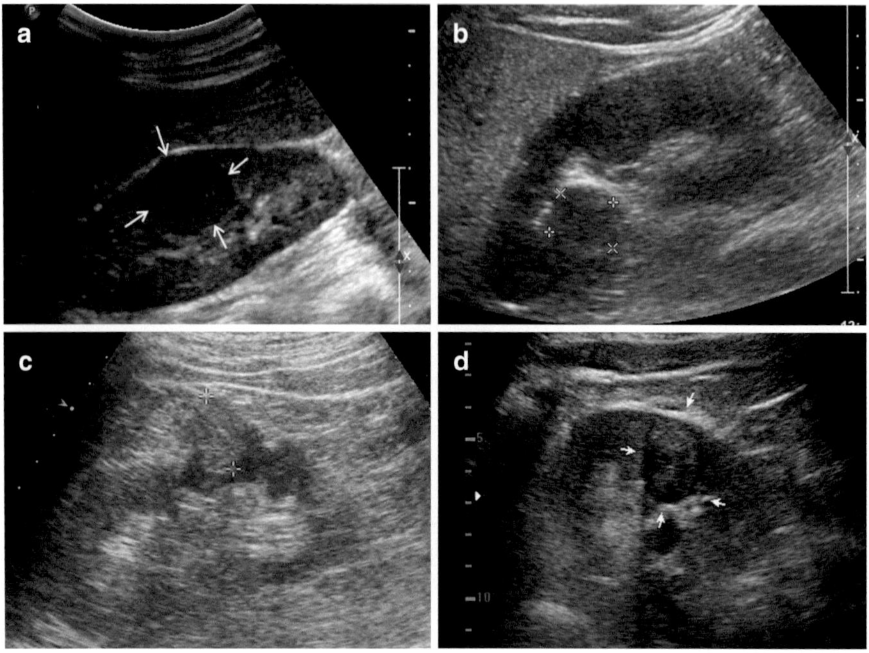

Fig. 17.10 Various appearances of RCCs on US. (**a**) Chromophobe RCC in 45-year-old woman. US shows a homogeneous hypoechoic mass (2.8 cm) in the right kidney (arrows, **a**). (**b**) Chromophobe RCC in 32-year-old man. US shows a homogeneous isoechoic mass (2.3 cm) in the right kidney renal sinus portion (cross marks, **b**). (**c**) Clear cell RCC in 38-year-old man. US showed a hyperechoic mass (2 cm) in the right kidney (cross marks, **c**). (**d**) Papillary RCC in 65-year-old man. US showed a heterogeneous echoic mass (2.3 cm) with an echoic rim in the left kidney (arrows, **d**)

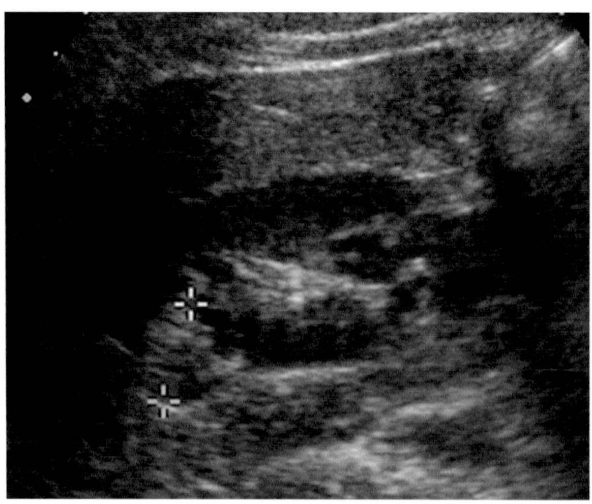

Fig. 17.11 US appearance of AML with minimal fat. AML with minimal fat in 51-year-old man. US showed a hyperechoic mass (2.8 cm) in the right kidney (cross marks, A)

to detect malignancies, most often papillary RCCs. If the contrast agent for CT or MR imaging is contraindicated due to concerns for renal damage or nephrogenic systemic fibrosis, CEUS can be used to confirm the solid nature of a renal mass. The differentiation of homogeneous T2 low signal intensity small renal masses on MRI is difficult due to overlapping features of AML with minimal fat and non-clear cell RCC. The most common sonographic feature of AML with minimal fat is marked hyperechogenicity, whereas no RCC with T2 low signal intensity on MR shows marked hyperechogenicity. Therefore, in small renal masses with low signal intensity on T2-weighted imaging, additional echogenicity information on US may aid differential diagnosis of AML with minimal fat and non-clear cell RCC [44].

Bosniak Classification for Complex Renal Cysts

Cystic renal masses are composed predominantly of fluid which does not enhance at imaging. Simple fluid attenuations show between 0 and 20 HU. If a cystic mass contains fluid higher attenuation than simple fluid, it probably has calcification within its walls or septa, has a thickened wall or septa, has hemorrhagic or proteinaceous component, or contains an enhancing soft-tissue component. This cystic mass may be benign or malignant depending on the degree of enhancement, thickness, and irregularity of the wall or septa. Cystic lesions with enhancing soft-tissue components are definitely malignant. On contrast-enhanced scan, greater than 20 HU increase indicates enhancement, and values of 10–20 HU increase on contrast-enhanced scan is regarded as equivocal enhancement [20]. In 1986, Bosniak proposed a renal cyst classification system based on CT findings, comprising distinct categories from I to IV, and this classification system has been widely used in the management of patients with cystic renal masses [45] (Figs. 17.12, 17.13, and 17.14). Contrast-enhanced CT is critical in the evaluation of complicated renal cysts with Bosniak classification [46]. During the last few decades, the Bosniak

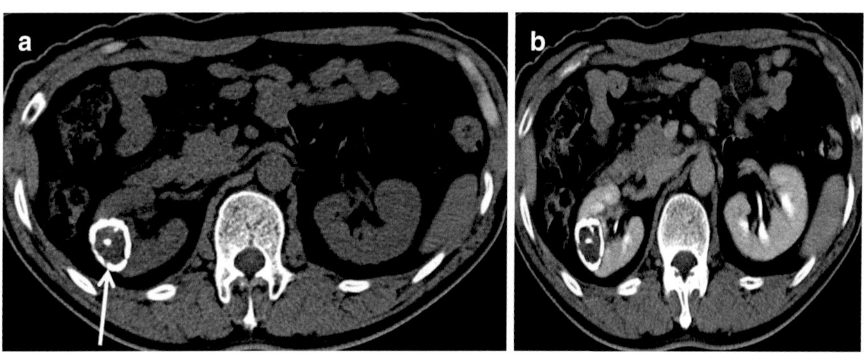

Fig. 17.12 CT appearance of Bosniak category IIF cyst. (**A**, **B**) Bosniak category IIF cyst in 58-year-old man. Contrast-enhanced transverse CT images at unenhanced (**a**) and excretory phases (**b**) show a cystic mass (3 cm) with thick and nodular calcifications in septa and wall (arrow **a**) without enhancement, in the right kidney. The lesion showed no change on follow-up

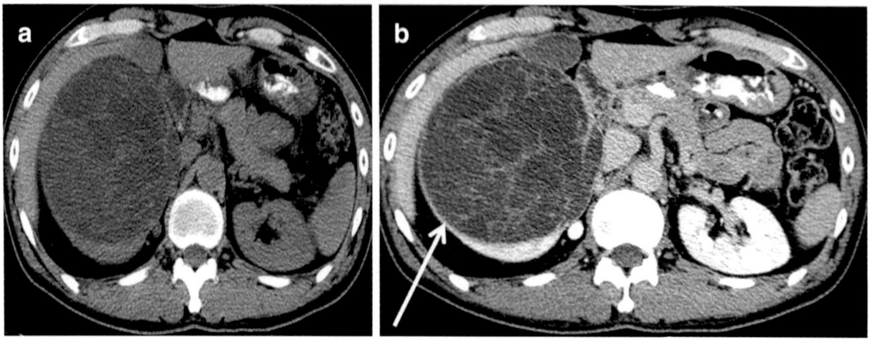

Fig. 17.13 CT appearance of Bosniak category III cyst. (**A**, **B**) Bosniak category III cyst in 38-year-old man. Contrast-enhanced transverse CT images at unenhanced (**a**) and excretory phases (**b**) show a multilocular cystic mass (10 cm) with multiple enhancing septa in the right kidney (arrow **b**). Patient underwent radical nephrectomy, and pathology confirmed cystic nephroma

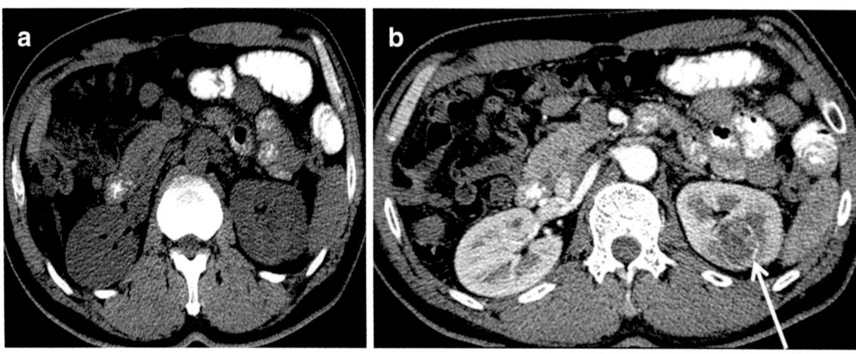

Fig. 17.14 CT appearance of Bosniak category III cyst. (**a**, **b**) Bosniak category III cyst in 53-year-old man. Contrast-enhanced transverse CT images at unenhanced (**a**) and corticomedullary phases (**b**) show a subtle high-density cystic mass (2.7 cm) with rim enhancement (arrow **b**) in the left kidney. Patient underwent partial nephrectomy, and pathology confirmed clear cell RCC

classification was modified [47]. Bosniak cysts (categories I and II) do not require follow-up or specific treatment. Bosniak category IIF cyst requires follow-up with probably benign imaging findings. Bosniak category III lesions present a broad spectrum from benign to malignant disease. Possible benign lesions of Bosniak category III cysts comprise chronic abscesses, chronically infected or hemorrhagic cysts, simple cysts after alcohol ablation, localized cystic disease, mixed epithelial and stromal tumors, and multilocular cystic nephromas [48, 49]. Bosniak category IV lesions are characterized by a solid enhancing component within the cyst on post-contrast images, and are highly suspicious for malignancy. Complex renal cysts categorized as Bosniak III and IV are considered malignant lesions, and surgical resection is recommended. According to previous reports [46, 50, 51], 25%, 54–72%, and 86–100% of type IIF, III, and IV Bosniak lesions, respectively, were diagnosed as RCCs. Schoots et al. [47] reported that the effectiveness of the Bosniak classification system for complex renal cysts was high in categories II, IIF, and IV, but low in category III, and about half of Bosniak III cysts were overtreated, as they turned out to be benign. In another report [52], two categories of IIF and III remained indeterminate and controversial. Although contrast-enhanced CT is the imaging modality of choice for the evaluation of complicated renal cysts with Bosniak classification, in the cases of IIF and III cysts, all available imaging techniques, including MRI, CEUS, and CT scanning, are recommended for accurate diagnosis. In addition, biopsy of IIF and IIII cystic lesions is not recommended, and thus the therapeutic decision for the best treatment strategy is based mainly on radiological findings without histological confirmation [53]. Therefore, accurate determination of the Bosniak category for complex renal cysts is very important, and this mainly depends on the expertise of the radiologist. Although size is not an important feature of the Bosniak classification, small cystic renal masses are more likely benign, but large ones are not necessarily more likely malignant [20]. Therefore, radiologists can lower the probability of malignancy for small-sized cysts, but cannot increase the probability of malignancy of large-sized cysts.

References

1. Siegel RL, Miller KD, Jemal A. Cancer statistics, 2018. CA Cancer J Clin. 2018;68(1):7–30.
2. Schieda N, Vakili M, Dilauro M, Hodgdon T, Flood TA, Shabana WM. Solid renal cell carcinoma measuring water attenuation (−10 to 20 HU) on unenhanced CT. Am J Roentgenol. 2015;205(6):1215–21.
3. Tsili AC, Argyropoulou MI, Gousia A, Kalef-Ezra J, Sofikitis N, Malamou-Mitsi V, et al. Renal cell carcinoma: value of multiphase MDCT with multiplanar reformations in the detection of pseudocapsule. Am J Roentgenol. 2012;199(2):379–86.
4. Gore ME, Larkin JM. Challenges and opportunities for converting renal cell carcinoma into a chronic disease with targeted therapies. Br J Cancer. 2011;104(3):399–406.
5. Moch H, Cubilla AL, Humphrey PA, Reuter VE, Ulbright TM. The 2016 WHO classification of tumours of the urinary system and male genital organs-part a: renal, penile, and testicular tumours. Eur Urol. 2016;70(1):93–105.
6. Sauk SC, Hsu MS, Margolis DJA, Lu DSK, Rao NP, Belldegrun AS, et al. Clear cell renal cell carcinoma: multiphasic multidetector CT imaging features help predict genetic karyotypes. Radiology. 2011;261(3):854–62.
7. Yamada T, Endo M, Tsuboi M, Matsuhashi T, Takase K, Higano S, et al. Differentiation of pathologic subtypes of papillary renal cell carcinoma on CT. Am J Roentgenol. 2008;191(5):1559–63.
8. Prasad SR, Humphrey PA, Catena JR, Narra VR, Srigley JR, Cortez AD, et al. Common and uncommon histologic subtypes of renal cell carcinoma: imaging spectrum with pathologic correlation. Radiographics. 2006;26(6):1795–806.
9. Raman SP, Johnson PT, Allaf ME, Netto G, Fishman EK. Chromophobe renal cell carcinoma: multiphase MDCT enhancement patterns and morphologic features. Am J Roentgenol. 2013;201(6):1268–76.
10. Amin MB, Edge SG, Greene FL, et al., editors. AJCC cancer staging manual. 8th ed. New York: Springer; 2017.

11. Kim C, Choi HJ, Cho KS. Diagnostic value of multidetector computed tomography for renal sinus fat invasion in renal cell carcinoma patients. Eur J Radiol. 2014;83(6):914–8.
12. Sheth S, Scatarige JC, Horton KM, Corl FM, Fishman EK. Current concepts in the diagnosis and management of renal cell carcinoma: role of multidetector CT and three-dimensional CT. RadioGraphics. 2001;21(suppl_1):S237–S54.
13. Remzi M, Marberger M. Renal tumor biopsies for evaluation of small renal tumors: why, in whom, and how? Eur Urol. 2009;55(2):359–67.
14. Frank I, Blute ML, Cheville JC, Lohse CM, Weaver AL, Zincke H. Solid renal tumors: an analysis of pathological features related to tumor size. J Urol. 2003;170(6 Pt 1):2217–20.
15. Remzi M, Katzenbeisser D, Waldert M, Klingler H-C, Susani M, Memarsadeghi M, et al. Renal tumour size measured radiologically before surgery is an unreliable variable for predicting histopathological features: benign tumours are not necessarily small. BJU Int. 2007;99(5):1002–6.
16. Frank I, Colombo JR, Rubinstein M, Desai M, Kaouk J, Gill IS. Laparoscopic partial nephrectomy for centrally located renal tumors. J Urol. 2006;175(3 Pt 1):849–52.
17. Jacobs BL, Tan HJ, Montgomery JS, Weizer AZ, Wood DP, Miller DC, et al. Understanding criteria for surveillance of patients with a small renal mass. Urology. 2012;79(5):1027–32.
18. Shikanov S, Lifshitz DA, Deklaj T, Katz MH, Shalhav AL. Laparoscopic partial nephrectomy for technically challenging tumours. BJU Int. 2010;106(1):91–4.
19. Kim MH. CT-guided biopsy of entirely endophytic small renal masses: diagnostic rates and complications using standard-dose and reduced-dose CT protocols. AJR Am J Roentgenol. 2017;208(5):1030–6.
20. Silverman SG, Israel GM, Herts BR, Richie JP. Management of the Incidental Renal Mass. Radiology. 2008;249(1):16–31.
21. Newatia A, Khatri G, Friedman B, Hines J. Subtraction imaging: applications for nonvascular abdominal MRI. Am J Roentgenol. 2007;188(4):1018–25.
22. Pedrosa I, Sun MR, Spencer M, Genega EM, Olumi AF, Dewolf WC, et al. MR imaging of renal masses: correlation with findings at surgery and pathologic analysis. Radiographics. 2008;28(4):985–1003.
23. Oliva MR, Glickman JN, Zou KH, Teo SY, Mortelé KJ, Rocha MS, et al. Renal cell carcinoma: T1 and T2 signal intensity characteristics of papillary and clear cell types correlated with pathology. Am J Roentgenol. 2009;192(6):1524–30.
24. Sasiwimonphan K, Takahashi N, Leibovich BC, Carter RE, Atwell TD, Kawashima A. Small (<4 cm) renal mass: differentiation of angiomyolipoma without visible fat from renal cell carcinoma utilizing MR imaging. Radiology. 2012;263(1):160–8.
25. Young JR, Coy H, Kim HJ, Douek M, Lo P, Pantuck AJ, et al. Performance of relative enhancement on multiphasic MRI for the differentiation of clear cell renal cell carcinoma (RCC) from papillary and chromophobe RCC subtypes and oncocytoma. Am J Roentgenol. 2017;208(4):812–9.
26. Sun MRM, Ngo L, Genega EM, Atkins MB, Finn ME, Rofsky NM, et al. Renal cell carcinoma: dynamic contrast-enhanced MR imaging for differentiation of tumor subtypes—correlation with pathologic findings. Radiology. 2009;250(3):793–802.
27. Woo S, Suh CH, Kim SY, Cho JY, Kim SH. Diagnostic performance of DWI for differentiating high- from low-grade clear cell renal cell carcinoma: a systematic review and meta-analysis. Am J Roentgenol. 2017:W1–8.
28. Hötker AM, Mazaheri Y, Wibmer A, Karlo CA, Zheng J, Moskowitz CS, et al. Differentiation of clear cell renal cell carcinoma from other renal cortical tumors by use of a quantitative multiparametric MRI approach. Am J Roentgenol. 2017;208(3):W85–91.
29. Rosenkrantz AB, Niver BE, Fitzgerald EF, Babb JS, Chandarana H, Melamed J. Utility of the apparent diffusion coefficient for distinguishing clear cell renal cell carcinoma of low and high nuclear grade. AJR Am J Roentgenol. 2010;195(5):W344–51.
30. Kim MH, Lee J, Cho G, Cho KS, Kim J, Kim JK. MDCT-based scoring system for differentiating angiomyolipoma with minimal fat from renal cell carcinoma. Acta Radiol. 2013;54(10):1201–9.

31. Murphy AM, Buck AM, Benson MC, McKiernan JM. Increasing detection rate of benign renal tumors: evaluation of factors predicting for benign tumor histologic features during past two decades. Urology. 2009;73(6):1293–7.
32. Kim JK, Park SY, Shon JH, Cho KS. Angiomyolipoma with minimal fat: differentiation from renal cell carcinoma at biphasic helical CT. Radiology. 2004;230(3):677–84.
33. Hosokawa Y, Kinouchi T, Sawai Y, Mano M, Kiuchi H, Meguro N, et al. Renal angiomyolipoma with minimal fat. Int J Clin Oncol. 2002;7(2):120–3.
34. Obuz F, Karabay N, Secil M, Igci E, Kovanlikaya A, Yorukoglu K. Various radiological appearances of angiomyolipomas in the same kidney. Eur Radiol. 2000;10(6):897–9.
35. Jinzaki M, Tanimoto A, Narimatsu Y, Ohkuma K, Kurata T, Shinmoto H, et al. Angiomyolipoma: imaging findings in lesions with minimal fat. Radiology. 1997;205(2):497–502.
36. Chung MS, Choi HJ, Kim MH, Cho KS. Comparison of T2-weighted MRI with and without fat suppression for differentiating renal angiomyolipomas without visible fat from other renal tumors. AJR Am J Roentgenol. 2014;202(4):765–71.
37. Park JJ, Kim CK. Small (< 4 cm) renal tumors with predominantly low signal intensity on T2-weighted images: differentiation of minimal-fat angiomyolipoma from renal cell carcinoma. Am J Roentgenol. 2016;208(1):124–30.
38. Ng CS, Wood CG, Silverman PM, Tannir NM, Tamboli P, Sandler CM. Renal cell carcinoma: diagnosis, staging, and surveillance. Am J Roentgenol. 2008;191(4):1220–32.
39. Forman HP, Middleton WD, Melson GL, McClennan BL. Hyperechoic renal cell carcinomas: increase in detection at US. Radiology. 1993;188(2):431–4.
40. Yamashita Y, Takahashi M, Watanabe O, Yoshimatsu S, Ueno S, Ishimaru S, et al. Small renal cell carcinoma: pathologic and radiologic correlation. Radiology. 1992;184(2):493–8.
41. Yamashita Y, Ueno S, Makita O, Ogata I, Hatanaka Y, Watanabe O, et al. Hyperechoic renal tumors: anechoic rim and intratumoral cysts in US differentiation of renal cell carcinoma from angiomyolipoma. Radiology. 1993;188(1):179–82.
42. Lindner JR. Microbubbles in medical imaging: current applications and future directions. Nat Rev Drug Discov. 2004;3(6):527–32.
43. Atri M, Tabatabaeifar L, Jang H-J, Finelli A, Moshonov H, Jewett M. Accuracy of contrast-enhanced US for differentiating benign from malignant solid small renal masses. Radiology. 2015;276(3):900–8.
44. Park KJ, Kim MH, Kim JK, Cho KS. Sonographic features of small (<4 cm) renal tumors with low signal intensity on T2-weighted MR images: differentiating minimal-fat angiomyolipoma from renal cell carcinoma. AJR Am J Roentgenol. 2018;211(3):605–13.
45. Bosniak MA. The current radiological approach to renal cysts. Radiology. 1986;158(1):1–10.
46. Song C, Min GE, Song K, Kim JK, Hong B, Kim CS, et al. Differential diagnosis of complex cystic renal mass using multiphase computerized tomography. J Urol. 2009;181(6):2446–50.
47. Schoots IG, Zaccai K, Hunink MG, Verhagen P. Bosniak classification for complex renal cysts reevaluated: a systematic review. J Urol. 2017;198(1):12–21.
48. Wood CG 3rd, Stromberg LJ 3rd, Harmath CB, Horowitz JM, Feng C, Hammond NA, et al. CT and MR imaging for evaluation of cystic renal lesions and diseases. Radiographics. 2015;35(1):125–41.
49. Israel GM, Bosniak MA. Pitfalls in renal mass evaluation and how to avoid them. Radiographics. 2008;28(5):1325–38.
50. Mousessian PN, Yamauchi FI, Mussi TC, Baroni RH. Malignancy rate, histologic grade, and progression of Bosniak category III and IV complex renal cystic lesions. AJR Am J Roentgenol. 2017;209(6):1285–90.
51. Smith AD, Remer EM, Cox KL, Lieber ML, Allen BC, Shah SN, et al. Bosniak category IIF and III cystic renal lesions: outcomes and associations. Radiology. 2012;262(1):152–60.
52. Ljungberg B, Bensalah K, Canfield S, Dabestani S, Hofmann F, Hora M, et al. EAU guidelines on renal cell carcinoma: 2014 update. Eur Urol. 2015;67(5):913–24.
53. Veltri A, Garetto I, Tosetti I, Busso M, Volpe A, Pacchioni D, et al. Diagnostic accuracy and clinical impact of imaging-guided needle biopsy of renal masses. Retrospective analysis on 150 cases. Eur Radiol. 2011;21(2):393–401.

Part IV
Molecular Pathology

Chapter 18
Molecular Pathology of Kidney Tumors

Seyda Erdogan, Ayhan Ozcan, and Luan D. Truong

Renal cell carcinoma (RCC) consists of various tumor types. Each type has distinct histological features, different genetic alterations, and variable clinical course including response to treatment. The variable histologic features are equaled by a complex spectrum of molecular changes. Much molecular insight has been gained by traditional molecular studies, and much more is expected with the advent of modern genetic techniques. Yet, the molecular basis for renal neoplasm is far from full understanding.

RCC may be hereditary or sporadic. The hereditary forms of RCC represent only 2–4% of all RCCs. However, the original studies on their molecular pathogenesis play the most important role in clarifying the molecular pathways of RCC in general. The morphologic spectrum of RCC in the hereditary and sporadic contexts overlaps to a significant extent. This histologic overlapping is also reflected by a shared molecular mechanism. In fact, several molecular changes originally identified in a histologic type in the hereditary context were later also found in its sporadic counterpart. Aside from this hereditary underpinning,

S. Erdogan (✉)
Department of Pathology, Cukurova University, School of Medicine, Adana, Turkey

A. Ozcan
Gulhane Military Medical Academy, School of Medicine, Department of Pathology, Ankara, Turkey

Yeni Yuzyil University Gaziosmanpasa Hospital, Department of Pathology, Istanbul, Turkey
e-mail: ayhan.ozcan@gophastanesi.com.tr

L. D. Truong
Department of Pathology and Genomic Medicine, The Houston Methodist Hospital, Houston, TX, USA

Department of Pathology and Laboratory Medicine, Weill Cornell Medical College of Cornell University, New York, NY, USA

Department of Pathology and Medicine, Baylor College of Medicine, Houston, TX, USA

M. K. Divatia et al. (eds.), *Kidney Cancer*, https://doi.org/10.1007/978-3-030-28333-9_18

derived mostly from narrowly targeted studies focusing on a limited number of putatively pathogenetic genes, more recent "whole-genome" studies have revealed additional pathogenetic genes or molecular pathways pertinent to both hereditary and sporadic RCC.

This chapter aims at a summary of a vast body of literature on the molecular pathology of RCC, with emphasis on the more frequent or the better-known tumor types. For each tumor type, molecular changes in the hereditary context were first described followed by those of the sporadic counterparts.

Clear Cell Renal Cell Carcinoma

Clear cell RCC can be hereditary or sporadic. Clear cell RCC is the typical and predominant histologic type of RCC in von Hippel–Lindau (VHL) disease, a hereditary disease due to mutation of the VHL gene. Clear cell RCC is the most frequent type of sporadic RCC (65–70%) (Table 18.1).

Table 18.1 The summary of molecular features of the RCC subtypes

Subtype of RCC	Molecular features
Clear cell RCC	Loss of chromosomes 3p, 14q, 9p, 4p, gain of 5q Loss of *VHL* gene Genetic alterations in the PI3/Akt pathway Mutations of *PBRM1, BAP1, SETD2, KDM5C, KDM6A*
Hereditary form VHL disease	Germline mutation of *VHL*
Papillary RCC	Trisomy 7, 17, loss of chromosome Y Loss of chromosomes 1p, 3p, 5q, 6, 8, 9p, 10, 11, 15, 18, and 22 Mutation of *MET, SETD2, CDKN2A* silencing
Hereditary papillary RCC	Germline mutation of *MET*
Chromophobe RCC	Loss of chromosomes 1,2,6,10,13,17,21, and Y Mutation of *TP53, PTEN* High TERT expression Mutation of *MT-NDS*, a member of electron transport chain complex I
Birt–Hogg–Dubé syndrome	The mutation of *FLCN*
MIT family tRCC	Xp11 tRCC; TFE3 rearrangement t(6,11)RCC; TFEB rearrangement
Succinate dehydrogenase RCC	Inactivation of *SDH* genes
Tubulocystic RCC	Gain of chromosomes 7, 17, loss of Y chr
Mucinous tubular and spindle cell carcinoma	Loss of chromosomes 1, 4, 6, 8, 9, 11, 13, 14, 15, 18, 22, and X Gain of chromosomes 2, 3, 4, 5, 7, 9, 10, 12, 15, 16, 17, 18, 19, 20, 22, and Y
Acquired cystic disease-associated RCC	Gain of chromosomes 3716, and 17Y
Clear cell papillary RCC	–

Hereditary Clear Cell RCC

Initial studies showed that deletion of chromosome 3 is the major event in the carcinogenesis of clear cell RCCs in both hereditary and sporadic contexts. Subsequent studies provided further genetic insight that mutations of *VHL* tumor suppressor gene located on the short arm of chromosome 3 are the cause of the renal tumors [1–4].

VHL disease is caused by germline mutations of the *VHL* gene, a tumor suppressor gene located on chromosome 3p25–26, encoding the VHL protein. Germline mutations of the *VHL* gene can be inherited or arise de novo in about 20% of patients. Sequence analysis detects mutations in about 72% of VHL family members. Southern blot analysis and/or quantitative polymerase chain reaction (PCR) detect partial or complete gene deletions in the remaining (28%) of VHL family members [5, 6]. Newer genetic techniques, such as array comparative genomic hybridization (array CGH) and next-generation sequencing, are more powerful tools, especially, in cases of suspected mosaicism with a negative VHL genetic test, for identifying genomic imbalances [7, 8]. So far, more than 500 different types of VHL mutation have been described in the Human Gene Mutation Database (www.hgmd.org) [8, 9]. Truncating mutation or deletion of the *VHL* gene is responsible for VHL type 1 disease with retinal and CNS hemangioblastomas and clear cell RCC, but no pheochromocytoma. In contrast, missense mutation of the *VHL* gene is responsible for VHL type 2 disease with the constant development of pheochromocytoma [8, 10]. VHL type 2 disease is subclassified into 2A, 2B, and 2C types, which, in addition to the common pheochromocytoma, differ in other tumor phenotypes. These observations suggest that aside from the type of the *VHL* gene mutation, mutation of other currently unknown genes, environmental influence, or epigenetic impact may also be responsible for the phenotype divergence [8].

The *VHL* gene was first described in 1988 [11] and cloned in 1993 [12]. The *VHL* gene is composed of three exons: exon 1 spans codons 1–113 (nucleotides 1–340), exon 2 spans codons 114–154 (nucleotides 341–463), and exon 3 spans codons: 155–213 (nucleotides 464–642). It is translated into two proteins: pVHL30, a 213 amino-acid protein with a molecular weight of 28–30 kDa; and pVHL19, a 160 amino-acid protein with a molecular weight of 18–19 kDa, synthesized by internal translation initiation from the codon 54 methionine. These two proteins seem to have the same functional properties and are widely expressed in both fetal and adult human tissues.

Since normal *VHL* gene is a tumor suppressor, its mutation results in a loss of function, leading to tumor development. Furthermore, the types of mutation may account for different tumor phenotypes [13]. Recent studies provided more in-depth pathogenetic insight, implying the crucial role of the VHL-hypoxia-inducible factor (HIF) pathway. The protein pVHL, encoded by the *VHL* gene, has multiple physiologic functions in many cellular pathways, especially, the oxygen-sensing pathway [6, 14–16]. These physiologic functions of pVHL protein involve its interaction with VCB-CUL2, HIF-1α and 2α, ubiquitin, and ubiquitin-mediated degradation in proteasomes [16]. pVHL protein, widely localized in the cytosol, but shuttling between the cytosol and nucleus, has α and β domains with different functions. VCB–CUL2 is a cytosolic multiprotein complex, which is consisted of elongin C, elongin B, Rbx1 (Roc1), NEDD8, and cullin 2 (CUL2), and collectively acts as an E3 ubiquitin ligase. HIF-1α or HIF-2α are transcription factors, which are composed of α and β subunits, and can induce transcription of several downstream genes with widespread tissue effects.

In physiologic condition, the α domain of pVHL protein binds and activates the VCB–CUL2 complex. This complex, acting as ubiquitin ligase, binds to α subunits of HIF-1α and HIF-2α and targets them for ubiquitinylation and proteasomal degradation (Fig. 18.1). Oxygen is crucial for this binding, since this binding requires hydroxylation of α subunit of both HIF-1α and HIF-2α, which in turn depends on oxygen-mediated activation of prolyl hydroxylases (PHD1–3). Especially, HIF1α activates genes involved in apoptotic and glycolytic pathways, whereas HIF2α promotes genes involved in cell proliferation and angiogenesis [17].

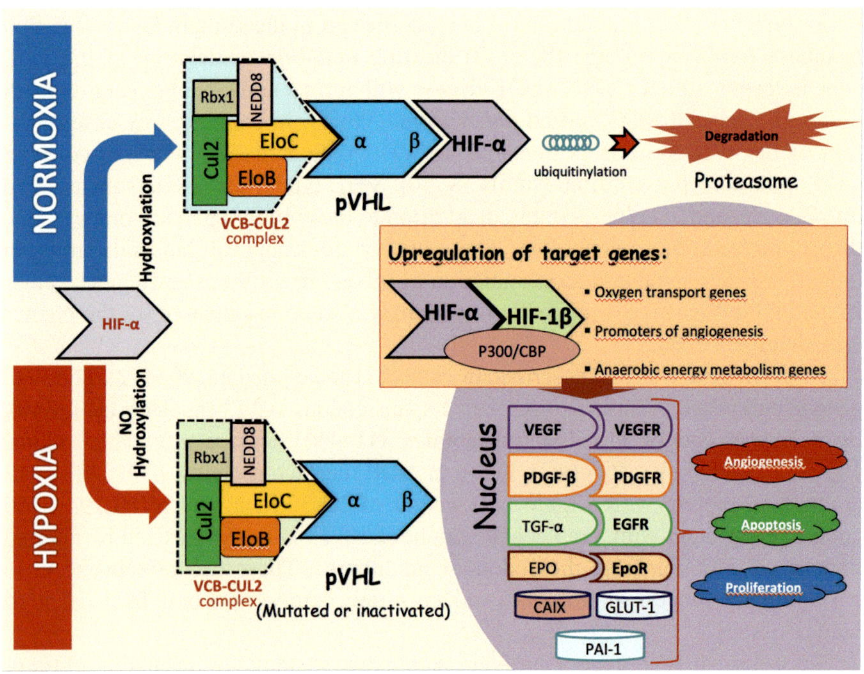

Fig. 18.1 The pathogenesis of clear cell RCC associated with VHL disease: α domain of pVHL protein binds and activates the VCB–CUL2 complex, which is acting as a ubiquitin ligase, binds to α subunits of HIF-1 and HIF-2 and targets them for ubiquitinylation and proteasomal degradation. Oxygen (normoxia) is crucial for this binding, since this binding requires hydroxylation of α subunit of both HIF-1 and -2, which in turn depends on oxygen-mediated activation of proline hydroxylase (blue pathway). In hypoxic condition, which is a common environment for a solid tumor, the physiologic degradation of HIF is inhibited (red pathway). The absence of pVHL due to mutation of the *VHL* gene further prevents this degradation. These effects collectively lead to induce the expression of several genes

In hypoxic condition, which is a common environment for a solid tumor, the physiologic degradation of HIF is inhibited. The functional absence of pVHL protein due to the mutation of the *VHL* gene further prevents this degradation. These effects collectively lead to the formation of the hetero-dimerized complex consisting of the stable HIF-α subunit and HIF-β subunit, which now can serve as an active transcription factor to induce the expression of several genes, such as vascular endothelial growth factor (VEGF), platelet-derived growth factor-β (PDGF-β), transforming growth factor-α (TGF-α), glucose transporter 1 (GLUT1), erythropoietin (EPO), plasminogen activator inhibitor-1 (PAI-1), carbonic anhydrase 9 (CA9), C-X-C chemokine receptor type 4, and c-mesenchymal-epithelial transition factor (c-MET) (Figs. 18.1 and 18.3). Many of these factors involved in diverse processes such as angiogenesis, proliferation, and apoptosis. Thus, they promote tumorigenesis, tumor invasion, and metastasis.

Recent studies suggest additional pathogenetic roles for pVHL [17–20]. These mechanisms may include the following:

1. Downregulation of VEGF production directly by binding it, or indirectly by inhibiting the transcription factor specificity protein 1 (Sp1).
2. Regulation of exit from the cell cycle and enter to the quiescent state.
3. Regulation of proper extracellular fibronectin matrix assembly by binding both fibronectin and hydroxylated collagen IV.
4. Regulation of the urokinase-type plasminogen activator (u-PA).
5. Degradation of some proteins such as TGFα, nuclear factor kappa beta 2 (NFKB2, which is also known as LYT10), TGFβ, and carbonic anhydrase 9 and 12 (CA9 and CA12).
6. Ubiquitination and degradation of various protein kinase C (PKC) family members, which play a role in the regulation of apoptosis.
7. Modulation of NFKB and p53, which are critical regulator proteins of apoptosis and they are involved in the development of RCC.
8. Induction of RCC invasion by inhibiting the hepatocyte growth factor (HGF).
9. Stabilization of microtubules and regulation of primary cilium. The lack of pVHL causes formation of the cystic lesion in VHL disease.

Sporadic Clear Cell RCC

Chromosome 3 and VHL gene

Deletion of chromosome 3 is also the major event in the carcinogenesis of clear cell RCCs in the sporadic context, and VHL gene is also implicated. Non-germline genetic alterations in the *VHL* gene are detected in up to 70–75% of sporadic clear cell RCC patients [5, 12, 13, 21]. In addition to genetic mutation, the *VHL* gene can be somatically inactivated by several mechanisms, including inactivation of wild-type copy, loss of heterozygosity (LOH), and promoter hypermethylation [5, 8, 12, 13, 21]. Hypermethylation of the *VHL* gene is observed in 10–20% of sporadic RCC patients. A recent genome-wide study showed a similar genomic profile for

VHL disease-associated clear cell RCCs and sporadic *VHL* gene-defective clear cell RCC [8].

Genome-wide sequencing studies revealed other genetic changes besides *VHL* mutations during carcinogenesis of ccRCC. These genes control chromatin remodeling, chromosomal alterations, PI3K/Akt/mTOR pathway, and tumor cell differentiation. These genetic changes are discussed below.

Chromatin-Remodeling Genes

Chromatin remodeling is an epigenetic mechanism, occurred by covalent histone modifications such as methylation, demethylation, or ATP-dependent remodeling complexes. This process is under the control of several genes, the mutations of which promote carcinogenesis.

Polybroma 1(PBRM1) gene, located on 3p21, is the second most commonly mutated gene (41%) after *VHL*. It encodes a histone nucleosome-remodeling complex named BAF 180 that belongs to the switch sucrose nonfermentable (SWI/SNF) chromatin-remodeling complexes. These are macromolecules located on different chromosomes, and have a role on chromatin remodeling by using ATP to mobilize nucleosome to regulate chromatin structure. Somatic, point, and truncating mutations of *PBRM1* result in protein loss, which promote carcinogenesis perhaps through perturbed cell motility and proliferation [22–26].

The BRCA1-associated protein-1 (BAP1) gene mutations were found in 10–15% of clear cell RCC. BAP1 protein is a member of the ubiquitin c-terminal hydrolase family which encodes a nuclear protein containing ubiquitin carboxy-terminal hydrolase domain that targets histone H2A. The mutation of *BAP1* causes the activation of phosphoinositide kinase-3 (PI3K) pathway and mTORC1 activation. *BAP1*-mutant tumors are often high-grade with poor prognosis [22, 26].

The *SETD2* gene is also found to be somatically mutated in clear cell RCC. It is the main methyltransferase that is responsible for histone 3 trimethylation. The mutation of *SETD2* gene causes the loss of H3K36me3, which physiologically help maintain DNA mismatch repair and control microsatellite instability [22, 26, 27].

KDM5C (also known as *JARID 1C*) and *KDM6A* (also known as *UTX*) are the other genes that located on chromosome 3p and act as tumor suppressor genes in clear cell RCC pathogenesis [22, 26].

Chromosomal Alterations

Allelic losses on chromosomes 14q, 9p, or 4p are also carcinogenic and may be related to poor prognosis. Loss of 14q and gain of 5q can be seen either alone or together in RCC [22, 26–29]. Loss of 14q, which houses the *HIF-1α* gene, portends an aggressive behavior. Recent studies showed that the gain of 5q promotes the oncogenic activity of the oncogene *SQSTM1* [22, 29].

Alterations in the Phosphoinositide Kinase-3/Akt/Mammalian Target of Rapamycin Pathway

Activation of the PI3K/Akt/mTOR pathway has been demonstrated in clear cell RCC.

Beside *PTEN* and *mTOR* mutations, alterations in several genes controlling the PI3K/Akt/mTOR pathway have been identified in 28% of clear cell RCC [22, 25–27, 30].

Differentiation

Differentiation is frequent in clear cell RCC, and can appear sarcomatoid or rhabdoid. Dedifferentiation, implying an aggressive behavior and a poor prognosis, has commanded much attention to its molecular mechanism.

Sarcomatoid change, developed in 1–8% of all clear cell RCC, fundamentally reflects an epithelial-to-mesenchymal transformation (EMT). EMT is a process in which epithelial cells lose polarity and contact with their underlying basement membrane, culminating in a mesenchymal-like phenotype [31–33]. The molecular control of EMT is complex. It is linked to the mutations of *TP53* gene, well identified in sarcomatoid RCC. It may be also under the guidance of microRNAs. MicroRNAs are endogenous small, single-stranded non-coding RNAs which control a wide swath of gene expression by binding to the mRNAs of the target genes. Within oncogenesis, they can act as tumor promoters or tumor suppressors. Several microRNAs have been studied in RCC, where increase is noted for some, but decrease is observed for others. The microRNA-200 family (microR-200s, miR-141, microR-429, miR-138, microR-218, microR-30c), which controls EMT, are downregulated in RCC, leading to EMT promotion. Thus far, it seems that microRNAs promote EMT, mostly through acting as tumor suppressors [33].

Recently, Agaimy et al. [32] reported that SWI/SNF complex proteins (SMARCB1, SMARCA2, SMARCA4, ARID1A, SMARCC1, and SMARCC2) are responsible for undifferentiated/rhabdoid phenotype in RCC.

Papillary Renal Cell Carcinoma, Type 1

Papillary RCC is the second-most common type of RCC. Two distinct subtypes, Type 1 and Type 2, have been described in 1997. These two types are encountered in both sporadic and hereditary contexts. Type 1 is prevalent in hereditary papillary RCC syndrome (HPRCC), whereas the hereditary leiomyomatosis and RCC syndrome features the Type 2. In spite of the morphologic restriction, the molecular changes of these two forms of papillary RCC are quite variable. This heterogeneous molecular mechanism calls for further investigations to identify specific targets for more efficient treatments.

The molecular changes of Type 1 papillary RCC, including both hereditary and sporadic forms, are herein described, and those for Type 2 papillary is reported in the next section on papillary RCC in hereditary leiomyomatosis and RCC syndrome.

The Papillary RCC in the HPRCC Syndrome

The papillary RCC in the HPRCC syndrome is caused by a germline *gain-of-function* mutation of the *MET* proto-oncogene located on chromosome 7q31.3. Most HPRCC patients have amplification of the mutated copy of the *MET* gene [34]. The patients and the affected members of their family harbor gain-of-function (activating) mutations of *MET*, usually accompanied by trisomy 7 with the nonrandom duplication and overexpression of the mutant allele of the *MET* proto-oncogene [35–39]. Family members with mutant *MET* gene develop multifocal and bilateral papillary renal tumors [39].

The mechanism by which the *MET* gene mutation leads to RCC involves mostly the MET–HGF pathway. *MET* proto-oncogene encodes a transmembrane protein (MET). Normally, MET is expressed by stem cells and progenitor cells, and is crucial for embryogenesis and organogenesis in embryonic life, and healing of damaged tissues in adult life. MET is a tyrosine kinase which serves as the receptor for and is activated by hepatocyte growth factor (HGF). The gain-of-function mutation of *MET* gene amplifies the MET–HGF signaling pathways leading to uncontrolled growth irrelevant of the surrounding environmental conditions, and tumorigenesis [34]. Specifically, multiple signal transduction pathways are activated including the RAS, phosphatidylinositol 3-kinase [PI3K], STAT, beta-catenin, and Notch pathways, which collectively plays a major role in epithelial–mesenchymal transition, cell proliferation, differentiation and migration in tissues, and tumor progression (Fig. 18.2) [13, 34, 40].

Other pathways are also involved. Growth signaling can be normally controlled by the growth factor receptor activity and the surrounding nutrient levels. LKB1-AMPK-mTOR is a nutrient and energy-sensing pathway, the deregulation of which causes HGF/MET activation [34, 41].

Sporadic Type 1 Papillary RC

The molecular mechanism of sporadic papillary RCC, Type 1, is less known. According to the Cancer Genome Atlas Research Network (TCGA), Type 1 tumors also harbor alteration of the MET gene in many cases (up to 81%). However, other genetic changes are also frequent, including a gain of chromosome 7 and chromosome 17. Trisomy chromosome 7 can be found in a variety of other neoplasms and normal cells, indicating that trisomy 17 is much more specific for papillary RCC than trisomy 7 [26, 31, 42–44]. CDKN2A alterations either by mutation or hypermethylation have also been studied in papillary RCC, but seem to be more important for Type 2 tumor (see below).

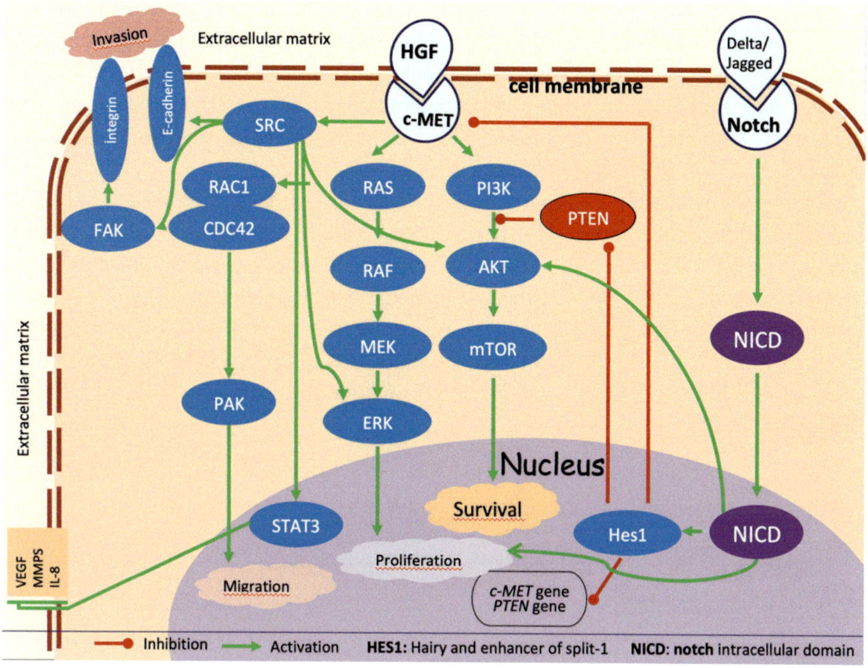

Fig. 18.2 The pathogenesis of hereditary papillary RCC: *MET* proto-oncogene encodes a transmembrane protein (MET). MET is a tyrosine kinase receptor for hepatocyte growth factor (HGF). The engagement of MET–HGF activates multiple signal transduction pathways (RAS, phosphatidylinositol 3-kinase [PI3K], STAT, beta-catenin, and Notch pathways) and activations of these pathways play a major role in epithelial mesenchymal transition, cell proliferation, differentiation and migration in tissues, and tumor progression

Some genetic differences between the hereditary and sporadic Type 1 papillary RCC were reported [13, 34, 45, 46], including the following: The mutation of *MET* gene has been identified in only a minority of type 1 sporadic papillary RCCs. Trisomy of chromosome 7, 16, or 17, and loss of chromosome Y (in men) are frequently observed in sporadic papillary RCC, but only trisomy 7 is found in hereditary papillary RCC, which accounts for duplication (and thus a double "dose") of the pathogenic mutant *MET* allele [13].

Type 2 Papillary RCC

Papillary RCC in the Hereditary Leiomyomatosis and Renal Cell Carcinoma (HLRCC) Syndrome

Type 2 papillary RCC is the principal renal tumor in the HLRCC syndrome. HLRCC is an autosomal dominant disease that is associated with germline mutation of the *fumarate hydratase* (*FH*) gene at chromosome 1q42.3-q43. Normally, cell respiration involves the tricarboxylic acid cycle. Abnormal function of the enzymes in this cycle may force cells to switch to glucose transport and aerobic glycolysis for survival. And this switching may be oncogenic. Normally, the *FH* gene codes fumarate hydratase, a tricarboxylic acid cycle enzyme, which converts fumarate to malate. Loss of fumarate hydratase due to *FH* gene mutation disrupts the tricarboxylic acid cycle and oxidative phosphorylation that causes a metabolic shift to aerobic glycolysis for the energy needs (Warburg effect).

The mutation-induced functional impairment of fumarate hydratase may also cause intracellular accumulation of fumarate, which may mediate inhibition HIF prolyl hydroxylases, reduction of AMPK and p53 levels, and activation of anabolic factors, such as acetyl-CoA carboxylase and ribosomal protein S6 [34, 47, 48]. Inhibition of HIF prolyl hydroxylases and reduction of AMPK level may lead to accumulation of HIF-1α, but not HIF-2α, and thus activation of HIF target genes such as VEGF and GLUT, an essential oncogenic pathway in VHL disease (Fig. 18.3) [47–49].

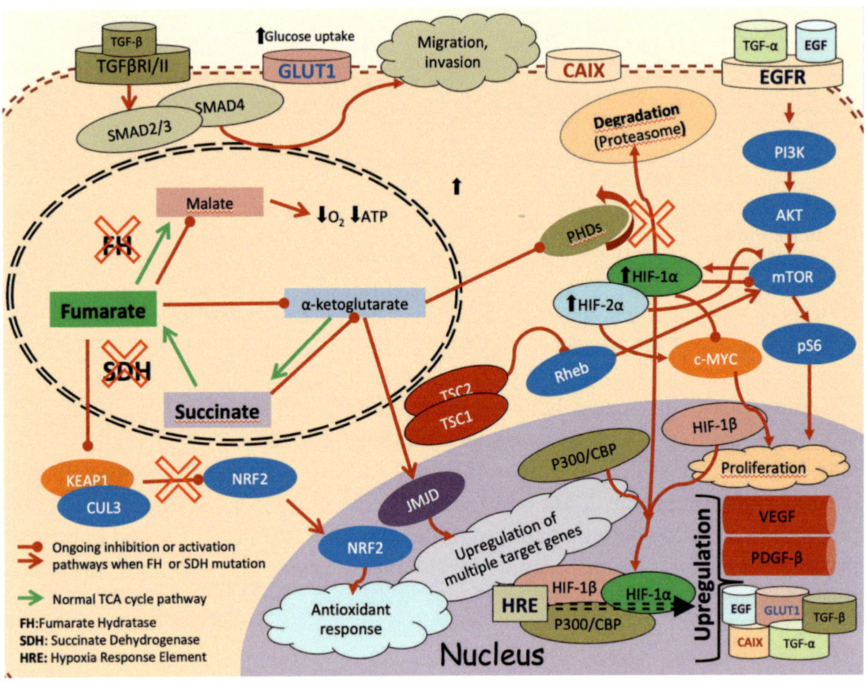

Fig. 18.3 The pathogenesis of type 2 PRCC in hereditary leiomyomatosis and renal cell carcinoma syndrome: Mutated fumarate hydratase may cause intracellular accumulation of fumarate, which may mediate inhibition HIF prolyl hydroxylases, reduction of AMPK and p53 levels, and activation of anabolic factors, such as acetyl-CoA carboxylase and ribosomal protein S6.This inhibition may lead to accumulation of HIF-1α, but not HIF-2α, and thus activation of HIF target genes such as VEGF and GLUT, an essential oncogenic pathway in VHL disease. In addition, increased fumarate inhibits KEAP1 (Kelch-like ECH-associated protein 1) and this inhibition causes upregulation of NRF2 and related multiple target genes involved in pseudohypoxia pathway

Increased cytosol fumarate is also oncogenic by other pathways. Nuclear factor, erythroid 2-like 2 (NRF2), a transcription factor, is a key regulator of the antioxidant response, with multiple-target genes including heme oxygenase-1, ferritin, NQO1, SOD1, GCLM, GCLC, GCS, GSR, G6PD, malic enzyme, GSTs, UGTs, GPX2, and peroxiredoxin [50]. NRF2 is regulated and inhibited by Kelch-like ECH-associated protein 1 (KEAP1), which is a substrate recognized by a subunit of a Cul3-based E3 ubiquitin ligase. Inhibition of KEAP1 by increased fumarate causes upregulation of NRF2and related multiple target genes involved in pseudohypoxia pathway (Fig. 18.3).

Other pathways independent from the tricarboxylic acid pathway may be involved. Reduction of AMPK results in the activation of mTOR signaling pathway, which is an important oncogenic pathway also for the RCCs in HPRCC and BHD syndromes. These observations indicate that different types of gene mutation can converge into a limited number of common downstream pathogenic signaling pathways, which should facilitate the design of target-directed therapy [48].

Sporadic Type 2 Papillary RCC

Type 2 papillary RCC can occur sporadically. The molecular changes of sporadic Type 2 papillary RCC are poorly understood. Molecular changes of the sporadic and hereditary forms overlap but not identical. Mutation of *FH* gene, which is noted in virtually all cases of hereditary Type 2 papillary RCC, is noted in only a subset of its sporadic counterpart (see below). However, other genetic changes have been described including LOH of chromosomes 1p, 3p, 5q, 6, 8, 9p, 10, 11, 15, 18, and 22, silencing the functions of *CDKN2A* gene, mutations of *SETD2* gene, and activation of the NRF2-antioxidant response (NRF2/ARE) pathway [26]. Silencing the functions of *CDKN2A* gene may be mediated by a loss of *CDKN2A* gene, or hypermethylation of the CDKN2A promoter, which is called CpG island methylator phenotype (CIMP). These silencing changes are not only pathogenetically important but also portend a poor prognosis (Table 18.1) [42, 44]. In addition, the CIMP tumors are affected by a marked metabolic dysregulation mediated indeed by somatic or germline mutations in the *FH* gene. Additionally, there are increasing studies which, based on molecular and survival features, proposed that papillary RCC Type 2 can be divided into three subgroups, one of which is the CIMP tumors [26].

Chromophobe Renal Cell Carcinoma

Chromophobe RCC can be either hereditary or sporadic. Chromophobe RCC, as a hereditary RCC, is the principal histologic type in Birt–Hogg--Dubé (BHD) syndrome. Sporadic chromophobe RCC constitutes 5–7% of all RCCs.

Hereditary Chromophobe RCC

The mutation of the *FLCN* gene (also known as *BHD* gene) is responsible for the BDH syndrome. The *FLCN* gene, which is located on chromosome 17p11.2, functions normally as a tumor suppressor gene, and encodes a protein known under two different names, that is, folliculin or FLCN protein [51, 52]. Folliculin forms a complex with two interacting/binding proteins, which are folliculin-interacting protein 1 (FNIP1) and 2 (FNIP2) [53–55]. FNIP1 and FNIP2 proteins are encoded by two different genes, *FNIP1* and *FNIP2* genes, which are located on chromosomes 5q23.3 and 4q32.1, respectively. In normal condition, folliculin regulates cell growth and serves as a tumor suppressor. FLCN is crucial for the differentiation of proximal and distal tubules and collecting ducts, and regulation of the composition of the extracellular matrix [56]. *FLCN* gene involves in energy and/or nutrient sensing 5'AMP activated protein kinase (AMPK)–mammalian target of rapamycin (mTOR) signaling pathway [53]. A protein complex of FLCN, FNIP1, and FNIP2 interacts with AMPK, which is a critical energy and nutrient sensor modulating ATP levels. This interaction negatively regulates the Akt–mTOR signaling pathway [34, 53–55]. In addition to keeping the AMPK–mTOR signaling pathway in check, FLCN may play a physiologic role in regulating cell growth, ciliogenesis, cell–cell adhesion and cell polarity, apoptosis, autophagy, TGF-β signaling, TFE3/TFEB transcriptional control, HIF transcriptional activity, PGC1-α (peroxisome proliferator-activated receptor-gamma coactivator 1-alpha)-driven mitochondrial biogenesis, and Rag GTPases for amino acid-dependent activation of mTOR at the lysosome (Fig. 18.4) [55, 57].

Germline mutation of the *FLCN* gene develops in the majority of patients with BDH syndrome and also often in family members. The mutation can be frame-shift, nonsense, insertion/deletion, or splice type. Sequence alterations or LOH of the somatic copy of *FLCN* gene were detected in 80–88% of BHD patients [34, 58–60]. Mutation of the FLCN genes produces a truncated nonfunctioning folliculin with a loss of its physiologic cell-regulatory and tumor suppressor function, leading to upregulation of oncogenic pathways and tumor formation [16, 51, 61, 62].

Sporadic Chromophobe RCC

Mutation of the *FLCN* gene is detected in a minority (<10%) of sporadic chromophobe RCCs. Recent studies, most thorough among which is that from the Cancer Genome Atlas Project, reveal several additional responsible chromosomal changes, genetic mutation, and deranged molecular pathways.

Chromophobe RCC shows loss of chromosomes 1, 2, 6, 10, 13, 17, 21, and Y [26]. These chromosomal losses are later account for several alterations at the gene level (see below).

One pathogenetic molecular pathway involves the *p53-axis and PTEN pathway*. Chromophobe RCC has prominent tumor suppressor gene alterations such

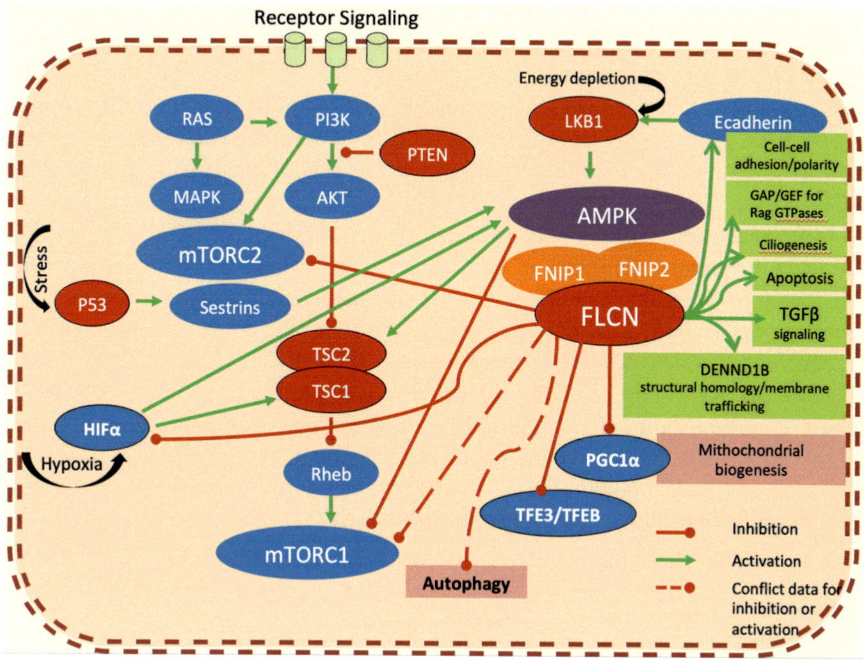

Fig. 18.4 The pathogenesis of hybrid tumors in Birt–Hogg–Dubé syndrome: A protein complex of FLCN, FNIP1, and FNIP2 interacts with AMPK and this interaction negatively regulates the Akt–mTOR signaling pathway. In addition to keeping the AMPK–mTOR signaling pathway in check, FLCN may play a physiologic role in regulating cell growth, ciliogenesis, cell–cell adhesion and cell polarity, apoptosis, autophagy, TGF-β signaling, TFE3/TFEB transcriptional control, HIF transcriptional activity, PGC1-α (peroxisome proliferator-activated receptor gamma coactivator 1-alpha)-driven mitochondrial biogenesis, and Rag GTPases for amino acid-dependent activation of mTOR at the lysosome

as *TP53* mutation (together with loss of chromosome 17) or *PTEN* mutation (together with loss of chromosome 10), which causes a break on the PI3K signaling pathway. Unlike other RCC types, chromophobe RCC is the only one that has *TP53* (32%) and *PTEN* (9%) mutations. Recently, HNF1B loss was shown in chromophobe RCC and, together with TP53 mutation, may cause an aggressive phenotype [26, 31, 63].

Pathogenesis also involves *the electron transport chain pathway and the Krebs cycle*. All genes encoding the enzymes of the Krebs cycle are overactivated in chromophobe RCC, resulting in more adenosine triphosphate (ATP) generation. *MT-ND*, one member of the genes for the electron transport chain complex I, is the most frequently altered gene. MT-ND5 is critical for the complex I, which is essential for electron transportation from NADH to ubiquinone. Loss of oxidative phosphorylation probably causes alternative pathways to supply the energy for tumor growth. But still studies are necessary to display the compensatory mechanisms [26, 63, 64]. Induction of oxidative stress due to the high level of reactive oxygen species or a higher resistance to apoptosis, which is induced by oxidative stress, were reported as the possible causes of tumor growth [65].

Whole genome sequencing studies of chromophobe RCC revealed genomic rearrangements in the *TERT* promoter area together with elevated *TERT* gene expression. Limited studies showed that high expression of TERT is associated with kataegis, a pattern of localized hypermutation, due to apolipoprotein B mRNA editing enzyme, catalytic polypeptide-like (APOBEC)–cystidine deaminase mutations. Further investigations are needed to highlight the role of kataegis in chromophobe RCC [25, 26, 63–65].

Molecular make-up may help with the differential diagnosis. Oncocytoma is in the main differential diagnosis of chromophobe RCC. Unlike chromophobe RCC, oncocytoma often exhibits a diploid karyotype, loss, or recurring rearrangements of chromosome 1 or 14. A subset of chromophobe RCC, the eosinophilic variant, can be confused histologically with oncocytoma or other RCC types with cytoplasmic eosinophilia. Recent findings showed that the eosinophilic variant displays the same losses of chromosomes 1, 2, 6, 10, and 17, as for the classic variant, supporting that these two variants belong to the same entity. Sarcomatoid change has been well documented for chromophobe RCC. It is now known that gain of chromosomes 1, 2, 6, 10 and 17 promotes this dedifferentiation [26, 31, 64].

MiT Family Translocation Renal Cell Carcinoma

Microphthalmia-associated transcription (MiT) family translocation RCC is newly described. The MiT family of transcription factors is TFE3, TFEB, MITF, and TFEC, all of which share the same binding domain and similar target genes. The physiologic function of these genes is tissue-specific and related to cell growth and differentiation. They play roles at melanocyte differentiation, and hematopoietic cell differentiation including macrophages, osteoclasts, lymphocytes, and mast cells. The fundamental molecular mechanism of this tumor family is the *translocation* of one of these genes to fuse with another gene in a different chromosome (thus the name "translocation RCC"), and this fusion is oncogenic. *TFE3* and *TFEB* fusion patterns have been elucidated. They account for most tumors in this family, are of sporadic nature, and are encountered in 1–5% of sporadic RCC of variably histologic patterns. *MITF* fusion is rare, its fusion partners are not known, and this fusion is described only in hereditary context [22, 66, 67]. *TFEC* gene has not been to be oncogenic. TFEC is most divergent member of the family and its activation domain is missing. *It appears to inhibit, rather than activate, transcription* [66].

Xp11 Translocation RCC (TF3 Gene-Mediated)

Xp11 translocation RCC was described as a RCC subtype by Argani et al. [68] and was first recognized in the 2004 WHO classification of the kidney tumors. Xp11 translocation RCC harbors fusion of *TFE3* gene residing on chromosome Xp11with other genes [69]. Five patterns of *TFE3* gene fusions (*PRCC–TFE3, ASPSCR1–TFE3, SFPQ–TFE3, NONO–TFE3*, and *CLTC–TFE3*) have been identified to date. The first identified gene fusion is the t(x;1) (p11.2;q21.2), *PRCC–TFE3* fusion that occurs between TFE3 on chromosome xp11.2 and a novel gene on chromosome 1q21.2 designated as *PRCC* [26, 69, 70]. Subsequent studies showed two more gene fusion patterns *SFPQ–TFE3* (also known as *PSF–TFE3*) and *NONO–TFE3* (also known as *p54nrb–TFE3*). These two new pathogenetic fusion patterns show that the critical oncogenic role resides on *TFE3* genes rather than *PRCC*. Argani et al. [71] identified two additional TFE3 fusions *ASPSCR1–TFE3* (also known as *ASPL–TFE3*) and *CLTC–TFE3*. *ASPSCR1* and *CLTC* genes are located on chromosome 17q. Among all these fusions, the two most common Xp11 translocation RCCs have t(X;1)(p11.2;q21) *PRCC–TFE3* fusion and t(X;17)(p11.2;q25) *ASPSCR1–TFE3* fusion. *TFE3* gene fusions can also be seen at other tumors such as alveolar soft part sarcoma (*ASPSCR1–TFE3*) and perivascular epithelioid cell neoplasm (PECOMA) (*SFPQ–TFE3*) [26, 70–72].

t(6;11) RCC (TFEB Gene-Mediated)

t(6;11) RCC is the second member of MiT family translocation RCC. Its development involves the fusion of the *TFEB* gene and the *MALAT1* gene [t(6;11)(p21;q12) translocation]. t(6;11) RCC was first described in 2001 and accepted as a RCC subtype under MiT family translocation RCC in the 2016 WHO classification. The Cancer Genome Atlas Research database helps identified three more novel fusion partners of the *TFEB* gene, including two fusion partners *COL21A1*and *CADM2* genes observed in papillary RCC, and *KHDRBS2* gene observed in clear cell RCC [66, 67, 69, 70–72].

The oncogenic effects of *TFE3* and *TFEB* gene fusions and their roles in renal cell tumor carcinogenesis remain unclear, but are summarized below [66, 67].

1. Activation of TGFβ pathways
2. Enhancing the activity of ETS-1 by binding
3. Transcription of E-cadherin; important for cancer cell–cell interactions
4. Expression of CD40 L which activates T-cell lymphocytes and plays a role in tumor immunoevasion
5. Enhancing the mTORC1 signaling that plays a role in protein synthesis which drives the tumor growth
6. Regulation of metabolic pathways. TFE3 affects insulin signaling and glucose metabolism by upregulation of IRS-2 and the hexokinase enzymes, decreasing lipogenesis and increasing glycogen synthesis
7. Preventing cell cycle arrest by interacting with the retinoblastoma protein

Succinate Dehydrogenase (SDH)-Deficient RCC

SDH-RCC is a recently described type of RCC with diverse histologic features, but the most characteristic among which is the presence of tumor cells with flocculent, pale staining cytoplasmic inclusions mostly representing damaged or dilated mitochondria.

SDH-RCC is caused by germline (hereditary) mutation of the succinate dehydrogenase (SDH) genes. Sporadic form has not been reported. These genes code for the SDH enzyme complex, which is a mitochondrial enzyme complex functional in the Krebs cycle. Five proteins constitute the SDH enzyme complex, SDHA, SDHB, SDHC, SDHD, and SDHAF2, and they are encoded by 5 genes, the *SDHx* genes/*SDH complex* genes, which consist of *SDHA* (5p15.33), *SDHB* (1p36.13), *SDHC* (1q23.3), *SDHD* (11q23.1), and *SDHAF2* (11q12.2). SDHAF2 protein, which is localized on the mitochondrial membrane, is essential for the assembling of subunits (SDHA, SDHB, SDHC, and SDHD) of SDH enzyme. The association of subunits of SDH and SDHAF2 protein is crucial for the formation of the Complex II of the electron transport chain, which is a critical component of the Krebs cycle. SDH catalyzes the oxidation of succinate to fumarate and transfers electrons to the respiratory chain ubiquinone pool [73, 74].

Mutational inactivation of *SDHx* genes result in a malfunctioning SDH, leading to accumulation of succinate first in the mitochondria, and then in the cytosol. Increased succinate can inhibit the prolyl hydroxylases, and leads to activation of HIF-1α. Activated HIF-1α may then in turn upregulate multiple downstream genes including CAIX (discussed in detail above). This effect may play an important role in tumorigenesis (Fig. 18.3) [34]. HIF1α inhibits c-MYC oncogene, mTOR, β-catenin, and activates p53, whereas HIF-2α activates c-MYC oncogene β-catenin, and inhibits p53 [75, 76].

Tuberous Sclerosis Complex

Tuberous sclerosis complex (TSC) is a hereditary disease characterized in part by neoplasms involving several organs, including kidney. The majority of TSC-associated renal tumors are angiomyolipoma, but RCC of diverse histology has been described in 2–4% of patients.

TSC result from loss-of-function or inactivating mutations of one of two tumor suppressor genes, *TSC1* and *TSC2*, locating on chromosomes 9q34 and 16p13.3, and encoding hamartin (TSC1) and tuberin (TSC2) proteins, respectively. In normal condition, hamartin and tuberin proteins combine to form a heterodimer (TSC protein complex), which controls several nutrient- and energy-sensing pathways, including those related to mTOR and AMPK. This physiologic effect is mediated at least in part by activation of Rheb, a Ras-family GTPase, which inhibits mTOR activity (Fig. 18.3 and 18.4). Mutation-mediated loss of functions of TSC protein complex leads to activation of several oncogenic pathways shared by several hereditary cancer syndromes. Thus the mTOR signaling pathway is activated by inhibiting Rheb, which in turn causes the production of VEGF, EPO, PDGF-β, and TGF-α, collectively favoring tumor formation by promoting cell growth and angiogenesis, and inhibition of apoptosis (Fig. 18.1). In addition, the loss of function TSC2 protein leads to accumulation of HIF1α and increasing of HIF-responsive genes such as *VEGF* (Fig. 18.3).

Mutation of *TSC1* or *TSC2* genes has not been described in sporadic RCC [77]. However, *TSC2* gene mutation, but not *TSC1*, may be seen in sporadic AML [78].

Recent studies suggested that additional genetic changes may play a role in at least some of RCCs in TSC patients [74]. Thus, TSC-associated papillary RCCs are rarely associated with gains of chromosomes 7 and 17 [74].

Molecular Changes of Other Types of Renal Neoplasm

Knowledge in this area is limited, reflecting both the rarity of these tumor types and limited pertinent studies.

Collecting Duct Carcinoma

Collecting duct carcinoma is a rare type of RCC that arise from the cells of distal tubules or collecting ducts. Its genetic mechanism is not fully understood, but clearly differs from the other types of RCC. Collecting duct carcinoma shares some molecular features with both urothelial carcinoma and RCC. Studies have shown that they have chromosomal losses like allelic loss of 1q, 6p, 8p, 13q, and 21q. LOH has been shown on 8p, 6p, 9p, 13q, and 21q. Monosomies of chromosomes 1, 6, 14, 15, and 22 have been also reported. Poor prognosis might be related to losses of 1p36, 3p, 6p, and 8p [26, 31].

Renal Medullary Carcinoma

Renal medullary carcinoma was firstly described by Davis et al. [79] in 1995. It is a poorly differentiated RCC that is associated with sickle cell trait or related hemoglobinopathy. These RCCs show loss of expression of the nuclear transcriptional regulator *SMARCB1 (INI1)* that is located on chromosome 22. Hemizygous deletions, LOH, and loss of chromosome 22 have been detected at the molecular studies [26, 31].

Mucinous Tubular and Spindle Cell Carcinoma

Mucinous tubular and spindle cell renal carcinoma is a rare type of RCC with diverse histological features. It is now accepted that they originated from proximal nephron and some reports suggested that it can be a variant of papillary RCC because of some histologic similarity. Genomic studies, however, show losses of chromosomes 1, 4, 6, 8, 9, 11, 13, 14, 15, 18, 22, and X. Gains of chromosomes 2, 3, 4, 5, 7, 9, 10, 12, 15, 16, 17, 18, 19, 20, 22, and Y have also been identified [26, 80].

Tubulocystic Renal Cell Carcinoma

It is an uncommon type of RCC that constitutes <1% of all RCC. The genomic features are similar to papillary RCC. They show gains of chromosomes 7 and 17 and loss of the Y chromosome [26].

Acquired Cystic Disease-Associated Renal Cell Carcinoma

There are two major types of renal neoplasm that have been described in end-stage renal disease: acquired cystic disease-associated RCC and clear cell papillary RCC. Acquired cystic disease-associated RCC shows gains of the chromosomes 3, 7, 16, 17, and sex chromosomes [26, 27, 31].

Clear Cell Papillary Renal Cell Carcinoma

This is a recently described variant of RCC, which is recognized in the 2016 WHO classification of renal tumors. It accounts for 1–4% of renal tumors and can develop from a background of end-stage renal disease or de novo. Although this RCC type displays histologic features of both clear cell RCC and papillary RCC, its molecular features are distinct from these two RCC types. Limited studies have revealed no gains of chromosome 7 and loss of Y, unlike papillary RCC; or 3p deletion which is typical for clear cell RCC [25].

Molecular Testing

Although much insight into the molecular mechanism of the renal tumor has been expeditiously gained, its clinical applications are still limited and molecular testing for patient care is still in its infancy. Guidelines for routine molecular testing in RCC have not been developed. In principle, molecular testing can be performed on tumor tissue in a sporadic context to detect clinically relevant genetic alterations, which are limited to the tumor tissue. Alternatively, it can be performed in blood samples to detect pathogenetic germline mutations responsible for hereditary tumors.

Several genetic mutations responsible for a specific tumor phenotype (e.g., sarcomatoid or rhabdoid) or an aggressive behavior have been identified. However, these molecular findings have not yet lead to routine clinical testing, perhaps because they offer no additional prognostic impact beyond routine histology and, furthermore, targeted therapy has not been developed for these genetic changes. Several targeted therapies for RCC have recently approved, each of which targets a few specific oncogenic molecular pathways. Yet, testing for these targets in tumor tissue is currently not a prerequisite for treatment, as is the histologic types of tumors. This approach is perhaps due, at least in part, to the observation that many of the same pathways are oncogenic across the border of histologic types.

On the other hand, molecular testing for germline mutations is clearly indicated. A recent study of 1235 blood or saliva samples from patients with renal tumor to evaluate 19 genes known to be pathogenetic for renal tumors reveals hereditary forms of RCC in 6.1%, a frequency comparable to the reported frequency of these tumor types [81]. Interestingly, hereditary RCC was first detected by molecular testing in several patients, who did not display other features of hereditary RCC. Furthermore, young age of patients (< 45 years) is the only predictor for a positive result [81, 82]. Molecular testing for germline mutations is currently available as not only a diagnostic test but also offers significant clinical utility.

Conclusion

Renal cell carcinomas are a heterogeneous group of tumors with different molecular backgrounds. Much insight has been gained into the molecular mechanism of these tumors and much more is expected thanks to the advent of sophisticated tools for genetic study. These findings should help connect histologic features with molecular landmarks and provide insights into the mechanism of renal neogenesis. These findings also begin to facilitate molecular diagnosis and prognostication. Of vital interest, they will help with the development and administration of molecular targeted therapy.

References

1. Alba AG, Arranzb JA, Puente J, Méndez-Vidal MJ, Gallardo E, Grande E, Pérez-Valderrama B, González-Billalabeitia E, Lázaro-Quintela M, Pintoj A, Lainez N, Piulats JM, Esteban E, Rey JPM, Garcíao JA, Suárezp C. Recent advances in genitourinary tumors: a review focused onbiology and systemic treatment. Crit Rev Oncol Hematol. 2017;113:171–90.
2. Costa WH, Netto GJ, Isabela WI. Urological cancer related to familial syndromes. Int Braz J Urol. 2017;43:192–201.
3. Favazza L, Chitale DA, Barod R, Rogers CG, Kalyana-Sunduram S, Palanisamy N, Gupta NS, Williamson SR. Renal cell tumors with clear cell histology and intact VHL and chromosome 3p: a histological review of tumors from the Cancer Genome Atlas database. Mod Pathol. 2017;30(11):1603–12.

4. Inamura K. Renal cell tumors: understanding their molecular pathological epidemiology and the 2016 WHO classification. Int J Mol Sci. 2017;18(10):2195.
5. Stolle C, Glenn G, Zbar B, Humphrey JS, Choyke P, Walther M, Pack S, Hurley K, Andrey C, Klausner R, Linehan WM. Improved detection of germline mutations in the von Hippel-Lindau disease tumor suppressor gene. Hum Mutat. 1998;12:417–23.
6. Hoebeeck J, van der Luijt R, Poppe B, De Smet E, Yigit N, Claes K, Zewald R, de Jong GJ, De Paepe A, Speleman F, Vandesompele J. Rapid detection of VHL exon deletions using real-time quantitative PCR. Lab Invest. 2005;85:24–33.
7. Coppin L, Grutzmacher C, Crépin M, Destailleur E, Giraud S, Cardot-Bauters C, Porchet N, Pigny P. VHL mosaicism can be detected by clinical next-generation sequencing and is not restricted to patients with a mild phenotype. Eur J Hum Genet. 2014;22:1149–52.
8. Nordstrom-O'Brien M, van der Luijt RB, van Rooijen E, van den Ouweland AM, Majoor-Krakauer DF, Lolkema MP, van Brussel A, Voest EE, Giles RH. Genetic analysis of von Hippel-Lindau disease. Hum Mutat. 2010;31:521–37.
9. Schmid S, Gillessen S, Binet I, Brändle M, Engeler D, Greiner J, Hader C, Heinimann K, Kloos P, Krek W, Krull I, Stoeckli SJ, Sulz MC, van Leyen K, Weber J, Rothermundt C, Hundsberger T. Management of von Hippel-Lindau disease: an interdisciplinary review. Oncol Res Treat. 2014;37:761–71.
10. Beroukhim R, Brunet JP, Di Napoli A, Mertz KD, Seeley A, Pires MM, Linhart D, Worrell RA, Moch H, Rubin MA, Sellers WR, Meyerson M, Linehan WM, Kaelin WG Jr, Signoretti S. Patterns of gene expression and copy-number alterations in von-Hippel lindau disease-associated and sporadic clear cell carcinoma of the kidney. Cancer Res. 2009;69:4674–81.
11. Seizinger BR, Rouleau GA, Ozelius LJ, Lane AH, Farmer GE, Lamiell JM, Haines J, Yuen JW, Collins D, Majoor-Krakauer D, Seizinger BR, et al. Von Hippel–Lindau disease maps to the region of chromosome 3 associated with renal cell carcinoma. Nature. 1988;332:268–9.
12. Latif F, Tory K, Gnarra J, Yao M, Duh FM, Orcutt ML, Stackhouse T, Kuzmin I, Modi W, Geil L, et al. Identification of the von Hippel-Lindau disease tumor suppressor gene. Science. 1993;260:1317–20.
13. Verine J, Pluvinage A, Bousquet G, Lehmann-Che J, de Bazelaire C, Soufir N, Mongiat-Artus P. Hereditary renal cancer syndromes: an update of a systematic review. Eur Urol. 2010;58:701–10.
14. Herring JC, Enquist EG, Chernoff A, Linehan WM, Choyke PL, Walther MM. Parenchymal sparing surgery in patients with hereditary renal cell carcinoma: 10-year experience. J Urol. 2001;165:777–81.
15. Housley SL, Lindsay RS, Young B, McConachie M, Mechan D, Baty D, Christie L, Rahilly M, Qureshi K, Fleming S. Renal carcinoma with giant mitochondria associated with germ-line mutation and somatic loss of the succinate dehydrogenase B gene. Histopathology. 2010;56:405–8.
16. Houweling AC, Gijezen LM, Jonker MA, van Doorn MB, Oldenburg RA, van Spaendonck-Zwarts KY, Leter EM, van Os TA, van Grieken NC, Jaspars EH, de Jong MM, Bongers EM, Johannesma PC, Postmus PE, van Moorselaar RJ, van Waesberghe JH, Starink TM, van Steensel MA, Gille JJ, Menko FH. Renal cancer and pneumothorax risk in Birt–Hogg–Dubé syndrome; an analysis of 115 FLCN mutation carriers from 35 BHD families. Br J Cancer. 2011;105:1912–9.
17. Zhang Q, Yang H. The roles of VHL-dependent ubiquitination in signaling and cancer. Front Oncol. 2012;2:35.
18. Weinmann M, Thews O, Schroeder T, Vaupel P. Expression pattern of the urokinase-plasminogen activator system in rat DS-sarcoma: role of oxygenation status and tumour size. Br J Cancer. 2002;86:1355–61.
19. Shuin T, Yamasaki I, Tamura K, Okuda H, Furihata M, Ashida S. Von Hippel-Lindau disease: molecular pathological basis, clinical criteria, genetic testing, clinical features of tumors and treatment. Jpn J Clin Oncol. 2006;36:337–43.
20. Richard S, Gardie B, Couvé S, Gad S. Von Hippel-Lindau: how a rare disease illuminates cancer biology. Semin Cancer Biol. 2013;23:26–37.

21. Pfaffenroth EC, Linehan WM. Genetic basis for kidney cancer: opportunity for disease-specific approaches to therapy. Expert Opin Biol Ther. 2008;8:779–90.
22. Moch H, Bonsib SM, Delahunt B, Eble J, Egevad L, Grignon DJ, Linehan WM, Reuter VE, Srigley JR, Sulser T, Tan PH. Clear cell carcinoma. In: Moch H, Humphrey PA, Ulbright TM, Reuter VE, editors. WHO classification of tumours of the urinary system and male genital organs. 4th ed. Lyon: IARC; 2016. p. 18–22.
23. Kim SH, Park WS, Park EY, Park B, Joo J, Joung JY, Seo HK, Lee KH, Chung J. The prognostic value of BAP1, PBRM1, pS6, PTEN, TGase2, PD-L1, CA9, PSMA, and Ki-67 tissue markers in localized renal cell carcinoma: a retrospective study of tissue microarrays using immunohistochemistry. PLoS One. 2017;12(6):e0179610.
24. Sato Y, Yoshizato T, Shiraishi Y, Maekawa S, Okuno Y, Kamura T, Shimamura T, Sato-Otsubo A, Nagae G, Suzuki H, Nagata Y, Yoshida K, Kon A, Suzuki Y, Chiba K, Tanaka H, Niida A, Fujimoto A, Tsunoda T, Morikawa T, Maeda D, Kume H, Sugano S, Fukayama M, Aburatani H, Sanada M, Miyano S, Homma Y, Ogawa S. Integrated molecular analysis of clear-cell renal cell carcinoma. Nat Genet. 2013;45(8):860–7.
25. Su D, Singer EA, Srinivasan R. Molecular pathways in renal cell carcinoma: recent advances in genetics and molecular biology. Curr Opin Oncol. 2015;27(3):217–23.
26. Haake SM, Weyandt JD, Rathmell WK. Insights into the genetic basis of the renal cell carcinomas from The Cancer Genome Atlas (TCGA). Mol Cancer Res. 2016;14(7):589–98.
27. Arai E, Kanai Y. Genetic and epigenetic alterations during renal carcinogenesis. Int J Clin Exp Pathol. 2011;4(1):58–73.
28. Kroeger N, Klatte T, Chamie K, Rao PN, Birkhäuser FD, Sonn GA, Riss J, Kabbinavar FF, Belldegrun AS, Pantuck AJ. Deletions of chromosomes 3p and 14q molecularly subclassify clear cell renal cell carcinoma. Cancer. 2013;119:1547–54.
29. Li L, Shen C, Nakamura E, Ando K, Signoretti S, Beroukhim R, Cowley GS, Lizotte P, Liberzon E, Bair S, Root DE, Tamayo P, Tsherniak A, Cheng SC, Tabak B, Jacobsen A, Hakimi AA, Schultz N, Ciriello G, Sander C, Hsieh JJ, Kaelin WG Jr. SQSTM1 is a pathogenic target of 5q copy number gains in kidney cancer. Cancer Cell. 2013;24(6):738–50.
30. Guo H, German P, Bai S, Barnes S, Guo W, Qi X, Lou H, Liang J, Jonasch E, Mills GB, Ding Z. The PI3K/AKT pathway and renal cell carcinoma. Genet Genomics. 2015;42(7):343–53.
31. Lopez-Beltran A, Montironi R, Egevad L, Caballero-Vargas MT, Scarpelli M, Kirkali Z, Cheng L. Genetic profiles in renal tumors. Int J Urol. 2010;17(1):6–19.
32. Agaimy A, Cheng L, Egevad L, Feyerabend B, Hes O, Keck B, Pizzolitto S, Sioletic S, Wullich B, Hartmann A. Rhabdoid and undifferentiated phenotype in renal cell carcinoma, analysis of 32 cases indicating a distinctive common pathway of dedifferentiation frequently associated with SWI/SNF complex deficiency. Am J Surg Pathol. 2017;41:253–62.
33. He H, Magi-Galluzzi C. Epithelial-to-mesenchymal transition in renal neoplasms. Adv Anat Pathol. 2014;21:174–80.
34. Linehan WM, Ricketts CJ. The metabolic basis of kidney cancer. Semin Cancer Biol. 2013;23:46–55.
35. Zbar B, Glenn G, Lubensky I, Choyke P, Walther MM, Magnusson G, Bergerheim US, Pettersson S, Amin M, Hurley K. Hereditary papillary renal cell carcinoma: clinical studies in 10 families. J Urol. 1995;153:907–12.
36. Zhuang Z, Park WS, Pack S, Schmidt L, Vortmeyer AO, Pak E, Pham T, Weil RJ, Candidus S, Lubensky IA, Linehan WM, Zbar B, Weirich G. Trisomy 7-harbouring non-random duplication of the mutant MET allele in hereditary papillary renal carcinomas. Nat Genet. 1998;20:66–9.
37. Fischer J, Palmedo G, von Knobloch R, Bugert P, Prayer-Galetti T, Pagano F, Kovacs G. Duplication and overexpression of the mutant allele of the MET proto-oncogene in multiple hereditary papillary renal cell tumours. Oncogene. 1998;17:733–9.
38. Singer EA, Bratslavsky G, Middelton L, Srinivasan R, Linehan WM. Impact of genetics on the diagnosis and treatment of renal cancer. Curr Urol Rep. 2011;12:47–55.
39. Coleman JA. Familial and hereditary renal cancer syndromes. Urol Clin North Am. 2008;35:563–72.

40. Linehan WM, Pinto PA, Srinivasan R, Merino M, Choyke P, Choyke L, Coleman J, Toro J, Glenn G, Vocke C, Zbar B, Schmidt LS, Bottaro D, Neckers L. Identification of the genes for kidney cancer: opportunity for disease-specific targeted therapeutics. Clin Cancer Res. 2007;13:671s–9s.
41. Linehan WM, Srinivasan R, Schmidt LS. The genetic basis of kidney cancer: a metabolic disease. Nat Rev Urol. 2010;7:277–85.
42. Saleeb RM, Plant P, Tawedrous E, Krizova A, Brimo F, Evans AJ, Wala SJ, Bartlett J, Ding Q, Boles D, Rotando F, Farag M, Yousef GM. Integrated phenotypic/genotypic analysis of papillary renal cell carcinoma subtypes: identification of prognostic markers, cancer-related pathways, and implications for therapy. Eur Urol Focus. 2018;4(5):740–8.
43. Modi PK, Singer EA. Improving our understanding of papillary renal cell carcinoma with integrative genomic analysis. Ann Transl Med. 2016;4(7):143.
44. Cancer Genome Atlas Research Network. Comprehensive molecular characterization of papillary renal cell carcinoma. N Engl J Med. 2016;374(2):135–45.
45. Cho E, Adami HO, Lindblad P. Epidemiology of renal cell cancer. Hematol Oncol Clin North Am. 2011;25:651–65.
46. Cohen D, Zhou M. Molecular genetics of familial renal cell carcinoma syndromes. Clin Lab Med. 2005;25:259–77.
47. Isaacs JS, Jung YJ, Mole DR, Lee S, Torres-Cabala C, Chung YL, Merino M, Trepel J, Zbar B, Toro J, Ratcliffe PJ, Linehan WM, Neckers L. HIF overexpression correlates with biallelic loss of fumarate hydratase in renal cancer: novel role of fumarate in regulation of HIF stability. Cancer Cell. 2005;8:143–53.
48. Tong WH, Sourbier C, Kovtunovych G, Jeong SY, Vira M, Ghosh M, Romero VV, Sougrat R, Vaulont S, Viollet B, Kim YS, Lee S, Trepel J, Srinivasan R, Bratslavsky G, Yang Y, Linehan WM, Rouault TA. Theglycolytic shift in fumarate-hydratase-deficient kidney cancer lowers AMPKlevels, increases metabolic propensities and lowers cellular iron levels. Cancer Cell. 2011;20:315–27.
49. Toro JR, Nickerson ML, Wei MH, Warren MB, Glenn GM, Turner ML, Stewart L, Duray P, Tourre O, Sharma N, Choyke P, Stratton P, Merino M, Walther MM, Linehan WM, Schmidt LS, Zbar B. Mutations in the fumarate hydratase gene cause hereditary leiomyomatosis and renal cell cancer in families in North America. Am J Hum Genet. 2003;73:95–106.
50. Giudice A, Arra C, Turco MC. Review of molecular mechanisms involved in the activation of the Nrf2-ARE signaling pathway by chemopreventive agents. Methods Mol Biol. 2010;647:37–74.
51. Toro JR, Wei MH, Glenn GM, Weinreich M, Toure O, Vocke C, Turner M, Choyke P, Merino MJ, Pinto PA, Steinberg SM, Schmidt LS, Linehan WM. BHD mutations, clinical and molecular genetic investigations of Birt-Hogg-Dube´ syndrome: a new series of 50 families and a review of published reports. J Med Genet. 2008;45:321–31.
52. Toro JR, Pautler SE, Stewart L, Glenn GM, Weinreich M, Toure O, Wei MH, Schmidt LS, Davis L, Zbar B, Choyke P, Steinberg SM, Nguyen DM, Linehan WM. Lung cysts, spontaneous pneumothrorax and genetic associations in 89 families with Birt-Hogg-Dube syndrome. Am J Respir Crit Care Med. 2007;175:1044–53.
53. Baba M, Hong SB, Sharma N, Warren MB, Nickerson ML, Iwamatsu A, Esposito D, Gillette WK, Hopkins RF 3rd, Hartley JL, Furihata M, Oishi S, Zhen W, Burke TR Jr, Linehan WM, Schmidt LS, Zbar B. Folliculin encoded by the BHD gene interacts with a binding protein, FNIP1, and AMPK, and is involved in AMPK and mTOR signaling. Proc Natl Acad Sci U S A. 2006;103:15552–7.
54. Hasumi H, Baba M, Hong SB, Hasumi Y, Huang Y, Yao M, Valera VA, Linehan WM, Schmidt LS. Identification and characterization of a novel folliculin-interacting protein FNIP2. Gene. 2008;415:60–7.
55. Schmidt LS. Birt-Hogg-Dubé syndrome: from gene discovery to molecularly targeted therapies. Fam Cancer. 2013;12:357–64.

56. Kuroda N, Furuya M, Nagashima Y, Gotohda H, Kawakami F, Moritani S, Ota S, Hora M, Michal M, Hes O, Nakatani Y. Review of renal tumors associated with Birt-Hogg-Dubé syndrome with focus on clinical and pathobiological aspects. Pol J Pathol. 2014;65:93–9.
57. Schmidt LS, Linehan WM. Clinical features, genetics and potential therapeutic approaches for Birt-Hogg-Dubé syndrome. Expert Opin Orphan Drugs. 2015;3:15–29.
58. Toro JR. Birt-Hogg-Dubé syndrome. 2006 Feb 27 [Updated 2014 Aug 7]. In: Pagon RA, et al., editors. GeneReviews® [Internet]. Seattle: University of Washington, Seattle; 1993–2015. Available from: http://www.ncbi.nlm.nih.gov/books/NBK1522/.
59. Vocke CD, Yang Y, Pavlovich CP, Schmidt LS, Nickerson ML, Torres-Cabala CA, Merino MJ, Walther MM, Zbar B, Linehan WM. High frequency of somatic frameshift BHD gene mutations in Birt–Hogg–Dubé-associated renal tumors. J Natl Cancer Inst. 2005;97:931–5.
60. Nickerson ML, Warren MB, Toro JR, Matrosova V, Glenn G, Turner ML, Duray P, Merino M, Choyke P, Pavlovich CP, Sharma N, Walther M, Munroe D, Hill R, Maher E, Greenberg C, Lerman MI, Linehan WM, Zbar B, Schmidt LS. Mutations in a novel gene lead to kidney tumors, lung wall defects,and benign tumors of the hair follicle in patients with the Birt-Hogg-Dube syndrome. Cancer Cell. 2002;2:157–64.
61. Schmidt LS, Nickerson ML, Warren MB, Glenn GM, Toro JR, Merino MJ, Turner ML, Choyke PL, Sharma N, Peterson J, Morrison P, Maher ER, Walther MM, Zbar B, Linehan WM. Germline BHD-mutation spectrum and phenotype analysis of a large cohort of families with Birt-Hogg-Dubé syndrome. Am J Hum Genet. 2005;76:1023–33.
62. Yusenko MV. Molecular pathology of chromophobe renal cell carcinoma: a review. Int J Urol. 2010;17:592–601.
63. Davis CF, Ricketts CJ, Wang M, Yang L, Cherniack AD, Shen H, Buhay C, Kang H, Kim SC, Fahey CC, Hacker KE, Bhanot G, Gordenin DA, Chu A, Gunaratne PH, Biehl M, Seth S, Kaipparettu BA, Bristow CA, Donehower LA, Wallen EM, Smith AB, Tickoo SK, Tamboli P, Reuter V, Schmidt LS, Hsieh JJ, Choueiri TK, Hakimi AA, The Cancer Genome Atlas Research Network, Chin L, Meyerson M, Kucherlapati R, Park WY, Robertson AG, Laird PW, Henske EP, Kwiatkowski DJ, Park PJ, Morgan M, Shuch B, Muzny D, Wheeler DA, Linehan WM, Gibbs RA, Rathmell WK, Creighton CJ. The somatic genomic landscape of chromophobe renal cell carcinoma. Cancer Cell. 2014;26(3):319–30.
64. Rathmell KW, Chen F, Creighton CJ. Genomics of chromophobe renal cell carcinoma: implications from a rare tumor for pan-cancer studies. Oncoscience. 2015;2:81–90.
65. Garcia-Heredia JM, Carnero A. Decoding Warburg's hypothesis: tumor-related mutations in the mitochondrial respiratory chain. Oncotarget. 2015;6(39):41582–99.
66. Medendorp K, van Groningen JJ, Schepens M, Vreede L, Thijssen J, Schoenmakers EF, van den Hurk WH, Geurts van Kessel A, Kuiper RP. Molecular mechanisms underlying the MiT translocation subgroup of renal cell carcinomas. Cytogenet Genome Res. 2007;118:157–65.
67. Kauffman EC, Ricketts CJ, Rais-Bahrami S, Yang Y, Merino MJ, Bottaro DP, Srinivasan R, Linehan WM. Molecular genetics and cellular features of TFE3 and TFEB fusion kidney cancers. Nat Rev Urol. 2014;11(8):465–75.
68. Argani P, Antonescu CR, Illei PB, Lui MY, Timmons CF, Newbury R, Reuter VE, Garvin AJ, Perez-Atayde AR, Fletcher JA, Beckwith JB, Bridge JA, Ladanyi M. Primary renal neoplasms with the ASPL-TFE3 gene fusion of alveolar soft part sarcoma: a distinctive tumor entity previously included among renal cell carcinomas of children and adolescents. Am J Pathol. 2001;159:179–92.
69. Argani P. MiT family translocation renal cell carcinoma. Semin Diagn Pathol. 2015;32(2):103–13.
70. Inamura K. Translocation renal cell carcinoma: an update on clinicopathological and molecular features. Cancers (Basel). 2017;9(9):E111.
71. Argani P, Lui MY, Couturier J, Bouvier R, Fournet JC, Ladanyi M. A novel CLTC-TFE3 gene fusion in pediatric renal adenocarcinoma with t(X;17)(p11.2;q23). Oncogene. 2003;22:5374–8.

72. Magers MJ, Udager AM, Mehra R. MiT family translocation-associated renal cell carcinoma a contemporary update with emphasis on morphologic, immunophenotypic, and molecular mimics. Arch Pathol Lab Med. 2015;139:1224–33.
73. Ricketts CJ, Shuch B, Vocke CD, Metwalli AR, Bratslavsky G, Middelton L, Yang Y, Wei MH, Pautler SE, Peterson J, Stolle CA, Zbar B, Merino MJ, Schmidt LS, Pinto PA, Srinivasan R, Pacak K, Linehan WM. Succinate Dehydrogenase Kidney Cancer (SDH-RCC): an aggressive example of the Warburg effect in cancer. J Urol. 2012;188:2063–71.
74. Yang P, Cornejo KM, Sadow PM, Cheng L, Wang M, Xiao Y, Jiang Z, Oliva E, Jozwiak S, Nussbaum RL, Feldman AS, Paul E, Thiele EA, Yu JJ, Henske EP, Kwiatkowski DJ, Young RH, Wu CL. Renal cell carcinoma in tuberous sclerosis complex. Am J Surg Pathol. 2014;38:895–909.
75. Dang CV, Kim JW, Gao P, Yustein J. The interplay between MYC and HIF in cancer. Nat Rev Cancer. 2008;8:51–6.
76. Gordan JD, Bertout JA, Hu CJ, Diehl JA, Simon MC. HIF-2alpha promotes hypoxic cell proliferation by enhancing c-myc transcriptional activity. Cancer Cell. 2007;11:335–47.
77. Parry L, Maynard JH, Patel A, Clifford SC, Morrissey C, Maher ER, Cheadle JP, Sampson JR. Analysis of the TSC1 and TSC2 genes in sporadic renal cell carcinomas. Br J Cancer. 2001;19:1226–30.
78. Qin W, Bajaj V, Malinowska I, Lu X, MacConaill L, Wu CL, Kwiatkowski DJ. Angiomyolipoma have common mutations in TSC2 but no other common genetic events. PLoS One. 2011;6(9):e24919.
79. Davis CJ Jr, Mostofi FK, Sesterhenn IA. Renal medullary carcinoma. The seventh sickle cell nephropathy. Am J Surg Pathol. 1995;19(1):1–11.
80. Zhao M, He XL, Teng XD. Mucinous tubular and spindle cell renal cell carcinoma: a review of clinicopathologic aspects. Diagn Pathol. 2015;10:168.
81. Nguyan KA, Syed JS, Espenschied CR, LaDuca H, Bhagat AM, Suarez-Sarmiento A, O'Rourke TK, Brierley KL, Hofstatter EW, Shuch B. Advances in the diagnosis of hereditary kidney cancer: Initial results of a multigene panel test. Cancer. 2017;123(22):4363–71.
82. Scelo G, et al. Genome-wide association study identifies multiple risk loci for renal cell carcinoma. Nat Commun. 2017;9(8):15724. https://doi.org/10.1038/ncomms15724.

Chapter 19
Targeted Treatment of Renal Cell Carcinoma

Matteo Santoni, Alessia Cimadamore, Liang Cheng, Antonio Lopez-Beltran, Marina Scarpelli, Nicola Battelli, and Rodolfo Montironi

Targeting VEGF/VEGFR

Angiogenesis represents the main objective of targeted approaches for patients with mRCC. These strategies are directed against the vascular endothelial growth factor (VEGFR) or its ligand (VEGF). A monoclonal antibody (mAb, bevacizumab) and several tyrosine kinase inhibitors (sorafenib, sunitinib, pazopanib, axitinib, cabozantinib, lenvatinib) or mammalian target of rapamycin (mTOR) inhibitors (everolimus and temsirolimus) have been approved for their clinical use in mRCC patients and are described in the sections below (Fig. 19.1).

M. Santoni · N. Battelli
Oncology Unit, Macerata Hospital, Macerata, Italy

A. Cimadamore
Institute of Pathological Anatomy and Histopathology, University of the Marche Region, Ancona, Italy

L. Cheng
Departments of Pathology, Urology, and Laboratory Medicine, Indiana University School of Medicine, Indianapolis, IN, USA

A. Lopez-Beltran (✉)
Department of Pathology and Surgery, Cordoba University School of Medicine, Córdoba, Spain

M. Scarpelli · R. Montironi
Institute of Pathological Anatomy and Histopathology, United Hospitals, Ancona, Italy

M. K. Divatia et al. (eds.), *Kidney Cancer*, https://doi.org/10.1007/978-3-030-28333-9_19

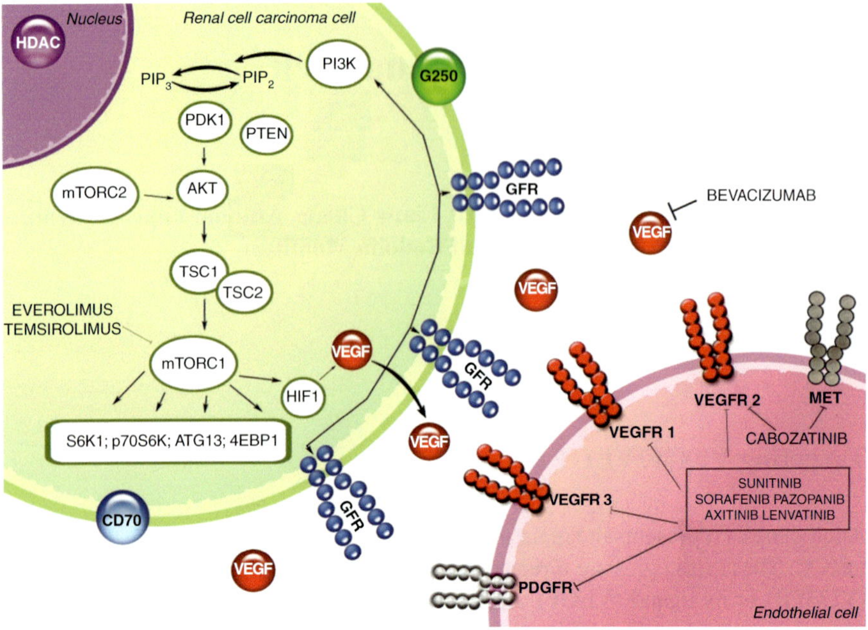

Fig. 19.1 Approved TKIs and mTOR inhibitors and their targets in metastatic renal cell carcinoma (mRCC)

Bevacizumab

Bevacizumab is a recombinant human mAb that binds and inhibits all the active isoforms of VEGF [1]. The combination of bevacizumab with interferon (IFN) alfa-2a as initial therapy was compared to IFN alone in two separate phase III clinical trials (CALGB 90206 and AVOREN) [2, 3]. In both studies, bevacizumab administered at 10 mg/kg every 2 weeks combined with IFN alfa-2a at 9 MU three times weekly showed longer median PFS (but not OS) compared to IFN. The most frequent AEs were anorexia, fatigue, proteinuria, and hypertension.

Based on these results, bevacizumab plus IFN was approved by the U.S. Food and Drug Administration (FDA) in August 2009 for untreated patients with mRCC classified at good or intermediate risk according to Memorial Sloan Kettering Cancer Center (MSKCC) model (Table 19.1). More recently, bevacizumab has been tested in combination with mTOR inhibitors, without showing clinical benefits and with a poor toxicity profile [4–7].

Table 19.1 Agents approved for the first-line therapy of advanced RCC

Agent	Target	Schedule	Administration	Progression-free survival
Bevacizumab	VEGF	Bevacizumab 10 mg/kg every 2 weeks + IFN 9MU 3 times per week for 1 year	Intravenous (Bevacizumab) and subcutaneous (IFN)	10.2 months (AVOREN); 8.5 months (CALGB)
Sunitinib	VEGFR 1–2- 3, PDGFR, c-Kit, Fit3	50 mg daily, 4 week on, 2 weeks off	Oral	11 months
Pazopanib	VEGFR 1–2- 3, PDGFR, c-Kit	800 mg daily	Oral	9.2 months
Temsirolimus	mTOR	25 mg weekly	Intravenous	5.5 months

Sorafenib

Sorafenib is an oral multitarget TKI that inhibits VEGFR 1–3, platelet-derived growth factor receptor (PDGFR), c-Kit, the serine–threonine Kinase Raf-1, and the stem cell factor (SCF) receptor. The efficacy and safety of sorafenib was first reported in the randomized phase III TARGET trial [8, 9] enrolling 905 patients with cytokine refractory metastatic RCC. In this study, patients with favorable or intermediate MSKCC features were treated with 800 mg of daily Sorafenib and showed a significant benefit in terms of progression-free survival (PFS) versus placebo (5.5 vs. 2.8 months; hazard ratio (HR) 0.44; p <0.01) but not of overall survival (OS). The most common grade 3 or 4 adverse events (AEs) correlated with the administration of sorafenib were hand–foot syndrome (86%), fatigue (5%), and hypertension (4%). On this scenario, sorafenib was approved by the FDA in December 2005, for cytokine refractory advanced RCC patients.

As for the second-line setting, the phase III INTORSECT trial randomized 512 mRCC patients previously treated with sunitinib to receive temsirolimus or sorafenib [10] (Table 19.2). The median PFS was not significantly different between the two arms (4.2 vs. 3.9 months, respectively). Interestingly, sorafenib showed longer median OS (16.6 vs. 12.3 months), which was a secondary endpoint in this study.

Recently, sorafenib has been tested as adjuvant therapy in the ASSURE study, without showing a significant advantage in terms of PFS and OS versus placebo [11]. In the same setting, the SORCE study is comparing sorafenib to placebo administered for 1 or 3 years after surgery (NCT00492258).

Table 19.2 Agents approved for the second-line therapy of advanced RCC

Agent	Target	Schedule	Administration	Progression-free survival
Sorafenib	VEGFR 1-2-3, PDGFR, c-Kit, Raf- 1	400 mg twice daily	Oral	5.5 months
Everolimus	mTOR	10 mg daily	Oral	4.9 months
Axitinib	VEGFR 1-2-3	10 mg twice daily	Oral	6.7 months
Cabozantinib	MET, VEGFR2, RET	60 mg daily	Oral	7.4 months
Lenvatinib + Everolimus	VEGFR1-3, FGFR1-4, PDGFRb, RET, KIT + mTOR	18 mg daily with EVEROLIMUS 5 mg daily	Oral	14.6 months

Sunitinib

Sunitinib is a multikinase inhibitor that targets VEGFR 1–3, c-Kit, PDGFR, and FMS-like tyrosine kinase-3 (Flt3). Motzer and his colleagues performed phase III trials comparing sunitinib versus IFN in 750 untreated patients with mRCC [12]. Sunitinib was administered at a dose of 50 mg once daily 4 weeks on/2 weeks off, while subcutaneous IFN was given at an increasing dose from 3 to 9 MU, 3 times weekly. This study reported a significant advantage in terms of both ORR (39% vs. 8%) and median PFS (11 vs. 5 months) for sunitinib, without differences in median OS, maybe due to the crossover occurred in >50% of control arm. Hypothyroidism (14%), hypertension (12%), and fatigue (11%) were the most frequent severe AEs. Sunitinib was first registered by the FDA in January 2006 for patients with mRCC refractory to cytokine therapy and in 2007 for untreated mRCC patients.

Concerning the adjuvant setting, the S-TRAC study, differently from the ASSURE trial, reported that 1-year treatment with sunitinib after nephrectomy for high-risk RCC increased by 1.2 years (6.8 vs. 5.6 years) the median disease-free survival (DFS) compared to placebo, with a good tolerability [13].

Pazopanib

Pazopanib is an oral multikinase inhibitor of VEGFR1–3, c-kit, and PDGFR. Sternberg and her colleagues led a placebo-controlled randomized phase III trial that included 435 cytokine-pretreated or treatment-naïve mRCC patients [14]. Study population was mainly composed of patients with good or intermediate MSKCC risk and the patients were 1:1 randomized to receive either pazopanib 800 mg daily or placebo. Pazopanib showed a significantly longer median PFS versus placebo in both treatment-naïve (11.1 vs. 2.8 months, HR 0.40, p <0.0001) and cytokine-pretreated patients. Otherwise, no advantage in terms of OS was registered in an updated OS analysis [15]. These data led to the approval of pazopanib by the FDA in October 2009 as first-line therapy in mRCC patients.

Successively, pazopanib was compared to sunitinib in terms of efficacy and patient preference, resulting not significantly inferior in terms of PFS (8.4 vs. 9.5 months, respectively) and showing a manageable safety profile [16]. Interestingly, pazopanib was also tested as second-line therapy, reporting an ORR of 27% and a median PFS of 7.5 months [17]. Additionally, this drug was also investigated as adjuvant therapy in the phase III PROTECT trial, including more than 1500 patients with high-grade pT2, pT3, or greater clear cell RCC who received pazopanib or placebo for 1 year. Thus, the study was successively emended by reducing pazopanib dose to 600 mg daily to increase tolerability. Liver toxicity was the main cause leading to treatment discontinuation [18]. The results of this study did not show any benefit over placebo in the adjuvant setting.

Axitinib

Axitinib is a TKI targeting VEGFR1–3 and was compared at a dose of 5 mg twice daily to sorafenib at standard dose in the phase III AXIS trial enrolling 723 mRCC patients previously treated with sunitinib (54%), cytokines (35%), and bevacizumab-IFN or temsirolimus (11%) [19]. The primary endpoint was PFS, which was significantly longer in the axitinib arm compared to sorafenib (6.7 vs. 4.7 months, HR 0.67, $p < 0.001$). In the same view, axitinib showed a higher ORR (19.4% vs. 9.4%, $p < 0.001$). Based on these findings, axitinib was approved in January 2012 by the FDA as second-line therapy for mRCC patients. An updated analysis of OS from the AXIS trial showed no difference between axitinib and sorafenib (20.1 vs 19.2, $p = 0.374$), respectively [20].

Axitinib was also compared to sorafenib as initial therapy. Axitinib showed increased PFS (10.1 vs. 6.5 months) and ORR (32.3% vs 14.6%) compared to Sorafenib. However, the superior results obtained by sunitinib and pazopanib have not allowed the approval of axitinib in this setting [21].

Axitinib at 5 mg twice daily given for 3 years has been also investigated as adjuvant therapy in a prospective, randomized, double blind placebo-controlled phase 3 study (the ATLAS trial, NCT01599754). The primary endpoint is increasing DFS in patients with high-risk RCC and results are awaited.

Cabozantinib

Cabozantinib is an oral TKI targeting MET, VEGFR2, AXL, and RET. In the METEOR randomized phase III study, RCC patients previously treated with antiangiogenics received cabozantinib at a dose of 60 mg daily or everolimus at a dose of 10 mg daily. Cabozantinib showed a longer median PFS (7.4 vs. 3.8 months), with an increased median OS at interim analysis (HR 0.67; 95% CI 0.51–0.89) and a manageable toxicity profile [22]. Based on these findings, in 2016, FDA approved cabozantinib at a dose of 60 mg daily for patients with an advanced RCC following treatment with antiangiogenics.

More recently, cabozantinib was compared to sunitinib as first-line therapy in a phase II study (CABOSUN) enrolling patients with intermediate or poor risk mRCC. Cabozantinib showed significantly higher median PFS (8.2 vs. 5.6 months) and overall response rate (46% vs. 18%), with a similar rate of grade 3–4 AEs [23], opening the way to its potential use in the first-line setting in future years.

Lenvatinib

Lenvatinib is a TKI targeting VEGFR1–3, FGFR1–4, PDGFRb, RET, and KIT. In 2014, Molina et al. led a phase Ib study to test lenvatinib in combination with everolimus in patients with pretreated mRCC [24]. They reported a response rate of 30% and a median PFS of 10.9 months. In the same view, a phase II study was performed comparing lenvatinib alone or in combination with everolimus to everolimus alone, showing that the combination reported 14.6 months of median PFS, which was the highest registered in clinical trials including patients progressed on VEGFR TKIs. This led to the approval of this combination by the FDA in March 2016. At present, a phase III trial is in course to compare lenvatinib in combination with everolimus to lenvatinib to anti-programmed death (PD)-1 pembrolizumab or sunitinib as first-line therapy (NCT02811861).

Targeting the mTOR Pathway

TORC1 and TORC2 are two distinct complexes that modulate several aspects of protein expression implicated in cell proliferation and survival, making them ideal candidate for targeted approaches in RCC.

Temsirolimus

Temsirolimus is an intravenous mTOR inhibitor administered at a dose of 25 mg in a weekly basis [25, 26]. Its approval derived from the results of a phase III randomized clinical study enrolling patients with untreated poor risk mRCC [27]. In this trial, patients were randomized to receive IFN, temsirolimus or their combination, showing a longer median OS in the temsirolimus arm (10.9 months) and a mild toxicity profile. In this study, approximately 20% of patients had a non-clear cell

RCC, which resulted responsive to temsirolimus. On this scenario, temsirolimus was approved by the FDA in 2007 as initial therapy in patients with untreated poor risk mRCC.

Everolimus

Everolimus is an oral mTOR inhibitor administered at 10 mg daily in mRCC patients following VEGFR inhibitors. Its approval followed the results of a randomized, double-blind phase III trial (RECORD-1) investigating everolimus versus placebo, which showed an advantage in terms of median PFS (4.9 vs. 1.9 months; HR 0.33; $p < 0.001$) but not of OS (14.8 vs. 14.4 months; HR 0.87; $p = 0.162$). The main AEs in the everolimus arm were rash, fatigue, stomatitis, and pneumonitis. In 2009, everolimus was approved by the FDA for the treatment of mRCC following antiangiogenics.

Successively, two phase II studies (RECORD-2 and RECORD-3) have investigated everolimus in different settings. RECORD-2 trial evaluated everolimus combined with bevacizumab versus IFN plus bevacizumab as first-line therapy, without demonstrating clinical benefit [28]. On the other hand, the RECORD-3 study compared the sequences sunitinib–everolimus versus Everolimus–Sunitinib, later supporting the use of TKIs as first-line therapy [29]. Finally, alternating anti-VEGFR TKIs with mTOR inhibitors is under evaluation in two separate phase II trials as first-line treatment: Sunitinib with temsirolimus (NCT01517243) and pazopanib with everolimus (NCT01408004).

Conclusions

The prognosis of patients with mRCC remains relatively poor, but the progress obtained in the last decade in the number of available drugs gives grounds for a moderate optimism. The introduction of targeted agents has represented a revolution in the therapeutic armamentarium for mRCC. This has been the result of the great enforces of worldwide researchers in understanding the biology of this complex disease. The successive results obtained by anti-PD-1 agent nivolumab, used alone in pretreated patients [30] or as first-line therapy in combination with anti-cytotoxic T-lymphocyte antigen (CTLA)-4 ipilimumab [31], have further changed this scenario, reopening the way to the extensive use of immunotherapy in these patients, in particular in dose without favorable prognosis. Nevertheless, targeted agents used in sequential or combined strategies with immunotherapies will represent a cornerstone of the therapeutic approach to mRCC patients in future years, even if further research efforts should be directed to maximize patient benefit and guarantee a sustainable system.

References

1. Presta LG, Chen H, O'Connor SJ, Chisholm V, Meng YG, Krummen L, et al. Humanization of an anti-vascular endothelial growth factor monoclonal antibody for the therapy of solid tumors and other disorders. Cancer Res. 1997;57:4593–9.
2. Escudier B, Bellmunt J, Negrier S, Bajetta E, Melichar B, Bracarda S, et al. Phase III trial of bevacizumab plus interferon alfa-2a in patients with metastatic renal cell carcinoma (AVOREN): final analysis of overall survival. J Clin Oncol. 2010;28:2144–50. https://doi.org/10.1200/JCO.2009.26.7849.
3. Rini BI, Halabi S, Rosenberg JE, Stadler WM, Vaena DA, Archer L, et al. Phase III trial of bevacizumab plus interferon alfa versus interferon alfa monotherapy in patients with metastatic renal cell carcinoma: final results of CALGB 90206. J Clin Oncol. 2010;28:2137–43. https://doi.org/10.1200/JCO.2009.26.5561.
4. Hainsworth JD, Spigel DR, Burris HA III, Waterhouse D, Clark BL, Whorf R. Phase II trial of bevacizumab and everolimus in patients with advanced renal cell carcinoma. J Clin Oncol. 2010;28:2131–6. https://doi.org/10.1200/JCO.2009.26.3152.
5. Negrier S, Gravis G, Perol D, Chevreau C, Delva R, Bay JO, et al. Temsirolimus and bevacizumab, or sunitinib, or interferon alfa and bevacizumab for patients with advanced renal cell carcinoma (TORAVA): a randomised phase 2 trial. Lancet Oncol. 2011;12:673–80. https://doi.org/10.1016/S1470-2045(11)70124-3.
6. Rini BI, Bellmunt J, Clancy J, Wang K, Niethammer AG, Hariharan S, et al. Randomized phase III trial of temsirolimus and bevacizumab versus interferon alfa and bevacizumab in metastatic renal cell carcinoma: INTORACT trial. J Clin Oncol. 2014;32:752–9. https://doi.org/10.1200/JCO.2013.50.5305.
7. Harshman LC, Barbeau S, McMillian A, Srinivas S. A phase II study of bevacizumab and everolimus as treatment for refractory metastatic renal cell carcinoma. Clin Genitourin Cancer. 2013;11:100–6. https://doi.org/10.1016/j.clgc.2012.12.002.
8. Escudier B, Eisen T, Stadler WM, Szczylik C, Oudard S, Siebels M, et al. Sorafenib in advanced clear-cell renal-cell carcinoma. N Engl J Med. 2007;356:125–34. https://doi.org/10.1056/NEJMoa060655.
9. Escudier B, Eisen T, Stadler WM, Szczylik C, Oudard S, Staehler M, et al. Sorafenib for treatment of renal cell carcinoma: final efficacy and safety results of the phase III treatment approaches in renal cancer global evaluation trial. J Clin Oncol. 2009;27:3312–8. https://doi.org/10.1200/JCO.2008.19.5511.
10. Hutson TE, Escudier B, Esteban E, Bjarnason GA, Lim HY, Pittman KB, et al. Randomized phase III trial of temsirolimus versus sorafenib as second-line therapy after sunitinib in patients with metastatic renal cell carcinoma. J Clin Oncol. 2014;32(8):760–7. https://doi.org/10.1200/JCO.2013.50.3961.
11. Haas NB, Manola J, Uzzo RG, Atkins MB, Wilding G, Pins M, et al. Initial results from ASSURE (E2805): adjuvant sorafenib or sunitinib for unfavorable renal carcinoma, an ECOG-ACRIN-led, NCTN phase III trial. J Clin Oncol. 2015;33. Suppl 7; abstr 403:403. https://doi.org/10.1200/jco.2015.33.7_suppl.403.
12. Motzer RJ, Hutson TE, Tomczak P, Michaelson MD, Bukowski RM, Oudard S, et al. Overall survival and updated results for sunitinib compared with interferon alfa in patients with metastatic renal cell carcinoma. J Clin Oncol. 2009;27:3584–90. https://doi.org/10.1200/JCO.2008.20.1293.
13. Ravaud A, Motzer RJ, Pandha HS, George DJ, Pantuck AJ, Patel A, et al., S-TRAC investigators. Adjuvant sunitinib in high-risk renal-cell carcinoma after nephrectomy. N Engl J Med. 2016;375:2246–2254. doi: https://doi.org/10.1056/NEJMoa1611406.
14. Sternberg CN, Davis ID, Mardiak J, Szczylik C, Lee E, Wagstaff J, et al. Pazopanib in locally advanced or metastatic renal cell carcinoma: results of a randomized phase III trial. J Clin Oncol. 2010;28:1061–8. https://doi.org/10.1200/JCO.2009.23.9764.

15. Sternberg CN, Hawkins RE, Wagstaff J, Salman P, Mardiak J, Barrios CH, et al. A randomised, double-blind phase III study of pazopanib in patients with advanced and/or metastatic renal cell carcinoma: final overall survival results and safety update. Eur J Cancer. 2013;49:1287–96. https://doi.org/10.1016/j.ejca.2012.12.010.
16. Escudier B, Porta C, Bono P, Powles T, Eisen T, Sternberg CN, et al. Randomized, controlled, double-blind, cross-over trial assessing treatment preference for pazopanib versus sunitinib in patients with metastatic renal cell carcinoma: PISCES Study. J Clin Oncol. 2014;32:1412–8. https://doi.org/10.1200/JCO.2013.50.8267.
17. Hainsworth JD, Rubin MS, Arrowsmith ER, Khatcheressian J, Crane EJ, Franco LA. Pazopanib as second-line treatment after sunitinib or bevacizumab in patients with advanced renal cell carcinoma: a Sarah Cannon Oncology Research Consortium Phase II Trial. Clin Genitourin Cancer. 2013;11:270–5. https://doi.org/10.1016/j.clgc.2013.04.006.
18. Motzer R, Haas NB, Donskov F, Gross-Goupil M, Varlamov S, Kopyltsov E,et al. Randomized phase III trial of adjuvant pazopanib versus placebo after nephrectomy in patients with locally advanced renal cell carcinoma (RCC) (PROTECT). J Clin Oncol. 2017;35 Suppl 15:abstr 4507. doi: https://doi.org/10.1200/JCO.2017.35.15_suppl.4507.
19. Rini BI, Escudier B, Tomczak P, Kaprin A, Szczylik C, Hutson TE, et al. Comparative effectiveness of axitinib versus sorafenib in advanced renal cell carcinoma (AXIS): a randomised phase 3 trial. Lancet. 2011;378:1931–9. https://doi.org/10.1016/S0140-6736(11)61613-9.
20. Motzer RJ, Escudier B, Tomczak P, Hutson TE, Michaelson MD, Negrier S, et al. Axitinib versus sorafenib as second-line treatment for advanced renal cell carcinoma: overall survival analysis and updated results from a randomised phase 3 trial. Lancet Oncol. 2013;14:552–62. https://doi.org/10.1016/S1470-2045(13)70093-7.
21. Hutson TE, Lesovoy V, Al-Shukri S, Stus VP, Lipatov ON, Bair AH, et al. Axitinib versus sorafenib as first-line therapy in patients with metastatic renal-cell carcinoma: a randomised open-label phase 3 trial. Lancet Oncol. 2013;14:1287–94. https://doi.org/10.1016/S1470-2045(13)70465-0.
22. Choueiri TK, Escudier B, Powles T, Tannir NM, Mainwaring PN, Rini BI, et al., METEOR investigators. Cabozantinib versus everolimus in advanced renal cell carcinoma (METEOR): final results from a randomised, open-label, phase 3 trial. Lancet Oncol 2016;17:917–927. doi: https://doi.org/10.1016/S1470-2045(16)30107-3.
23. Choueiri TK, Halabi S, Sanford BL, Hahn O, Michaelson MD, Walsh MK, et al. Cabozantinib versus sunitinib as initial targeted therapy for patients with metastatic renal cell carcinoma of poor or intermediate risk: the alliance A031203 CABOSUN trial. J Clin Oncol. 2017;35:591–7. https://doi.org/10.1200/JCO.2016.70.7398.
24. Molina AM, Hutson TE, Larkin J, Gold AM, Wood K, Carter D, et al. A phase 1b clinical trial of the multi-targeted tyrosine kinase inhibitor lenvatinib (E7080) in combination with everolimus for treatment of metastatic renal cell carcinoma (RCC). Cancer Chemother Pharmacol. 2014;73:181–9. https://doi.org/10.1007/s00280-013-2339-y.
25. Atkins MB, Hidalgo M, Stadler WM, Logan TF, Dutcher JP, Hudes GR, et al. Randomized phase II study of multiple dose levels of CCI-779, a novel mammalian target of rapamycin kinase inhibitor, in patients with advanced refractory renal cell carcinoma. J Clin Oncol. 2004;22:909–18. https://doi.org/10.1200/JCO.2004.08.185.
26. Raymond E, Alexandre J, Faivre S, Vera K, Materman E, Boni J, et al. Safety and pharmacokinetics of escalated doses of weekly intravenous infusion of CCI- 779, a novel mTOR inhibitor, in patients with cancer. J Clin Oncol. 2004;22:2336–47. https://doi.org/10.1200/JCO.2004.08.116.
27. Hudes G, Carducci M, Tomczak P, Dutcher J, Figlin R, Kapoor A, et al. Temsirolimus, interferon alfa, or both for advanced renal-cell carcinoma. N Engl J Med. 2007;356:2271–81. https://doi.org/10.1056/NEJMoa066838.
28. Ravaud A, Barrios CH, Alekseev B, Tay MH, Agarwala SS, Yalcin S, et al. RECORD-2: phase II randomized study of everolimus and bevacizumab versus interferon a-2a and bevacizumab as

first-line therapy in patients with metastatic renal cell carcinoma. Ann Oncol. 2015;26:1378–84. https://doi.org/10.1093/annonc/mdv170.

29. Motzer RJ, Barrios CH, Kim TM, Falcon S, Cosgriff T, Harker WG, et al. Phase II randomized trial comparing sequential first-line everolimus and second-line sunitinib versus first-line sunitinib and second-line everolimus in patients with metastatic renal cell carcinoma. J Clin Oncol. 2014;32:2765–72. https://doi.org/10.1200/JCO.2013.54.6911.
30. Motzer RJ, Escudier B, McDermott DF, et al. Nivolumab versus everolimus in advanced renal-cell carcinoma. N Engl J Med. 2015;373:1803–13. https://doi.org/10.1056/NEJMoa1510665.
31. Hammers HJ, Plimack ER, Infante JR, et al. Safety and efficacy of nivolumab in combination with ipilimumab in metastatic renal cell carcinoma: the CheckMate 016 Study. J Clin Oncol. 2017;35:3851–8. https://doi.org/10.1200/JCO.2016.72.1985.

Part V
Specimen Handling, Staging and Reporting

Chapter 20
Specimen Handling: Radical and Partial Nephrectomy Specimens

Antonio Lopez-Beltran, Maria R. Raspollini, Liang Cheng, Marina Scarpelli, Alessia Cimadamore, Silvia Gasparrini, and Rodolfo Montironi

This chapter is devoted to specimen handling of radical and partial nephrectomies (including tumorectomy specimens). The main issues to be considered have been discussed thoroughly in the literature. In particular, we have followed the conclusions raised by the International Society of Urologic Pathology 2012 Consensus Conference on renal cancer, through working group 3, focused on the issues of staging and specimen handling of renal tumors and reported by Trypkov et al. [1]. Proper consideration is also given to the most recent *AJCC/UICC TNM Cancer Staging Manual* [2], and the most recent World Health Organization Classification of Tumours of the Urinary System and Male Genital Organs [3].

The proper handling of renal specimens provides the pathologists a guide to accurate staging of renal tumors. Several experts and expert groups have published recommendations on handling and dissection strategies, and have produced widely used protocols for the evaluation of renal cell carcinoma (RCC), which have proved

A. Lopez-Beltran (✉)
Department of Pathology and Surgery, Cordoba University School of Medicine, Córdoba, Spain

M. R. Raspollini
Histopathology and Molecular Diagnostics. University Hospital Careggi, Florence, Italy

L. Cheng
Departments of Pathology, Urology, and Laboratory Medicine, Indiana University School of Medicine, Indianapolis, IN, USA

M. Scarpelli · R. Montironi
Institute of Pathological Anatomy and Histopathology, United Hospitals, Ancona, Italy

A. Cimadamore
Institute of Pathological Anatomy and Histopathology, University of the Marche Region, Ancona, Italy

S. Gasparrini
Section of Pathological Anatomy, Polytechnic University of the Marche Region, School of Medicine, Ancona, Italy

M. K. Divatia et al. (eds.), *Kidney Cancer*, https://doi.org/10.1007/978-3-030-28333-9_20

their utility in practice [1–39]. Likewise, most previously published protocols reflect personal practice preferences of dedicated pathologists [1–39]. In fact, very limited objective data exist regarding handling and organ dissection protocols in the current literature despite widespread implementation of some of them in practice [4–39]. Therefore, in the absence of supporting data on this issue, as a practical rule, most available handling protocols of RCC specimens are acceptable if they provide enough information allowing the assessment of prognostic/predictive parameters relevant in clinical practice. Adherence to International Society of Urologic Pathology recommendation on handling RCC samples [1] will provide a standardized approach which is in use by most Uropathologists around the world.

Specimen Sectioning and Inking

Radical or partial nephrectomies are the standard surgical procedures for localized renal cell carcinoma. The specimen dissection is required to achieve proper fixation of tissue and to allow gross evaluation of tumor extension into the perinephric fat, renal sinus, renal vein, and/or adrenal gland [1–3] (Table 20.1).

The preferred method of dissection is to make an initial section into radical nephrectomy specimens along the long axis (Fig. 20.1); this is frequently followed by additional perpendicular or parallel cuts to evaluate the greatest tumor dimension and other tumor characteristics including extension [1, 2]. Other methods are acceptable in practice as no data actually exist to indicate the superiority of any method and therefore the use of one over the other frequently reflects practice preferences. Partial nephrectomy specimens should be sectioned perpendicularly to the inked marginal surface; if a portion of perinephric fat is present in the specimen, this margin should also be assessed (Fig. 20.2).

Ink should be used for margin assessment in radical nephrectomies following either localized use of ink restricted only to the areas suspicious for the presence of tumor (most commonly applied), or by inking of the entire external surface of the specimen. Most pathologists also use ink for partial nephrectomies, either localized use of ink or by inking of the entire external surface of the specimen. Selective inking of partial nephrectomies primarily relates to inking of the renal parenchymal margins, as margin status is of clinical importance [1].

Tumor Measurement

No validated data exist in the literature as to how tumor size should be measured [1]. Since it is a relevant practice parameter, the size should be estimated after sectioning of the entire tumor at regular intervals, and the greatest tumor dimension should be recorded. Special attention should be given to size determination in and around cutoff points of 4, 7, and 10 cm, which are important for accurate staging [1–3]. The

Table 20.1 Key points relevant to handling kidney specimens with cancer

Radical nephrectomy: The initial cut should be made along the long axis
Radical/partial nephrectomy specimens should be inked
Partial nephrectomy specimens should be sectioned perpendicularly to the inked marginal surface
General guideline: Sampling 1 block per cm of the tumor with a minimum of 3 blocks
The length of a renal vein/caval thrombus should not be part of the measurement of the renal tumor
Sampling should include at a minimum of the 5 largest tumors, when multiple tumors
Perinephric fat invasion assessment: Examining multiple perpendicular sections of the tumor/perinephric fat interface Sampling areas suspicious for invasion
Perinephric fat invasion defined as: Tumor touching the fat Tumor extending as irregular tongues/nests into the perinephric tissue Invading tumor with or without desmoplasia
Renal sinus invasion is present when the tumor is: Direct contact with the sinus fat Direct contact with loose connective tissue of the sinus, clearly beyond the renal parenchyma, There is involvement of any endothelium-lined spaces within the renal sinus, regardless of the size
Assessing renal sinus, submit: 3 blocks (at least) of the tumor–renal sinus interface when invasion of the renal sinus is uncertain Submit only 1 block if invasion is grossly evident, or obviously not present (small peripheral tumor)
The renal vein margin: Positive only when there is adherent tumor visible microscopically at the actual margin
Submitted caval thrombus: Take 2 or more sections to look for the adherent caval wall tissue.
Adrenal with tumor: Submitted sections should reflect whether this represents contiguous spread (pT4) or a metastasis (pM1). *Adrenal without tumor:* Submit a section of the adrenal gland.
Uninvolved renal parenchyma sampling: Normal parenchyma with tumor Normal parenchyma distant from the tumor
To identify lymph nodes by dissection/palpation of the fat in the hilar area (lymph nodes are found in <10% of radical nephrectomy specimens).

Based on the consensus conclusions raised by the International Society of Urologic Pathology 2012 Consensus Conference on renal cancer through working group 3. Trypkov et al. [1]

kidney is typically bivalved (sectioned along the long axis) and the greatest dimension is based on the two-dimensional assessment of the highest tumor length. Frequently, after bivalving the kidney, additional perpendicular or parallel cuts may be required to accurately evaluate the greatest tumor dimension [1].

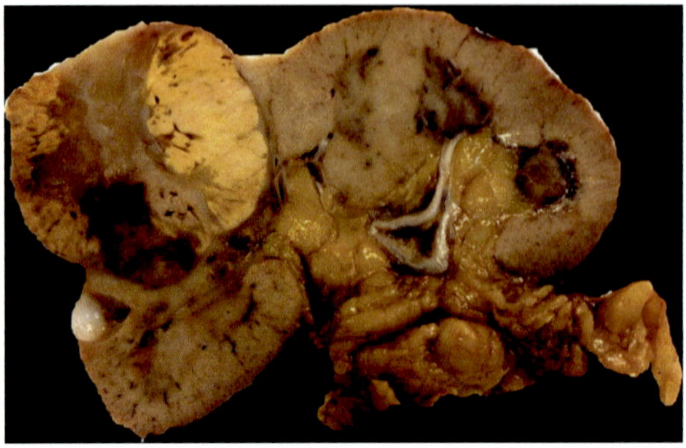

Fig. 20.1 Radical nephrectomy specimen sectioned along the long axis. Note the typical yellow color that characterizes clear cell renal cell carcinoma

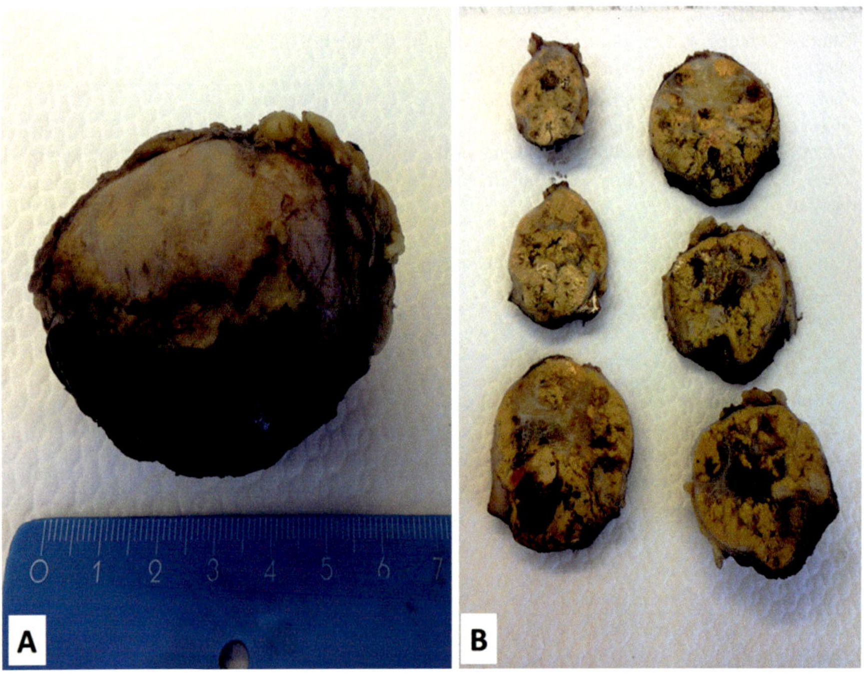

Fig. 20.2 (**a**, **b**) Partial nephrectomy with inked surgical edge. Partial nephrectomy specimen step-sectioned perpendicularly to the inked edge

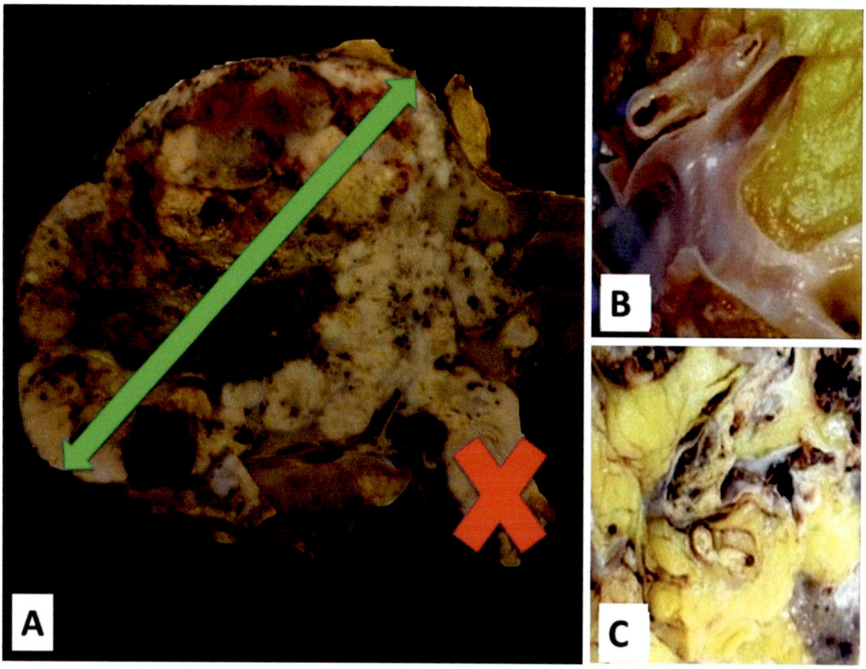

Fig. 20.3 Tumor measurement should include the greatest dimension; however, the length of a renal vein/caval thrombus should not be part of the main tumor mass measurement (**a**). Renal sinus interface with renal vein and its branches (**b**) with invasion seen grossly (**c**)

The main tumor should be measured with the inclusion, when present, of any tumor invading into the peripheral extracapsular tissue and the renal sinus; however, renal vein or caval thrombus should not be measured and reported as part of the main tumor dimension (Fig. 20.3). Similarly, smaller satellite nodules should not be included in the estimation of the greatest size of a dominant tumor mass. When multiple tumors are present in the kidney, it has been suggested to report the tumor dimensions for all tumors up to some designated maximum such as 5 [1–3].

Number of Blocks for Sampling

The optimal sampling strategy for a renal tumor has not been established so far, but however, it should allow for determination of tumor stage, histologic type/subtype, surgical margin status, assessment of pathologic grade, tumor multifocality, or to illustrate underlying incidental renal pathology [1–39]. To date, however, no study has addressed the appropriate number of sections needed to evaluate a renal tumor. A reasonable sampling strategy to address key parameters is to focus on the tumor interface with renal sinus, perirenal fat, renal vein, adjacent nonneoplastic parenchyma, and areas of tumor showing differing gross appearances. In partial nephrectomies, it is relevant to adequately sample the tumor–normal renal parenchyma margin interface. A section of the adrenal gland, if present, should also be included, as should sections of the vascular and ureteric surgical margins. A general guideline provided by the International Society of Urologic Pathology [1] favors sampling 1 block/cm of tumor with a minimum of 3 blocks (subject to modification as individual cases may require) (Fig. 20.4). This approach was previously suggested in published recommendations for both pediatric and adult renal tumors [1, 9–11]. Modifications of the sampling should allow for appropriate assessment of invasion into the renal sinus, perinephric fat, adrenal gland, or renal pelvis, when necessary.

Sampling Multiple Renal Tumors

Multiple tumors are most frequently encountered in the setting of hereditary RCC (von Hippel–Lindau disease, hereditary papillary RCC, tuberous sclerosis, hereditary leiomyomatosis/RCC syndrome, and Birt–Hogg–Dube syndrome) [3, 5, 10, 39]. Multifocality also occurs in acquired cystic kidney disease and hybrid oncocytic/chromophobe tumor (HOCT; also known as renal oncocytosis). Sporadic multifocal RCC tumors are less often seen in practice (range 4%–5% of specimens) with higher incidence reported in papillary RCC. The International Society of Urologic Pathology recommended sampling at a minimum the 5 largest tumors (Fig. 20.5). One may assess only the 5 largest tumors when >5 tumors are present, particularly if the remaining, smaller tumors show similar gross features [1]. However, additional sampling can always be performed in case of uncertainty or at the discretion of the pathologist.

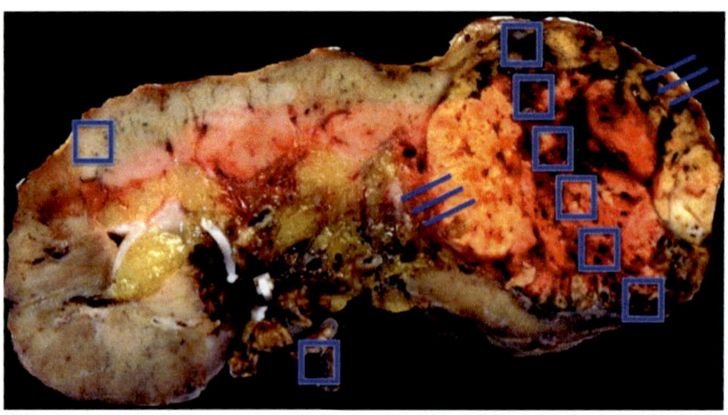

Fig. 20.4 Renal cell carcinoma showing multiple satellite nodules

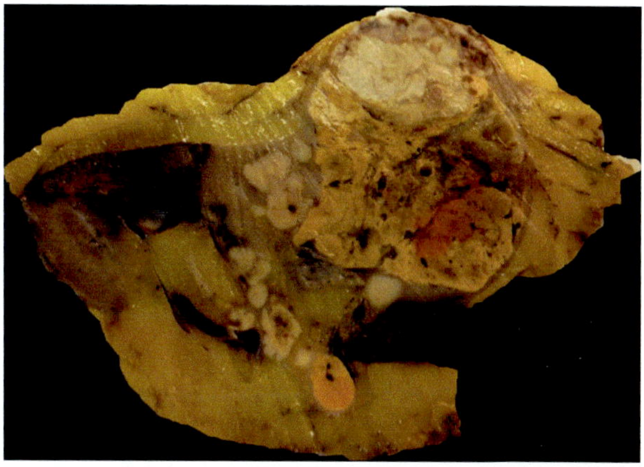

Fig. 20.5 The sampling method should focus on the interface between tumor and perinephric fat, renal sinus, renal vein. Tumor sampling should include at least one block per cm of the tumor mass

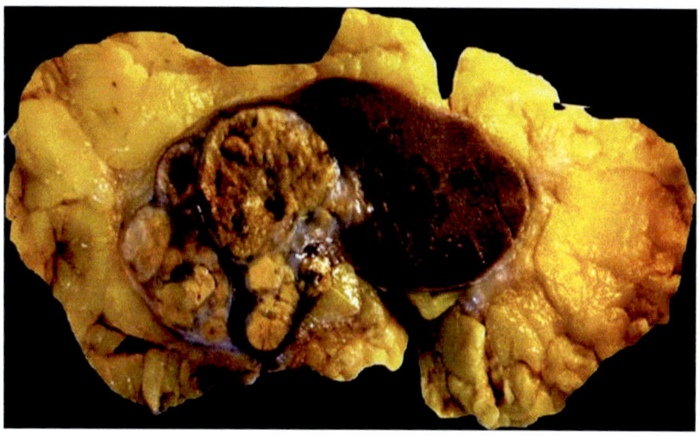

Fig. 20.6 The presence of a circumscribed pushing border close to perinephric fat is not diagnostic of fat invasion

Perinephric Fat Invasion

The quantity of perinephric fat largely varies in nephrectomy specimens; typically, the adrenal gland is seen within the fat at the inner aspect of the upper pole of the kidney. The perinephric fat is therefore located outside of the renal capsule and within the confines of the Gerota fascia [1–39].

A number of RCCs grow pushing into the perinephric fat, which distort the renal contour resulting in a circumscribed pushing border, a fact which should not be mistaken as perinephric fat invasion (Fig. 20.6). Infiltration into the perinephric fat can be established on gross examination when the tumor loses its rounded and smooth interface with the capsule and the perinephric fat or when visible as nodules or irregular tumor masses protruding within the perinephric fat (Fig. 20.7). Perinephric fat invasion is best determined by gross examination of multiple perpendicular sections of the tumor–perinephric fat interface followed by microscopic confirmation of invasion which includes the tumor either touch the fat or extend as irregular tongues into the perinephric tissue; desmoplasia may be present at the invasive edge in some cases [1–39].

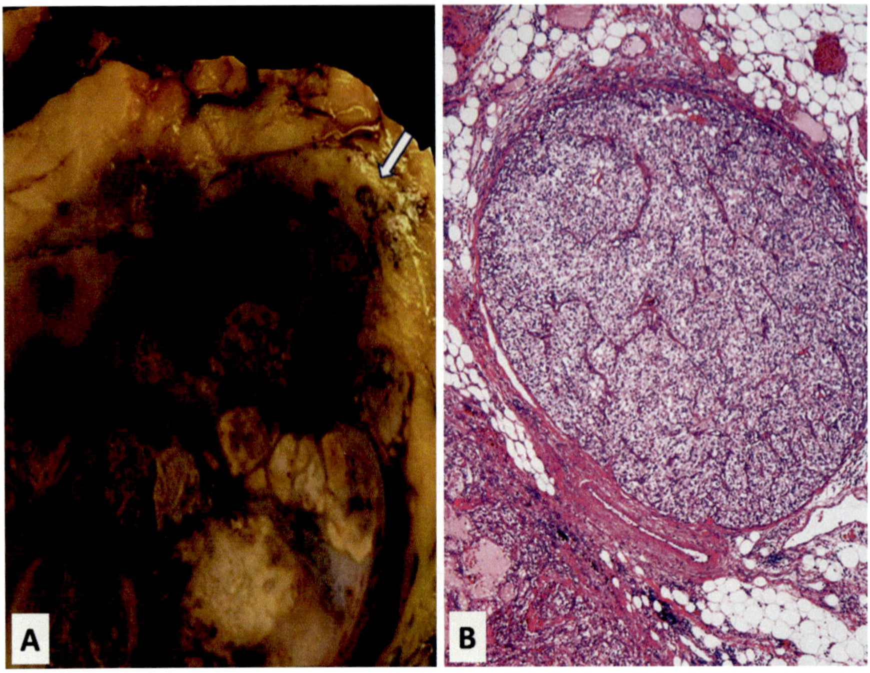

Fig. 20.7 Perinephric fat invasion is determined by gross careful examination of multiple perpendicular sections of the tumor–perinephric fat interface (**a**) and with histologic confirmation (**b**)

Assessment of Renal Sinus Invasion

Renal sinus fat is located between the pelvi-calyceal system and the renal parenchyma and contains the main lympho-vascular supply of the kidney [2, 4, 6, 8–10, 16, 17, 21]. Some studies have demonstrated that renal sinus invasion is the principal route for extrarenal extension of the tumor [8–10, 16, 17, 21].

Renal sinus invasion is an important prognostic parameter needing to be specifically assessed in nephrectomy specimens. In cases when there is uncertainty as to the presence of renal sinus invasion, at least 3 blocks of the tumor–renal sinus interface should be submitted (Fig. 20.8). If sinus invasion is grossly evident, or obviously not present, only 1 block would be needed to confirm the gross impression that renal sinus invasion is present or absent [1, 2, 4, 6, 8–10, 16, 17, 21]. Renal sinus invasion can be established by histologic examination when the tumor is in direct contact with the sinus fat, in the loose connective tissue beyond the renal parenchyma, or when there is involvement of any endothelium-lined spaces within the renal sinus, regardless of the size [1].

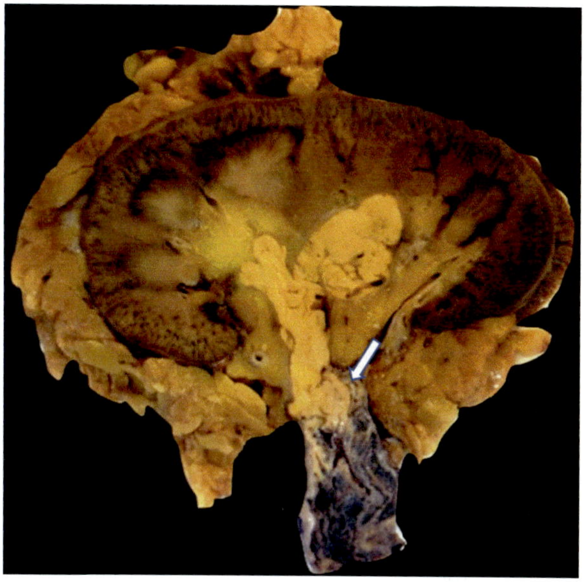

Fig. 20.8 Renal sinus and renal vein invasion

Sampling of Renal Vein, Vena Cava Invasion, and Renal Vein Margin

Renal vein invasion is defined as a tumor that "grossly extends into the renal vein or its segmental (muscle-containing) branches" [2]. Therefore, a careful gross examination of the renal vein and its major branches is a relevant component of the dissection of radical nephrectomy specimens (Fig. 20.3).

Another question that arises is when the renal vein margin should be considered positive. As recommended by the International Society of Urologic Pathology, the margin is considered positive only if there is an adherent tumor at the actual margin, which has been confirmed microscopically [1]. Vena cava wall invasion is defined as a tumor that invades the wall of the vena cava. When a specimen is submitted separately as "caval thrombus," the pathologist's role is to confirm that the thrombus contains tumor and to establish whether there is adherent caval wall tissue. The most appropriated sampling strategy in this setting would be to include ≥2 sections to search for adherent caval wall tissue and possible caval vein invasion. Sometimes, however, the thrombus is received piecemeal and can be assessed only for the presence of tumor [1].

Sampling of Uninvolved Renal Parenchyma

In addition to sampling of the tumor, the uninvolved renal parenchyma should also be routinely evaluated by including both normal parenchyma with (or adjacent to) the tumor and renal parenchyma distant from the tumor (see Chap. 21 for details) [1].

Adrenal Gland Involvement

When the adrenal gland is involved by RCC, gross examination is relevant in determining whether this represents contiguous spread (pT4 disease) or a metastasis (pM1) in the current AJCC/UICC TNM staging system [2]. The gross description and submitted sections should specifically address the conclusion in this regard [1].

Lymph Nodes Assessment

To assess lymph nodes, radical nephrectomy specimens should be examined by palpation and dissection of the renal hilar area fat, rather than all the fat in the nephrectomy specimen. Nodes are seen in <10% of the cases and are mostly located in the renal hilar fat [36–38].

Concerning lymphadenectomy samples, once the specimen is properly fixed, the pathologist should retrieve and examine all lymph nodes from the submitted tissue, which is important for accurate nodal staging; limited evidence suggests that 12–13 nodes are currently acceptable as a minimum for accurate pN staging [36–38].

References

1. Trpkov K, Grignon DJ, Bonsib SM, Amin MB, Billis A, Lopez-Beltran A, Samaratunga H, Tamboli P, Delahunt B, Egevad L, Montironi R, Srigley JR, members of the ISUP Renal Tumor Panel. Handling and staging of renal cell carcinoma. The International Society of Urological Pathology Consensus (ISUP) conference recommendations. Am J Surg Pathol. 2013;37:1505–17.
2. Amin, MB, Edge S, Greene F, Byrd DR, Brookland RK, et al., editors. American Joint Committee on Cancer (AJCC) staging manual. 8th ed. Switzerland: Springer; 2017.
3. Moch H, Humphrey PA, Ulbright TM, Reuter VE. World Health Organization (WHO) classification of Tumours of the urinary system and male genital organs, vol. 8. 4th ed; 2016.
4. Bonsib S. Renal veins and venous extension in clear cell renal carcinoma. Mod Pathol. 2007;20:44–53.
5. Srigley JR, Delahunt B, Eble JN, et al. The International Society of Urological Pathology (ISUP) Vancouver classification of renal neoplasia. Am J Surg Pathol. 2013;37:1469–89.
6. Bonsib SM. Macroscopic assessment, dissection protocols and histologic sampling strategy for renal cell carcinomas. Diagn Pathol. 2008;14:151–6.

7. Novara G, Ficarra V, Antonelli A, et al. Validation of the 2009 TNM version in a large multi-institutional cohort of patients treated for renal cell carcinoma: are further improvements needed? Eur Urol. 2010;58:588–95.
8. Griffiths DF, Nind N, O'Brien CJ, et al. Evaluation of a protocol for examining nephrectomy specimens with renal cell carcinoma. J Clin Pathol. 2003;56:374–7.
9. Fleming S, Griffiths DF. Best practice no 180. Nephrectomy for renal tumour; dissection guide and dataset. J Clin Pathol. 2005;58:7–14.
10. Lopez-Beltran A, Scarpelli M, Montironi R, Kirkali Z. WHO classification of the renal tumors of the adults. Eur Urol. 2006;49:798–805.
11. Algaba F, Trias I, Scarpelli M, et al. Handling and pathology reporting of renal tumor specimens. Eur Urol. 2004;45:437–43.
12. Higgins JP, McKenney JK, Brooks JD, et al. Recommendations for the reporting of surgically resected specimens of renal cell carcinoma: the Association of Directors of Anatomic and Surgical Pathology. Hum Pathol. 2009;40:456–63.
13. Lopez-Beltran A, Suzigan S, Montironi R, et al. Multilocular cystic renal cell carcinoma: a report of 45 cases of a kidney tumor of low malignant potential. Am J Clin Pathol. 2006;125:217–22.
14. Srigley JR, Amin MB, Delahunt B, et al. Protocol for the examination of specimens from patients with invasive carcinoma of renal tubular origin. Arch Pathol Lab Med. 2010;134: e25–30.
15. Eble JN. Recommendations for examining and reporting tumorbearing kidney specimens from adults. Semin Diagn Pathol. 1998;15:77–82.
16. Bonsib SM, Gibson D, Mhoon M, et al. Renal sinus involvement in renal cell carcinomas. Am J Surg Pathol. 2000;24:451–8.
17. Bonsib SM. The renal sinus is the principal invasive pathway: a prospective study of 100 renal cell carcinomas. Am J Surg Pathol. 2004;28:1594–600.
18. Thompson RH, Leibovich BC, Cheville JC, et al. Is renal sinus fat invasion the same as perinephric fat invasion for pT3a renal cell carcinoma? J Urol. 2005;174:1218–21.
19. Grignon D, Paner GP. Renal cell carcinoma and the renal sinus. Adv Anat Pathol. 2007;14: 63–8.
20. Montironi R, Cheng L, Scarpelli M, Lopez-Beltran A. Pathology and genetics: tumours of the urinary system and male genital system: clinical implications of the 4th edition of the WHO classification and beyond. Eur Urol. 2016;70(1):120–3. https://doi.org/10.1016/j.eururo.2016.03.011.
21. Bonsib SM. Renal lymphatics, and lymphatic involvement in sinus vein invasive (pT3b) clear cell renal cell carcinoma: a study of 40 cases. Mod Pathol. 2006;19:746–53.
22. Bonsib SM. Renal veins and venous extension in clear cell renal cell carcinoma. Mod Pathol. 2007;20:44–53.
23. Lopez-Beltran A, Cheng L, Raspollini MR, Montironi R. SMARCB1/INI1 genetic alterations in renal medullary carcinomas. Eur Urol. 2016;69(6):1062–4. https://doi.org/10.1016/j.eururo.2016.01.002.
24. Thompson RH, Blute ML, Krambeck AE, et al. Patients with pT1 renal cell carcinoma who die from disease after nephrectomy may have unrecognized renal sinus fat invasion. Am J Surg Pathol. 2007;31:1089–93.
25. Lopez-Beltran A, Montironi R, Carazo JL, Vidal A, Cheng L. Primary renal osteosarcoma. Am J Clin Pathol. 2014;141(5):747–52. https://doi.org/10.1309/AJCPM86FVHAMWJSR.
26. Frank I, Blute ML, Cheville JC, et al. Solid renal tumors: an analysis of pathological features related to tumor size. J Urol. 2003;170:2217–20.
27. Qualman SJ, Bowen J, Amin MB, et al. Protocol for the examination of specimens from patients with Wilms tumor (nephroblastoma) or other renal tumors of childhood. Arch Pathol Lab Med. 2003;127:1280–9.
28. Lopez-Beltran A, Kirkali Z, Montironi R, Blanca A, Algaba F, Scarpelli M, Yorukoglu K, Hartmann A, Cheng L. Unclassified renal cell carcinoma: a report of 56 cases. BJU Int. 2012;110(6):786–93. https://doi.org/10.1111/j.1464-410X.2012.10934.x.

29. Verine J, Pluvinage A, Bousquet G, et al. Hereditary renal cancer syndromes: an update of a systematic review. Eur Urol. 2010;58:701–10.
30. Richstone L, Scherr DS, Reuter VR, et al. Multifocal renal cortical tumors: frequency, associated clinicopathological features and impact on survival. J Urol. 2004;171:615–20.
31. Zini L, Destrieux-Garnier L, Leroy X, et al. Renal vein ostium wall invasion of renal cell carcinoma with an inferior vena cava tumor thrombus: prediction by renal and vena caval vein diameters and prognostic significance. J Urol. 2008;179:450–4.
32. Han KR, Bui MH, Pantuck AJ, et al. TNM T3a renal cell carcinoma: adrenal gland involvement is not the same as renal fat invasion. J Urol. 2003;169:899–903.
33. Conti A, Santoni M, Sotte V, Burattini L, Scarpelli M, Cheng L, Lopez-Beltran A, Montironi R, Cascinu S, Muzzonigro G, Lund L. Small renal masses in the era of personalized medicine: tumor heterogeneity, growth kinetics, and risk of metastasis. Urol Oncol. 2015;33(7):303–9.
34. Thompson RH, Leibovich BC, Cheville JC, et al. Should direct ipsilateral adrenal invasion from renal cell carcinoma be classified as pT3a? J Urol. 2005;173:918–21.
35. Raspollini MR, Castiglione F, Martignoni G, Lapini A, Cheng L, Montironi R, Lopez-Beltran A. Multiple and bilateral kidney tumors with clear cells of three different histotypes: a case report with clinicopathologic and molecular study. APMIS. 2016;124(7):619–23.
36. Mehta V, Mudaliar K, Ghai R, et al. Renal lymph nodes for tumor staging: appraisal of 861 adult nephrectomies with microscopic examination of hilar fat. Arch Pathol Lab Med. 2013;137:1584.
37. Terrone C, Guercio S, De Luca S, et al. The number of lymph nodes examined and staging accuracy in renal cell carcinoma. BJU Int. 2003;91:37–40.
38. Crispen PL, Breau RH, Allmer C, et al. Lymph node dissection at the time of radical nephrectomy for high-risk clear cell renal cell carcinoma: indications and recommendations for surgical templates. Eur Urol. 2011;59:18–23.
39. Shuch B, Amin A, Armstrong AJ, Eble JN, Ficarra V, Lopez-Beltran A, Martignoni G, Rini BI, Kutikov A. Understanding pathologic variants of renal cell carcinoma: distilling therapeutic opportunities from biologic complexity. Eur Urol. 2015;67(1):85–97.

Chapter 21
Staging and Reporting of Renal Cell Carcinomas

Antonio Lopez-Beltran, Maria R. Raspollini, Liang Cheng, Marina Scarpelli, Alessia Cimadamore, Matteo Santoni, Silvia Gasparrini, and Rodolfo Montironi

This chapter is devoted to staging and reporting renal cell carcinoma (RCC) specimens and applies to both radical nephrectomy and partial nephrectomy (including tumorectomy) specimens [1–4]. Main issues to be considered have been covered thoroughly in the literature with significant differences between different AJCC classifications [1–39] (Fig. 21.1). Since January 2018 is the official call for implementing the *AJCC Cancer Staging System*, 8th Edition, in practice, we will provide along the next pages, a brief discussion of relevant changes incorporated in the 8th Edition as compared to the previous one.

Concerning reporting RCC specimens, we have followed the conclusions raised by ICCR initiative on cancer reporting, which incorporates specific protocols developed to report RCC specimens [4]. The ICCR is supported by the College of American

A. Lopez-Beltran (✉)
Department of Pathology and Surgery, Cordoba University School of Medicine, Córdoba, Spain

M. R. Raspollini
Histopathology and Molecular Diagnostics. University Hospital Careggi, Florence, Italy

L. Cheng
Departments of Pathology, Urology, and Laboratory Medicine, Indiana University School of Medicine, Indianapolis, IN, USA

M. Scarpelli · R. Montironi
Institute of Pathological Anatomy and Histopathology, United Hospitals, Ancona, Italy

A. Cimadamore
Institute of Pathological Anatomy and Histopathology, University of the Marche Region, Ancona, Italy

M. Santoni
Oncology Unit, Macerata Hospital, Macerata, Italy

S. Gasparrini
Section of Pathological Anatomy, Polytechnic University of the Marche Region, School of Medicine, Ancona, Italy

M. K. Divatia et al. (eds.), *Kidney Cancer*, https://doi.org/10.1007/978-3-030-28333-9_21

	AJCC 2002	AJCC 2009	AJCC 2016
pT1a	Tumor 4 cm or less, limited to the kidney	Tumor 4 cm or less, limited to the kidney	Tumor 4 cm or less, limited to the kidney
pT1b	Tumor 4 to 7 cm, limited to the kidney	Tumor 4 to 7 cm, limited to the kidney	Tumor 4 to 7 cm, limited to the kidney
pT2	> 7 cm, limited to the kidney	pT2a – Tumor 7 to 10 cm, limited to the kidney	pT2a - Tumor 7 to 10 cm, limited to the kidney
		pT2b - Tumor > 10 cm, limited to the kidney	pT2b - Tumor >10 cm, limited to the kidney
pT3a		Tumor grossly extends into the renal vein or its segmental ("muscle containing") branches or invades perirenal and/or renal sinus fat	Tumor extends into the renal vein or its segmentat branches or invades the pelycaliceal system, or invades perirenal and/or renal sinus fat, but not beyond Gerota's fascia
pT3b	Renal vein, includes "muscular" sinus veins, vena cava below diaphragm	Tumor grossly extends into the vena cava below the diaphragm	Tumor grossly extends into the vena cava below the diaphragm
pT3c	Vena cava above diaphragm Wall of vena cava	Tumor grossly extends into the vena cava above the diaphragm or invades the wall of the vena cava	Tumor grossly extends into the vena cava above the diaphragm or invades the wall of the vena cava
pT4	Tumor invades beyond Gerota's fascia	Tumor invades beyond Gerota's fascia, including contiguous extension into ipsilateral adrenal gland	Tumor invades beyond Gerota's fascia, including contiguous extension into ipsilateral adrenal gland

Fig. 21.1 Comparison of 6–7 and 8 editions of the AJCC/TNM staging systems for renal cell carcinoma

Pathologists, the Royal College of Pathologists of Australasia, and the Royal College of Pathologists of the United Kingdom. It also counts with the support by the European Society of Pathology. The ICCR protocols can be accessed following the link www.iccr-cancer.org and then datasets can be followed; this will bring the reader to RCC datasets under the heading of "invasive carcinoma of renal tubular origin."

Proper consideration along the text, in this chapter, is also given to the International Society of Urologic Pathology 2012 Consensus Conference on renal cancer, through working group 3, focused on the issues of staging and specimen handling of renal tumors [2], the *AJCC TNM Cancer Staging Manual*, 8th Edition [1], and the most recent World Health Organization Classification of Tumours of the Urinary System and Male Genital Organs [3].

Adherence to the ICCR reporting datasets [4] will provide a standardized approach which is in use by most Uropathologists around the world.

Staging of Kidney Specimens with Cancer: Radical Nephrectomy and Partial Nephrectomy

The recent publication of the AJCC TNM 8th Edition [1] has introduced minor changes on RCC when compared to the 7th Edition [7]. This is due to the fact that major changes had been actually made in the 7th Edition [7], and data related to

Table 21.1 Renal carcinoma pathologic staging

Definition of the primary tumor (T category)
TX Primary tumor cannot be assessed
T0 No evidence of primary tumor
T1 Tumor ≤7 cm in greatest dimension, limited to the kidney
T1a Tumor ≤4 cm in greatest dimension, limited to the kidney
T1b Tumor more than 4 cm but ≤7 cm in greatest dimension, limited to the kidney
T2 Tumor more than 7 cm in greatest dimension, limited to the kidney
T2a Tumor more than 7 cm but ≤10 cm in greatest dimension, limited to the kidney
T2b Tumor more than 10 cm, limited to the kidney
T3 Tumor extends into major veins or perinephric tissues but not into the ipsilateral adrenal gland and not beyond Gerota's fascia
T3a Tumor extends into the renal vein or its segmental branches, or invades the pelvi-calyceal system, or invades perirenal and/or renal sinus fat but not beyond Gerota's fascia
T3b Tumor extends into vena cava below diaphragm
T3c Tumor extends into the vena cava above the diaphragm or invades the wall of the vena cava
T4 Tumor invades beyond Gerota fascia (including contiguous extension into the ipsilateral adrenal gland)
Regional lymph nodes (N)
NX Regional lymph nodes cannot be assessed.
N0 No regional lymph node metastasis
N1 Regional lymph node metastasis
Definition of distant metastasis (M)
M0 No distant metastases
M1 Distant metastasis

Modified from the AJCC TNM 8th Edition

these novelties are still accruing. In AJCC TNM 8th Edition [1] T3 category, further clarifications were made in T3a disease classification concerning involvement of the renal vein and its tributaries (Table 21.1). T3a criteria in the AJCC TNM 7th Edition have been redefined since it is not uncommon that tumor involvement of renal vessels can be missed grossly in both radical and partial nephrectomy specimens (Fig. 21.2). The thickness of renal vein and its branches is considered by most authorities a poor identification method as it largely varies between specimens, but also, because with certain frequency may be thin with minimal muscular wall and therefore cannot be accurately identified macroscopically [5]. Another factor is that histologic examination of small tumor nodules within the renal sinus most frequently reveal intravascular tumor (Fig. 21.3). Thus, the word "grossly" to describe invasion of renal vein and its segmental branch for T3a is now removed, and therefore, a constellation of gross and microscopic features can be used to define pT3a staging according to the AJCC TNM 8th Edition [1].

An important addition in the 8th Edition [1] is the invasion of the pelvi-calyceal system, which has been placed in T3a. The renal sinus has being recognized as the

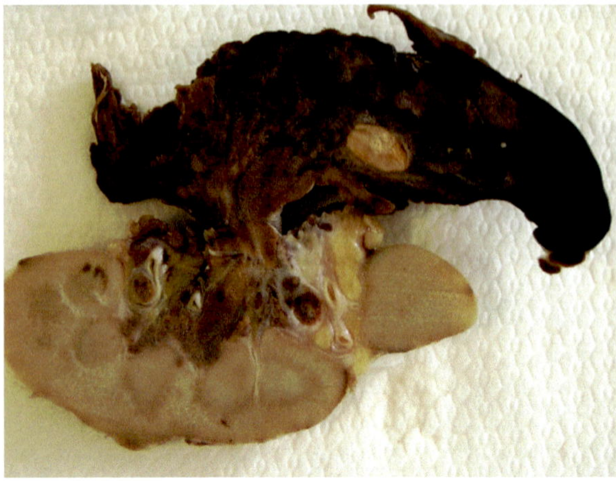

Fig. 21.2 Tumor invasion is seen in the renal vein also invading the vena cava as a neoplastic thrombus

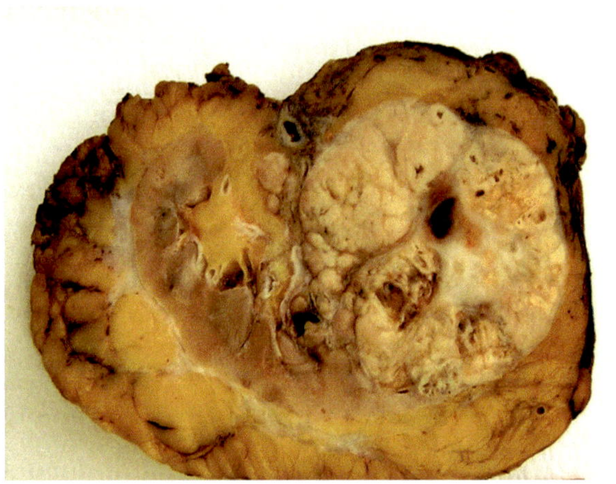

Fig. 21.3 Small tumor nodules seen in the renal sinus frequently represent vascular extension

main route for extrarenal extension, and chances of sinus invasion increases with larger tumor size particularly for tumors larger than 4 cm [5–17]. Renal sinus invasion is most commonly seen in clear cell renal cell carcinoma. Of note is the fact that in clear cell renal cell carcinomas ≥7 cm in greatest dimension, renal sinus invasion is seen in more than 90% of cases [5, 15–17]. Sampling the renal hilum by pathologists for microscopic examination of vessel involvement is emphasized in the AJCC TNM 8th Edition [1, 2]. There are some reports suggesting that renal sinus fat involvement by RCC predicts a more aggressive outcome than peripheral perinephric fat invasion by RCC (Fig. 21.4). Involvement of the renal sinus by tumor is a feature of pT3a tumor staging category of the AJCC/TNM classification. It is likely that renal sinus invasion is preceded by involvement of renal sinus veins, an issue still under discussion.

In addition to the novelties described above, other relevant classic parameters are needed to provide the proper pathologic staging according to AJCC TNM 8th

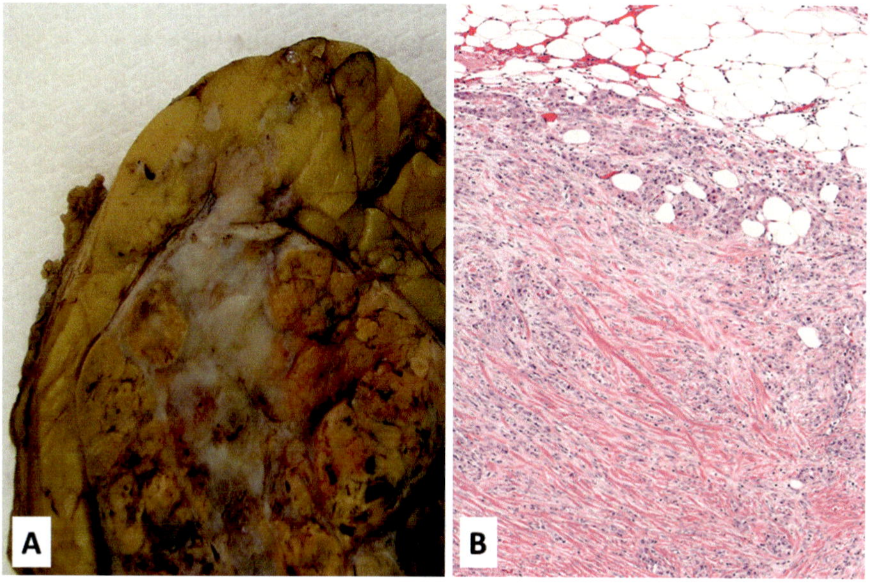

Fig. 21.4 Renal cell carcinoma may present perinephric fat invasion grossly (**a**) and microscopically (**b**)

Edition. These are presented in Table 21.1, as they are typically part of the AJCC/TNM categories [1–39]. Special care should be given to measure the greatest dimension of the tumor, in particular measurement in and around 4, 7, and 10 cm are particularly sensitive since they are used to establish T1 and T2 disease. Also, when renal carcinoma involves the adrenal gland, it is important to document whether the involvement is contiguous spread of tumor, which is considered as pT4, or a separate/noncontiguous nodule of carcinoma, which represents metastatic disease (pM1) (Fig. 21.5). Extension of tumor beyond Gerota's fascia is a feature of the pT4 staging category of the 8th Edition of the AJCC/TNM staging system [1–3].

It is curious, however, the fact that the UICC virtually left the 7th TNM staging system for kidney cancer unchanged for its 8th Edition, and this has created problems in the implementation of the new AJCC that it expected to be use in daily practice in January 2018.

Reporting of Kidney Specimens with Cancer: Radical Nephrectomy and Partial Nephrectomy

Concerning reporting RCC specimens, we have followed the conclusions raised by ICCR initiative on cancer reporting, therefore incorporating the specific protocols developed to report RCC specimens [4]. The ICCR protocols can be accessed following the link www.iccr-cancer.org and then follow the datasets, which will bring

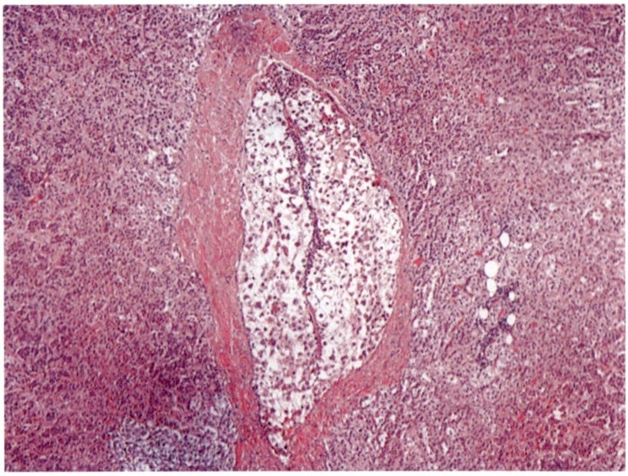

Fig. 21.5 Renal cell carcinoma may infiltrate the ipsilateral adrenal gland

the reader to RCC-related datasets under the title "invasive carcinoma of renal tubular origin." The ICCR is supported by the College of American Pathologists, the Royal College of pathologists of Australasia, and the Royal College of Pathologists of the United Kingdom. It also accounts with the support by the European Society of Pathology. The dataset also incorporate consensus documents such as the International Society of Urologic Pathology 2012 Consensus Conference on Renal Cancer [2], the most recent World Health Organization Classification of Tumours of the Urinary System and Male Genital Organs [3] and run parallel to the implementation of the *AJCC TNM Cancer Staging Manual*, 8th Edition [1].

In the ICCR protocols, the dataset has been developed for excision specimens of the kidney. Urothelial carcinoma arising from the upper renal tract, Wilms tumors, and other nephroblastic and mesenchymal tumors are not included in scope. Also worth to remember is that the dataset is designed for the reporting of a single laterality of specimen (left or right). If both are submitted as it might happen in bilateral tumors, then separate datasets should be completed for left or right specimens [4].

Another important novelty is the inclusion of the new four-tiered WHO/ISUP nucleolar grade, which has been adopted to replace the traditional Fuhrman nuclear grade in the AJCC TNM 8th Edition (Fig. 21.6). It has also been incorporated into the most recent World Health Organization Classification of Tumours of the Urinary System and Male Genital Organs [3] and by the novel ICCR reporting of invasive carcinoma of renal tubular origin, and therefore is part of the reporting items to be included in practice [3, 36]. In contrast to Fuhrman nuclear grade, which assesses a combination of nuclear and nucleolar features, the WHO/ISUP nucleolar grading for its first three grades relies exclusively on the degree of nucleolar prominence, thus providing better objectivity in the pathologist's interpretation (Table 21.2). Other known aggressive histologic features such as sarcomatoid and rhabdoid differentiation are incorporated into WHO/ISUP as grade 4 disease (Figs. 21.7, 21.8, and 21.9). Recent studies have shown that WHO/ISUP nucleolar grade provides

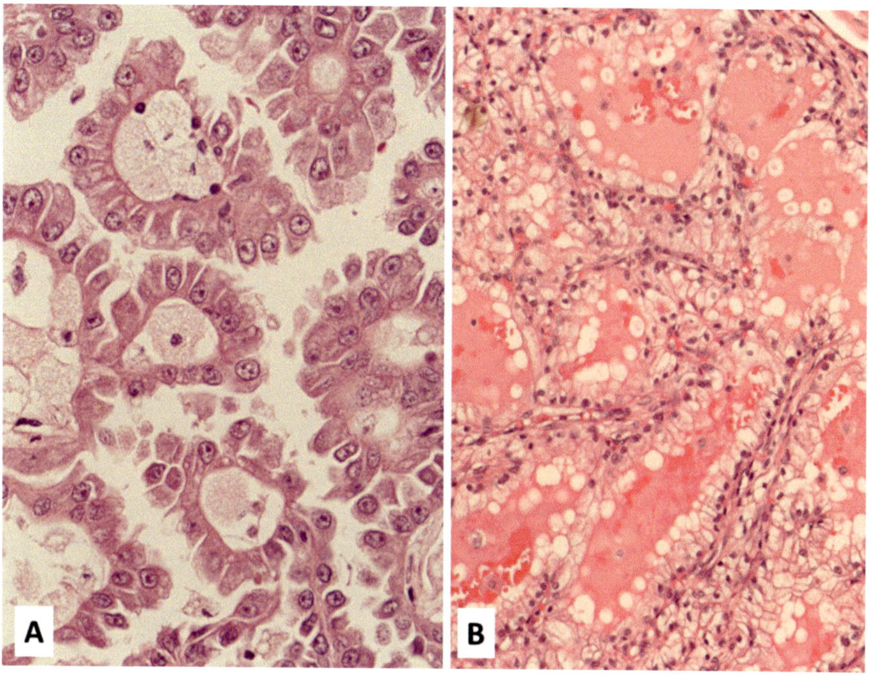

Fig. 21.6 Nucleolar prominence is characteristic of grade 3 WHO/ISUP grading system (**a**) as compares with lack of nucleolar prominence seen in grade 1 WHO/ISUP (**b**)

Table 21.2 Histologic nucleolar grade

ISUP nucleolar grade	Histological features
Grade 1	Nucleoli absent or inconspicuous and basophilic at 400× magnification
Grade 2	Nucleoli conspicuous and eosinophilic at ×400 magnification, visible but not prominent at ×100 magnification
Grade 3	Nucleoli conspicuous and eosinophilic at ×100 magnification
Grade 4	Extreme nuclear pleomorphism and/or multi nuclear giant cells and/or rhabdoid and/or sarcomatoid differentiation

better grade separation in intermediate categories, and the main benefit is to separate grades 2 and 3 (a problem with Fuhrman grading), and this separation has stronger association with patient outcome [36]. Reportedly, the WHO/ISUP grade is best applied for clear cell and papillary subtypes of RCC. Chromophobe RCC subtype does not benefit by this novel grading system [4–36]. Rhabdoid differentiation, characterized by tumor cells resembling rhabdomyoblasts (Fig. 21.7), is emphasized in the AJCC TNM 8th manual as a poor prognostic indicator of RCC [24, 35–38]. Rhabdoid differentiation, may occur across any of the RCC subtypes, predicts poor outcome independent of histologic subtype, grade, and stage, and there-

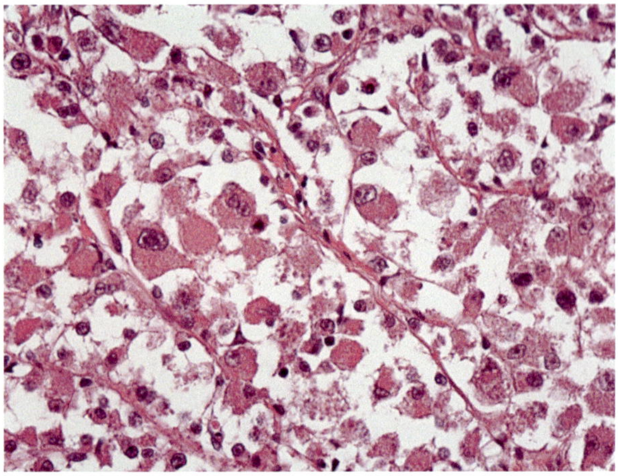

Fig. 21.7 Rhabdoid differentiation is an important prognostic factor in renal cell carcinoma

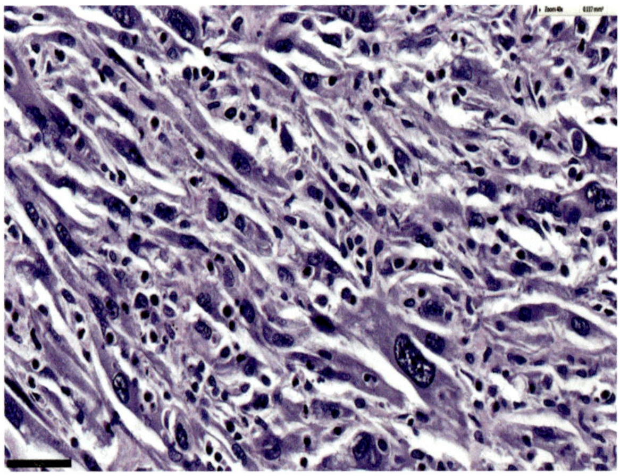

Fig. 21.8 Sarcomatoid differentiation is an important prognostic factor in renal cell carcinoma

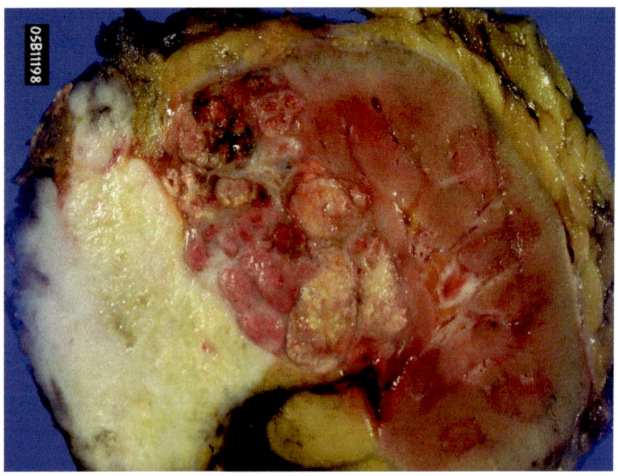

Fig. 21.9 The presence of sarcomatoid differentiation may be identified grossly due to is whitish firm appearance

fore is one of the features that need to be reported together with the presence of sarcomatoid differentiation, also known as an aggressive feature in RCC (Table 21.3) [24, 35–37].

The histologic tumor subtype is also an important contribution to the pathology report (Table 21.4). The classification of tumor subtypes is based on the Fourth Edition World Health Organization classification of renal cell tumors and the International Society of Urological Pathology Vancouver classification of renal neoplasia [2–4, 8]. In the rare case of more than one histologic type of carcinoma occur-

Table 21.3 Main variables to be assessed in RCC

Histologic tumor type (WHO classification)
Histologic tumor grade (ISUP nucleolar grade)
Presence and percentage of sarcomatoid and/or rhabdoid differentiation
Presence or absence of tumor necrosis
Tumor dimension (greatest dimension)
Tumor site
Tumor involvement of renal sinus and/or of perinephric fat
Tumor involvement of adrenal gland (contiguous = pT4 or noncontiguous M1)
Tumor involvement of margins (vascular margin in radical nephrectomy specimens or renal margin in partial nephrectomy specimens)

Table 21.4 Reporting of renal cell carcinoma following the ICCR dataset (www.iccr-cancer.org)

Preoperative treatment (not specified, tumor embolization, cryoablation, radio frequency ablation, external-beam radiation therapy, Tyrosine kinase inhibitors, immunotherapy, and other)
Specimen laterality (left/right)
Surgical procedure (partial/radical nephrectomy)
Accompanying/attached structures (adrenal, lymph nodes)
Tumor site(s) (upper or lower pole, medulla)
Tumor focality (uni/multifocal)
Maximum tumor dimension (if multiple tumors the maximum dimension of the largest five should be recorded)
Macroscopic extent of invasion (tumor confined to kidney or extent into perinephric fat, renal sinus fat, beyond Gerota's fascia, major veins, pelvi-calyceal system, ipsilateral adrenal contiguous or noncontiguous, other organs)
Histological tumor type (WHO 2016) [3]
Clear cell renal cell carcinoma
Multilocular clear cell renal cell neoplasm of low malignant potential
Papillary renal cell carcinoma
Type 1 or type 2
Oncocytic subtype
NOS
Chromophobe renal cell carcinoma
Hybrid oncocytic chromophobe tumor

(continued)

Table 21.4 (continued)

Collecting duct carcinoma
Renal medullary carcinoma
MiT family translocation renal cell carcinoma
Xp11 translocation renal cell carcinoma
t(6;11) renal cell carcinoma
Other, specify
Mucinous tubular and spindle cell carcinoma
Tubulocystic renal cell carcinoma
Acquired cystic disease-associated renal cell carcinoma
Clear cell papillary/tubulopapillary renal cell carcinoma
Hereditary leiomyomatosis and renal cell carcinoma-associated renal cell carcinoma
Succinate dehydrogenase (SDH) deficient renal carcinoma
Renal cell carcinoma, unclassified
Other, specify
Histological tumor grade (World Health Organization/ International Society of Urological Pathology (WHO/ISUP) nucleolar grading system) [3]
Sarcomatoid morphology (if present give %)
Rhabdoid morphology (if present give %)
Microscopic extent of invasion (if present in fat, vascular spaces or both, beyond Gerota's fascia, pelvi-calyceal system, renal vein or renal vein wall, adrenal gland, in other organs/structures)
Tumor necrosis (present/absent, macro or microscopic [add % as an option])
Lymphovascular invasion (present/absent)
Lymph node status (number of lymph nodes examined and number of positives)
Margin status (specify sites)
Coexisting pathology in non-neoplastic kidney (glomerular or tubule-interstitial disease, cysts, adenomas)
Ancillary studies if performed
Pathologic staging (AJCC/TNM 8th edition) (see Table 21.1)

ring within the same kidney specimen, it is recommended to separately record each tumor type and to provide their relative percentage [2–4, 8].

Most subtypes of renal epithelial carcinoma exhibit differing clinical behavior and prognosis; a fact that has been confirmed in large single and multicenter studies, and in particular for clear cell, papillary, and Chromophobe RCC. Of relevance, the observation that many of the newly described entities of RCC have a prognosis that differs from that of clear cell renal cell carcinoma, and therefore are worth to be reported. However, the overall information available on these categories is still limited and there is much need of larger reported series (Table 21.4) [2–4, 8].

The 2013 International Society of Urological Pathology Vancouver Classification of adult renal tumors identified a group of renal cell carcinomas currently placed as emerging/provisional category of RCC [2–4, 8]. This category was also included in the fourth edition of the World Health Organization classification of renal neoplasia. While appearing distinctive, these rare tumors had not been fully characterized by morphology, immunohistochemistry, and molecular studies. Examples of this category include oncocytoid RCC after neuroblastoma (neuroblastoma-associated RCC), thyroid-like follicular RCC, anaplastic lymphoma kinase (ALK) rearrangement-associated RCC, and RCC with (angio) leiomyomatous stroma. Although initially included in this category, oncocytic papillary RCC has been included in the fourth edition of the World Health Organization renal tumor classification [3] as a specific category; therefore, we suggest that tumors showing typical features should be included in this category instead of as an emerging/provisional category [1–39].

Papillary RCC is associated with a more favorable outcome than CCRCC, collecting duct carcinoma, and HLRCC. Papillary RCC has been subdivided into type 1 and type 2, with recent studies showing these tumors to be biologically and clinically distinct. Papillary subtyping is also of prognostic significance with type 1 tumors having a better prognosis than those with type 2 morphology. Type 1 tumors are associated with alterations in the MET pathway while type 2 tumors are associated with activation of the NRF2–ARE pathway. Molecular features suggest that type 2 tumors may be subdivided into at least three subtypes, a fact that produces certain confusion on how to report these cases. Type 1 and type 2 tumors show differing immunohistochemical staining with type 1 tumors more frequently expressing cytokeratin 7 in comparison to type 2 [1–39].

An overview of other topics to be reported is presented on Table 21.4 (Figs. 21.10 and 21.11). To fully benefit from the ICCR reporting, the reader is invited to visit the www.iccr-cancer.org which will give a detailed landscape of the different parameters to be reported and the rationale behind [4].

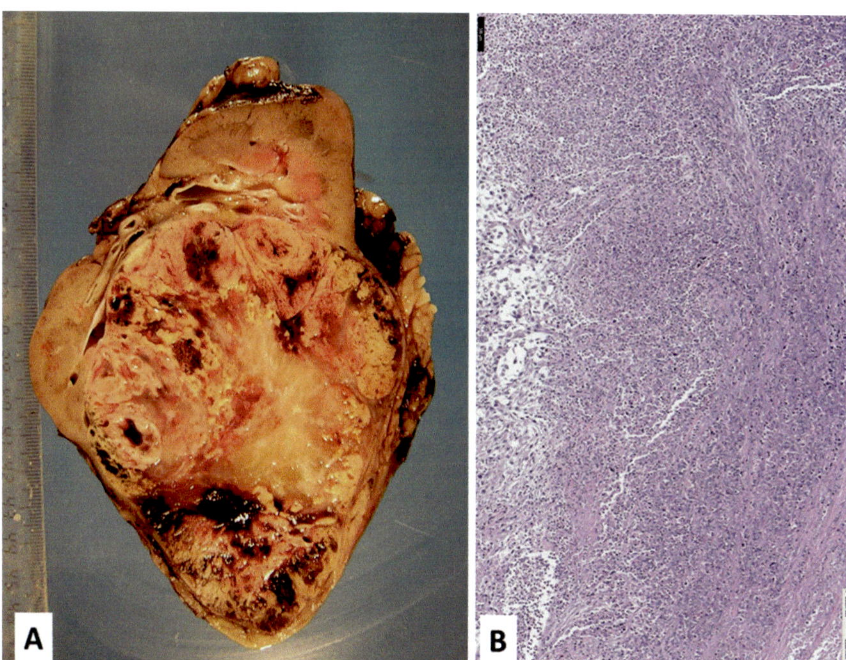

Fig. 21.10 Tumor necrosis is an important prognostic factor in renal cell carcinoma, both grossly (**a**) and microscopically (**b**)

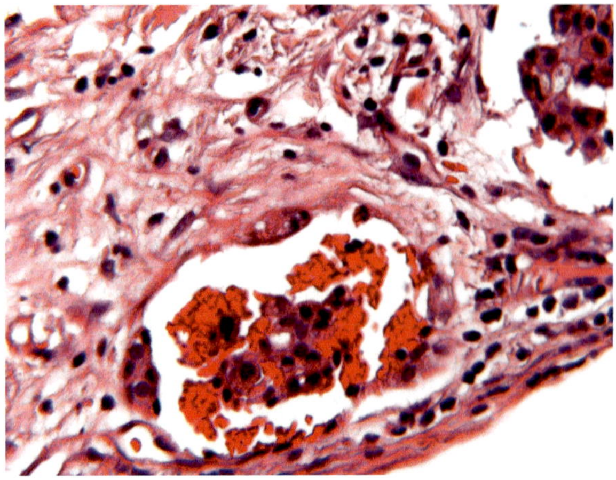

Fig. 21.11 Lymphovascular invasion may be present upon histologic examination of renal cell carcinoma

References

1. Amin MB, Edge S, Greene F, Byrd DR, Brookland RK et al., editors. American Joint Committee on Cancer (AJCC) staging manual. 8th ed. Switzerland: Springer; 2017.
2. Trpkov K, Grignon DJ, Bonsib SM, Amin MB, Billis A, Lopez-Beltran A, Samaratunga H, Tamboli P, Delahunt B, Egevad L, Montironi R, Srigley JR, members of the ISUP Renal Tumor Panel. Handling and staging of renal cell carcinoma. The International Society of Urological Pathology Consensus (ISUP) conference recommendations. Am J Surg Pathol. 2013;37:1505–17.
3. Moch H, Humphrey PA, Ulbright TM, Reuter VE. World Health Organization (WHO) classification of tumours of the urinary system and male genital organs, vol. 8. 4th ed. Lyon: International Agency for Research on Cancer, cop.; 2016.
4. Delahunt B, Srigley JR, Amin MB, Billis A, Camparo P, Evans AJ, Fleming S, Griffiths D, Lopez-Beltran A, Martignoni G, Moch H, Nacey JN, Zhou M. Invasive carcinoma of renal tubular origin, histopathology reporting guide. 1st ed. Sydney: International Collaboration on Cancer Reporting; 2017. isbn:978-1-925687-00-2.
5. Bonsib S. Renal veins and venous extension in clear cell renal carcinoma. Mod Pathol. 2007;20:44–53.
6. Greene F, Page D, Fleming I. American Joint Committee on cancer staging manual. 6th ed. New York: Springer; 2002. p. 131–44.
7. Edge SB, Byrd DR, Compton CC, Fritz AG, Greene FL, Trotti A. American Joint Committee on Cancer (AJCC) cancer staging manual. 7th ed. Chicago: Springer, Inc; 2010.
8. Srigley JR, Delahunt B, Eble JN, et al. The International Society of Urological Pathology (ISUP) Vancouver Classification of renal neoplasia. Am J Surg Pathol. 2013;37:1469–89.
9. Novara G, Ficarra V, Antonelli A, et al. Validation of the 2009 TNM version in a large multi-institutional cohort of patients treated for renal cell carcinoma: are further improvements needed? Eur Urol. 2010;58:588–95.
10. Lopez-Beltran A, Scarpelli M, Montironi R, Kirkali Z. WHO classification of the renal tumors of the adults. Eur Urol. 2006;49:798–805.
11. Algaba F, Trias I, Scarpelli M, et al. Handling and pathology reporting of renal tumor specimens. Eur Urol. 2004;45:437–43.
12. Higgins JP, McKenney JK, Brooks JD, et al. Recommendations for the reporting of surgically resected specimens of renal cell carcinoma: the Association of Directors of Anatomic and Surgical Pathology. Hum Pathol. 2009;40:456–63.

13. Lopez-Beltran A, Suzigan S, Montironi R, et al. Multilocular cystic renal cell carcinoma: a report of 45 cases of a kidney tumor of low malignant potential. Am J Clin Pathol. 2006;125:217–22.
14. Eble JN. Recommendations for examining and reporting tumor-bearing kidney specimens from adults. Semin Diagn Pathol. 1998;15:77–82.
15. Bonsib SM. The renal sinus is the principal invasive pathway: a prospective study of 100 renal cell carcinomas. Am J Surg Pathol. 2004;28:1594–600.
16. Thompson RH, Leibovich BC, Cheville JC, et al. Is renal sinus fat invasion the same as perinephric fat invasion for pT3a renal cell carcinoma? J Urol. 2005;174:1218–21.
17. Grignon D, Paner GP. Renal cell carcinoma and the renal sinus. Adv Anat Pathol. 2007;14:63–8.
18. Montironi R, Cheng L, Scarpelli M, Lopez-Beltran A. Pathology and genetics: tumours of the urinary system and male genital system: clinical implications of the 4th Edition of the WHO classification and beyond. Eur Urol. 2016;70(1):120–3. https://doi.org/10.1016/j.eururo.2016.03.011.
19. Bonsib SM. Renal lymphatics, and lymphatic involvement in sinus vein invasive (pT3b) clear cell renal cell carcinoma: a study of 40 cases. Mod Pathol. 2006;19:746–53.
20. Bonsib SM. Renal veins and venous extension in clear cell renal cell carcinoma. Mod Pathol. 2007;20:44–53.
21. Lopez-Beltran A, Cheng L, Raspollini MR, Montironi R. SMARCB1/INI1 genetic alterations in renal medullary carcinomas. Eur Urol. 2016;69(6):1062–4. https://doi.org/10.1016/j.eururo.2016.01.002.
22. Thompson RH, Blute ML, Krambeck AE, et al. Patients with pT1 renal cell carcinoma who die from disease after nephrectomy may have unrecognized renal sinus fat invasion. Am J Surg Pathol. 2007;31:1089–93.
23. Frank I, Blute ML, Cheville JC, et al. Solid renal tumors: an analysis of pathological features related to tumor size. J Urol. 2003;170:2217–20.
24. Lopez-Beltran A, Kirkali Z, Montironi R, Blanca A, Algaba F, Scarpelli M, Yorukoglu K, Hartmann A, Cheng L. Unclassified renal cell carcinoma: a report of 56 cases. BJU Int. 2012;110(6):786–93. https://doi.org/10.1111/j.1464-410X.2012.10934.x.
25. Verine J, Pluvinage A, Bousquet G, et al. Hereditary renal cancer syndromes: an update of a systematic review. Eur Urol. 2010;58:701–10.
26. Richstone L, Scherr DS, Reuter VR, et al. Multifocal renal cortical tumors: frequency, associated clinicopathological features and impact on survival. J Urol. 2004;171:615–20.
27. Zini L, Destrieux-Garnier L, Leroy X, et al. Renal vein ostium wall invasion of renal cell carcinoma with an inferior vena cava tumor thrombus: prediction by renal and vena caval vein diameters and prognostic significance. J Urol. 2008;179:450–4.
28. Han KR, Bui MH, Pantuck AJ, et al. TNM T3a renal cell carcinoma: adrenal gland involvement is not the same as renal fat invasion. J Urol. 2003;169:899–903.
29. Conti A, Santoni M, Sotte V, Burattini L, Scarpelli M, Cheng L, Lopez-Beltran A, Montironi R, Cascinu S, Muzzonigro G, Lund L. Small renal masses in the era of personalized medicine: tumor heterogeneity, growth kinetics, and risk of metastasis. Urol Oncol. 2015;33(7):303–9.
30. Thompson RH, Leibovich BC, Cheville JC, et al. Should direct ipsilateral adrenal invasion from renal cell carcinoma be classified as pT3a? J Urol. 2005;173:918–21.
31. Raspollini MR, Montagnani I, Montironi R, Cheng L, Martignoni G, Minervini A, Serni S, Nicita G, Carini M, Lopez-Beltran A. A contemporary series of renal masses with emphasis on recently recognized entities and tumors of low malignant potential: A report based on 624 consecutive tumors from a single tertiary center. Pathol Res Pract. 2017;213(7):804–8.
32. Mehta V, Mudaliar K, Ghai R, et al. Renal lymph nodes for tumor staging: appraisal of 861 adult nephrectomies with microscopic examination of hilar fat. Arch Pathol Lab Med. 2013;137:1584.
33. Terrone C, Guercio S, De Luca S, et al. The number of lymph nodes examined and staging accuracy in renal cell carcinoma. BJU Int. 2003;91:37–40.
34. Crispen PL, Breau RH, Allmer C, et al. Lymph node dissection at the time of radical nephrectomy for high-risk clear cell renal cell carcinoma: indications and recommendations for surgical templates. Eur Urol. 2011;59:18–23.

35. Shuch B, Amin A, Armstrong AJ, Eble JN, Ficarra V, Lopez-Beltran A, Martignoni G, Rini BI, Kutikov A. Understanding pathologic variants of renal cell carcinoma: distilling therapeutic opportunities from biologic complexity. Eur Urol. 2015;67(1):85–97.
36. Delahunt B, Cheville JC, Martignoni G, et al. The International Society of Urological Pathology (ISUP) grading system for renal cell carcinoma and other prognostic parameters. Am J Surg Pathol. 2013;37:1490–504.
37. Przybycin CG, McKenney JK, Reynolds JP, et al. Rhabdoid differentiation is associated with aggressive behavior in renal cell carcinoma: a clinicopathologic analysis of 76 cases with clinical follow-up. Am J Surg Pathol. 2014;38:1260–5.
38. Reuter VE, Argani P, Zhou M, Delahunt B, Amin MB, Epstein JI, Ulbright TM, Humphrey PA, Egevad L, Montironi R, Grignon D, Trpkov K, Lopez-Beltran A, Berney DM, Srigley JR. Best practice recommendations in the application of immunohistochemistry in kidney tumors; report for the International society of Urological Pathology consensus conference. Am J Surg Pathol. 2014;38:e35–49.
39. Bijol V, Mendez GP, Hurwitz S, Rennke HG, Nose V. Evaluation of the non-neoplastic pathology in tumor nephrectomy specimens: predicting the risk of progressive failure. Am J Surg Pathol. 2006;30:575–84.

Index

M. K. Divatia et al. (eds.), *Kidney Cancer*, https://doi.org/10.1007/978-3-030-28333-9

C

D

E

J

K

L

S

MIX
Papier aus verantwortungsvollen Quellen
Paper from responsible sources
FSC® C105338

If you have any concerns about our products,
you can contact us on
ProductSafety@springernature.com

In case Publisher is established outside the EU,
the EU authorized representative is:
Springer Nature Customer Service Center GmbH
Europaplatz 3, 69115 Heidelberg, Germany

Printed by Libri Plureos GmbH
in Hamburg, Germany